Wiedemann • Kunze • Grosse • Dibbern

Clinical Syndromes

Atlas of
Clinical Syndromes
A Visual Aid to Diagnosis
for Clinicians and Practicing Physicians

Professor H.R. Wiedemann MD Kiel
Professor J. Kunze MD Berlin
Dr F.-R. Grosse Osterholz-Scharmbeck
Herta Dibbern Kiel

Third, fully revised, substantially enlarged German edition
Second edition, English translation

This book appeared in the first edition under the title
'An Atlas of Characteristic Syndromes'

English translation by Dr Mary F. Passarge

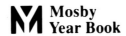

Mosby Year Book

St. Louis   Baltimore   Boston   Chicago   London   Philadelphia   Sydney   Toronto

*In grateful remembrance of forerunners, whose
analyses and descriptions of disease
were exemplary, including:*

Johann Friedrich Meckel Jr. (1781–1833)
August von Rothmund Jr. (1830–1906)
Friedrich Daniel von Recklinghausen
(1833–1910)
Heinrich Ernst Albers-Schönberg (1865–1921)
Meinhard von Pfaundler (1872–1947)
Georg Benno Gruber (1884–1977)
Ernst Hanhart (1891–1973)
Guido Fanconi (1892–1979) and
Otto Ullrich (1894–1957)

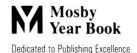

Mosby Year Book

Dedicated to Publishing Excellence

Mosby–Year Book, Inc.
11830 Westline Drive
St. Louis, MO 63146

Authorized translation of the 3rd German language edition 'Atlas der
Klinischen Syndrome' by H.-R. Wiedemann, F.-R. Grosse,
H. Dibbern, 1989

ISBN 0-8151-9331-9

English edition first published by Wolfe Publishing Ltd,
2–16 Torrington Place, London WC1E 7LT, UK.

**Library of Congress Cataloging in Publication Data has been applied
for.**

Preface to the Third German Edition

This *Atlas of Clinical Syndromes* was preceded by *Characteristic Syndromes*, in two editions, five languages, and 15,000 copies distributed around the world. Stimulated by readers and reviewers, the new publication is presented herewith, through the efforts of the editor, his former longtime co-worker Professor Jürgen Kunze, Berlin, and his clinical photographer, Mrs Herta Dibbern.

Compared with its predecessor, the *Atlas of Clinical Syndromes* deals more extensively with the stages of life of adolescence and adulthood, and it includes clinical disorders in which visual signs do not play a prominent role. It presents over 260 disease entities or processes in texts and illustrated plates (with a total of almost 1,700 single pictures) and a further 11 conditions without illustrations. These are preceded by five photographic plates to demonstrate characteristic 'minor anomalies, malformations, and unusual characteristics of man' (69 individual pictures).

In the texts we employ the more recently accepted international nomenclature, although neither rigidly nor exclusively. The nomenclature is briefly presented immediately after the table of contents, before the 'Diagnostic Overview' intended for medical practise. Each section of text has been signed by its author. Literature up to 1989, the year of publication, was taken into consideration. Special attention was devoted to the index.

Warm thanks are due to our numerous colleagues for their energetic and unselfish support of this and, in part, the preceding works. These colleagues include

M. Bauer, Gießen (a.d.L.)
F.A. Beemer, Amsterdam-Utrecht
G. Beluffi, Pavia
C.-G. Bennholdt-Thomsen†, Cologne
A. Blankenagel, Heidelberg
W. Blauth, Kiel
G.R. Burgio, Pavia
O. Butenandt, Munich
E. Christophers, Kiel
E. Dieterich, Kiel-Heide
H. Doose, Kiel
C. Fauré, Paris
J.P. Fryns, Leuven

A. Fuhrmann-Rieger, Gießen
W. Fuhrmann, Gießen
E. Gladtke, Cologne
W. Grote, Kiel
M. Habedank, Aachen
F. Hanefeld, Berlin-Göttingen
H.-G. Hansen, Lübeck
R. Happle, Njmwegen
H. Hauss, Kiel
P. Heintzen, Kiel
H. Helge, Berlin
M. Hermanussen, Kiel
U. Hillig, Marburg
D. Hosenfeld, Kiel
E. Jiminez, Berlin
H.J. Kaufmann, Berlin
H. Kemperdick, Düsseldorf
C. v. Klinggräff, Kiel
D. Knorr, Munich
K. Kruse, Würzburg-Lübeck
T. Kushnick, Greenville, U.S.A.
B. Leiber, Frankfurt a. M.
W. Lenz, Münster i.W.
F. Majewski, Düsseldorf
H. Manzke, Kiel-Norderney
P. Maroteaux, Paris
P. Meinecke, Hamburg-Altona
T. Michael, Berlin
C. Mietens†, Bochum
J. Murken, Munich
G. Neuhäuser, Gießen
M. Obladen, Bochum-Berlin
J.W. Oorthuys, Amsterdam
H.-C. Oppermann, Kiel
E. Passarge, Essen
W. Plenert, Jena
A. Proppe, Kiel
H. Reich, Münster i. W.
A. Rett, Vienna
A. Rütt, Cologne-Würzburg
J. Schaub, Kiel
A. Schinzel, Zürich
H. Schönenberg, Aachen
M. Seip, Oslo
W. Sippell, Kiel
H.-L. Spohr, Berlin
J. Spranger, Mainz
E. Stephan†, Kiel
G. Stickler, Rochester, U.S.A.
R. B. Stolowsky, Berlin

B. Stück, Berlin
M. Vogel, Berlin
R.-D. Wegner, Berlin
U. Wendel, Düsseldorf-Hilden
G.G. Wendt†, Marburg a.d.L.
E. Werner, Berlin
K. Zerres, Bonn

Furthermore, we would like to thank Mrs Yvonne Heitmann, Kiel and Mrs Erika Schäfer, Berlin, for their efforts. And last but not least we thank Mr Dieter Bergemann, our publisher, and his experienced co-workers from Schattauer Publishers for their kind criticism and fine work.

In the name of all authors,
Hans-Rudolf Wiedemann
Kiel

From the Preface to the Second German Edition

Characteristic Syndromes has met with much interest and approval; the first reprinting was required after two years, and foreign-language editions have appeared. Reviewers have consistently commended the atlas, not only for its basic format and the 'information density' of the texts, but also for the quality of the illustrations. Encouraged by this, and stimulated by frequently expressed wishes that further syndromes be included, we now present a new edition. The basic idea and purpose of this book and its organization have remained unchanged: it is meant for medical practise. (Please refer to the Preface to the first edition.)

In the first edition the photographic material came almost without exception from the archives of the pediatric department of the University of Kiel or from the private files of the first author. In this edition 204, instead of 97, syndromes are illustrated—thus more than doubling the content of the book. This has required 'material help' on the part of kind colleagues. We are grateful for the photographs and clinical data for more than 50 of the newly included malformation complexes and hereditary syndromes. Again, color photographs have been intentionally excluded.

More than 170 acknowledged and generally familiar syndromes are presented here with the goal of 'visual recognition' or tentative diagnosis from appearance. Additionally about 30 further singular clinical pictures have been included which were apparently previously unknown. These have come almost exclusively from the collected observations of the first author, and for the time being represent special cases or 'personal syndromes'. In our experience the study of this kind of presentation by colleagues frequently leads to their 'recognizing' earlier analogous observations they themselves have made or to helpful associations from other fields—and so to closer definition and classification. Thus, the inclusion of these cases is 'for the good of the cause'. The texts and some of the photographic plates of the first edition have been revised. In addition to a table of contents, a diagnostic overview (which has been expanded to include new groups), and an alphabetical index of the syndromes (including the most important synonyms), the present edition offers a table of particularly noteworthy signs.

In conclusion, clinical genetics has become greatly differentiated and continues to become more so at an increasing rate. As a result, a book such as this contains many, albeit well-deliberated, simplifications. This was unavoidable in order to stay within the prescribed framework.

Finally, we would like to acknowledge the slide collection 'Syndromes' ROCOM/Roche 1982, which supplemented the present edition of the atlas.

Hans-Rudolf Wiedemann
Kiel

From the Preface to the First German Edition

*Was ist das Schwerste von allem? Was dir das
  Leichteste dünket.
Mit den augen zu sehn, was vor den Augen dir
  liegt.**

(J.W. v. Goethe, Xenia**, from the literary
remains)

'Syndromes' are plentiful in modern medicine.
According to G. Fanconi, more than six times as
many syndromes can be tabulated now than
could be at the beginning of the century. Essentially, this is an effect of advances in research
and, therefore, may be viewed positively.

It is important to diagnose syndromes early
and to draw the necessary conclusions from the
diagnosis. Many syndromes are easy for the
physician with a trained eye to recognize. The
intention of this book is to aid in this training.
Almost one hundred syndromes that can be
partially or totally visually comprehended have
been presented here, each with an illustrated
plate. Most of them represent so-called dys-
morphosis syndromes, whereby the manifestations may be present at birth, but also may not
be apparent until later. Since this book is meant
to be of practical use, the authors have neither
followed the strict definition of syndromes nor
limited themselves to a sharply delineated
category of syndromes.

Blickdiagnosen (diagnoses from appearance)
are not to be taken literally to mean 'on sight'
or 'instant' diagnoses. To be sure, most of the
syndromes presented can be identified by an
experienced observer with a physician's eye
alone and do not require extensive laboratory
tests, which unfortunately and unjustifiably are
often given priority by young physicians. But in
many cases, a careful history to supplement the
impression, and a thorough clinical examination to substantiate the tentative diagnosis, will
be required. The text accompanying each of the
photographic plates gives the basic guidelines
and additional information, concisely formu-
lated.

The frequencies of the syndromes are to be
understood within the framework of dysmor-
phosis syndromes in general. Several stand out,
especially Down's syndrome (1 in approx. 650
births), but also neurofibromatosis, Noonan
syndrome, Prader–Willi syndrome, Turner syndrome, and several others, perhaps including
the newly recognized fetal alcohol syndrome.
For the patient at hand and his family it is of no
particular consolation that his condition is
rare. To him the frequency of his disorder is
'100%', and he expects his physician to be well
informed about it. Furthermore, 'the rare
things in medicine are *not rare*, only observers
are rare' (H.R. Clouston, 1939).

Patients with the syndromes presented here
will be taken to general practitioners and to
colleagues of the most diverse specialities—
ophthalmologists and radiologists, dermatolo-
gists and psychiatrists, human geneticists and
otologists, internists and orthopaedic surgeons,
pediatricians and neurologists. This atlas is
meant to serve all of them. The diagnostic
overview following the table of contents is
intended to facilitate locating syndromes that
come into question.

Hans-Rudolf Wiedemann
Kiel

---

* Roughly:
  What is the hardest of all? What you as easiest would deem,
    To see with your eyes, what lies before your eyes.

** Satirical epigrams

Contents

Nomenclature of Syndromes

In 1982, a clinical genetics working group (Spranger, Benirschke, J.G. Hall, Lenz, Lowry, Opitz, Pinsky, Schwarzacher, and D.W. Smith) published their recommendations for an international nomenclature to describe patients with morphological anomalies. With these recommendations, clinical syndromologists are obliged to orient their thinking pathogenetically. In addition, classification using the new concepts has important practical significance: it says something about prognosis, recurrent risk, and diagnostic measures.

However, the definitions are not to be followed rigidly. Today, no one refers to Marfan 'dysplasia', and even the diagnosis Potter 'syndrome' is clinically widespread. As a further example, a syndrome-like picture in genetically heterogeneous patients is called Pena–Shokeir phenotype.

The following concepts shall be described according to their strict definitions:

Single morphological defects are divided into malformations, disruptions, deformities, and dysplasias.

A *malformation* is an anomaly resulting when the anlage of an organ, part of an organ, or a body region is defective. It arises 'ab ovo'. Thus, malformations are of genetic origin.

A *disruption* is a morphological defect resulting from the effects of exogenic factors on an organ with an initially normal anlage and development. Thus, disruptions are of a non-genetic nature.

A *deformity* is an anomaly of form and position of part of the body caused by mechanical influences. It may also arise postnatally. Deformities, too, are of a non-genetic nature and are accessible to therapy.

A *dysplasia* is a defect of tissue, whether localized or generalized, that leads to morphological anomalies. Generalized dysplasias are genetic in nature.

Multiple morphological defect patterns are defined as follows:

Polytopic field defects are topically differentiable anomalies due to disturbance of a single embryonal 'developmental field'. Polytopic means: widely separated structures.

A *sequence* is a pattern of congenital malformations that can be attributed to a single factor. The main disturbance can be a morphological defect or a mechanical influence.

A *syndrome* is a pattern of pathogenetically connected anomalies. The pathogenetic mechanism of origin itself is unknown. If the pathogenesis is defined in part, the clinical picture is designated avoiding the term syndrome (mucopolysaccharidosis).

J.K.

References:

Spranger, J., Benirschke, K., Hall, J.G., Lenz, W., Lowry, R.B., Opitz, J.M., Pinsky, L., Schwarzacher, H.G., Smith, D.W. Errors of morphogenesis: concepts and terms. Recommendations of an international working group. *J. Pediatr.*, 100, 160–165 (1982).

Diagnostic Overview

I. Syndromes with prominent anomalies of the cranium and/or face

II. Syndromes in which tall stature is a (possibly transient) prominent feature

But see also:

III. Syndromes with prominent short stature (primordial and/or postnatal, proportionate or disproportionate)

IV. Syndromes with prominent aged appearance

V. Syndromes with prominent thinness or emaciation

VI. Syndromes with prominent obesity

XII. Syndromes with prominent connective tissue weakness

XIII. Syndromes with prominent spontaneous fractures

XIV. Syndromes with prominent anomalies of the extremities

XXIV. Syndromes with hematological signs

See under:

XXV. Syndromes with muscular hypotonia and/or neurological signs (apart from seizures, seizure disorders, or isolated mental retardation)

But see also:

XXVI. Syndromes with obligatory or possible visual impairment

XXVII. Syndromes with possible hearing impairment or deafness

See under:

XXVIII. Syndromes regularly or possibly with mental retardation and/or behavioral disorders

See under:

H.-R.W.

1. Minor Anomalies, Malformations, and Unusual Physical Features in Man

1. Bilateral epicanthus
2. Epicanthus inversus
3. Mongoloid slant of the palpebral fissures (up-slanting palpebral fissures)
4. Antimongoloid slant of the palpebral fissures (down-slanting palpebral fissures)
5. Brushfield's spots
6. Epibulbar dermoid
7. Synophrys (eyebrows meeting across the midline)
8. Hypotelorism; coloboma of the iris, left; broad nasal root
9. Megalocornea ('beautiful large eyes')
10. Megalocornea, lateral view
11. Long eyelashes
12. Hypertelorism

J.K./H.-R.W.

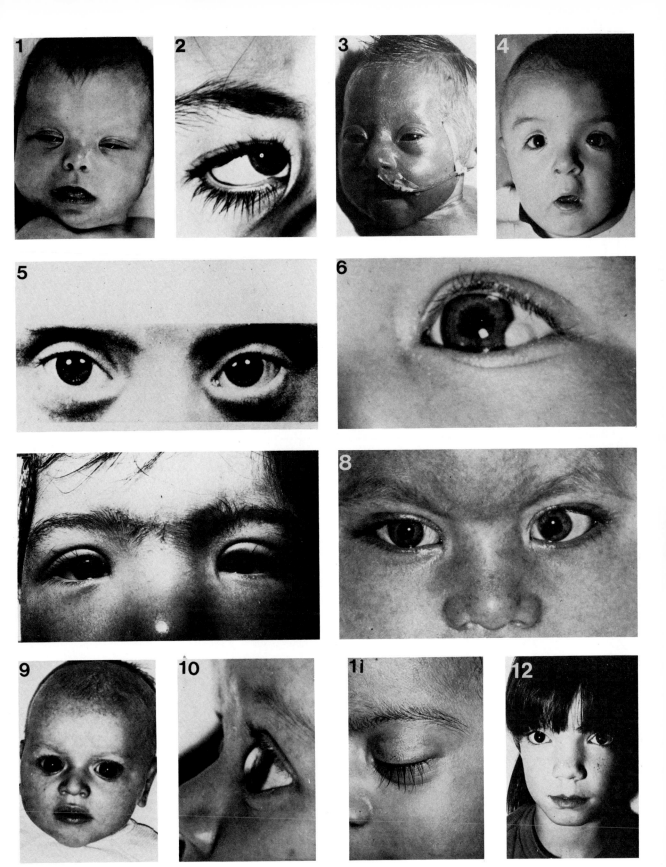

2. Minor Anomalies, Malformations, and Unusual Physical Features in Man (cont.)

1. Nevus flammeus = port-wine stain = capillary hemangioma (also: 'stork mark'; Bossard spot, frontal)
2. Nevus flammeus = port-wine stain = capillary hemangioma ('stork mark'; Unna–Politzer nevus, nuchal)
3. Depressed nasal root
4. Pterygium colli, short neck, low nuchal hairline
5. Prognathism
6. Micrognathia
7. Transverse facial and orbital clefts
8. Lisch nodules (pigmented hamartomas of the iris) (Recklinghausen's disease, neurofibromatosis)
9. Vertical median cleft lip with median cleft face syndrome
10. Interocular blind-ending sinus
11. Stenosis of the lacrimal ducts
12. Conjunctival telangiectasis (e.g., Louis–Bar syndrome)

J.K./H.-R.W.

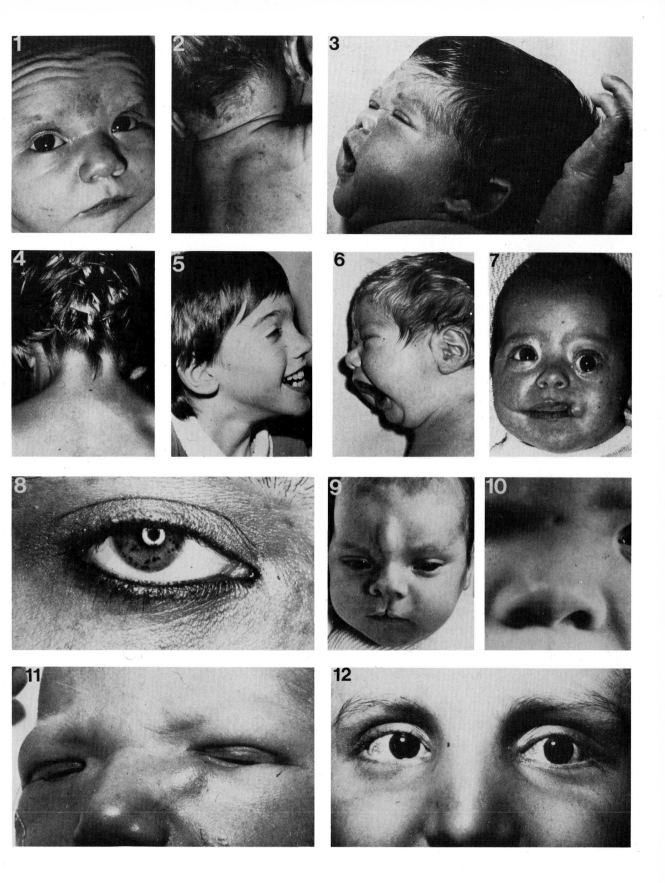

3. Minor Anomalies, Malformations, and Unusual Physical Features in Man (cont.)

1. Protruding ears
2. Auricular tag, dysplasia of the helix
3. Preauricular tag, dysplasia of the helix
4. Preauricular tags
5. Preauricular blind-ending sinus
6. Auricular tubercle
7. Inclusion of cystic masses in the helix (diastrophic dysplasia)
8. Grooved or notched ear (Wiedemann–Beckwith syndrome)
9. Bipartite tongue
10. Fissured tongue
11. Macroglossia
12. Pilonidal sinus
13. Nevus flammeus as a cutaneous marker for spina bifida occulta
14. Sacral skin tag as a cutaneous marker for 'tethered cord syndrome'

J.K./H.-R.W.

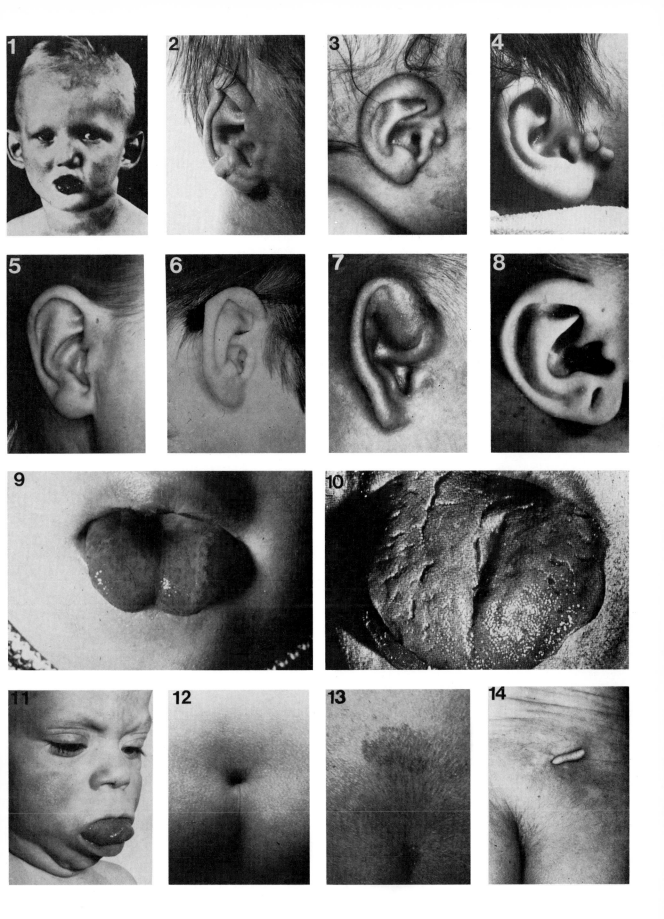

4. Minor Anomalies, Malformations, and Unusual Physical Features in Man (cont.)

1. Café au lait spots
2. Pigmented nevi with mucous membrane involvement (Peutz–Jeghers syndrome)
3. Multiple neurofibromas
4. 'White spots' (tuberous sclerosis)
5. Mongolian spot
6. Accessory nipples
7. Subungual tumor = Koenen tumor in tuberous sclerosis
8. Clinodactyly of the distal phalanges of both fifth fingers
9. Simian crease and single crease of the fifth finger
10. Absence of the large flexion creases of the fingers
11. Acromial dimple
12. Benign ring-shaped constrictions of the skin
13. Shawl scrotum

J.K./H.-R.W.

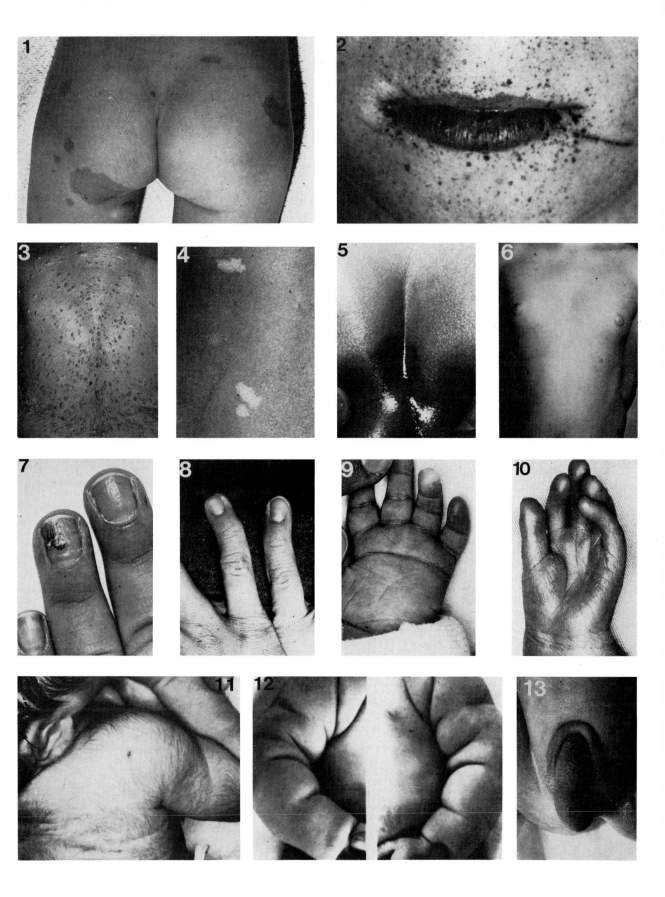

5. Minor Anomalies, Malformations, and Unusual Physical Features in Man (cont.)

1. 'Hitch-hiker thumb' (e.g., diastrophic dysplasia)
2. Partial cutaneous syndactyly
3. Preaxial hexadactyly (duplication of the thumb)
4. Flexion contractures of the fingers (e.g., trisomy 18 syndrome, distal arthrogryposis type I, Freeman–Sheldon syndrome)
5. Partial rudimentary postaxial hexadactyly (duplication of the little finger)
6. Camptodactyly
7. Hypoplasia of the thumb and clino- camptodactyly
8. Triphalangeal thumb
9. Reduction of the fourth metatarsal, corresponding to that of the fourth toe (e.g., pseudohypoparathyroidism)
10. Hypoplasia of the big toe
11. Partial syndactyly of the second and third toes
12. Deep crease between the big and second toes ('sandal-gap')
13. Partial postaxial hexadactyly of the fifth toe in the form of a bifid nail
14. Parietal foramina (foramina parietalia)
15. Fenestra parietales

J.K./H.-R.W.

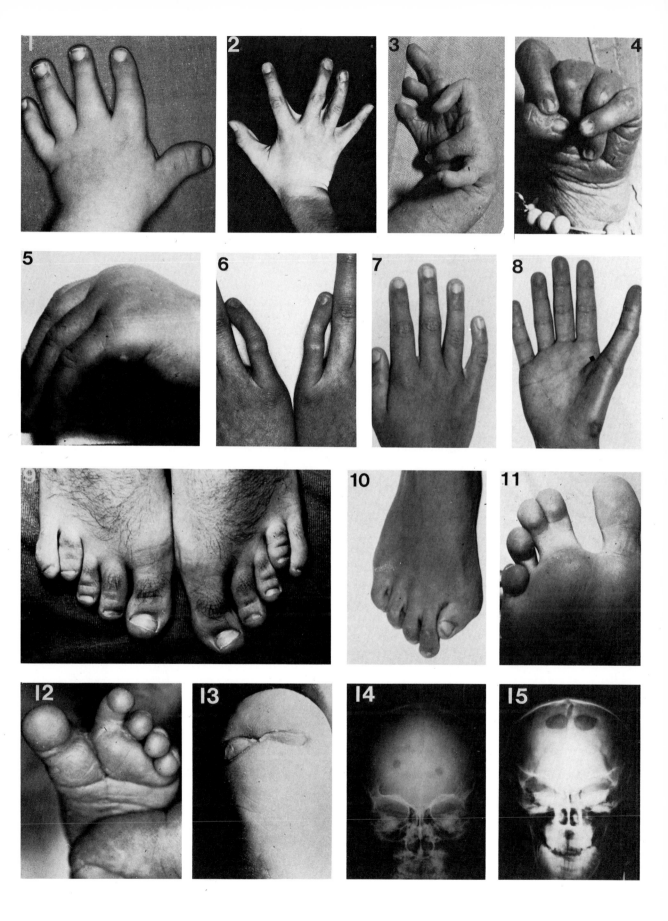

6. Crouzon Syndrome

(Craniofacial dysostosis)

A characteristic syndrome with oxycephaly (turricephaly).

Main signs:
1. Oxycephaly (acrocephaly) with a high wide forehead, sometimes with pronounced bulging of the anterior fontanelle region; flat occiput (1–3, 5, 6).
2. Exophthalmos (with flat orbits); hypertelorism. Convergence of the globes difficult or impossible; divergent strabismus. Slight antimongoloid slant of the palpebral fissures. Possible ptosis. (1–6)
3. Maxillary hypoplasia with 'parrot-beak' nose, short upper lip, high narrow palate, narrowly spaced teeth; prognathism. (2, 3c, 6a, 6c, 7b)

Supplementary findings: Frequent mild to moderate mental retardation. In some cases signs of craniostenosis and/or optic atrophy with decreased visual acuity. Exceptionally, impaired hearing.

Radiologically, craniosynostosis, especially of the coronal and lambdoid sutures; short anterior, deep middle and posterior cranial fossae; often very pronounced digital markings of the skull. (7a, 7c)

Manifestation: At birth.

Etiology: An autosomal dominant condition with 100% penetrance but variable expression. Increased paternal age; germinal mosaicism.

Frequency: Relatively low, but most observations are no longer published (in 1966 somewhat more than 100 published cases were counted).

Course, prognosis: Mainly dependent on the presence and degree of mental retardation and/or optic nerve damage.

Differential diagnosis: Chotzen syndrome (p.14).

Treatment: Symptomatic. Early craniotomy, performed in the first months of life, even in the absence of signs of craniostenosis, suited to the individual's condition and revised at regular intervals. Cosmetic surgery may be indicated eventually to mitigate facial deformity.

Illustrations:
1 A newborn.
2 An infant.
3 and 5 Young preschool children.
4 and 7 A 6-year-old girl.
6 A 10-year-old girl.
7a and 7c Digital markings of the skull of the child in 4 and 7b at age 10 years.

Some of these children represent definite hereditary cases; the others, sporadic cases (interpreted as new mutations).

H.-R.W.

References:

Vulliamy, D.G. and Normandale, P.A. Craniofacial dysostosis in a Dorset family. *Arch. Dis. Childh.*, 41, 375 (1966).

Kushner, J., Alexander, E., Davies, C.H., Jr. et al. Crouzon's disease (craniofacial dysostosis). Modern diagnosis and treatment. *J. Neurosurg.*, 37, 434 (1972).

Cohen, M.M. Jr. Craniosynostosis . . . *Birth Defects Orig. Art. Ser.*, XV, 5B, 13–63 (1979).

Kreiborg, S. Crouzon syndrome . . . *Scand. J. Plast. Reconstruct. Surg. (Suppl.)*, 18 (1981).

Marchac, D. and Renier, D. *Craniofacial Surgery for Craniosynostosis.* Little, Brown and Co, Boston, 1982 (211 pp).

Cohen, M.M. Jr. Syndromes with craniosynostosis. In: *Craniosynostosis* . . . Raven Press, New York, (1986).

Rollnick, B.R. Germinal mosaicism in Crouzon syndrome. *Clin. Genet.*, 33, 145–150 (1988).

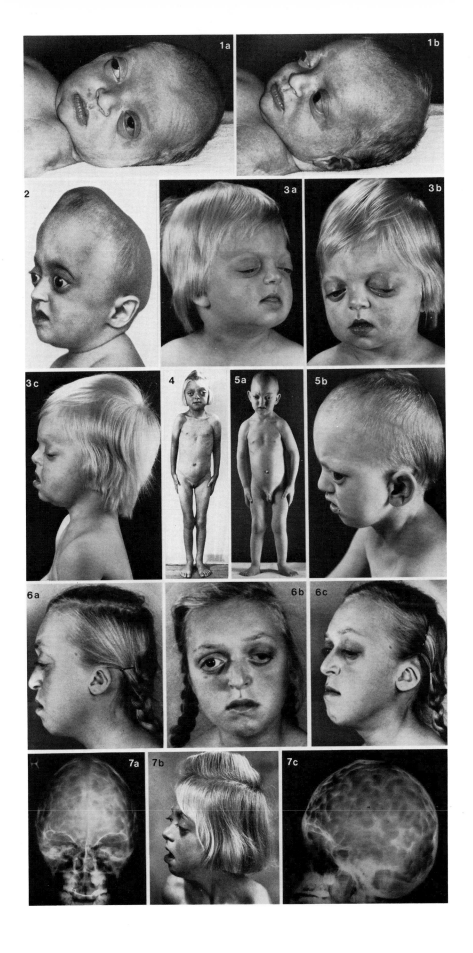

13

7. Saethre–Chotzen Syndrome

(ACS Type III, Acrocephalosyndactyly Type Chotzen, Chotzen Syndrome)

A syndrome comprising acrocephaly, quite characteristic facies, mild to moderate syndactyly of the hands and feet, and possible mental retardation.

Main signs:
1. Relatively mild acrocephaly with a broad forehead (1–3).
2. Face: Often markedly asymmetric. Frequently low anterior hairline. Hypertelorism, broad flat nasal root, antimongoloid slant of the palpebral fissures, often highly arched eyebrows, possible mild exophthalmos. Ptosis, strabismus. Tear ducts may be narrowed, dystopia canthorum. Beaklike curve of the nose with deviated septum. Possibly low-set ears. Hypoplasia of the maxilla, narrow palate; prognathism (1–3, 4, 6).
3. Relatively short stubby fingers (frequently inturned little fingers); exclusively soft-tissue syndactyly between the proximal segments principally of digits II and III of the hands (5), but also of other digits. Normal number of fingers and toes; normal thumbs and big toes. Cutaneous syndactyly of the toes.

Supplementary findings: Frequent mental retardation. Often mild hearing impairment.
 Small stature.
 Possible cryptorchidism.
 Radiologically craniosynostosis of the coronal suture.

Manifestation: At birth.

Etiology: Autosomal dominant disorder. Variable expression; occasionally incomplete penetrance.

Frequency: Low, but substantially higher than that of the Apert syndrome (p.18).

Course, prognosis: Principally dependent on whether mental retardation is present.

Differential diagnosis: Crouzon syndrome (p. 12).

Treatment: Early neurosurgical intervention should considerably improve the patient's later appearance.

Illustrations:
1–6 The same boy at ages 4 months and 2 years. Acrocephaly with premature closure of the coronal suture. Characteristic facies (including mild ptosis, right convex facial scoliosis, deviated septum, and low-set ears). Short, stubby fingers with bridges of soft tissue between digits II and III (5), radial deviation of the little fingers; soft-tissue syndactyly between toes III and IV bilaterally. Slight shortness of stature. Psychomotor retardation.

H.-R.W.

References

Kreiborg, S., Pruzansky, S., Pashayan, H. The Saethre–Chotzen syndrome. *Teratology*, 6, 287 (1972).
Pantke, O.A., Cohen, M.M. Jr., Witkop, C.R. Jr. The Saethre–Chotzen syndrome. *Birth Defects*, 11, 190 (1975).
Friedman, J.M., Hanson, J.W. et al. Saethre–Chotzen syndrome . . . *J. Pediatr.*, 91, 929–933 (1977).
Thompson, E.M., Baraitser, M. et al. Parietal foramina in Saethre–Chotzen syndrome. *J. Med. Genet.*, 21, 369–372 (1984).
Bianchi, E., Arico, M. et al. A family with the Saethre–Chotzen syndrome. *Am. J. Med. Genet.*, 22, 649–658 (1985).

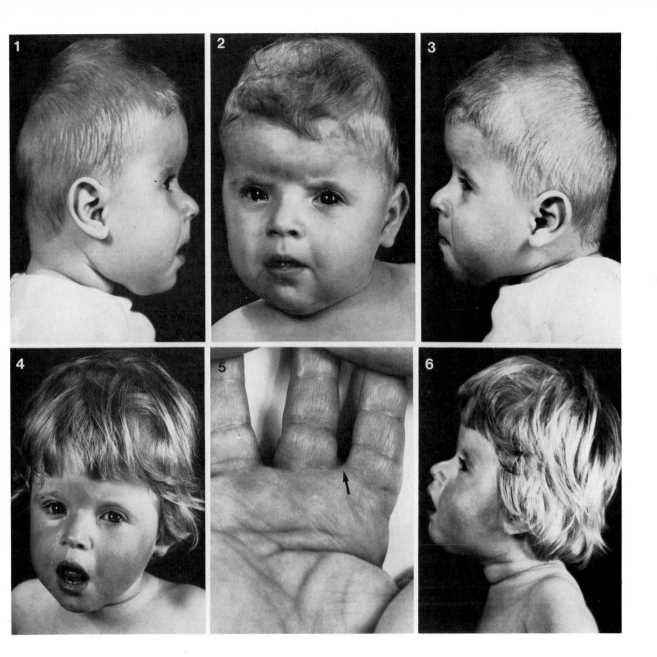

15

8. Pfeiffer Syndrome

(ACS Type V, Acrocephalosyndactyly Type Pfeiffer)

A syndrome of acrocephaly; facial dysmorphism; broad stubby thumbs and halluces; and syndactyly of a mild to moderate degree.

Main signs:
1. Acrobrachycephaly (1–3).
2. Face: Broad with a flat profile; hypertelorism; broad low nasal root; antimongoloid slant of the palpebral fissures; high arched palate; small upper and, in some cases, lower jaw. (1, 2)
3. Big toes (4) and thumbs broad and short and usually deviated. Various degrees of soft-tissue syndactyly.

Supplementary findings: Possible small stature.
  On X-ray, the anterior fontanelle may be enlarged (3), with premature closure especially of the coronal suture; various malformations, especially of the first rays of the hands and feet, e.g., trapezoidal first phalanges of the big toes.

Manifestation: At birth.

Etiology: Autosomal dominant disorder; markedly variable expression. Occurrence of germinal mosaics?

Frequency: Low.

Course, prognosis: On the whole, favorable.

Differential diagnosis: Other acrocephalosyndactyly syndromes. Among other questions open to discussion is whether Pfeiffer syndrome and Saethre–Chotzen or Apert syndrome (pp. 14 and 18) represent different grades of severity of a single hereditary defect.

Treatment: Corrective surgical measures for the cranium and/or hands may be indicated.

Illustrations:
1–5 A 2-month-old girl. Acrobrachycephaly with flat occiput; distinct interparietal bone; wide open anterior fontanelle with premature ossification of the coronal suture and part of the sagittal suture (3). Hypertelorism, antimongoloid slant of the palpebral fissures, strabismus. Broad, fat thumbs and halluces with mild cutaneous syndactyly.
  Unremarkable female chromosome complement. The mental development of this girl, who underwent early cranial surgery and whose progress has been followed for years, is within normal limits.

H.-R.W.

References:

Naveh, S. and Friedman, A. Pfeiffer syndrome: report of a family and review of the literature. *J. Med. Genet.*, 13, 277 (1976).
Bull, M.J., Escobar, V., Bixler, D. et al. Phenotype definition and occurrence risk in the acrocephalosyndactyly syndromes. *Birth Defects*, 15/5B, 65 (1979).
Sanchez, J.M. and de Negrotti, T.C. Variable expression in Pfeiffer syndrome. *J. Med. Genet.*, 18, 73 (1981).
Vaněk, J. and Losǎn F. Pfeiffer's type of acrocephalosyndactyly in two families. *J. Med. Genet.*, 19, 289–292 (1982).
Rasmussen, S.A. and Frias, J.L. Mild expression of the Pfeiffer syndrome. *Clin. Genet.*, 33, 5–10 (1988).
Hall, J.G. Mild expression of the Pfeiffer syndrome. *Clin. Genet.*, 34, 144 (1988).

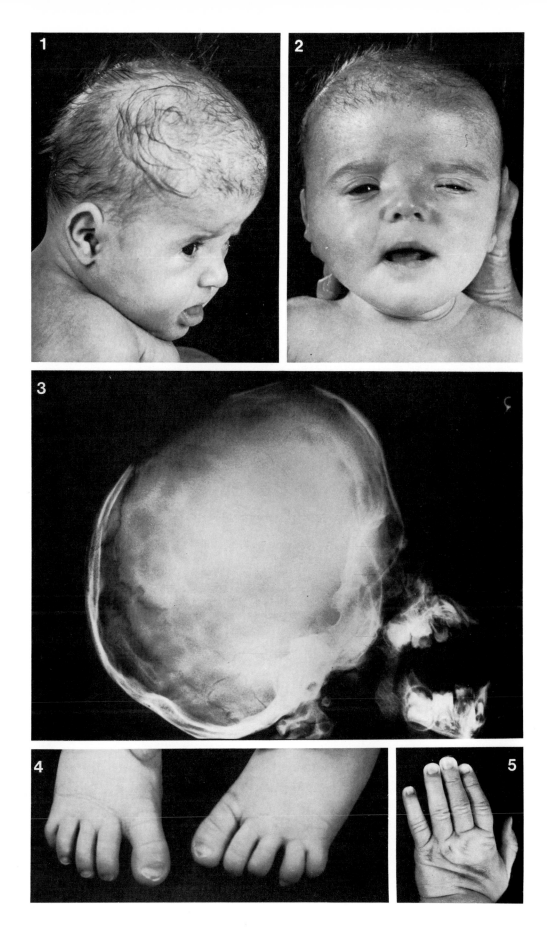

9. Apert Syndrome

(ACS Type I, Acrocephalosyndactyly Type I)

A characteristic syndrome comprising acrocephaly, facial dysmorphism, and extensive symmetrical syndactyly of the fingers (including osseous) and toes.

Main signs:
1. Acrocephaly with high prominent forehead, flat occiput (**1, 2, 4, 6**).
2. Flattish face with a horizontal supraorbital groove, hypertelorism, flat orbits with exophthalmos, strabismus, slight antimongoloid slant of the palpebral fissures, and often a small up-turned (sometimes beaklike) nose and low-set ears. Maxillary hypoplasia. Narrow palate (sometimes cleft); narrowly spaced teeth (**1, 2, 4, 6**).
3. Extensive syndactyly to almost complete spoonlike deformity of the hands (**4–7**), generally with bony fusion of the second to fourth fingers (**10**), which often share a common nail (**5**). Fingers often short (**4**). Ends of the thumbs frequently broad and distorted (**7**). Soft-tissue syndactyly of many or all toes. Big toes stubby and deformed (**8, 9, 11, 12**).

Supplementary findings: Abnormally short upper extremities (**4**), impaired mobility of the elbow and shoulder joints, anomalies of the shoulder girdle.

Not infrequently mental retardation, which may be severe; however, in about 80% of the patients an IQ of >50 to >70 can be expected.

Radiologically, irregular craniosynostosis, especially of the coronal, and often of the lambdoid, sutures; short anterior and deepened middle and posterior cranial fossae; maxillary hypoplasia, possible digital markings of the skull (**3**).

Numerous other possible associated malformations (gastrointestinal or urinary tract, cardiac, etc.).

Manifestation: At birth.

Etiology: An autosomal dominant disorder. However, the vast majority of cases are sporadic and represent new mutations (such as occur more frequently with increased paternal age); significance of germinal mosaics not yet certain.

Frequency: Low (in 1960, 150 published cases were counted).

Course, prognosis: Essentially dependent on the severity of the typical malformations, the presence or development of mental impairment, and the possible manifestations and consequences of additional defects in other organ systems. Relatively high mortality in the first years of life. Sonography and CT of the skull immediately after birth are recommended.

Treatment: Symptomatic. Early neurosurgical intervention for acrocephaly (in the first months of life), even in the absence of signs and symptoms of craniostenosis. Corrective surgery of the extremities should be undertaken sufficiently early, at a time determined in consultation with the hand surgeon. Psychological guidance and all necessary handicap aids.

Illustrations:
1, 2 and 6 Newborns.
4 A 5-year-old child.
12 A 3-year-old boy.
2, 5 and 9 The first child of a 33-year-old father. Craniosynostosis of the coronal suture, bifid uvula, suspected cardiac defect, mild mental retardation at follow-up.
3, 7, 8, 10 and 11 X-rays and close-ups of the child in 4.

H.-R.W.

References:

Spranger, J.W., Langer, L.O. Jr., Wiedemann, H.-R. *Bone Dysplasias. An Atlas of Constitutional Disorders of Skeletal Development.* G. Fischer and W.B. Saunders, Stuttgart and Philadelphia, 1974.

Stewart, R.E., Bixon, G., Cohen, A. The pathogenesis of premature craniosynostosis in acrocephalosyndactyly (Apert's syndrome). *Plast. Reconst. Surg.,* 59, 699 (1977).

Beligere, N., Harris, V., Pruzansky, S. Progressive bone dysplasia in Apert syndrome. *Radiology,* 139, 593 (1981).

Allanson, J.E. Germinal mosaicism in Apert syndrome. *Clin. Genet.,* 29, 429–433 (1986).

Kim, H., Uppal, V. et al. Apert syndrome and fetal hydrocephaly. *Hum. Genet.,* 73, 93–95 (1986).

Patton, M.A., Goodship, J. et al. Intellectual development in Apert's syndrome . . . *J. Med. Genet.,* 25, 164–167 (1988).

Rollnick, B.R. Male transmission of Apert syndrome. *Clin. Genet.,* 33, 87–90 (1988).

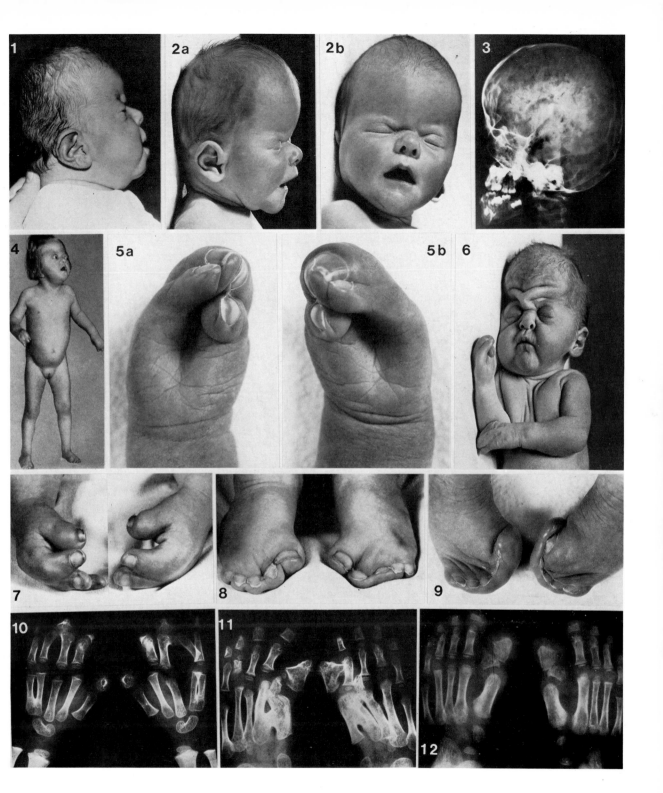

10. Opitz Trigonocephaly Syndrome

(C Syndrome [after the initial of the family name of the first cases described])

A genetic syndrome with characteristic facies, peculiar conformation of the palate, short neck, cutis laxa, joint disorders, microcephalic mental retardation, and in some cases polysyndactyly.

Main signs:
1. A somewhat triangular-shaped cranium, narrowing at the top (trigonocephaly) with the forehead showing a prominent median ridge and in some cases bitemporal depressions (1, 4). In some cases nevus flammeus of the glabella, hypertrichosis of the forehead. Hypotelorism. Mongoloid slant of the palpebral fissures. Strabismus, epicanthal folds (1, 2), and other eye anomalies; broad short nasal bridge, pug nose; long philtrum; and diverse anomalies of the external ears (low-set or rotated ears, soft pinnae due to paucity of cartilage, and others). High palate, very narrow especially anteriorly, between abnormally wide alveolar ridges (sometimes with frenulae between the latter and the buccal mucous membrane). Macrostomia, micrognathia.
2. Loose skin, especially of the neck. Widely spaced nipples. Hyperextensibility, dislocation, or contractures of the large joints.
3. Failure to thrive in most cases. Hypotonia. Increasing tendency to microcephaly with corresponding psychomotor retardation.
4. In some cases short hands and/or fingers (possible aplasia of phalanges of the fingers and/or toes), club feet; postaxial, less frequently preaxial hexadactyly; curved little fingers, and cutaneous syndactyly.

Supplementary findings: Possible cardiovascular defects. Lung, kidney, or other internal malformations. Deformities of the thorax, genital anomalies, short extremities, short stature.

Manifestation: At birth.

Etiology: This syndrome, which is phenotypically very variable, apparently can occur as the expression of an autosomal recessive gene or as the result of anomalies of chromosome 3. Careful, sometimes repeated, chromosome analysis is indicated, especially in the light of the great difference in recurrence risks!

Frequency: Barely 35 cases have been described to date. However, the syndrome is probably not extremely rare.

Course, prognosis: After initial, usually severe, failure to thrive, frequently death in early infancy. Surviving children are usually severely retarded.

Differential diagnosis: The Gruber–Meckel and the Smith–Lemli–Opitz syndromes should be considered in some cases, as well as a number of chromosome aberrations that may be accompanied by trigonocephaly.

Treatment: Conservative, symptomatic.

Illustrations: 1–8 A 5-month-old boy. Microdolichotrigonocephaly (1–4). Bilateral buphthalmos, pug nose. Long philtrum. Macrostomia (1 and 2); high narrow palate; preauricular pits (5). Short neck, deformation of the thorax, ventricular septal defect; cryptorchidism. Laxity of the skin and musculature. Short hands with bilateral fifth-finger clinodactyly and simian crease (6 and 7); club feet with hypoplasia of rays III–V. A repeated chromosome analysis (after an initial 'normal' result) demonstrated a pericentric inversion of chromosome 3.

H.-R.W.

References:
Oberklaid, E. and Danks, M. The Opitz trigonocephaly syndrome. *Am. J. Dis. Child.*, 129, 1348 (1975).
Antley, R.M., Sung Hwang, D., Theopold, W., Gorlin, R.J., Steeper, T., Pitt, D., Danks, M., McPherson, E., Bartels, H., Wiedemann, H.-R., Opitz, J.M. Further delineation of the C (trigonocephaly) syndrome. *Am. J. Med. Genet.*, 9, 147–163 (1981).
Flatz, S.D., Schinzel, A., Doehring, E. Opitz trigonocephaly syndrome: report of two cases. *Eur. J. Pediatr.*, 141, 183–185 (1984).
Fryns, J.P., Snoeck, L., Kleczkowska, A. et al. Opitz trigonocephaly syndrome and terminal transverse limb reduction defects. *Helv. Paed. Acta*, 40, 485–488 (1985).
Sargent, C., Burn, J., Baraitser, M. et al. Trigonocephaly and the Opitz C syndrome. *J. Med. Genet.*, 22, 39–45 (1985).
Reynolds, J.F., Johnston, K.M. et al. Nosology of the C syndrome. *Abstracts of the 10th anniversary David W. Smith Workshop on Malformations and Morphogenesis.* Madrid, May 1989, p. 34.

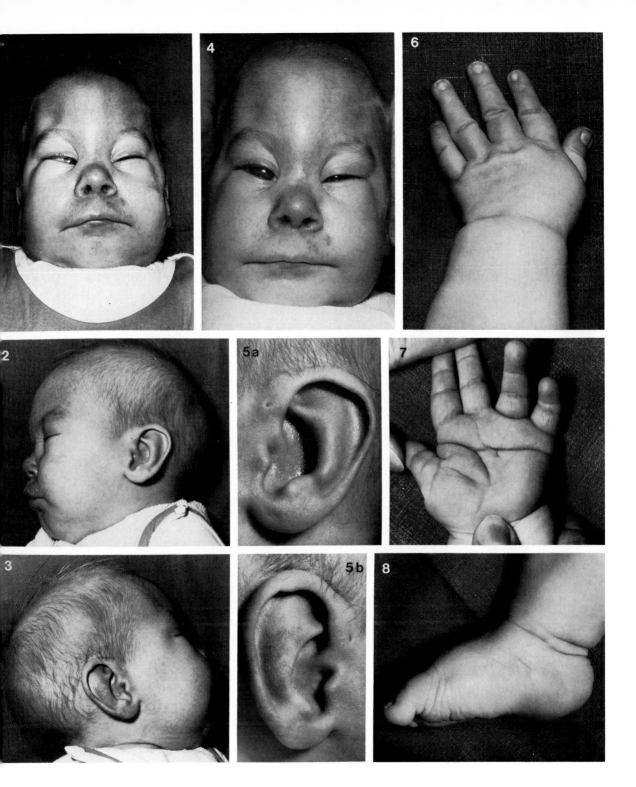

21

11. Carpenter Syndrome

(ACPS Type II, Acrocephalopolysyndactyly Type Carpenter)

A syndrome of acrocephaly, facial dysmorphism, brachyclinosyndactyly of the hands and polysyndactyly of the feet.

Main signs:
1. Oxy- and acrobrachycephaly with bulging fontanelle (1). In some cases marked bulging of the temporal areas, symmetrically or asymmetrically (1, 3), with resemblance to or actual formation of a cloverleaf skull (p.24).
2. Face broad and flat with exophthalmos, dystopia canthorum, possible mongoloid or antimongoloid slant of the palpebral fissures and epicanthal folds, low-set and posteriorly rotated ears, high-arched palate and micrognathia (1, 2). Broad, thick neck.
3. Short hands; brachy-, campto-, and clinodactyly; broad thumbs; cutaneous syndactyly between the middle and ring fingers, in some cases more fingers are involved (1, 2). Short and very wide halluces, may appear bifid, with various degrees of syndactyly of the toes.

Supplementary findings: Frequently cardiac defects, mild mental retardation, anomalies of the cornea, truncal obesity, also small stature, urogenital anomalies.

Coxa valga, genu valgum, lateral dislocation of the patella, pes varus.

Radiologically, characteristic configuration, deviation and duplication in the thumb and big toe regions (4 and 5). Brachy- or amesophalangia of the fingers and toes.

Manifestation: At birth.

Etiology: Autosomal recessive disorder; variable expression.

Frequency: Rare (40 reported cases up to 1987).

Course, prognosis: Mainly dependent on the presence and degree of primary mental retardation and on early surgical treatment of the cranium and, in some cases, the heart.

Diagnosis, differential diagnosis: Greig's cephalopolysyndactyly syndrome (p. 414) can be easily ruled out by the mild cranial dysmorphism; in addition, it is transmitted by autosomal dominant inheritance.

A Bardet–Biedl syndrome (p. 288), suggested by the obesity, hypogenitalism, mental retardation, and polydactyly, can be excluded by the shape of the skull, the facies, the duplication of the halluces, and syndactyly of the Carpenter syndrome, and by the absence of tapetoretinal degeneration. The ACPS observations of Goodman et al. and Summit et al. probably fall within the domain of the Carpenter syndrome.

Treatment: Surgical measures, as required, on the cranium, the extremities, and the heart.

Illustrations:
1–5 A female infant with the Carpenter syndrome. Cutaneous syndactyly of the third and fourth fingers and of the first to third toes bilaterally; broad, stubby thumbs and halluces. Radiologically, deviation of the hypoplastic proximal phalanx of the thumb and hypo- and aplasia of various middle phalanges. Coarse broadening of the first ray in both feet, with duplication of the proximal and distal phalanges of the halluces.

H.-R.W.

References:
Pfeiffer, R.A., Seemann, K.B., Tünte, W. et al. Akrozephalopolysyndaktylie. *Klin. Pädiatr.*, 189, 120 (1977).
Verdy, M., Dussault, R.G. et al. Carpenter's syndrome . . . *Acta Endocrinol.*, 104, 6–9 (1983).
Robinson, L.K., James, H.E. et al. Carpenter syndrome: natural history and clinical spectrum. *Am. J. Med. Genet.*, 20, 461–469 (1985).
Cohen, D.M., Green, J.G. et al. Acrocephalopolysyndactyly type II—Carpenter syndrome . . . *Am. J. Med. Genet.*, 28, 311–324 (1987).

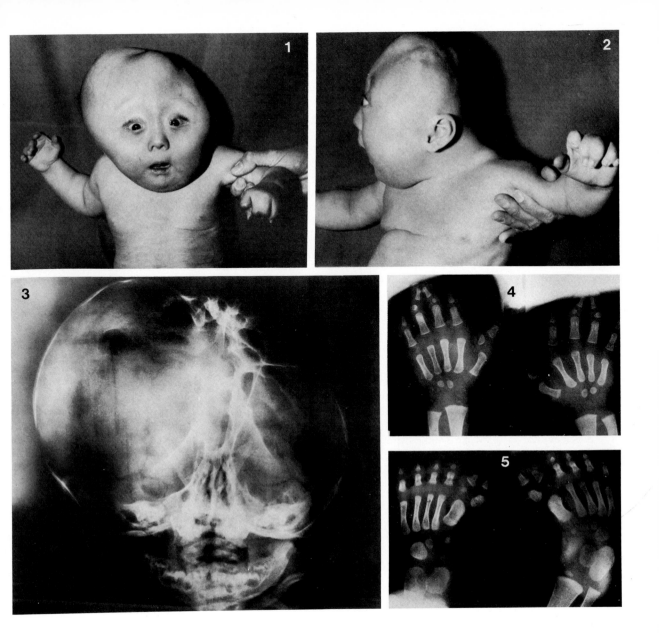

12. Cloverleaf skull

(Kleeblattschädel, Crâne en Trèfle)

A cloverleaf-like deformity of the skull resulting from premature closure of the cranial sutures, occurring alone or as part of a number of fairly extensive and well-defined clinical syndromes.

Main signs: Marked bubble-like outpouching of the cranium upwards and bilaterally outwards at the temporal areas, with downward displacement of the ears to an almost horizontal position, depressed nasal root, and exophthalmos (1, 2). Hydrocephalus (3).

Supplementary findings: Increased intracranial pressure, muscle wasting, impaired psychomotor development.

Manifestation: At birth.

Etiology: Etiologically and pathogenetically heterogeneous. Cloverleaf skull can occur in the Apert, Carpenter, Crouzon, and Pfeiffer syndromes; with camptomelic dysplasia (p. 232), thanatophoric dysplasia type II (p. 216), and some other skeletal dysplasias; with certain chromosomal aberrations, in combination with impaired mobility of the large joints (especially the elbows); and as an apparently isolated finding.

Frequency: Low (120 case reports in the literature).

Course, prognosis: Unfavorable; early death.

Treatment: Symptomatic neurosurgical measures may be indicated.

Illustrations:
1 and 2 A 2-month-old infant with cloverleaf skull as an isolated finding. Normally proportioned trunk and extremities. At examination, no anomalies apart from the cranial. No joint disorders.
3 The pneumoencephalogram shows markedly dilated lateral ventricles in the protruding temporal areas. (Child died at age 5 months.)

H.-R.W.

References:
Holtermüller, K. and Wiedemann, H.-R. Kleeblattschädel-Syndrom. *Med. Mschr.*, 14, 439 (1960).
Wiedemann, H.-R. and Ostertag, B. Kleeblattschädel und allgemeine Mikromelie. *Klin. Pädiatr.*, 186, 261 (1974).
Aksu, F. and Mietens, C. Kleeblattschädel-Syndrom. *Klin. Pädiatr.*, 191, 418 (1979).
Cohen, M.M. Jr. Craniosynostosis . . . *Birth Defects, Orig. Art. Ser.*, XV, 5B, 13–63 (1979).
Banna, M., Omaloja, M.E. et al. The cloverleaf skull. *Br. J. Radiol.*, 53, 730–732 (1980).
Turner, P.T. and Reynolds, A.F. Generous craniectomy for Kleeblattschädel anomaly. *Neurosurg.*, 6, 555–558 (1980).
Kremens, B., Kemperdick, H. et al. Thanatophoric dysplasia with cloverleaf skull. *Eur. J. Pediatr.*, 139, 298–303 (1982).
Zuleta, A. and Basauri, L. Cloverleaf skull syndrome. *Child's Brain*, 11, 418–427 (1984).
Kozlowski, K., Warren, P.S. et al. Cloverleaf skull with generalized bone dysplasia. *Pediatr. Radiol.*, 15, 412–414 (1985).
Gathmann, H.A., Vitzthum, H., Aksu, F. Zur Klinik und Pathogenese der 'Kleeblattschädel-Anomalie'. In: *Entwicklungsstörungen des Zentralnervensystems.* Neuhäuser, G. (ed.). Kohlhammer, Stuttgart p. 90–98 (1986).
Kroczek, R.A., Mühlbauer, W. et al. Cloverleaf skull associated with Pfeiffer syndrome . . . *Eur. J. Pediatr.*, 145, 442–445 (1986).
Benallègue, A., Lacette, F. et al. Crâne en trèfle . . . *Ann. Génét.*, 30, 113–117 (1987).
Dambrain, R. Fround, M. et al. Considerations about the cloverleaf skull. *J. Craniofac. Genet. Develop. Biol.*, 7, 387–401 (1987).
Say, B. and Poznanski, A.K. Cloverleaf skull . . . *Pediatr. Radiol.*, 17, 93–96 (1987).
Cohen, M.M. Jr. Craniosynostosis update 1987. *Am. J. Med. Genet.* (Suppl.), 4, 99–148 (1988).

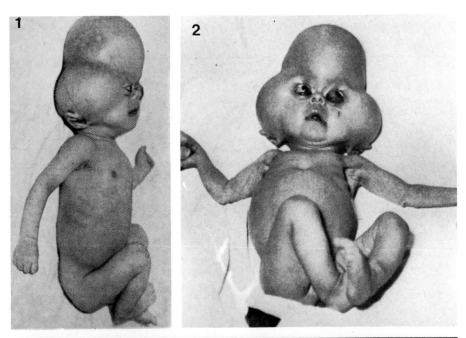

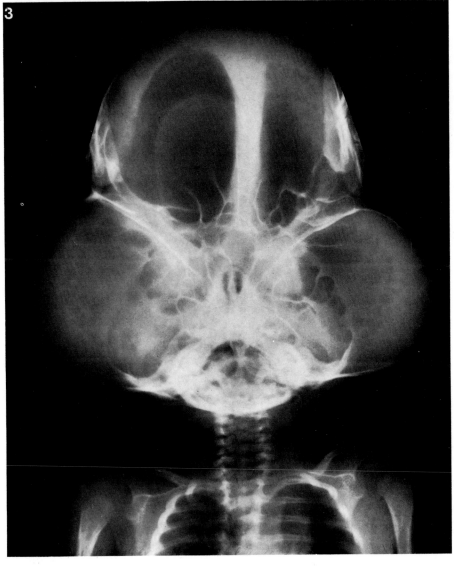

13. Oto-palato-digital Syndrome

A malformation syndrome with typical facial dysmorphism; signs of bone dysplasia, particularly in the form of 'frog hands and frog feet'; cleft palate; and impaired hearing.

Main signs:

1. Characteristic facies with broad prominent forehead, hypertelorism, antimongoloid slant of the palpebral fissures, marked supraorbital bulging, broad root of the nose, flat midface, and microstomia with down-turned corners of the mouth (3, 4, 11, 12). Prominent occiput. Low-set ears. Micrognathia and cleft palate.

2. Broad and short distal phalanges of the hands and feet, particularly of the first ray, the shortness of which is due mainly to hypoplasia of the metacarpal or first metatarsal and the proximal phalanx. Frequent clinodactyly of the little finger. Partial syndactyly. All in all, reminiscent of a 'frog hand' or 'frog foot' (5–8). Enlargement and limited movement of the large joints.

3. Frequently moderate conductive hearing impairment. Tendency to otitis, sinusitis, and mastoiditis. Frequent mild mental retardation.

Supplementary findings: Slight shortness of stature. Dental anomalies.

Fusion and deformity of the metacarpals and metatarsals with additional ossification centers and ossicles. Incomplete fusion of the neural arches generally involving several vertebrae. Vertical clivus.

Manifestation: At birth.

Etiology: Hereditary disorder, with the mode of inheritance not yet definitely established. X-linked recessive is probably the predominant type, but X-linked dominant and autosomal dominant with sex-limited expression have also been suggested. Females usually are much less severely affected.

Frequency: Including the children shown here, 69 cases in males and 34 in females were known up to 1981.

Course, prognosis: Normal life expectancy.

Diagnosis, differential diagnosis: Other syndromes with broad, short halluces and thumbs, such as the Munchmeyer (p. 444) or the Rubinstein–Taybi syndrome (p. 162), etc., can easily be excluded by the total picture. The same should be true for the Larsen syndrome (p. 404), which also includes the flat facies and joint deformities.

An X-ray of the feet is especially valuable in confirming a tentative clinical diagnosis of oto-palato-digital syndrome.

Comment: A further X-linked disorder, which has similar facial dysmorphism, has been designated oto-palato-digital syndrome type II. This is distinguishable by more extensive skeletal changes (narrowed thorax; marked bowing of long bones of the extremities; absence of the fibulae, etc.), a hearing defect as a constant feature, and a much less favorable prognosis.

Treatment: Symptomatic.

Illustrations:

1–6 The index case at age 7 years. Birth measurements and present size within normal limits. Tetralogy of Fallot, totally corrected. Bifid uvula, slightly impaired hearing, frequent otitis. Intellect in the low normal range. Limited motion of the large joints; thenar hypoplasia. Anomalies in the carpal and tarsal regions with synostoses in the latter. Wide defect of the neural arches from the lower thoracic to the sacral vertebrae.

7–12 The brother of the index patient at age 12 years. Birth measurements and present size within normal limits. Essentially the same somatic findings; however, complete median cleft of the soft palate (surgically corrected), no cardiac defect; no X-rays of the vertebral column.

13 and 14 The sister of the two brothers at age 13 years. On the basis of her similar facial features, she may be regarded as a gene carrier. Except for slightly limited motion at her wrists, she has no further anomalies.

H.-R.W.

References:

Spranger, J.W., Langer, L.O. Jr., Wiedemann, H.-R. *Bone Dysplasias. An Atlas of Constitutional Disorders of Skeletal Development.* G. Fischer and W.B. Saunders, Stuttgart and Philadelphia, 1974.

André, M., Vigneron, J. et al. Abnormal facies, cleft palate, and generalized dysostosis: a lethal X-linked syndrome. *J. Pediatr.,* 98, 747–752 (1981).

Fitch, N., Jequier, S. et al. The oto-palato-digital syndrome, proposed type II. *Am. J. Med. Genet.,* 15, 655–664 (1983).

Kaplan, J. and Maroteaux, P. Syndrome oto-palato-digital de type II. *Ann. Génét.,* 27, 79–82 (1984).

Brewster, T. G., Lachmann, R.S. et al. Oto-palato-digital syndrome, type II . . . *Am. J. Med. Genet.,* 20, 249–254 (1985).

Pazzaglia, U.E. and Beluffi, G. Oto-palato-digital syndrome in four generations . . . *Clin. Genet.,* 30, 338–344 (1986).

Marec, B. le, Odent, S. et al. Syndrome oto-palato-digital de type I . . . *Ann. Génét.,* 31, 155–171 (1988).

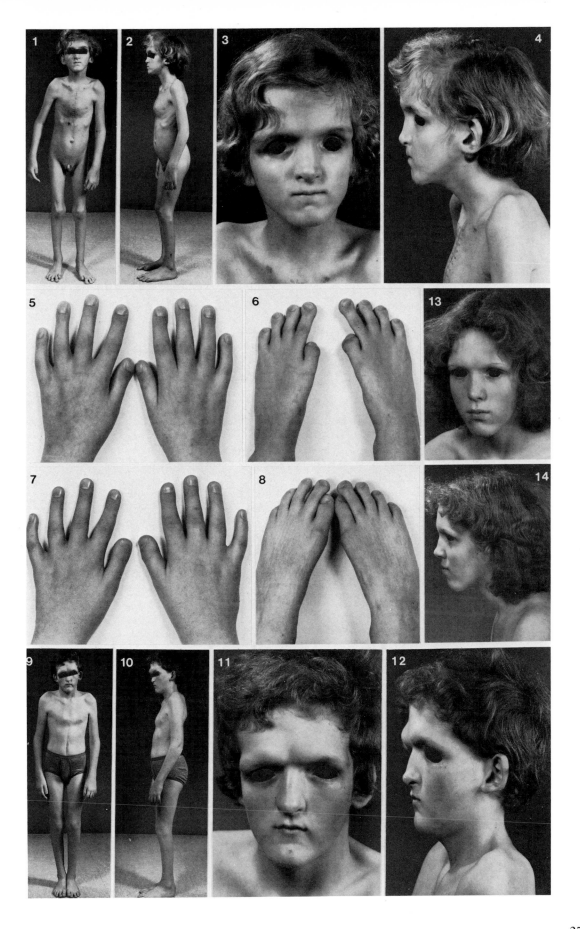

14. Coffin–Lowry Syndrome

A syndrome comprising unusual coarse facies, mental retardation, small stature, generalized hypotonia, and characteristic hands — with males far more severely affected than females.

Main signs:

1. Narrow, rectangular protruding forehead appearing bitemporally compressed; prominent supraorbital ridges, hypertelorism, antimongoloid slant of the palpebral fissures, thick upper eyelids, sometimes ptosis; broad nasal root and short broad pug nose with a thick septum and alae; pouting lower lip, prognathism, mouth usually open; hypodontia, dysodontiasis; and unusual ears (2, 4–7).
2. Mental retardation, considerable in males (IQ usually below 50), less severe in females.
3. Small stature, variously severe, height possibly below the third percentile.
4. 'Full' forearms. Plumpish, lax, soft hands with tapered, hyperextensible fingers (8). Short halluces.

Supplementary findings: Laxity of the joints and ligaments. Cutis laxa and poor muscle performance (1). Frequently kyphoscoliosis (3), pectus carinatum or excavatum, and pes valgus. Clumsy wide-based gait. (These findings especially pronounced in males.)

Radiologically: distal phalanges of the fingers short and distally distended ('tufted'); dysplastic middle phalanges; short rays of the big toes; coxa valga; and other signs.

Possible convulsive disorder.

Manifestation: At birth or later (increasing coarseness of facial features; increasingly apparent short stature).

Etiology: Possibly a systemic connective tissue disorder; anomalies of proteoglycan metabolism in cultured fibroblasts and other abnormalities have been described. The syndrome is X-linked (no male-to-male transmission), with diminished expression in females. The gene appears to be located on the short arm of the X chromosome. Female 'carriers' can be recognized mainly by facial characteristics or peculiarities of the hands and fingers (see above).

Frequency: Low; to date about 60 case reports.

Course, prognosis: The signs become more marked with age.

Differential diagnosis: Other forms of mental retardation and short stature with coarse facies, especially fragile X syndrome (p. 100), Sotos syndrome (p. 138) and Williams–Beuren syndrome (p. 484).

Treatment: Symptomatic. Handicap aids. Genetic counseling for the parents.

Illustrations:

1–8 A proband with typical signs of the syndrome.

H.-R.W.

References:

Tentamy, S.A., Miller, D., Hussels-Maumenee, I. The Coffin–Lowry syndrome: an inherited faciodigital mental retardation syndrome. *J. Pediatr.*, 86, 724 (1975).

Fryns, J.P., Vinken, L., Berge, H. van den. The Coffin syndrome. *Hum. Genet.*, 36, 271 (1977).

Wilson, W.G. and Kelly, T.E. Early recognition of the Coffin–Lowry syndrome. *Am. J. Med. Genet.*, 8, 215–220 (1981).

Hunter, A.G.W., Partington, M.W. et al. The Coffin–Lowry syndrome . . . *Clin. Genet.*, 21, 321–335 (1982).

Beck, M., Glössl, J. et al. Abnormal proteodermatan sulfate in three patients with Coffin–Lowry syndrome. *Ped. Res.*, 17, 926–927 (1983).

Machin, G.A., Walther, G.L. et al. Autopsy findings in two adult siblings with Coffin–Lowry syndrome. *Am. J. Med. Genet.* (Suppl.), 3, 303–309 (1987).

Gilgenkrantz, S., Mujica, P. et al. Coffin–Lowry syndrome: a multicenter study. *Clin. Genet.*, 34, 230–245 (1988).

Partington, M.W., Mulley, J.C. et al. A family with the Coffin–Lowry syndrome revisited . . . *Am. J. Med. Genet.*, 30, 509–521 (1988).

Hanauer, A., Alembik, Y. et al. Probable localization of the Coffin–Lowry locus . . . *Am. J. Med. Genet.*, 30, 523–530 (1988).

Young, I.D. The Coffin–Lowry syndrome. *J. Med. Genet.*, 25, 344–348 (1988).

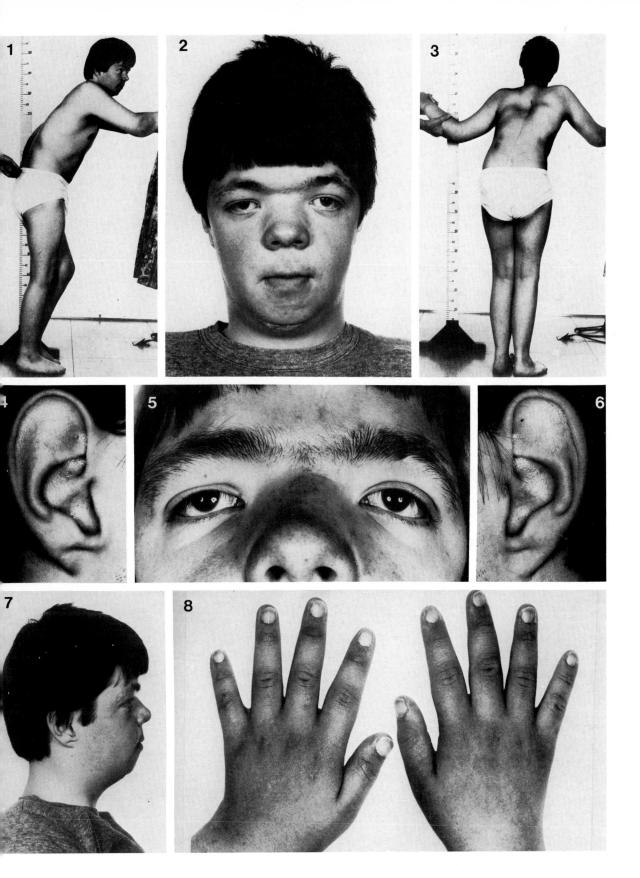

15. Melnick–Needles Syndrome

(Osteodysplasty)

A highly characteristic syndrome mainly of the skeletal system, the affected having a typical facial appearance.

Main signs:
1. Relatively large cranium with high prominent forehead and generally marked delay in closure of the anterior fontanelle. Facial part of the skull small with exophthalmos, hypertelorism, fleshy nose, full cheeks, relatively large ears, micrognathia of the lower jaw, malalignment of the teeth, malocclusion (1).
2. Some degree of bowing of the arms and legs with cubitus valgus and genu valgum positions. Slight shortening of the distal phalanges of the hands and feet, especially of the thumbs.
3. Bizarre, characteristic radiological changes (especially cortical irregularities and narrowing of the diaphyses) of the long bones (2), the ribs (4), clavicles, shoulder blades, and the pelvis (5) with severe coxa valga; other areas also affected in this generalized skeletal dysplasia.

Supplementary findings: Narrow thorax with possible impairment of respiration; hip dysplasia not infrequent; club feet may be present. Hyperextensibility of the joints and skin, diastasis recti abdominis, hernias. Mental development not affected.

A possible hearing defect or anomalies of the urinary tract must be ruled out.

Manifestation: Pre- and postnatally. Apart from the abnormal facies and delayed closure of the anterior fontanelle, the patients usually come to attention because of an abnormal gait and 'bowed' limbs.

Etiology: Monogenic hereditary disease, autosomal dominant or X-linked dominant, with possible lethality in males and survival in females.

Frequency: Very low (about 65 observations have been reported in the literature).

Course, prognosis: Not infrequently initial failure to thrive and increased susceptibility to infections of the upper respiratory tract and the middle ear in the first years of life.

As a rule, normal adult height. Normal life expectancy. Possible difficulties with child bearing due to pelvic deformity. Premature arthrosis.

Diagnosis, differential diagnosis: Prenatal recognition of skeletal changes on X-ray possible. Some superficial similarities to, e.g., pyknodysostosis (p. 200), craniometaphyseal dysplasia (p. 104), or Engelmann–Camurati syndrome (p. 520), which can be immediately ruled out radiologically. Partially expressed forms of the syndrome may be recognized only by chance.

Treatment: Symptomatic. Orthopedic treatment, as required, especially for the spinal column, the hips, and the feet. Dental and orthodontic care.

Illustrations:
1–5 An 8-year-old patient with the fully expressed syndrome. Note in addition the disease-related sclerosis of the base of the skull (3).

H.-R.W.

References:

Spranger, J.W., Langer, L.O. Jr., Wiedemann, H.-R. *Bone Dysplasias. An Atlas of Constitutional Disorders of Skeletal Development.* G. Fischer and W.B. Saunders, Stuttgart and Philadelphia, 1974.
Leiber, B., Olbrich, G., Moelter, N. et al. Melnick–Needles-Syndrom. *Monatschr. Kinderheilkd.,* 123, 178 (1975).
Fryns, J.P., Maertens, R., Berghe, H. van den. Osteodysplastia—a rare skeletal dysplasia. *Acta Pediatr. Belg.,* 32, 65 (1979).
Dereymaeker, A.M., Christens, J. et al. Melnick-Needles syndrome (osteodysplasty). Clinical and radiological heterogeneity. *Helv. Pediatr. Acta,* 41, 339–351 (1986).
Donnenfeld, A.E., Conard, A.K. et al. Melnick–Needles syndrome in males: a lethal multiple congenital anomalies syndrome. *Am. J. Med. Genet.,* 27, 159–173 (1987).
Krajewska-Walasek, M., Winkielman, J. et al. Melnick–Needles syndrome in males. *Am. J. Med. Genet.,* 27, 153–158 (1987).
Fryns, J.P., Schinzel, A. et al. Hyperlaxity in males with Melnick–Needles syndrome. *Am. J. Med. Genet.,* 29, 607–611 (1988).
Sauter, R., Klemm, T. et al. Melnick–Needles-Syndrom. *Pädiatr. Prax.,* 37, 173–180 (1988).

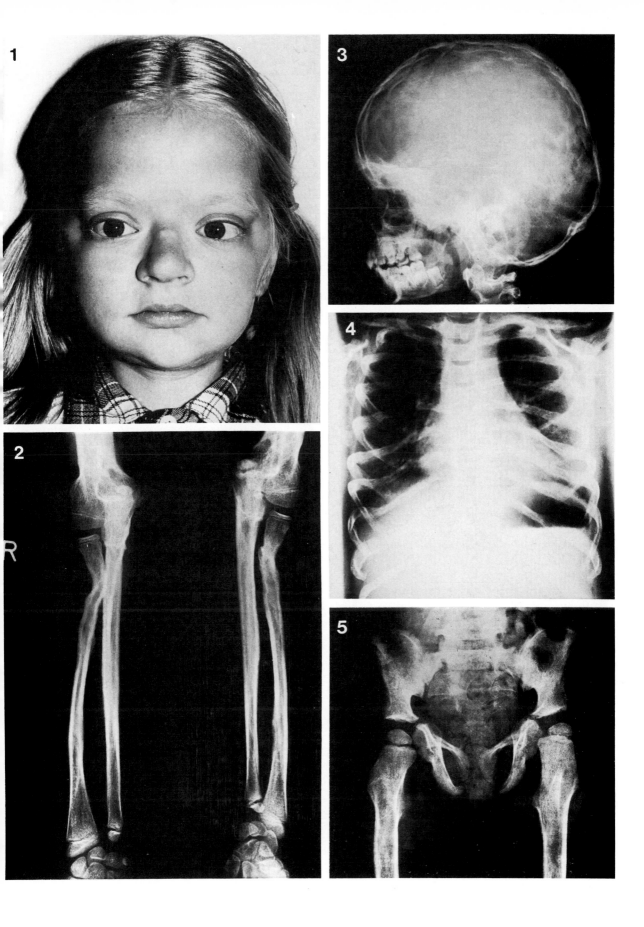

31

16. Cleidocranial Dysplasia

(Scheuthauer–Marie Syndrome)

A characteristic hereditary disorder especially of the skeleton (cranium, clavicles, pelvis) with typical physical appearance.

Main signs:
1. Large, broad, and short cranium with frontal and parietal bossing and a supraglabellar depression (**1, 3**), persistence of the fontanelles and open sutures for years (**7**); facial part of the cranium relatively small with hypertelorism, broad depressed nasal root, in some cases anteverted nares (**2**), and mild exophthalmos.
2. Upper thorax narrow with absent or poorly defined superior and inferior clavicular depressions and drooping, angular shoulders (**2, 4, 5**) with a-, hypo-, or dysplasia of the clavicles (**8**). Hypermobility of the shoulders (**3, 6**)!

Supplementary findings: Narrow pelvis, slender extremities, slight shortness of stature possible after infancy. Dysodontiasis (delay of both dentitions, supernumerary teeth) (**9**). Nails may be hypoplastic and brittle (**10**).

Radiologically, numerous wormian bones (**7**), markedly delayed ossification of the bony pelvis, especially the pubic bones.

Manifestation: At birth.

Etiology: Monogenic hereditary disorder, autosomal dominant, with quite variable expression. Isolated occurrence of a case in a kindred with no signs of the condition suggests a new mutation. However, the occurrence of an autosomal recessive form has recently been under discussion.

Frequency: Not so rare. By 1962, about 700 cases in the literature.

Course, prognosis: Life expectancy normal or slightly reduced. Developmental defects of the teeth and jaws are frequent and may be very troublesome. Tendency to dislocations. Narrowness of the pelvis may necessitate caesarean deliveries.

Differential diagnosis: In newborn and young infants, possible erroneous initial diagnosis of hydrocephalus or osteogenesis imperfecta. Later, possible confusion with the much less frequently occurring pyknodysostosis (p. 200; having distinct growth deficiency, absence of the supraglabellar depression, clavicular ridges usually normal, no comparable ossification defect of the pelvic bones; but above all, osteosclerosis, tendency to fractures, poorly defined submaxillary angle. Autosomal recessive transmission.).

Treatment: Early dental and orthodontic care as needed. Orthopedic treatment may be indicated.

Illustrations:
1 A 2½-year-old.
2 and 3 5-year-old children.
4–6 A 1½-year-old.
7 Skull X-ray of a 4-year-old child: open fontanelles and sutures, markedly widened frontal suture, numerous wormian bones.
8 Chest X-ray of an 8-year-old child: aplasia of the clavicles and abnormally positioned scapulae.
9 Supernumerary incisors in both the upper and lower jaws between persisting deciduous teeth in a 9-year-old child.
10 Hypoplastic, brittle nails in a 5-year-old child.

H.-R.W.

References:

Wiedemann, H.-R. Gestörte Ossifikation besonders der bindegewebig präformierten Belegknochen: Die Dysostosis cleidocranialis. *Handbuch der Kinderheilkunde*, vol. 6, p. 128 ff. Heidelberg, Springer 1967.

Spranger, J.W., Langer, L.O. Jr., Wiedemann, H.-R. *Bone Dysplasias. An Atlas of Constitutional Disorders of Skeletal Development.* G. Fischer and W.B. Saunders, Stuttgart and Philadelphia, 1974.

Goodman, R.M., Tadmor, R., Zaritsky, A. et al. Evidence for an autosomal recessive form of cleidocranial dysostosis. *Clin. Genet.*, 8, 20 (1975).

Fleischer-Peters, A. and Schuch, P. Befindlichkeit und Lebensschicksal von Patienten mit Dysostosis cleidocranialis. *Der Kinderarzt*, 14, 1059–1067 (1983).

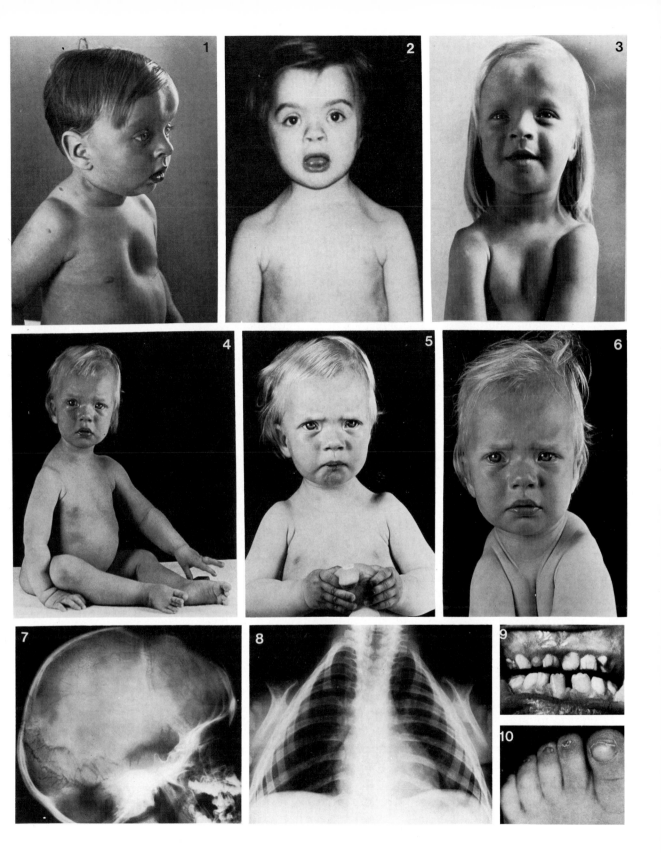

33

17. Syndrome of Increasing Macrocephaly with Signs of Cardiac Overload from Intracranial A-V Shunt

Progressive macrocephaly (with or without definite hydrocephalus) and signs of cardiac overload (in the absence of congenital heart defect) with intracranial A-V fistula (usually an aneurysm of the vein of Galen).

Main signs:
1. Abnormal growth of the cranium (**1, 2**) with development of some degree of dilatation of the ventricular system and with minimal to definite signs of increased intracranial pressure.
2. Signs of cardiac failure without demonstrable congenital heart disease.
3. In most (but not 100% of) cases a continuous or systolic vascular murmur can be detected over all or part of the cranium; in some cases increased vascularity, pulsations, etc. Usually visible pulsations of the cervical vessels, with thrills and murmurs.

Supplementary findings: Demonstration of an intracranial A-V fistula (A-V aneurysm, generally involving the great vein of Galen) (**3, 4**).

Manifestation: Macrocephaly apparent congenitally or postnatally. Signs of cardiac overload become manifest sooner or later depending on the size of the shunt.

Etiology: Uncertain.

Frequency: Not so rare; probably quite a few go unrecognized.

Course, prognosis: In view of the precarious cerebral and cardiac problems, always dubious.

Diagnosis: Initially, cranial sonography, perhaps computer tomography or subtraction-angiography; subsequently usually angiography of the carotid and vertebral arteries bilaterally.

Differential diagnosis: Intracranial A-V fistula in Osler disease. Family history.

Treatment: The cardiac insufficiency may not respond to medical treatment. Possibly surgery, if necessary, as a last resort, at a time very carefully chosen by the neurosurgeon and cardiologist in consultation together.

Comments:
1. In any location of the body an extracardiac A-V shunt can, depending on the size, lead to signs of cardiac overload and possibly to life-threatening decompensation.
2. Intracranial shunts of a given size frequently manifest immediately post partum with severe cyanotic cardiac insufficiency. When not manifest until later in infancy or thereafter, developing hydrocephalus and convulsions or subarachnoid hemorrhages and neurological defects may dominate the picture. The 'craniomegalic' form presented here is one particular, unusual form.

Illustrations:
1 and 3 A 5-year-old boy with congenital, progressive macrocephaly (at birth, 39 cm; 11 months, 52.8 cm; 13 months, 54 cm; 4 years, 58 cm). Signs of cardiac overload without evidence of heart defect, due to an extracardial left-to-right shunt. Continuous vascular murmur together with distended veins over the scalp; low-voltage EEG, dilated ventricles, and papilledema. Otherwise normal development for age, with no neurological deficits. On angiogram, a large aneurysm of the great vein of Galen; aneurysmal enlargement of the confluence of the sinuses and adjacent vessels due to A-V shunts to both posterior cerebral arteries; numerous angiomas.
2a, b, and c Another patient at ages 5, 7, and 8 years. Congenital progressive macrocephaly (at birth, 38 cm; 5 years, 60 cm). Signs of cardiac overload without evidence of heart defect, due to an extracardiac left-to-right shunt. Continuous vascular murmur and prominent veins and pulsations on the scalp; low-voltage EEG, secondary internal hydrocephalus (Pudenz–Heyer catheter). Otherwise normal development for age, with no neurological deficits. On angiogram, large aneurysm of the great vein of Galen with some angioma-like enlargement of adjacent vessels due to A-V shunts with both posterior cerebral arteries.
4 Successful operative closure at age 7 years of most of the pathological anastomoses, without neurological sequelae (Professor Yasargil, Zürich).

H.-R.W.

References:
Gold, A.P., Ransohoff, J., Carter, S. Vein of Galen malformation. *Acta Neurolog. Scand.*, 40 (Suppl. 11), 1 (1964).
Amacher, A.L. and Shillito, J. Jr. The syndromes and surgical treatment of aneurysms of the great vein of Galen. *J. Neurosurg.*, 39, 89 (1973).
Cuncliffe, P.N. Cerebral arteriovenous aneurysm presenting with heart failure. *Brit. Heart J.*, 36, 919 (1974).
Kelly, J.J. Jr., Mellinger, J.F., Sundt, T.M. Jr. Intracranial arteriovenous malformations in childhood. *Ann. Neurol.*, 338, 314 (1978).
Benz-Bohm, G., Neufang, K.F.R. et al. A. v. Mißbildung im Bereich der Vena Galeni . . . *Fortschr. Röntgenstr.*, 142, 579–581 (1985).

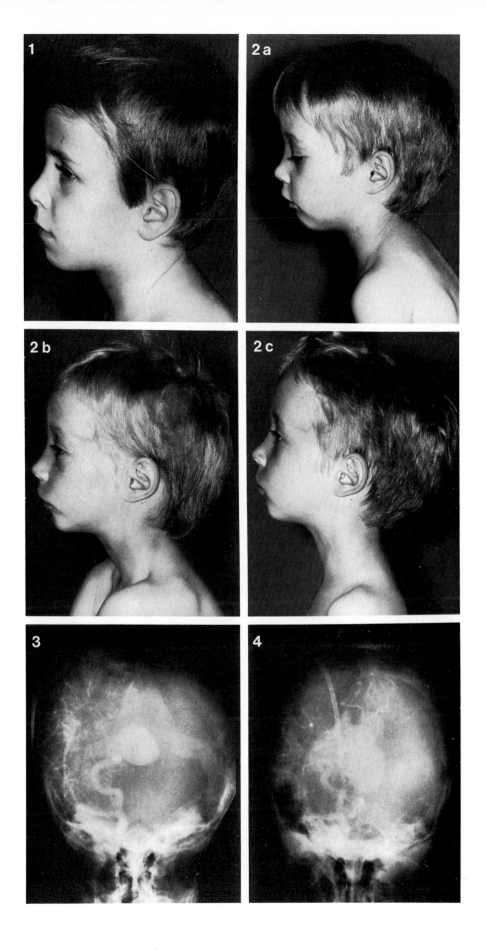

18. Megalencephaly

A condition with primary megalencephaly, occasionally associated with primary developmental retardation, hypotonia, epilepsy, or other anomalies, such as cardiac defects.

Main signs:
1. Macrodolichocephaly (head circumference increasingly above the 98th percentile, beginning at an early age). Prominent occiput, markedly delayed closure of the anterior fontanelle, which is neither bulging nor tense, prominent forehead. In the children presented here: strikingly deep-set eyes, broad nose, and pointed receding chin (**1, 2**).
2. In individual cases, primary psychomotor retardation, hypotonia, epilepsy (in up to 10% of cases).

Supplementary findings in the patients presented:
Normal height. Short neck; trunk and extremities somewhat obese and short (**1, 2**). Heart murmur. Large genitalia (**1a**); testicular volume of the older boy at 20 months, 3–4 ml; at 4 years and 5 months, 5–6 ml.

No evidence of intracranial vascular malformation nor of hydrocephalus (quite unremarkable ventricular system on repeated echoencephalography; transillumination and bilateral cerebral angiography negative). Ophthalmological examination normal, as were extensive neurological examinations, endocrinological studies, specific tests for storage diseases and other hereditary degenerative diseases, and chromosomal analysis.

Skull X-rays: elongated cranium, markedly delayed closure of the fontanelles, somewhat poorly defined and deeply serrated sutures, elongated flat sella turcica, numerous bony lacunae in the lambdoid suture (**3, 4**). Further X-rays of the skeleton: discordant bone maturation (areas of distinctly delayed, together with areas of partially accelerated, ossification). Normal-size heart with left-sided prominence in both brothers; in the older boy, possible atrial septal defect and idiopathic dilatation of the pulmonary artery.

Manifestation: Birth or shortly thereafter.

Etiology: Autosomal dominant condition with development of signs much more likely in males (4:1).

Course, prognosis: Occasionally complicated by cases with mental retardation (about 5–8%) or with epilepsy. No mental deterioration.

Diagnosis, differential diagnosis: Conditions with increased intracranial pressure and the syndrome described on p.34 must be ruled out. Macrocephaly, without signs of increased intracranial pressure, in a neurologically and developmentally normal child should, especially with familial occurrence, suggest megalencephaly and obviate the use of invasive methods of examination.

Treatment: None, or symptomatic.

Illustrations:
1–4 Two siblings, both with psychomotor retardation, the second and third children of young, healthy, nonconsanguineous parents after a girl and two abortions. Others with a large head in the family. The first child is—to a lesser degree—likewise macrodolichocephalic (at 5½ months, 44 cm; at 4 years 5 months, 55 cm) and has a cardiac defect (persistent ductus arteriosus, corrected; ventricular septal defect; anomalies of the pulmonary artery), completely normal psychomotor development, and slight obesity. Pregnancy and delivery were normal with both brothers. Birth measurements of the older: 4.3 kg, 59 cm, 38.5 cm. Head circumference of the younger (**2**) at 13 months, 53 cm (**3**); of the older at 10 months, 52 cm; 20 months, 57 cm; 2½ years, 59 cm; and 3 years 2 months (**4**), 61.5 cm. Obesity in the older brother. Resemblance of the brothers increasing.

H.-R.W./J.K.

References:
DeMyer, W. Megalencephaly in children. *Neurology*, 22, 634 (1972).
Jennings, M.T., Hall, J.G., Kukolich, M. Endocardial fibroelastosis, neurologic dysfunction, and unusual facial appearance in two brothers, coincidentally associated with dominantly inherited macrocephaly. *Am. J. Med. Genet.*, 5, 271 (1980).
Pettit, R.E., Kilroy, A.W., Allen, J.H. Macrocephaly with head growth parallel to normal growth pattern. *Arch. Neurol.*, 37, 518 (1980).
Priestly, B.L. and Lorber, J. Primary megalencephaly. *Z. Kinderchirur.*, 31, 335 (1980).
Lorber, J. and Priestly, B.L. Children with large heads ... 109 children with megalencephaly. *Develop. Med. Child. Neurol.*, 23, 494–504 (1981).

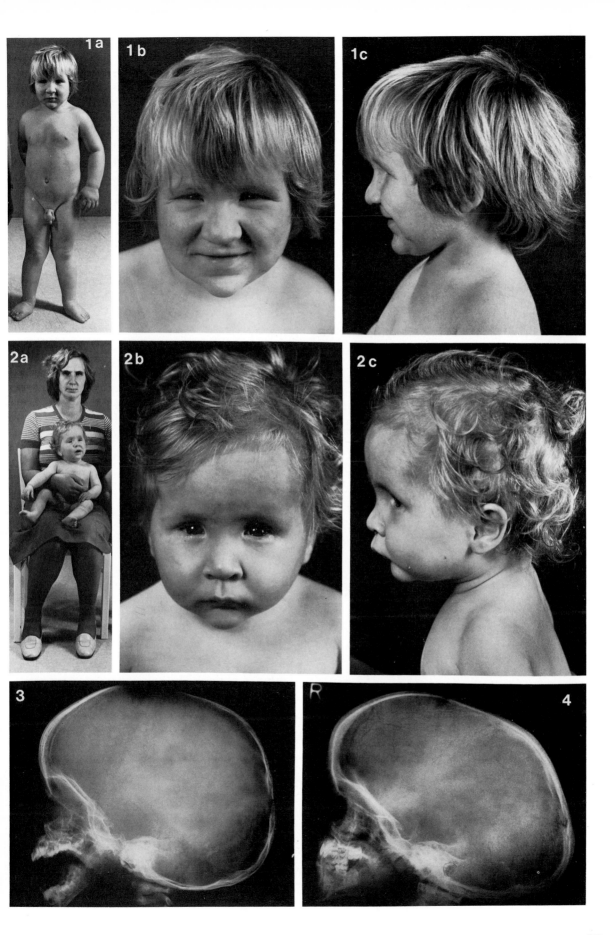

19. Alexander's Disease

A progressive, fatal leukodystrophy with megalencephaly, loss of neurological function, and mental deterioration

Main signs:
1. Megalencephaly with normal or enlarged ventricles.
2. Progressive psychomotor retardation.
3. Loss of speech.
4. Seizures, spastic tetraparesis, opisthotonus, contractures, pseudobulbar palsy, ataxia.

Supplementary findings: Increasing intracranial pressure, hyperpyrexia, attacks of vomiting, fluctuating course. Examination of the cranium with ultrasound can be diagnostically helpful.

Histologically, characteristic Rosenthal fibers, progressive fibrinoid degeneration of the fibril-rich astrocytes, demyelinating leukodystrophy, hyaline panmyelopathy.

Manifestation: Three forms with different ages of onset: infantile, juvenile, and adult.

Etiology: Autosomal recessive disorder. To date, only one family with three siblings of different sex has been described; otherwise only sporadic cases.

Frequency: Very rare. To date, only 20 known patients.

Course, prognosis: Progressive, with fatal outcome, which, with the early form, can occur between the fifth month and the fifth year of life.

Treatment: Symptomatic.

Differential diagnosis: Other megalencephalies. Multiple sclerosis.

Illustrations:
1 Three siblings with progressive macrocephaly (normocephalic at birth; crossing the 97th percentile by the end of the first year of life, then a parallel course above the 97th percentile).
2 The three siblings at ages 14, 15, and 17 years, confined to wheelchairs due to spastic quadriplegia; mental function still well preserved.

J.K.

References:

Russo, L.S., Aron, A., Anderson, P.J. Alexander's disease. A report and reappraisal. *Neurology* (Minneap), 26, 607–614 (1976).
Borrett, D. and Becker, L.E. Alexander's disease. A disease of astrocytes. *Brain*, 108, 367–385 (1985).
Harbord, M.G. and LeQuesne, G.W. Alexander's disease: cranial ultrasound findings. *Pediatr. Radiol.*, 18, 227–228 (1988).

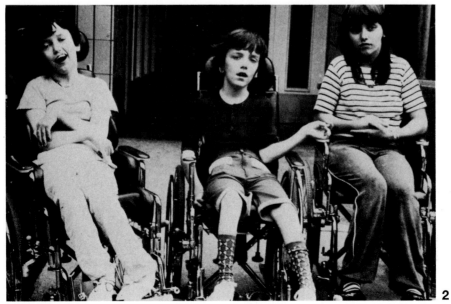

HEAD CIRCUMFERENCE, BOYS

Circumference (cm)

Thomas E.
*21.8.1968

Months — Years

HEAD CIRCUMFERENCE, GIRLS

Circumference (cm)

Petra E.
*23.2.1967

Angela E.
*23.1.1966

Months — Years

1

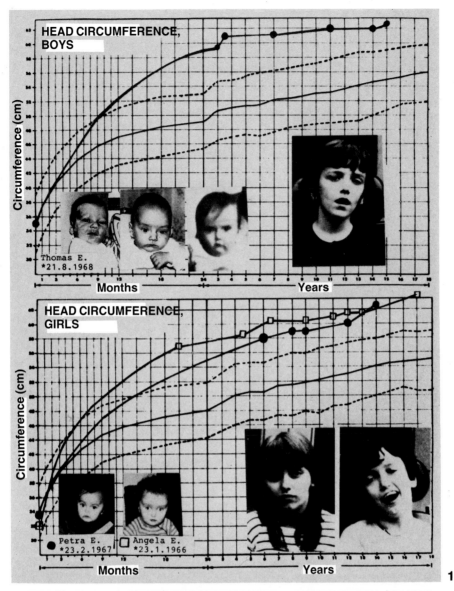

2

20. Frontonasal Dysplasia

(Median cleft face syndrome, craniofrontonasal dysplasia; Greig's hypertelorism syndrome?)

A developmental field defect of heterogeneous etiology with the signs hypertelorism, brachycephaly, prominent forehead, broad nasal root, and partial or complete bifid nose.

Main signs:
1. Hypertelorism (measure interpupillary distance), prominent forehead with wide bridge of the nose, which may be sagitally grooved or even cleft (then frequently associated with anterior cranium bifidum occultum and/or median cleft of the face), frequently wide open fontanelles with open metopic suture and coronary suture synostosis. Brachycephaly. Facial asymmetry.
2. Low nuchal hairline. Widow's peak.
3. High palate, widely spaced teeth.

Further signs: Broad neck, possibly pterygium colli; shoulder girdle anomalies with Sprengel's deformity, pseudarthrosis of the clavicles, scoliosis. Longitudinally grooved nails, preaxial polydactyly, syndactyly, clinodactyly, abnormalities of the distal phalanges of the fingers and toes, deep crease between hallux and second toe ('sandal-gap'). Infrequently, small stature and mental retardation.

Manifestation: At birth.

Etiology: Frontonasal developmental field defect of heterogeneous causes: sporadically occurring, autosomal dominant and autosomal recessive (the latter with severe craniofacial malformations). Females predominate over males 6:1. No transmission has been observed in male lines. Girls are also severely affected. Genetic transmission by an affected woman must be assumed to be 50%.

Frequency: Low. 1:250,000?

Course, prognosis: Dependent on the degree of severity. As a rule, normal life expectancy.

Differential diagnosis: Frontonasal dysplasia must be phenotypically and genetically differentiated (?) from Greig's hypertelorism syndrome (may be very difficult) and from the familial form of bifid nose occurring as an isolated defect.

Treatment: Symptomatic; plastic surgery may be indicated. Ultrasonographic and fetoscopic diagnosis in familial cases with female fetuses.

Illustrations:
1–4 Children affected to various degrees.
1 A 1-year-old male with median nasal cleft, broad nasal root, median cleft lip, and bilateral coloboma of the iris; sister and mother similarly affected.
3 A 3-year-old girl with cranial prominences, colobomas of the alae nasi notches, and severe neurological deficit due to malformation of the brain.

J.K.

References:

Gollop, T.R., Kiota, M.M., Martins, R.M.M. et al. Frontofacialnasal dysplasia: evidence for autosomal recessive inheritance. *Am. J. Med. Genet.*, 19, 301–305 (1984).

Anyane-Yeboa, K., Raifman, M.A., Berant, M. et al. Dominant inheritance of bifid nose. *Am. J. Med. Genet.*, 17, 561–563 (1984).

Toriello, H.V., Higgins, J.V., Walen, A. et al. Familial occurrence of a developmental defect of the medial nasal process. *Am. J. Med. Genet.*, 21, 131–133 (1985).

Bömelburg, T., Lenz, W., Eusterbrock, T. Median cleft face syndrome in association with hydrocephalus, agenesis of the corpus callosum, holoprosencephaly and choanal atresia. *Eur. J. Pediatr.*, 146, 301–302 (1987).

Morris, C.A., Palumbos, J.C., Carey, J.C. Delineation of the male phenotype in craniofrontonasal syndrome. *Am. J. Med. Genet.*, 27, 623–632 (1987).

Young, I.D. Craniofrontonasal dysplasia. *J. Med. Genet.*, 24, 193–196 (1987).

Meinecke, P. and Blunck, W. Frontonasal dysplasia, congenital heart defect, and short stature . . . *J. Med. Genet.*, 26, 408–409 (1989).

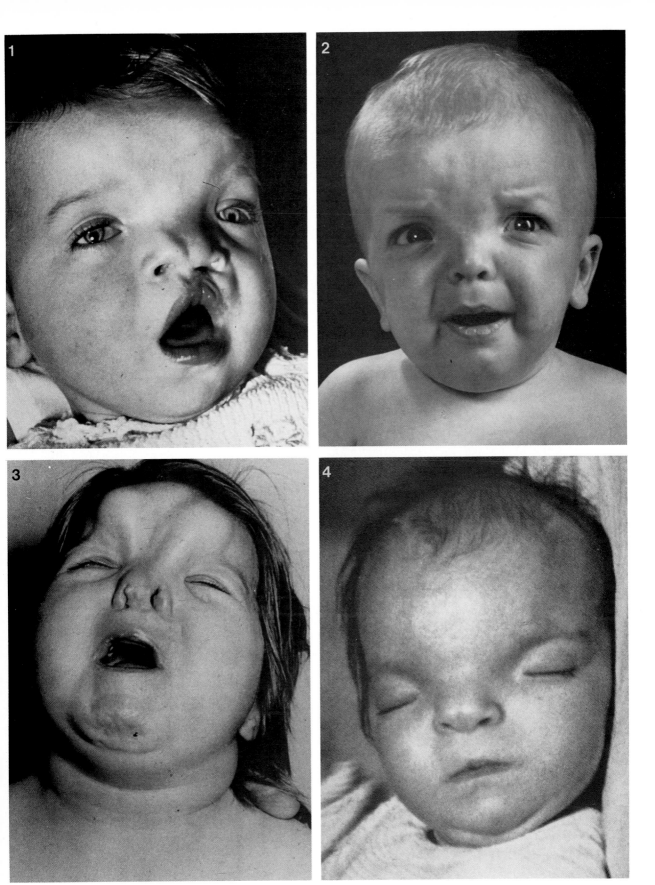

21. Holoprosencephaly

A disorder of prechordal development with cyclopia, arhinencephaly, absent bilobar development of the brain, and facial clefts, of varied etiology.

Main signs:
1. Cyclopia: medial monophthalmia, synophthalmia, or anophthalmia. Proboscis (tubular appendage). Nose duplicated, solitary with a single opening, or absent (arhinia).
2. Ethmocephaly: ocular hypotelorism with or without a proboscis.
3. Cebocephaly: ocular hypotelorism with only one nasal opening.
4. Premaxillary agenesis: ocular hypotelorism, flat nose, median cleft of the upper lip.
5. Minimal facial dysmorphism: variable phenotype with ocular hypotelorism, flat nose, uni- or bilateral cleft lip, and coloboma of the iris. Hypertelorism may also occur.
6. Alobar, semilobar, or lobar holoprosencephaly, monoventricular forebrain, rudimentary lobulation of the brain, posterior fissure of the hemispheres.

Supplementary findings: Absence of the ethmoid, mid-section of the sphenoid, vomer, intermaxilla, nasal bones, and lacrimal duct system. Hypo- or aplasia of the turbinates. Divided tongue or microglossia, possibly aglossia. Microstomia to astomia. Polydactyly, syndactyly, hypoplastic or absent thumbs, myelomeningocele, club feet.

Cardiovascular, urogenital, and many other internal malformations. Omphalocele. Anal stenosis.

Manifestation: Primary defect of the prechordal mesoderm. Disturbance during the 21st–25th weeks of pregnancy. Ultrasonography makes prenatal diagnosis possible. Otherwise diagnosis at birth.

Etiology: Heterogeneous causes. Different structural chromosomal disorders including trisomies 13 and 18 and triploidy. Recently several observations of deletions of the long arm of chromosome 7. Rarely familial translocations. As a rule sporadic occurrence.

Rarely observations in siblings or transmission with diminished expression over generations. Beware of confusing with Meckel syndrome.

Frequency: Lobar and alobar holoprosencephaly about 1 in 16,000 live births. With alobar holoprosencephaly female to male 3:1; with lobar form 1:1.

Course, prognosis: Severely affected infants usually do not survive beyond the sixth month of life.

Differential diagnosis: Asymmetric monophthalmus (**4**) and otocephaly (microstomia, agnathia, synotia). Arhinencephaly may also occur in the Kallmann syndrome and trisomy 13. Greig's hypertelorism or frontonasal dysplasia, the blepharophimosis-ptosis-epicanthus inversus syndrome, and the double nose syndrome may have to be ruled out.

Treatment: Symptomatic.

Illustrations:
1 Newborn with intrauterine growth retardation (46 cm, 2800 g, 28 cm head circumference). Convulsions, fluctuating temperature, tachypnea, dysphagia. Monoventricular prosencephalon, synostoses of the cranial sutures. Death at 5½ months.
2a and b Prematurely born (31st week of pregnancy) male with cyclopia: centrally located, 1 cm orbital cavity with rudimentary eye beneath a 1.8 cm long proboscis. Severe microstomia. Distinct medial groove of the flap-like upper lip. Low-set ears, dysplastic pinnae. Low nuchal hairline. Rudimentary tongue. Arhinencephaly, holoprosencephaly. Absence of the cribriform area, only one hemisphere. Double outlet right heart, malrotation. Partial trisomy for the short arm of one chromosome 3 with balanced parental translocation (3p−: 7q+).
3 Newborn with cebocephaly: microphthalmia, ocular hypotelorism, nose with a single opening.
4 Asymmetrical monophthalmia: one healthy eye, one malformed eye with proboscis. Not cyclopia.

J.K.

References:
Gorlin, R.J., Pindborg, J.J., Cohen, M.M. Jr. (eds.) *Syndromes of the Head and Neck.* McGraw-Hill, New York, 1976.
Schinzel, A. A further case of cyclopia due to unbalanced segregation of a previously reported rcp (1;7) (q23;q24) familial translocation. *Am. J. Med. Genet.*, 24, 205–206 (1986).
Smart, R.D., Ross, J., Amann, G. et al. Brief clinical report: cyclopia as a result of an unbalanced familial translocation rcp (7;18) (q34;q21). *Am. J. Med. Genet.*, 24, 269–272 (1986).
Suslak, L., Mimms, G.M., Desposito, F. Letter to the editor: monozygosity and holoprosencephaly: cleavage disorders of the 'midline field'. *Am. J. Med. Genet.*, 28, 99–102 (1987).
Hattori, H., Okuno, T., Momoi, T. et al. Brief clinical report: single central maxillary incisor and holoprosencephaly. *Am. J. Med. Genet.*, 28, 483–487 (1987).
Townes, P.L., Reuter, K., Rosquete, E.E. et al. XK Aprosencephaly and anencephaly in sibs. *Am. J. Med. Genet.*, 29, 523–528 (1988).

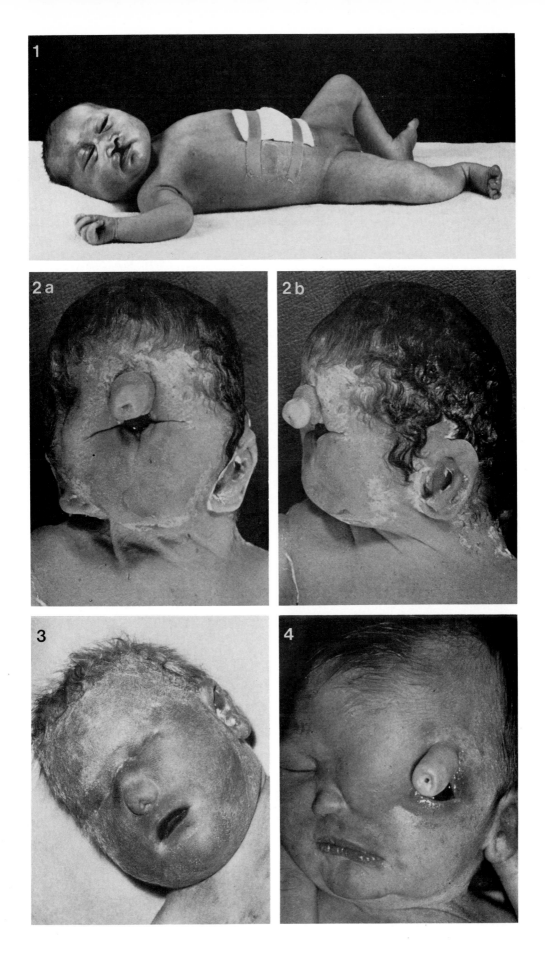

22. An Unknown Syndrome with Cleft Lip and Cleft Palate

A syndrome of cleft lip and palate, severe psychomotor retardation, and internal malformations.

Main signs:
1. Bilateral cleft lip; complete cleft maxilla on the left, wide cleft of the palate, incomplete cleft maxilla on the right (1–5). Abnormalities of the skull: acrocephalic cranium with anterior bulge of the right side of the forehead (1–5); delayed closure of the sutures and fontanelles. Low-set ears, dysplastic pinnae (5–8). Complete paralysis of the right facial nerve (2, 3, 5). Abnormal hairline.
2. Severe psychomotor retardation.
3. Cardiac defect.

Supplementary findings: Short neck with loose nuchal skin. Barrel-shaped chest. Limited motion of the shoulder joints. Retarded bone age.

Left-sided inguinal hernia. Bilateral cryptorchidism.

Manifestation: At birth.

Etiology: Undetermined.

Course: Early death of the child from renal insufficiency (see below).

Illustrations:
1–8 The above-described child at 7 and 8½ months. The boy was the second child of healthy young parents (first child healthy); no evidence of parental consanguinity. Child born 6 weeks prematurely (2130 g, 43 cm). Early signs of renal insufficiency; persistent anemia; no evidence of tubular pathy. Normal male karyotype on chromosome analysis (banding technique). Death at age 18 months. At autopsy, *diffuse angiomatosis of the leptomeninges over the frontal lobes* of both cerebral hemispheres. No hydrocephalus. Dilatation of the pulmonary artery. Right-sided *renal aplasia*.

H.-R.W.

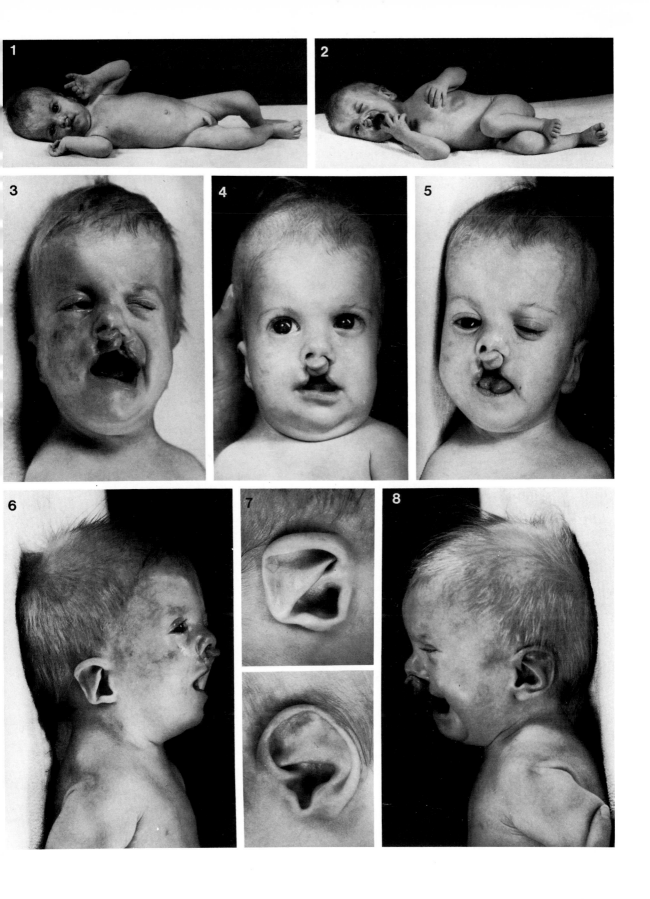

23. Freeman–Sheldon Syndrome

(Craniocarpotarsal dysplasia; whistling face syndrome)

A highly characteristic syndrome with mask-like 'whistling' face, hypoplastic alae nasi, ulnar deviation of the hands, flexion contractures of the fingers, and club feet.

Main signs:
1. Face: round, full-cheeked; mask-like immobility with deep-set, relatively widely spaced eyes, narrow palpebral fissures with slight antimongoloid slant, convergent strabismus; wide, low-set nasal root; epicanthus; small nose with hypoplastic alae nasi; long philtrum and small mouth, which is difficult to open, with, quite distinctly, pursed lips as though whistling. Paramedian grooves or dimples between the lower lip and the tip of the chin (1–3).
2. Ulnar deviation of the hands and flexion contractures of the fingers, especially the thumbs (4). Therapy-resistant club feet with contractures of the toes.

Supplementary findings: Transverse ridge across the lower forehead or supraorbital soft tissue furrow (3). Ptosis in some cases, high palate, usually not cleft; occasional hearing impairment. Normal mental development.

Short neck (sometimes with mild pterygium). Usually markedly short stature. Frequent development of marked scoliosis.

Manifestation: At birth.

Etiology: Hereditary disorder with autosomal dominant transmission. Also, apparent occurrence of an autosomal recessive type in, up to now, five families. X-linked recessive transmission also possible. Heterogeneity.

Frequency: Low. About 100 cases have been described.

Course, prognosis: Life expectancy is not affected.

Diagnosis, differential diagnosis: Exclusion of arthrogryposis (p. 402) should not cause problems. In children beyond infancy, Schwartz–Jampel syndrome (p. 508) may be difficult to rule out. The signs overlap considerably—thus, in 'true' cases of Freeman–Sheldon syndrome extra-facial disturbance of muscle tone may be seen at an early age, frequent contractures of the large joints observed later on, and mild skeletal dysplasias determined. However, in the Schwartz–Jampel syndrome as a rule no congenital manifestations; demonstrable myotonia (on EMG); and recessive transmission.

Treatment: Surgical treatment of club feet, the fingers, strabismus, the mouth, etc. as needed. Psychological guidance. Genetic counseling of the family.

Illustrations:
1–4 A 1-year-old boy from a healthy family (probable new mutation) with the full clinical picture at birth. Unremarkable psychomotor development. Extreme malpositioning of all fingers (4). The left second and right fourth toes are displaced proximally (shortened metatarsals).

H.-R.W.

References:
Antley, R.M., Uga, N., Burzynski, N.J. et al. Diagnostic criteria for the whistling face syndrome. *Birth Defects*, 11/5, 161 (1975).
Vaitiekaitis, A.S., Hornstein, I., Neale, H.W. A new surgical procedure for correction of lip deformity in cranio-carpo-tarsal dysplasia (whistling face syndrome). *J. Oral Surg.*, 37, 699 (1979).
Hall, J.G., Reed, S.D. et al. The distal arthrogryposes . . . *Am. J. Med. Genet.*, 11, 185–239 (1982).
Kousseff, B.G., McConnachie, P., Hadro, T.A. Autosomal recessive type of whistling face syndrome. *Pediatrics*, 69, 328 (1982).
Wang, T.R. and Lin, S.-J. Further evidence for genetic heterogeneity of whistling face or Freeman–Sheldon syndrome . . . *Am. J. Med. Genet.*, 28, 471–475 (1987).
Illum, N., Reske-Nielsen, E. et al. Lethal autosomal recessive arthrogryposis multiplex congenita with whistling face . . . *Neuropediatrics*, 19, 186–192 (1988).

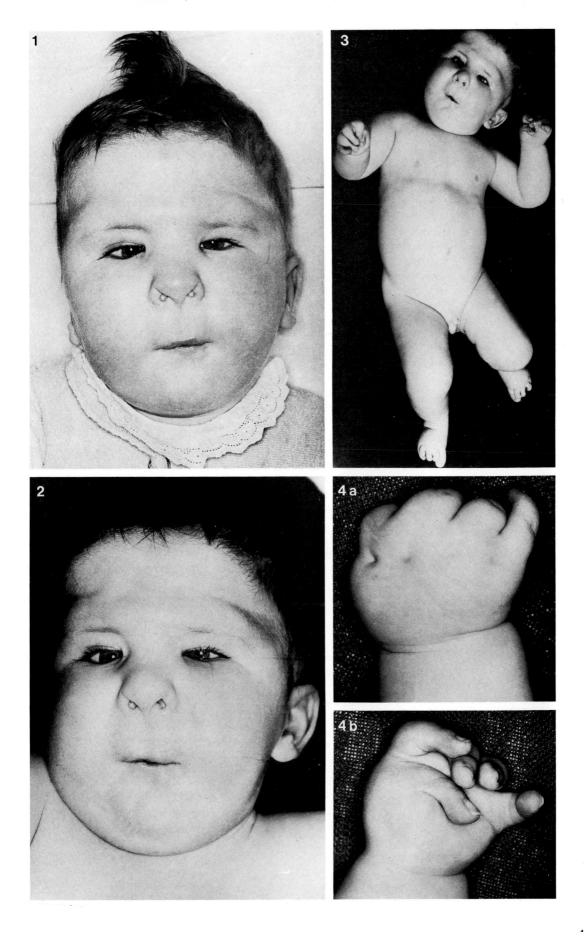

24. Mandibulofacial Dysostosis

(Franceschetti–Zwahlen Syndrome; Treacher Collins Syndrome)

A malformation syndrome with very characteristic facial dysmorphism.

Main signs:
1. Antimongoloid slant of the (possibly abnormally short) palpebral fissures with usually distinct coloboma (possibly only indentation) in the lateral half of the lower eyelids (from which the eyelashes may be absent)—rarely also of the upper lids (**1–4**).
2. Frontonasal angle often flat (**1–3**). Possibly aquiline and/or large-looking nose, sometimes with narrow nostrils (**1–4**).

Hypoplasia of the zygomata and of the upper and lower jaws with the cheeks appearing sunken (see especially **3a**); narrow, receding chin.

Frequent macrostomia (**1b**) with high, narrow or cleft palate and dental anomalies.
3. Usually considerable malformation of the external ear (microtia; stenosis or atresia of the auditory canal) (**1–4**). Not infrequently defects of the middle and/or inner ear; these are more likely, the more severe the external ear deformity. Possible atrophic areas of skin, blind fistulas, or skin tags between the corner of the mouth and the ear (**1c**).

(The appearance has been described as fish- or bird-like facies, (**1 and 2**)
4. Frequent conductive hearing impairment or deafness.

Supplementary findings: Abnormal hair growth from the temples on to the lateral cheeks, towards the corners of the mouth (**1a, 3b, 4a**).

The facial anomalies can, exceptionally, be asymmetric or even unilateral. Malformations of the eyes such as microphthalmos or coloboma of the iris are unusual. Choanal atresia in isolated cases.

Diverse extracranial malformations, e.g., cardiac defects, may occur. Intelligence normal as a rule (in case of doubt, allow for the patient's psychological handicap and for the possibility of a hearing defect).

Manifestation: At birth; hearing impairment later, if present.

Etiology: Autosomal dominant disorder with complete penetrance, but variable expression. High proportion of new mutations. Possibly also an autosomal recessive form.

Frequency: Not so rare (in 1964 it was possible to compare 200 cases from the literature).

Course, prognosis: Growth of the facial skeleton during childhood may bring some improvement in appearance.

Differential diagnosis: The Goldenhar syndrome (p.52), the Hallermann–Streiff–François syndrome (p.530), hemifacial microsomia (p.54), Nager acrofacial dysostosis (p.50), postaxial acrofacial dysostosis syndrome (p.418), and the Wildervanck syndrome (p.298) should not be particularly difficult to rule out.

Treatment: Symptomatic. Early evaluation of hearing and prompt application of appropriate aids when needed. Plastic surgery and orthodontic and dental treatment as indicated. Genetic counseling. Prenatal diagnosis possible.

Illustrations:
1 and 3 Two different newborn infants.
2 and 4 Two 3-month-old infants.

The child in **3** represents a hereditary case (father: full clinical picture of the syndrome); the other three children represent probable new mutations. The infants in **1, 2,** and **4** show bilateral atresia of the auditory canal; the child in **4** does not react at all to noises. Child in **1**: cleft palate. Child in **2**: bifid uvula, cardiac defect.

H.-R.W.

References:

Rogers, B.O. Berry–Treacher Collins syndrome: a review of 200 cases. *Brit. J. Plast. Surg.*, 17, 109 (1964).

Lowry, R.B., Morgan, K. et al. Mandibulofacial dysostosis in Hutterite sibs: a possible recessive trait. *Am. J. Med. Genet.*, 22, 501–512 (1985).

Crane, J.P. and Beaver, H.A. Midtrimester sonographic diagnosis of mandibulofacial dysostosis. *Am. J. Med. Genet.*, 25, 251–255 (1986).

Marsh, J.L. and Scott, E.C. The skeletal anatomy of mandibulofacial dysostosis . . . *Plast. Reconstr. Surg.*, 78, 460–468 (1986).

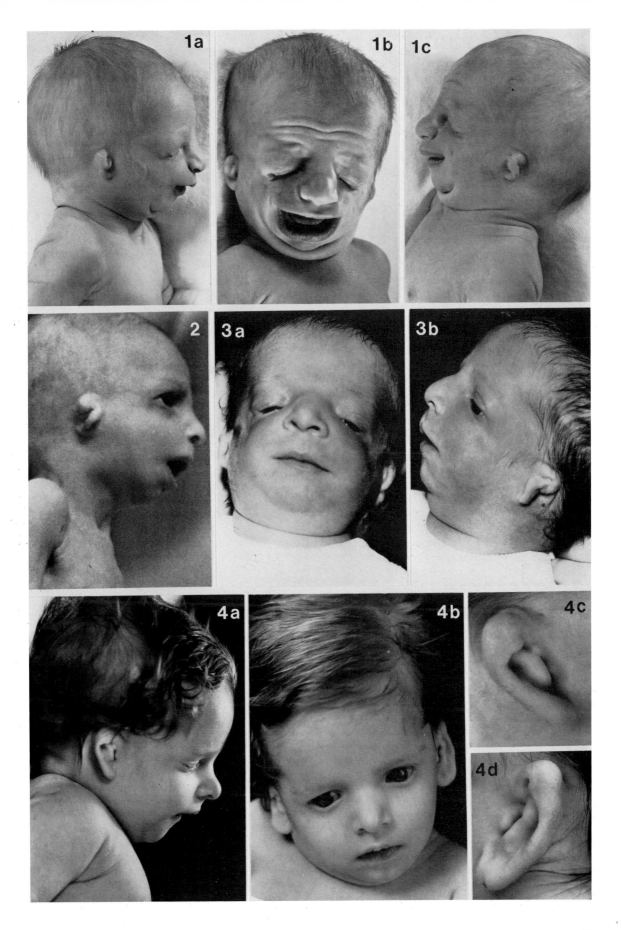

25. Nager Acrofacial Dysostosis

(Nager–de Reynier Type Acrofacial Dysostosis)

A hereditary mandibulofacial dysostosis with hypoplasia of the limbs, especially of the first rays of the upper extremities.

Main signs:
1. Facial dysmorphism similar to mandibulofacial dysostosis (p.48) (**1, 2**). Frequent conductive hearing defect.
In addition:
2. Anomalies of the thumbs (triphalangism, hypoplasia, aplasia) and in some cases of the neighboring ray or possibly of the bones of the forearms (hypoplasia of the radius, radioulnar synostosis, etc.) (**3, 4**). Hypoplasia may also occur in the lower extremities.

Supplementary findings: Initial difficulties with sucking and swallowing are not unusual (as with the Robin sequence, p.68). Small stature appears to be common. Cryptorchidism and dysplastic mamillae may occur, cardiac defects are rare.
Possible mental retardation.

Manifestation: At birth; hearing defect later, if present.

Etiology: A genetic basis certain, but the precise situation has not been adequately clarified. Autosomal recessive inheritance seems to be predominant, but apparently autosomal dominant inheritance occurs too. Thus, probable heterogeneity. Basic defect unknown.

Frequency: Low (about 30 case reports).

Course, prognosis: Growth of the facial skeleton during childhood may bring about improvement in appearance.

Differential diagnosis: Acrofacial dysostosis of the mainly postaxial type (p.418) should not be difficult to rule out because of the different location of the defects. However, there are additional, very rare and in some cases more severe, mandibulo- and acrofacial dysostoses that have not yet been further classified.

Treatment: Symptomatic. Early hearing tests and immediate special hearing and speech aids when required. Corrective surgery of the hands and corrective orthopedic, plastic-cosmetic, or orthodontic procedures may be indicated.

Illustrations:
1–4 A child of healthy nonconsanguineous parents. Bilateral triphalangeal thumb, no radial dysplasia. High palate without cleft; marked mandibular hypoplasia, also on X-ray; hearing apparently not affected. Heart and lower extremities unremarkable.

H.-R.W.

References:
Burton, B.K. and Nadler, H.L. Nager acrofacial dysostosis. *J. Pediatr.*, 91, 84 (1977).
Meyerson, M.D., Jensen, K.M., Meyers, J.M. et al. Nager acrofacial dysostosis: early intervention and long-term planning. *Cleft Palate J.*, 14/1, 35 (1977).
Halal, F., Hermann, J. et al. Differential diagnosis of Nager acrofacial dysostosis syndrome . . . *Am. J. Med. Genet.*, 14, 209–224 (1983).
Pfeiffer, R.A. and Stoess, H. Acrofacial dysostosis (Nager syndrome): synopsis . . . *Am. J. Med. Genet.*, 15, 255–260 (1983).
Thompson, E., Cadbury, R. et al. The Nager acrofacial dysostosis syndrome with the tetralogy of Fallot. *J. Med. Genet.*, 22, 408–410 (1985).
Chemke, J., Mogilner, B.M. et al. Autosomal recessive inheritance of Nager acrofacial dysostosis. *J. Med. Genet.*, 25, 230–232 (1988).

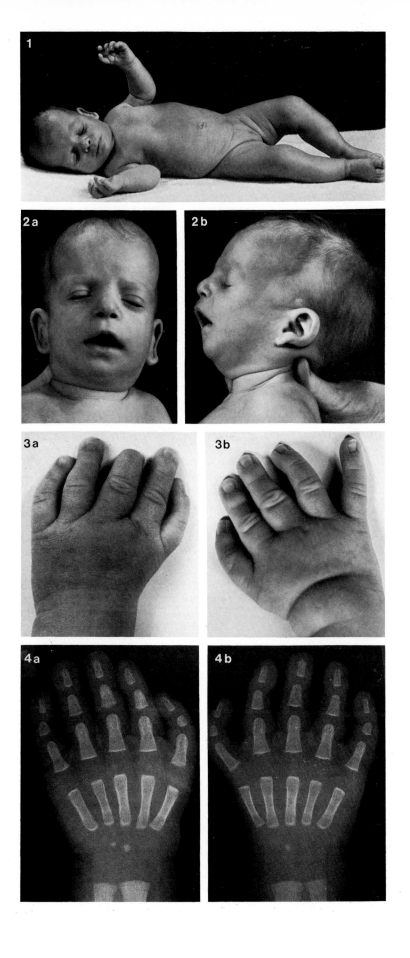

26. Goldenhar 'Syndrome'

(Goldenhar Anomaly, Goldenhar–Gorlin 'Syndrome', Goldenhar Sequence, Oculoauricular 'Dysplasia', Oculoauriculovertebral 'Dysplasia')

A very variable but relatively characteristic malformation complex of eye, ear, malar, and vertebral anomalies.

Main signs:
1. Often marked facial asymmetry due to unilateral hypoplasia (**2, 4**); usually prominent forehead (**1, 4**), hypoplasia of the zygomatic region and of the mandible, receding chin.
2. Epibulbar dermoid or lipodermoid (usually occurring bilaterally on the lateral corneoscleral junction); coloboma of the upper lid (usually unilateral). Occurrence also of other ocular anomalies.
3. One or more preauricular tags, uni- or bilateral, on a line between the tragus and the corner of the mouth (**1, 3, 4, 7**). Blind fistulas may also be located here. As a rule, microtia or other malformations of the external ear (**7a**).
4. Frequent macrostomia due to a transverse malar cleft (**2, 4**).
5. Usually marked malformations (often hemivertebrae) of the (especially upper) spine, frequently demonstrable only by X-ray (**5**); occasionally scoliosis.

Supplementary findings: Possible cleft lip and/or palate. Frequent dental anomalies.
　Possible conductive hearing defect.
　Occasional mental retardation.
　Lipomas of the corpus callosum may occur (ultrasonography, CT scan).
　Cardiac, pulmonary, and other anomalies also possible.

Manifestation: At birth; hearing defect later, if present.

Etiology: A causally heterogeneous and complex developmental field defect in which the manifestations vary markedly in severity. Usually sporadic occurrence (in some cases based on *in utero* interference of the blood supply). Evidence for autosomal dominant as well as for autosomal recessive inheritance. The majority of affected patients are males. The risk of recurrence after one affected child is about 3%, sibling risk is about 6%.

Frequency: About 1:3,000–5,000 newborns. Hundreds of cases have been documented.

Course, prognosis: Favorable.

Diagnosis, differential diagnosis: No single sign can be considered obligatory. Differentiation from typical mandibulofacial dysostosis (p.48) should not be particularly difficult, but from hemifacial microsomia (p.54) and from Wildervanck syndrome (p.298) can be practically impossible.

Treatment: Removal of preauricular tags and larger dermoids. Closure of malar cleft when present (**6**). Cosmetic surgery may be indicated. Dental care. Early hearing test as a precaution in every case. Hearing aids from early childhood, when needed.

Illustrations:
1–3 and 6 An affected infant at 8 and 9 months. Macrocephaly, mild facial asymmetry favoring the left side with distinct hypoplasia of the right mandible. Right lateral epibulbar lipodermoid, right palpebral fissure narrower than the left. One preauricular tag on the right, three small tags on the left, one of which lies between the ear and the corner of the mouth. Transverse buccal cleft on the right. Capillary angiomas of the midface and occiput. Scoliosis; 13 pairs of ribs. Mental development and hearing apparently unimpaired.
4 and 5 Newborn girl. Facial asymmetry. Three preauricular tags on the right; hypoplasia of the zygoma; macrostomia due to small transverse buccal cleft on the right, receding chin; anomalies of the vertebral bodies.
7a and b Newborn girl with left epibulbar dermoid; low-set ears; right microtia with atresia of the auditory canal (left canal abnormally narrow); bilateral preauricular tags; macrostomia (without buccal cleft); anomalies of the vertebral bodies (hemi- and block vertebrae); 10 ribs on the right, 11 on the left.

H.-R.W./J.K.

References:
Shokeir, M.H.K. The Goldenhar syndrome: a natural history. *Birth Defects,* 13/3C, 67 (1977).
Feingold, M. and Baum, J. Goldenhar's syndrome. *Am. J. Dis. Child.,* 132, 136 (1978).
Setzer, E.S., Ruiz-Castaneda, N. et al. Etiologic heterogeneity in the oculoauriculovertebral syndrome. *J. Pediatr.,* 98, 88 (1981).
Regenbogen, L., Godel, V., Goya, V. et al. Further evidence for an autosomal dominant form of oculoauriculovertebral dysplasia. *Clin. Genet.,* 21, 161 (1982).
Boles, D.J., Bodurtha, J. et al. Goldenhar complex in discordant monozygotic twins . . . *Am. J. Med. Genet.,* 28, 103–109 (1987).
Rollnick, B.R., Kaye, C.I. et al. Oculoauriculovertebral dysplasia and variants . . , *Am. J. Med. Genet.,* 26, 361–375 (1987).
Beltinger, C. and Saule, H. Imaging of lipoma of the corpus callosum . . . in the Goldenhar syndrome. *Pediatr. Radiol.,* 18, 72–73 (1988).
Rollnick, B.R. Oculoauriculovertebral anomaly . . . *Am. J. Med. Genet.* (Suppl.), 4, 41–53 (1988).
Ryan, C.A., Finer, N.N. et al. Discordance of signs in monozygotic twins concordant for the Goldenhar syndrome. *Am. J. Med. Genet.,* 29, 755–761 (1988).

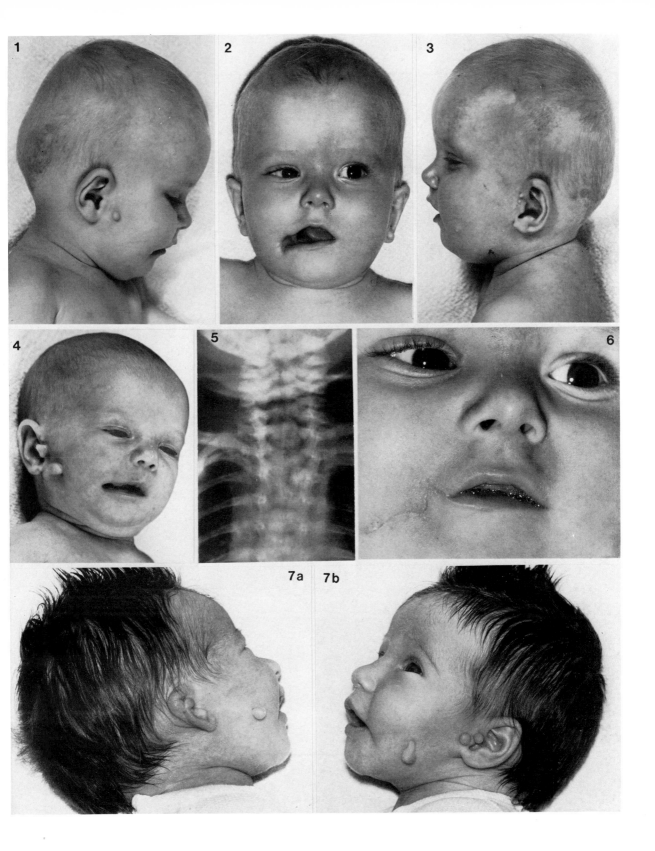

27. Hemifacial Microsomia

A clinical picture comprising unusual facial asymmetry with unilateral malformation of the ear and ipsilateral hypoplasia especially of the mandibular ramus and condyle.

Main signs:
1. Usually less marked facial asymmetry due to unilateral hypoplasia of the jaw, receding chin (1–3).
2. Preauricular tags or abnormality of the external ear (2). Aplasia in some cases.
3. Malocclusion on the affected side.

Supplementary findings: Rather as an exception: anomalies of the eye on the affected side of the face (and usually *no* dermoid, lipodermoid, or coloboma of the upper eyelid).
Possible hearing impairment.

Manifestation: At birth; hearing defect later, if present.

Etiology: Not uniform; cf. Goldenhar 'syndrome' (p.52), of which this clinical picture can be considered a favorable variant. Sporadic occurrence as a rule.

Frequency: Not so rare.

Course, prognosis: Favorable.

Diagnosis, differential diagnosis: Differentiation from mandibulofacial dysostosis (p.48) easy; from Goldenhar 'syndrome' (p.52) difficult or impossible.

Treatment: Corrective cosmetic surgery in some cases. Dental and orthodontic care. Early hearing test. Hearing aids, if indicated, from early childhood onward.

Illustrations:
1–3 A 5-year-old boy from a healthy family. Malformation of the right ear (2: the patient's appearance after two operations to reconstruct his—now less conspicuous—right ear) and hypoplasia of the right mandible.
Marked, probably combined hearing defect on the right. Normal psychomotor development. Additional abnormalities: limited ability to turn the head to the extreme right, low nuchal hairline, hypoplastic accessory mamilla on the right.

H.-R.W.

References:

Pashayan, H., Pinsky, I. and Fraser, F.C. Hemifacial microsomia: oculo-auriculo-vertebral dysplasia: a patient with overlapping features. *J. Med. Genet.*, 7, 185 (1970).
Stewart, R.E. Craniofacial malformations. *Pediatric Clinics of North America*, 25, 500 (1978).
Feingold, M. Hemifacial microsomia. In: *Birth Defects Compendium*, 2nd edn., p.511 (1979).
Burck, U. Genetic aspects of hemifacial microsomia. *Hum. Genet.*, 64, 291–296 (1983).
Rollnick, B.R. and Kaye, C.I. Hemifacial microsomia and variants. *Am. J. Med. Genet.*, 15, 233–253 (1983).
Kay, E.D. and Kay, C.N. Dysmorphogenesis of the mandible, zygoma, and middle ear ossicles in hemifacial microsomia . . . *Am. J. Med. Genet.*, 32, 27–31 (1989).

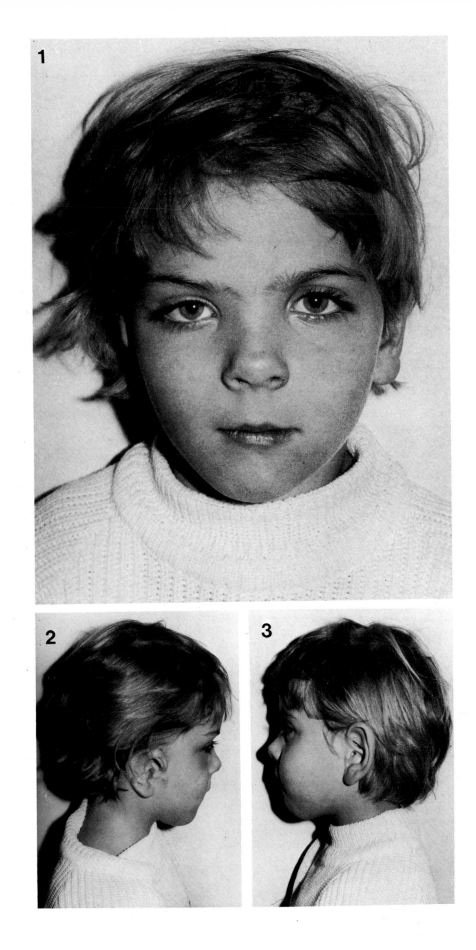

28. Syndrome of Progressive Hemifacial Atrophy

(Romberg Syndrome)

Localized facial atrophy, possibly associated with heterochromia iridis complex.

Main signs: Progressive atrophy of some or all of the tissues on one half of the face. The whole side of the face may be involved (early stage shown in **1**; further progression since). Or patchy or stripe-like areas are affected, such that the changes resemble a sword wound—'en coup de sabre' (**2**).

Supplementary findings: Frequent pigmentation changes in the affected skin areas; also, discoloration and later loss of hair (eyebrows, eyelashes, etc.). Sensation remains intact on the affected side of the face; motor function barely affected despite muscular involvement.

Involvement of the eye in some cases: sinking in of the eyeball, heterochromia iridis with iridocyclitis, strabismus.

Headaches or trigeminal neuralgia possible. In some cases contralateral disturbance of neurological function (e.g., focal epilepsy with contralateral expression).

Manifestation: Mainly in the first two decades of life.

Etiology: Uncertain. Uniformity of the syndrome questionable. Occasional familial occurrence suggests genetic factors in these cases.

Frequency: Low.

Course, prognosis: The atrophic process frequently comes to a halt after a course of several years.

Differential diagnosis: Hemifacial microsomia (p.54) and sometimes Goldenhar syndrome (p.52).

Treatment: Symptomatic. Cosmetic surgery may be indicated at a later date.

Illustrations:
1 A 2½-year-old, normally developed girl from a healthy family. Since the end of her first year of life, increasing 'sinking in' of the whole right side of her face, including soft tissue, bony parts, and the eye, with unaltered toddler-like fullness of the left side of the face.

Intermittent strabismus on the right. Tongue normal; no depigmentation of the skin; no heterochromia; no neurological findings. Symmetrical development of the remainder of the body, as judged by appearance and measurements.
2 A 7¼-year-old boy, tall and slightly obese, from a healthy family: underdevelopment of the left side of the face noted since infancy; distinct underdevelopment of the maxillary sinus and teeth on the left as compared with the right. On the forehead, two parallel vertical pigmented atrophic areas of skin about 4 cm long and barely a fingerbreadth wide, with bony involvement as in localized scleroderma of the 'en coup de sabre' type, the one median, the other 2 cm to the left. Development of these areas in the last few years. Intermittent left-sided headaches. Signs of a mild right-sided spastic hemiparesis with left-sided focal findings in EEG; no seizure disorder. Mild retardation. Ophthalmological examinations normal to date.

H.-R.W.

References:

Franceschetti, A. and Koenig, H. L'importance du facteur hérédo-dégénératif dans l'hémiatrophie faciale progressive (Romberg). Étude des complications oculaires dans ce syndrome. *J. Génét. Hum.*, 1, 27 (1952).

Fulmek, R. Hemiatrophia progressiva faciei (Romberg-Syndrom) mit gleichseitiger Heterochromia complicata (Fuchs-Syndrom). *Klin. Mbl. Augenheilkd.*, 164, 615 (1974).

Muchnick, R.S., Sherrell, J.A. and Rees, T.D. Ocular manifestations and treatment of hemifacial atrophy. *Am. J. Ophthalmol.*, 88, 889 (1979).

Goldhammer, Y. Progressive hemifacial atrophy (Parry–Romberg's disease) principally involving bone. *J. Laryng.*, 95, 643–647 (1981).

Asher, St.W. and Berg, B.O. Progressive hemifacial atrophy. *Arch. Neurol.*, 39, 44 (1982).

Lewkonia, R.M. and Lowry, R.B. Progressive hemifacial atrophy (Parry–Romberg syndrome); report with review of genetics and nosology. *Am. J. Med. Genet.*, 14, 385–390 (1983).

Küster, W., Kries, R.v. et al. Lineare zirkumskripte Sklerodermie unter dem Bilde einer Hemiatrophia faciei. *Pädiatr. Prax.*, 36, 131–136 (1987/88).

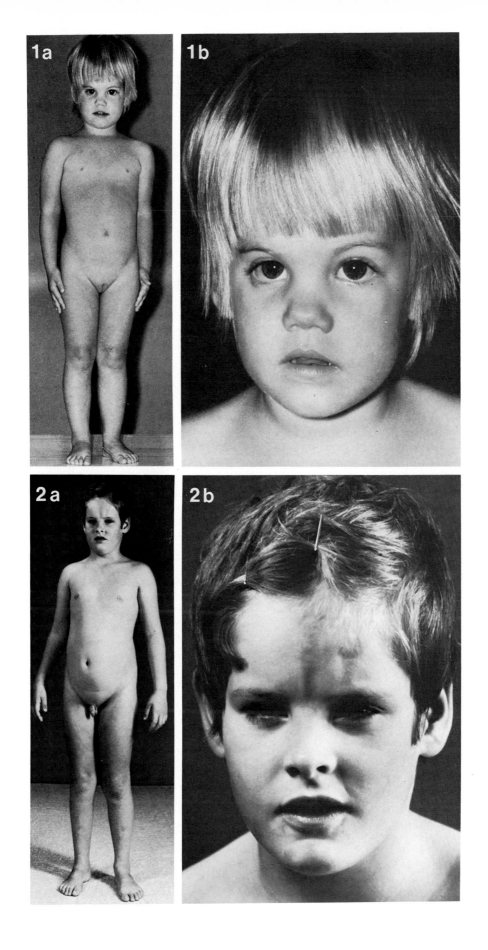

57

29. Anomalies in the Mid Anterior Neck Region

(Pterygium Colli Medianum, Raphe Mediana Supraumbilicalis—With or Without Vascular Nevi)

A number of rare anomalies occurring sporadically, alone or in combination, in the anterior midline region.

Main signs:
1. Median pterygium colli between the chin and jugular fossa (**1, 2**). Double origin from the protuberances of the chin (**1b, 2**); variably firm skin folds, which are scar-like in some areas; frequent micrognathia and limited extension of the neck.
2. Supraumbilical cicatricial raphe between the navel and the xiphoid (or extending even further upwards) (**3, 4**).
3. In some cases, a vascular nevus or cavernous hemangioma (the latter not infrequently ulcerating) on the neck and/or face, possibly also in the larynx (**4**).

Supplementary findings: In some cases a median fissure of the throat, characterized by a superficial scar (sometimes up to a full 1 cm wide) with subcutaneous connective tissue strands between the hyoid or chin (in this case originating from the paramedian tuberosities of the chin) and jugular fossa, where a depression can lead further into a fistula to the superior mediastinum. Infrequently, a median 'cleft' or cleft residue extends deeper or further caudally: cleft of the lower lip, tongue, lower jaw, or chin (possibly also just a Pierre–Robin sequence); anomalies of the sternum ranging from split sternum to aplasia with respiration-dependent median retraction and billowing of the anterior thorax, in some cases with an extensive ectopia cordis.

Manifestation: At birth and thereafter.

Etiology: Sporadic occurrence. Developmental field defect of the anterior midline. Practically no risk of recurrence.

Frequency: Rare.

Course, prognosis: Basically favorable.

Diagnosis: Not difficult. In the newborn the mid-abdominal raphe and the eventual pterygium initially appear as fine, delicate linear scars and only later, with time, become increasingly distinct and firmer. X-ray examination of the thorax and its organs is imperative. In case of stridor, intralaryngeal hemangiomas must be ruled out.

Treatment: Adequate treatment of progressive hemangiomatosis as required. In addition, cosmetic procedures may be indicated.

Illustrations:
1 A 17-year-old girl, otherwise completely normally developed, with median pterygium colli. Sternum and the rest of the bony thorax and internal organs unremarkable.
2 A similarly affected 4-year-old boy, otherwise normally developed and without further anomalies.
3 A 1¾-year-old with an upper mid-abdominal raphe, a defect of the manubrium of the sternum, and herniation of the lung. Widely spaced nipples.
4 A 3-month-old infant with an upper mid-abdominal raphe, a soft-tissue tag in the region of the jugular fossa, widely spaced nipples, facial hemangiomatosis. X-ray of the sternum and the rest of the thorax and thoracic organs unremarkable.

H.-R.W.

References:

Gotlieb, A., Hanukoglu, A., Fried, D. et al. Micrognathia associated with asternia and teleangiectatic skin lesion. *Syndrome identification (March of Dimes Birth Defects Foundation)*, 8, 1:10–13 (1982).

Leiber, B. Angeborene supraumbilikale Mittelbauchrhaphe (SMBR) und kavernöse Gesichtschämangiomatose—ein neues Syndrom? *Monatschr. Kinderheilkd.*, 130, 84–90 (1982).

Waldschmidt, J., Ribbe, R., Weineck, J. Diagnose und Differentialdiagnose der angeborenen Fisteln und Zysten des Halses. *Z. Kinderchir.*, 42, 271–278 (1987).

Godbersen, S., Heckel, V., Wiedemann, H.-R. Pterygium colli medianum and midline cervical cleft: Midline anomalies in the sense of a developmental field defect. *Am. J. Med. Genet.*, 27, 719–723 (1987).

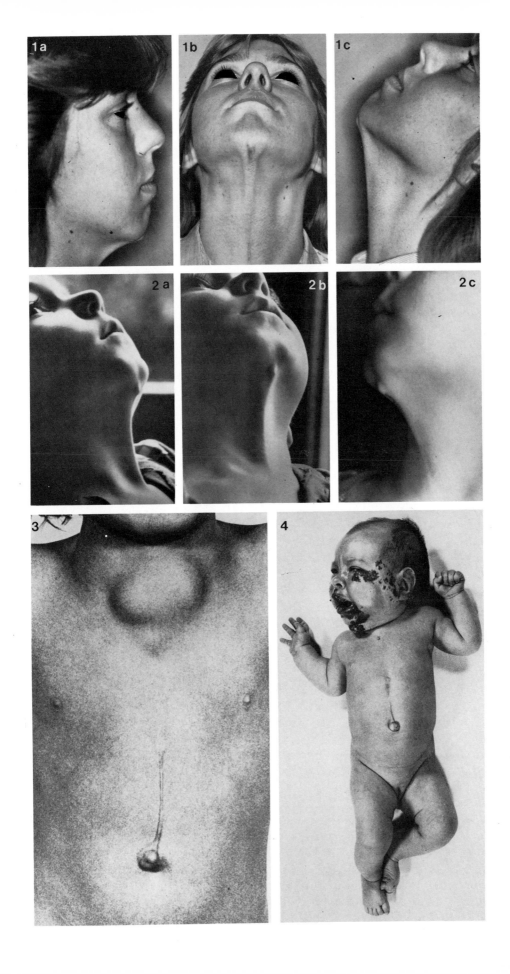

30. Van der Woude Syndrome

(Lower Lip Pits, Cleft Lip and Palate Syndrome)

A characteristic syndrome of pits of the lower lip and cleft lip/palate.

Main signs:
1. Generally symmetrical paramedian pits or protuberances of the lower lip ('fistulae labii inferioris') in over 80% of the cases (1–4).
2. Cleft lip and/or palate (in around 60%) (1a).
3. Hypodontia (usually with respect to the second incisors and second molars).

Manifestation: At birth (dental anomalies later).

Etiology: Autosomal dominant disorder with at least 90% penetrance. Numerous cases probably represent new mutations.

Frequency: Relatively high; about 1,000 or more cases in the literature. Estimation: 1 case in about 40,000 live births.

Course, prognosis: Good.

Diagnosis, differential diagnosis: The occurrence of weak forms should be kept in mind. Differentiation from the OFD syndrome type I and from the popliteal pterygium syndrome, which also can occur with lower lip pits and clefts.

Treatment: Operative correction of the cleft lip and/or palate is foremost.

Illustrations:
1–4 Two affected sisters.
1a and 1b The younger girl at 5 months and 3½ years (here, after surgical correction of the cleft lip and palate; before correction of the lower lip).
4 The older sister after cleft palate surgery; before correction of the lower lip. The previous four generations have been similarly affected.

H.-R.W.

References:
Van der Woude, A. Fistula labii inferioris congenita and its association with cleft lip and palate. *Am. J. Hum. Genet.*, 6, 244–256 (1954).
Schinzel, A. and Kläusler, M. The Van der Woude syndrome . . . *J. Med. Genet.*, 23, 291–294 (1986).
Wienker, T.F., Hudek, G. et al. Linkage studies in a pedigree with Van der Woude syndrome. *J. Med. Genet.*, 24, 160–162 (1987).
Küster, W. and Lambrecht, J.T. Cleft lip and palate, lower lip pits, and limb deficiency defects. *J. Med. Genet.*, 25, 565–572 (1988).

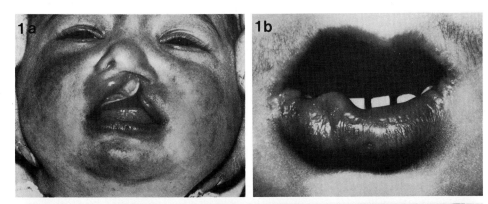

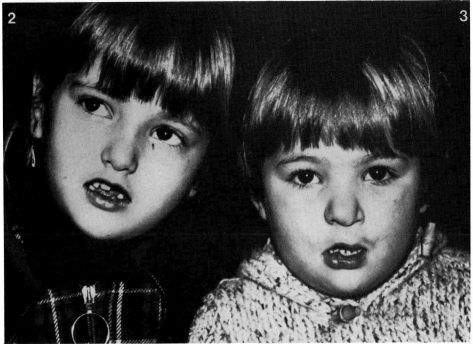

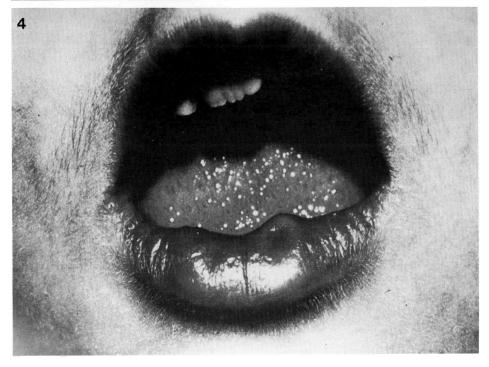

31. Orofaciodigital Syndrome Type I

(OFD Syndrome I, Papillon–Léage–Psaume Syndrome)

A hereditary syndrome in females, with lobulated tongue, hyperplastic frenula, notched alveolar crests, unusual facies, and anomalies of the hands and feet.

Main signs:
1. Lobulation of the tongue into two or more lobes (5). Multiple intraoral hyperplastic frenula, frequently with extensive fixation of the tongue and/or upper lip. Lateral notching of the alveolar ridge of the upper jaw (8), notches also possible in the anterior alveolar ridge of the lower jaw. High or cleft palate.
2. Unusual facies (1–3): frontal bossing, broad nasal root, hypertelorism or telecanthus, hypoplasia of the alae nasi, hypoplasia in the jaw region with dysodontiasis (lower lateral incisors frequently absent), possible median cleft of the upper lip. Milia of the ears and face in infancy, later receding. Dry skin and alopecia of the scalp in some cases.
3. Clino-, brachy-, and syndactyly of the hands and feet (7, 9, 10–12). Exceptionally, duplication of the big toes.

Supplementary findings: About half of the cases are mentally retarded (with an average IQ of about 70); malformations of the brain not uncommon.

Hamartoma of the tongue in a proportion of the cases.

Occasional short stature or deafness. Polycystic kidneys apparently frequent, sometimes with adult-type manifestation.

Manifestation: At birth.

Etiology: Hereditary disorder, X-linked dominant. Since the gene is completely lethal in males, only females are clinically affected (except in Klinefelter's syndrome).

Frequency: Low; estimated 1:50,000.

Course, prognosis: Dependent on the mental development of the patient. Life expectancy is probably essentially normal.

Differential diagnosis: Orofaciodigital syndrome type II (p.416) occurs in both sexes (autosomal recessive inheritance); the main differentiating characteristics are bilateral postaxial polydactyly of the hands (less frequently of the feet), hypoplasia of the alae nasi, broad tip of the nose, and absence more frequently of the middle than the lateral incisors.

Comment: This sharply outlined syndrome is only *one* representative of a probably relatively large, still provisionally classified, heterogeneous, and varied group of OFD syndromes (at least six types), for some of these there are only a few relevant observations.

Treatment: Closure of clefts, removal of hypertrophic frenula, orthodontic and dental care, etc. Surgical correction of the hands and special schooling may be indicated. Genetic counseling.

Illustrations:
1–12 A 10-year-old girl with the full syndrome (after operative correction of the inner canthi, upper lip, tongue, palate, and hands). Mild mental retardation. Height below the tenth percentile. Flat midface, thin hair.

H.-R.W.

References:
Melnick, M. and Shields, E.D. Orofaciodigital syndrome, Type I: a phenotypic and genetic analysis. *Oral Surg.*, 40, 599 (1975).
Annerén, G., Arvidson, B. et al. Orofaciodigital syndromes I and II . . . *Clin. Genet.*, 26, 178–186 (1984).
Baraitser, M. The Orofaciodigital (OFD) syndromes. *J. Med. Genet.*, 23, 116–119 (1986).
Connacher, A.A., Forsyth, C.C. et al: Orofaciodigital syndrome type I . . . *J. Med. Genet.*, 24, 116–122 (1987).
Donnai, D., Kerzon-Storrar, L. et al. Familial orofaciodigital syndrome type I . . . *J. Med. Genet.*, 24, 84–87 (1987).
Toriello, H.V. Heterogeneity and variability in the oral-facial-digital syndromes. *Am. J. Med. Genet. Suppl.*, 4, 149–159 (1988).

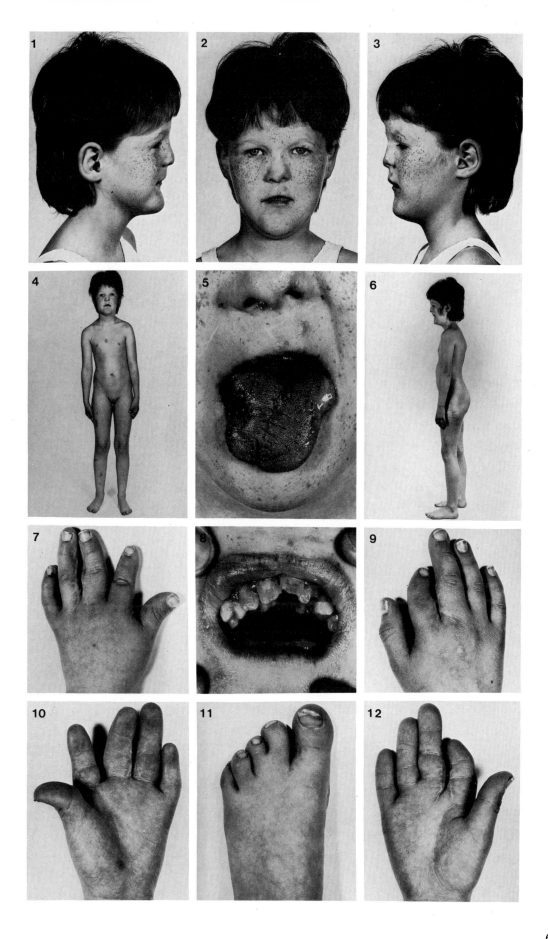

63

32. Syndrome of Microcephaly and Intraoral (Fibro-) Lipomatous Hamartomatosis

A syndrome of congenital microcephaly, polypoid (fibro-) lipomatous hamartomas of the oral mucous membranes, and mild mental retardation.

Main signs:
1. Congenital microcephaly (head circumference of the younger child at birth 33 cm, with birth length of 51 cm; head circumference thereafter always below the third percentile, at 3½ years 45 cm; in her older sibling 48 cm at 5 years) (1–5). Closure of fontanelles normal for ages.
2. Congenital polypoid (fibro-) lipomatous hamartomas of the oral mucosa (multiple tumorlike whitish to yellow-brown growths, rounded to lobular, on the tip, back, and edges of the tongue and on the alveolar processes, some removed shortly after birth and some later in infancy; no recurrence). In addition, long tongue, with furrow-like grooving, especially in the younger child (1, 2, 4, 5); residua on the tongue of the older girl (6).
3. Slight delay of gross motor development of the older girl (walking unsupported at 18 months), considerable delay in the younger child (walking without support, still somewhat unstable, at 3 years); relatively good mental development of the younger sister and practically normal mental development of the older.

Supplementary findings: Small stature (older girl below the tenth percentile, younger below the third).

In both girls, skin dimples above the knee bilaterally (1). Bluish sclera and hyperextensible joints; muscular hypotonia.

Skin, ocular fundi, neurological examination (in the younger child including CT scan, echocardiogram, EEG), alveolar processes, dentition, and hands and feet unremarkable. Blood biochemistry, endocrinological examinations (and chromosome analysis in the younger girl) normal.

Manifestation: At birth.

Etiology: Unknown; genetic basis probable.

Frequency: Unknown.

Course, prognosis: Apparently relatively favorable.

Comment: In the differential diagnosis, an atypical orofaciodigital syndrome type I (p. 62) was especially considered, but had to be rejected here. It appears to be a 'new syndrome'.

Illustrations:
1–6 The only children to date of young, healthy, nonconsanguineous parents.

H.-R.W.

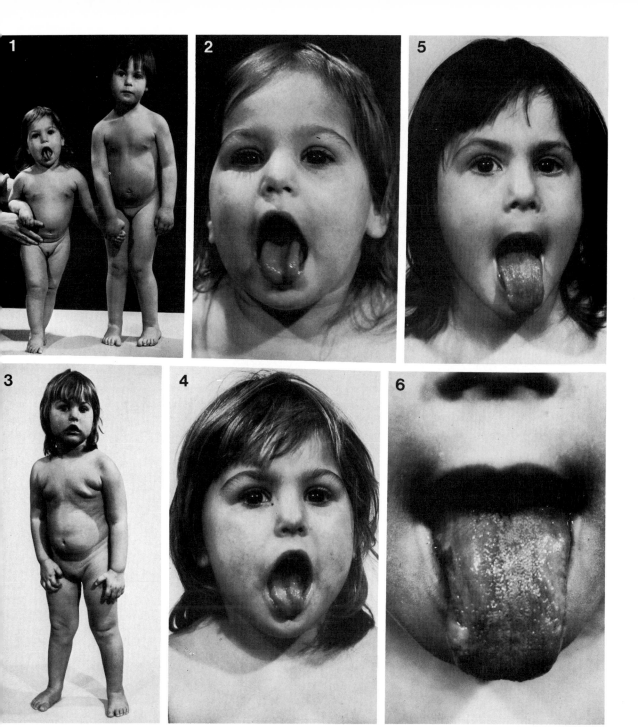

65

33. Cat-Eye Syndrome

(Coloboma-Anal Atresia Syndrome)

A syndrome of unusual facies, preauricular tags and/or fistulas, coloboma of the iris, anal atresia, other malformations, and mental retardation.

Main signs:
1. Facies characterized by hypertelorism, antimongoloid slant of the palpebral fissures, low nasal root (**1, 2**). Preauricular tags and/or fistulas (**3, 4**). Generally bilateral coloboma of the iris (retina, choroid) (**2**). Possible microphthalmos.
2. Anal atresia with or without rectovaginal or rectoperineal fistula.
3. Mental retardation not unusual, but generally mild.

Supplementary findings: Various malformations of the kidneys and urinary tract.
 Cardiac defects.
 Chromosome complement shows an extra small chromosome.

Manifestation: At birth.

Etiology: With *in situ* hybridization it could be unequivocally demonstrated that the extra marker chromosome allows the diagnosis of partial trisomy of the long arm of chromosome 22 (22 pter $\rightarrow$ q 11 : : q 11 $\rightarrow$ 22 pter). Sporadic duplication; rarely the result of a balanced parental translocation.

Frequency: Low. About 60 or more cases have been described.

Prognosis: Dependent on the presence and degree of mental retardation and on the severity of heart and kidney malformations and whether they are correctable.

Differential diagnosis: There is a further 'cat-eye syndrome' with normal chromosomes, positional anomalies of the hands and feet, and strikingly large thumbs.

Treatment: Operative correction of the anomalies amenable to surgical treatment and all appropriate handicap aids. Genetic counseling for the parents.

Illustrations:
1–4 A 5½-year-old girl after surgery for anal atresia and for partial removal of preauricular tags. Duplication of the renal pelves and ureters on pyelography. Development only initially delayed. IQ at 3½ years, 118.

H.-R.W./J.K.

References:
 Schinzel, A., Schmid, W., Fraccaro, M. et al. The 'Cat-Eye Syndrome': . . . *Hum. Genet.*, 57, 148 (1981).
 Duncan, A.M.V., Rosenfeld, W. et al. Re-evaluation of the supernumerary chromosome in an individual with cat eye syndrome. *Am. J. Med. Genet.*, 27, 225–227 (1987).

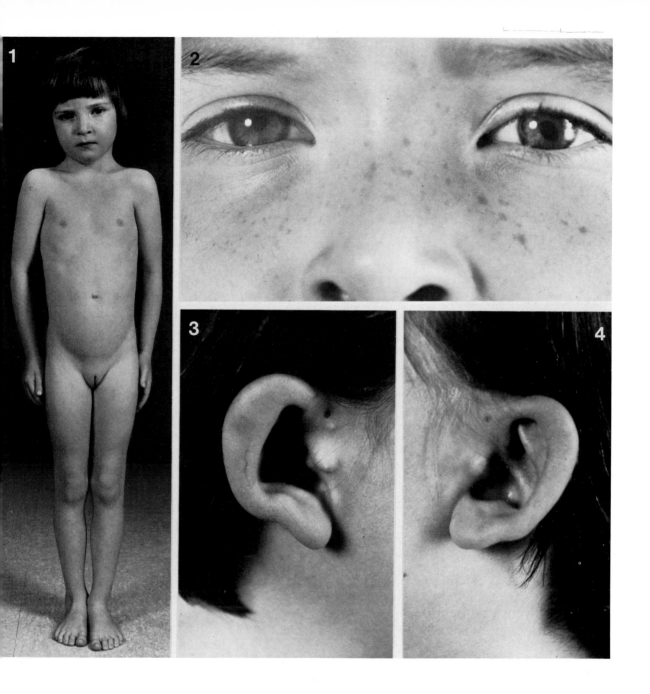

34. Pierre Robin Sequence

(Pierre Robin Anomaly, Pierre Robin Complex, Pierre Robin Syndrome, Pierre Robin Triad)

A characteristic combination of hypoplasia of the lower jaw, glossoptosis, and cleft palate.

Main signs:
1. Usually marked, sometimes extreme, micrognathia (1, 2, 4). As a result, retroglossia, glossoptosis with narrowing of the airway, corresponding stridor, and in some cases signs of hypoxia.
2. Cleft palate (3), possibly only very high palate or bifid uvula.

Supplementary findings: Bulging of the upper rib cage (5) as a result of obstructed respiration. Not infrequently mental retardation, whether as a result of hypoxic episodes, or of other causes, e.g., brain anomalies.

In the literature, the Robin sequence has been described in association with malformations of a great variety of other organs. Some of these cases can be further classified, e.g., as cerebrocostomandibular syndrome (p.72), trisomy 18 syndrome (p.88), oroacral syndrome (p.380), and a good 15 other clinical conditions, but some of them, up to now, cannot be further classified. For this reason and because of its heterogeneous etiology, the Robin triad is considered as a sequence, which can occur alone or as a component of a syndrome. In every newborn with Robin complex, arthro-ophthalmopathy (Stickler syndrome p.532) must be ruled out, especially when there is a family history of hereditary myopia, with or without retinal detachment, of cleft palate, and of spondyloepiphyseal dysplasia. Examination by a qualified ophthalmologist.

Manifestation: At birth.

Etiology: Not genetically uniform; predominantly sporadic occurrence. The primary defect is probably the failure of the mandible to attain the proper size during the second embryonal month, so that the tongue is not brought down and forward, and closure of the palate is impeded (sequence).

Frequency: Not rare.

Prognosis: For isolated Robin triad, dependent on the extent of the malformations. Danger of suffocation and of hypoxic brain damage. After survival of the first two months of life, prognosis good as a result of development of the mandible (4 and 5: the same child at ages 6 weeks and 18 months).

Treatment: Nurse prone, glossoplexy, procedures to extend the lower jaw; tracheostomy should be reserved as a last resort. Tube feeding, possibly gastrostomy. Surgery for cleft palate.

Illustrations:
1–3 A 4-week-old infant. Frequent asphyxial episodes. Aspiration pneumonia. Treated by nursing prone and tube feeding.
4 and 5 A patient at ages 6 weeks and 18 months. Dyspnea, stridor, frequent episodes of asphyxia in the first three weeks of life. Treatment by nursing prone and tube feeding. Note development of the mandible!

H.-R.W.

References:

Grimm, G., Pfefferkorn, A., Taatz, H. Die klinische Bedeutung des Pierre Robin-Syndroms und seine Behandlung. *Dtsch. Zahn-, Mund-, und Kieferheilkd.*, 43, 169 (1964).

Opitz, J.M. Familial anomalies in the Pierre-Robin syndrome. *Birth Defects*, 5, 119 (1969).

Cohen, M.M., Jr. The Robin anomaly—its nonspecificity and associated sydromes. *J. Oral. Surg.*, 34, 587 (1976).

Williams, A.J., Williams, M.A., Walker, C.A. et al. The Robin anomalad (Pierre Robin syndrome)—a follow up study. *Arch. Dis. Child.*, 56, 633 (1981).

Carey, J.C., Fineman, R.M. et al. The Robin sequence . . . *J. Pediatr.*, 101, 858–864 (1982).

Heaf, D.R., Helms, P.J., Dinwiddie, R. et al. Nasopharyngeal airways in Pierre Robin syndrome. *J. Pediatr.*, 100, 698 (1982).

Couly, G. Les formes graves néo-natales du syndrome de Pierre Robin. *Arch. Fr. Pédiatr.*, 41, 591–594 (1984).

Cozzi, F. and Pierro, A. Glossoptosis-apnea syndrome. *Pediatrics*, 75, 836–843 (1985).

Sheffeld, L.J., Reiss, J.A. et al. A genetic follow-up study of 64 patients with the Pierre Robin complex. *Am. J. Med. Genet.*, 28, 25–36 (1987).

Couly, G., Cheron, G. et al. Le syndrome de Pierre Robin. *Arch. Fr. Pédiatr.*, 45, 553–559 (1988).

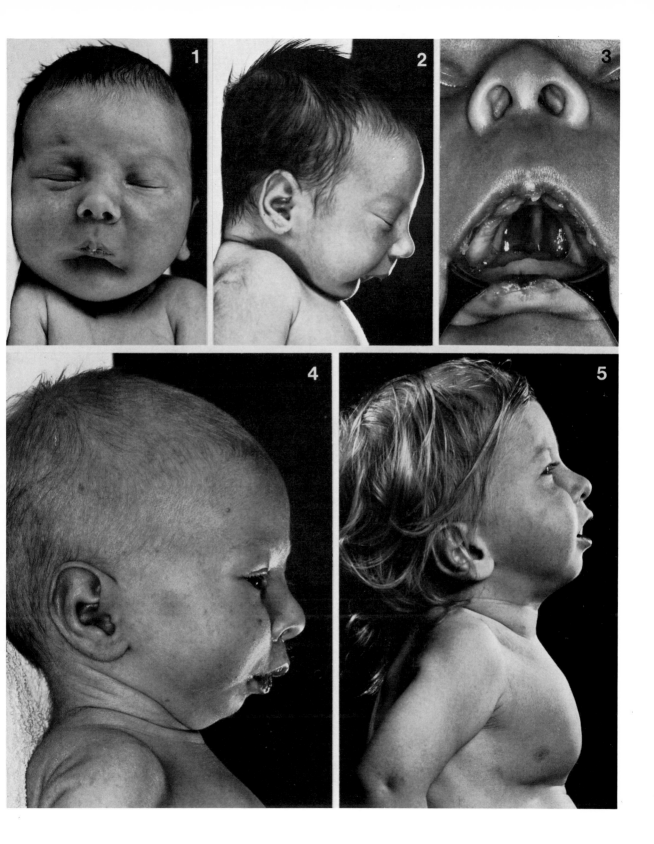

35. Catel–Manzke Syndrome

(Pierre Robin Complex with Accessory Metacarpal of the Index Finger)

A characteristic combination of the Pierre Robin complex and a peculiar finger malformation.

Main signs:
1. The more or less completely expressed Pierre Robin complex (mandibular hypoplasia, retroglossia, cleft palate); this holds true for all of the cases described to date (15:15) (1).
2. Position anomalies of both index fingers, due to a radiologically demonstrable accessory ossicle (rudimentary metacarpal?) between the—sometimes shortened—second metacarpal and the proximal phalanx (13 or 14:1). Usually radial deviation of the index fingers at the metacarpophalangeal joint and possible ulnar deviation at the first interphalangeal joint (2–4).
3. Clinodactyly of the little finger (7:15), and in some cases of the other fingers also; possible camptodactyly.
4. Congenital cardiac anomalies (8:15; atrial septal defect, ventricular septal defect, and others).

Supplementary findings: Possible club feet, small stature, dislocatable knees or other joints.

Manifestation: At birth.

Etiology: Not established. Sex ratio to date 11 male : 2 female (in 2 cases the sex was not given). Several sibling cases and striking family histories. Genetic syndrome of very variable expression.

Frequency: To date, 15 cases are known from the literature.

Course, prognosis: Dependent on the severity of the Pierre Robin complex and how prompt and effective its treatment; in addition, on the type, severity, and treatment of possible cardiac defects.

Diagnosis: Not difficult in typical cases.

Treatment: As in isolated Pierre Robin complex. In addition, care for the cardiac and other anomalies when present. Early consultation with an experienced hand surgeon!

Illustrations:
1 A case of Catel–Manzke syndrome, a boy, at age 6 weeks: hypoplasia of the mandible (with microglossia, glossoptosis, and a widely cleft palate); dyspnea on inspiration and expiration, secondary to the glossoptosis, distended barrel-shaped thorax.
2–4 X-rays of the hands of the proband at 6 weeks, 6½ years, and 26 years. Accessory bone (metacarpal?) between the second metacarpal and the proximal phalanx of the index finger bilaterally. Eventual fusion of the accessory part with the proximal phalanx and, on the left side, also with the second metacarpal. Radial deviation of both index fingers. Slight brachymesophalangy and clinodactyly of the fifth fingers.

No consanguinity of the proband's parents; several cases of mandibular hypoplasia without further abnormalities in the mother's family.

H.-R.W.

References:

Manzke, H. Symmetrische Hyperphalangie des zweiten Fingers durch ein akzessorisches Metacarpale. *Fortschr. Röntgenstr.*, 105, 425–427 (1966).

Sundaram, V., Taysi, K., Hartmann, A.F., Jr. et al. Hyperphalangy and clinodactyly of the index finger with Pierre Robin anomaly: Catel–Manzke syndrome . . . *Clin. Genet.*, 21, 407–410 (1982).

Brude, E. Pierre Robin sequence and hyperphalangy—a genetic entity (Catel–Manzke syndrome). *Eur. J. Pediatr.*, 142, 222–223 (1984).

Dignan, P.S.J., Martin, L.W. and Zenni, E.J., Jr. Pierre Robin anomaly with an accessory metacarpal of the index fingers. The Catel–Manzke syndrome. *Clin. Genet.*, 29, 168–173 (1986).

Thompson, E.M., Winter, R.M. and Williams, M.J.H. A male infant with the Catel–Manzke syndrome and dislocatable knees. *J. Med. Genet.*, 23, 271–274 (1986).

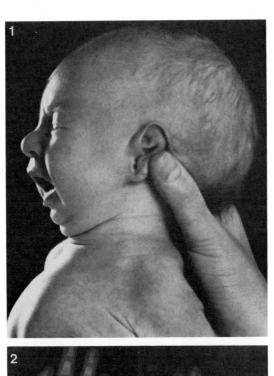

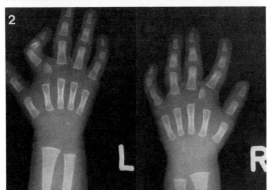

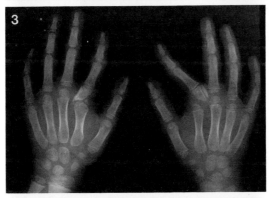

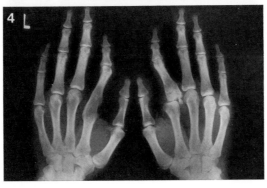

36. (Cerebro-)costo-mandibular Syndrome

(Smith–Theiler–Schachenmann Syndrome)

A syndrome of Robin sequence (micrognathia-glossoptosis-cleft palate), multiple dorsal rib defects, and, occasionally, microcephaly and mental retardation.

Main signs:
1. Dorsal rib defects (frequently absence of the twelfth rib) and possible vertebral anomalies; the former most frequently of the fifth and sixth ribs and usually symmetrical.
2. Robin sequence, with the mandibular defect being the most constant.
3. Microcephaly (or microbrachycephaly) in at least one-third of the cases. Mental retardation in about one-third of the surviving patients; functional central nervous system disorders also not infrequent.

Supplementary findings: hydrocephalus, porencephaly, spina bifida cystica, and other anomalies of the CNS may occur.

Short neck with nuchal skin fold and Sprengel's deformity in some patients. Possible development of scoliosis.

Occasionally hearing defects.

Polyhydramnios in some cases.

Manifestation: At birth and subsequently.

Etiology: A monogenic disorder with variable penetrance and expression can be assumed. Since there is evidence for autosomal recessive as well as for autosomal dominant transmission, heterogeneity is likely. (Mild signs of the disorder, including those on chest X-ray, should be sought in members of the proband's immediate family.)

Frequency: Low. About 40 cases known to date.

Course, prognosis: Only about half of the patients observed to date have survived the initial respiratory, feeding, and associated problems, and of these, about half have had diverse CNS disorders. The latter can, in some cases, be regarded as resulting from early postnatal hypoxic damage.

Treatment: Initially, that of the Robin complex or respiratory insufficiency. Later, any appropriate handicap aids. Genetic counseling. Prenatal diagnosis by ultrasonography or X-ray in some cases.

Illustrations:
1–6 A patient, the second child of healthy, young, nonconsanguineous parents (after a healthy boy).
1 and 2 Microretrognathia with the complete Robin sequence.
5 The multiple rib defects neonatally.
3 and 4 The bell-shaped deformity of the thorax of the now 2-year-old boy, with completely normal psychomotor development.
6 Marked narrowing of the upper thorax; some of the earlier rib defects have been bridged by bone.

The father of the proband shows mild micrognathia and a high narrow palate.

H.-R.W.

References:

McNicholl, B., Egan-Mitchell, B., Murray, J.P. et al. Cerebro-costo-mandibular syndrome . . . *Arch. Dis. Child.*, 45, 421–424 (1970).

Hennekam, R.C.M., Beemer, F.A., Huijbers, P.A. et al. The cerebro-costo-mandibular syndrome: third report of familial occurrence. *Clin. Genet.*, 28, 118–121 (1985).

Trautman, M.S., Schelley, S.L., Stevenson, D.K. et al. Cerebro-costo-mandibular syndrome: a familial case consistent with autosomal recessive inheritance. *J. Pediatr.*, 107, 990–991 (1985).

Meinecke, P., Wolff, G. and Schaefer, E. Cerebro-costo-mandibuläres Syndrom ohne cerebrale Beteiligung bei einem 4jährigen Jungen. *Monatschr. Kinderheilkd.*, 135, 54–58 (1987).

Merlob, P., Schonfeld, A., Grunebaum, M. et al. Autosomal dominant cerebro-costo-mandibular syndrome: ultrasonic and clinical findings. *Am. J. Med. Genet.*, 26, 195–202 (1987).

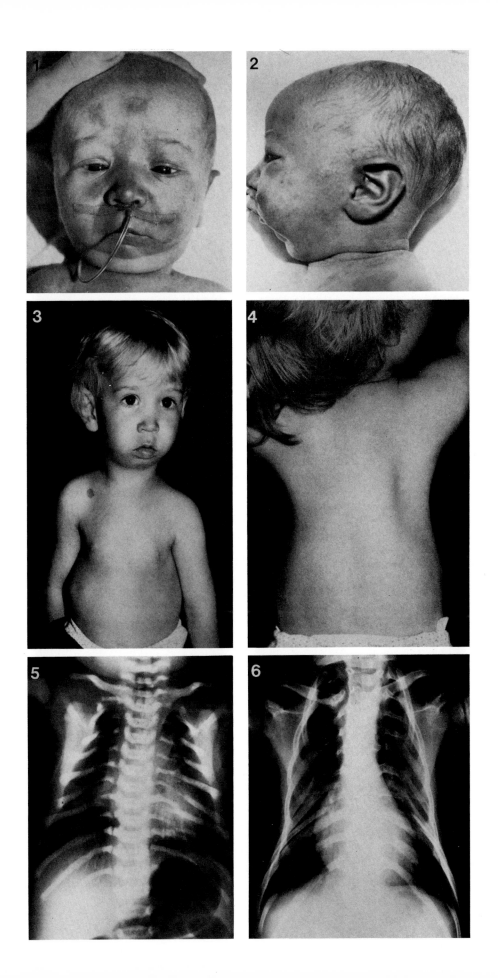

37. Fraser Syndrome

(Cryptophthalmos-Syndactyly Syndrome, Cryptophthalmos Syndrome)

Syndrome of absence of the palpebral fissure(s)—usually with partial or complete absence of eyelids and eyebrows and with defects of the eyes, especially the anterior segment—combined with anomalies of the ears, nose, limbs, urogenital system, and other areas.

Main signs:
1. Bi- or unilateral absence of the palpebral fissure (the normal lid structure is replaced by a skin-fold covering that originates from the forehead), with defects of the lids and eyebrows and anomalies of the eyes (defects of the anterior segment; microphthalmia, anophthalmia). Projections of scalp hair extending from the low-lying temples to the lateral eyebrow region (1–4, 6). Cryptophthalmos is not an obligatory feature (10).
2. Broad nasal root, hypoplasia and notching of alae nasi (1–4, 6, 10).
3. Variable dysplasia of the external (possibly also of the inner and middle) ears (2, 3, 6).
4. Partial cutaneous syndactyly and more extensive anomalies of the extremities (7–9, 11).
5. Bi- or unilateral agenesis or hypoplasia of the kidneys; genital malformations (hypospadias, vaginal atresia, pseudohermaphroditism) (10).

Supplementary findings: Possible anomalies of the cranial vault, encephalocele or other malformations of the brain, facial clefts (10), stenosis or atresia in the laryngeal region, anal atresia, malformations of the heart and/or lungs, anomalies of the efferent urinary tract.

Manifestation: At birth.

Etiology: Autosomal recessive disorder with variable expression; this mode of inheritance can be regarded as certain when ultrasonography (or autopsy) demonstrates a- or hypoplasia of the kidneys.

(Isolated cryptophthalmos does not signify Fraser syndrome and may follow autosomal dominant transmission.)

Frequency: Low. About 110 observations in the literature.

Course, prognosis: With cryptophthalmos, dubious to poor with regard to sight. Otherwise dependent on the type and severity of associated defects.

Diagnosis: Cryptophthalmos, anomalies of the ears and nose, syndactyly, and urogenital anomalies are the cardinal features; when cryptophthalmos is not present, the spectrum of the other signs should suggest the true diagnosis. Rule out renal anomalies.

Treatment: Rehabilitation, and cosmetic surgery if possible. Genetic counseling. Prenatal diagnosis (ultrasonography, fetoscopy).

Illustrations:
1, 2, 4–9 A newborn, the third child of healthy parents after two healthy children. The eyeballs are readily palpable bilaterally; median notch of the nose; syndactyly of the hands and feet with hypoplasia of the distal phalanges; ambiguous external genitalia (normal female karyotype); malformations of internal organs.
3 A 10-year-old girl, the second child of consanguineous parents (two healthy siblings). Small eyeball palpable on the left; mixed hearing loss and stenosis of the auditory canal bilaterally; partial cutaneous syndactyly of the hands and feet; vaginal atresia.
10 and 11 A newborn girl who died shortly after birth, the first child of healthy parents. Fraser syndrome without cryptophthalmos.

H.-R.W.

References:

Burn, J. and Marwood, R.P. Fraser syndrome presenting as bilateral renal agenesis in three sibs. *J. Med. Genet.*, 19, 360–361 (1982).
Lurie, J.W. and Cherstvoy, E.D. Renal agenesis as a diagnostic feature of cryptophthalmos-syndactyly syndrome. *Clin. Genet.*, 25, 528–532 (1984).
Mortimer, G., McEwan, H.P., Yates, J.R.W. Fraser syndrome presenting as monozygotic twins with bilateral renal agenesis. *J. Med. Genet.*, 22, 76–78 (1985).
Koenig, R. and Spranger, J. Cryptophthalmos-syndactyly syndrome without cryptophthalmos. *Clin. Genet.*, 29, 413–416 (1986).
Thomas, I.T., Frias, J.L., Felix, V. et al. Isolated and syndromic cryptophthalmos. *Am. J. Med. Genet.*, 25, 85–98 (1986).
Gattuso, A., Patton, M.A., Baraitser, M. The clinical spectrum of the Fraser syndrome . . . *J. Med. Genet.*, 24, 549–555 (1987).
Bialer, M.G. and Wilson, W.G. Syndromic cryptophthalmos. *Am. J. Med. Genet.*, 30, 385–387 (1988).
Boyd, P.A., Keeling, J.W. et al. Fraser syndrome . . . *Am. J. Med. Genet.*, 31, 159–168 (1988).

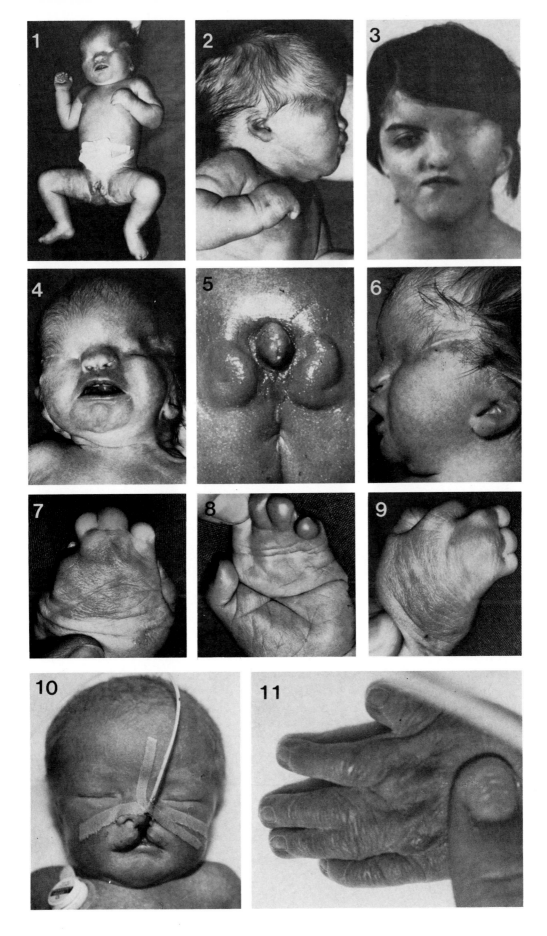

38. 'Potter Syndrome'

An etiologically heterogeneous, but clinically essentially uniform, sequence.

The term 'Potter syndrome' (oligohydramnios sequence) refers to the effect of prolonged amniotic fluid deficiency on the fetus, with hypoplasia of the lungs, facial dysmorphism, and skeletal changes, usually of renal origin. The degree to which the various features are expressed depends mainly on the degree and duration of the oligo-/anhydramnios.

The renal causes include bilateral agenesis of the kidneys, and the various different forms of polycystic kidney disease (see table). Also due to the same pathogenesis: various combinations of renal agenesis; renal dysplasia (polycystic kidneys Potter type II); the end-result of early acting obstructive processes (polycystic kidneys Potter type IV); and, as a later manifestation, hydronephrosis of different origins.

In a proportion of the cases, the kidney changes occur as a part of one of numerous syndromes (e.g., cerebro-oculo-facio-skeletal syndrome, Fraser-cryptophthalmos syndrome, caudal regression syndrome, Meckel syndrome, brachio-oto-renal syndrome, prune belly syndrome, VATER association, and chromosome disorders).

Main signs: Hypoplasia of the lungs, 'Potter' facies: hypertelorism, prominent skin folds originating from the inner corner of the eye, retrognathia, large dysplastic low-set ears with deficient cartilage formation. Additional malformations in more than 50% of cases: vertebral anomalies, club feet, joints contractures of variable severity, large hands, and caudal regression anomalies including sirenomelia.

Supplementary findings: Gonadal dysgenesis, pseudohermaphroditism, anorectal malformations, tracheoesophageal malformations (often within the spectrum of the VATER association), cardiovascular malformations.

Manifestation: The Potter phenotype in its various forms is always evident at birth; evidence of the underlying disorder may appear later in the less severe forms.

Frequency: About 1:3,000. The various underlying disorders are much less frequent individually (see table).

Characteristics of the most important forms of polycystic kidney disease which may also lead to Potter phenotype.

	Autosomal recessive form (Potter type I)	Autosomal dominant form (Potter type III)	Dysplasia (Potter type II)
Frequency	c. 1:40,000	c. 1:1,000	All forms c. 1:1,000
Pathology of the kidneys: Shape	Retains the kidney shape.	Kidney shape retained.	Usually loss of kidney form.
Size	Enlarged; initially normal size.	Enlarged; initially normal size.	Enlarged or hypoplastic.
Symmetry	Symmetrical.	Symmetrical; initally, may be asymmetrical for years.	Often asymmetrical.
Localization of cysts	Collecting tube.	Cysts in all parts of the nephron and collecting tube.	Usually complete loss of the kidney structure; classification often not possible.
Further malformations of the urogenital tract	None.	None.	Additional malformations frequent; usually obstruction.
Liver changes	Congenital fibrosis of the liver a constant feature.	In about a third of the adult cases.	None.
Additional signs	Pancreatic cysts (rare).	Aneurysms of the base of the brain.	Very frequently various malformations.
Main signs	Neonatal period: respiratory insufficiency. With increasing age of survival, renal insufficiency and portal hypertension.	Onset in the third to fifth decades of life, or during childhood; in rare cases in infancy with respiratory problems; renal insufficiency, pain, organomegaly, hypertension, hematuria, urinary tract infections.	Variable; either no signs (unilateral), or Potter sequence. Frequently signs due to additional malformations.
Frequency of the Potter sequence	Low.	Very low.	High.
Inheritance	Autosomal recessive.	Autosomal dominant.	Heterogeneous; multifactorial inheritance; empirical risk of recurrence usually low.

Course, prognosis: Fully expressed signs occur when the amniotic fluid deficiency has been marked and prolonged, and the prognosis is usually unfavorable. In the less severe forms, the prognosis may occasionally be more favorable, depending on the underlying disorder.

Differential diagnosis: Exclusion of chronic hydrorrhea gravidarum and diagnosis of the underlying disorder (ultrasonographic examination of the parents) should be carried out in every case.

Treatment: As a rule, none possible; with less prolonged obstructive processes, operative correction may help preserve (remaining) renal function.

Illustrations:
1 A child with 'classic Potter syndrome': Potter facies, malformations of the hands, genital anomalies.
2a and 2b Amnion nodosum (plain and enlarged views).

K. Zerres

References:
Zerres, K. Genetics of cystic kidney diseases. Criteria for classification and genetic counseling. *Pediatr. Nephrol.*, 1, 397–404 (1987).

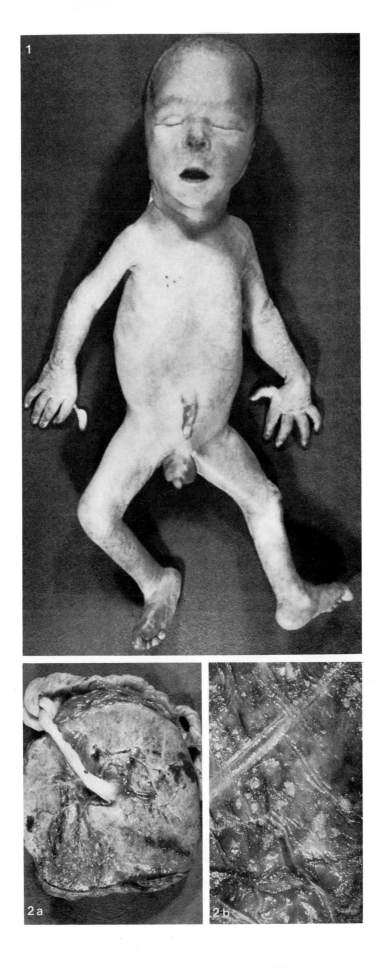

39. Sirenomelia

A characteristic malformation syndrome (sequence) with fused lower extremities, external and dorsal rotation of this symmelian extremity, dorsally located patellae and ventrally located popliteal fossae, absent external genitalia, anal atresia, renal anomalies, and hypoplasia of the lungs.

Main signs:
1. Fusion of the lower extremities with absence of one or both feet. The legs and feet are often rotated, with the extensors and flexors reversed in the lower extremities, so that the patellae are dorsal and the popliteal fossae medial.
2. Absence of the external genitalia, imperforate anus, absent rectum.
3. Vertebral anomalies, sacral agenesis, pelvic malformations (caudal regression syndrome).
4. Renal agenesis (oligohydramnios) or cystic renal dysplasia; horseshoe kidneys; hypoplasia or aplasia of the ureters, urinary bladder, and urethra. Asplenia. Single umbilical artery.
5. Pulmonary hypoplasia. Cardiac defects, tracheoesophageal fistula.
6. Potter facies: low-set large dysplastic ears; flattened nose; receding chin; old-appearing, wrinkled face.

Supplementary findings: Intrauterine growth retardation.

External genitalia sometimes represented by small skin tags.

Medial position and malformations of the fibulae. Occasionally phocomelia of the upper extremities unilaterally or bilaterally. Anomalies of the radius, club hand (talipomanus), absent or extra fingers, syndactyly.

Manifestation: At birth. Should be suspected in pregnancies with oligohydramnios; diagnosis by ultrasonography.

Etiology: Primary defect of the caudal axis skeleton during the third embryonal week. Damage to the primitive streak. Exogenous factors? One hundred times more frequent with uniovular twins than with single births. Ratio of males to females 2.7:1.

Frequency: Low. About 1 in 60,000 births. To date, over 300 classic cases reported.

Course, prognosis: Stillbirth or death within a few hours *post partum* (bilateral renal agenesis, pulmonary hypoplasia). In one case, the infant lived for 63 hours.

Differential diagnosis: With atypical cases, a smooth transition to VACTERL syndrome (*V*ertebral anomalies, *A*nal atresia, *C*ardiac anomalies, *T*racheo-*E*sophageal fistulas, *R*adial deformities, *L*ung hypoplasia) of varied etiology. Caudal regression syndrome in children of diabetic mothers, rarely autosomal dominant.

Treatment: No therapeutic efforts known to date can ensure survival. Prenatal diagnosis with ultrasonography in women with oligohydramnios and intrauterine growth retardation.

Illustrations:
1a–1d A prematurely born (33rd week) male infant (46 XY) who lived for 2 hours: Potter facies, large ears lying close to the head; helices dysplastic, with the upper edge folded in; fused lower extremities in external and dorsal rotation (patellae dorsal, popliteal fossae ventral); dorsolaterally lying dysplastic fibulae with sharp lateral tapering of the bone (1d). Absence of external genitalia in the expected location; para-anal 2 cm-long skin tag corresponded histologically to a primitive penis.
2a–2c The first born of male twins (brother free of external malformations); survival for 30 minutes. Potter facies; fusion of the lower extremities even more extensive than in 1.

J.K.

References:

Smith, D.W., Bartlett, C., Harrah, L.M. Monozygotic twinning and the Duhamel anomalad (imperforate anus to sirenomelia): a non-random association between two aberrations in morphogenesis. *Birth Defects*, XII, 5, 53–63 (1976).
Temtamy, S. and McKusick, V. The genetics of hand malformations. *Birth Defects*, XIV, 3, 181–184 (1978).
Stevenson, R.E., Jones, K.L., Phelan, M.C. Vascular steal: the pathogenetic mechanism producing sirenomelia and associated defects of the viscera and soft tissues. *Pediatrics*, 78, 451–457 (1986).
Duncan, P.A. and Shapiro, L.R. Sirenomelia and VATER association . . . *Dysmorphol. Clin. Genet.*, 2, 96 (1989).

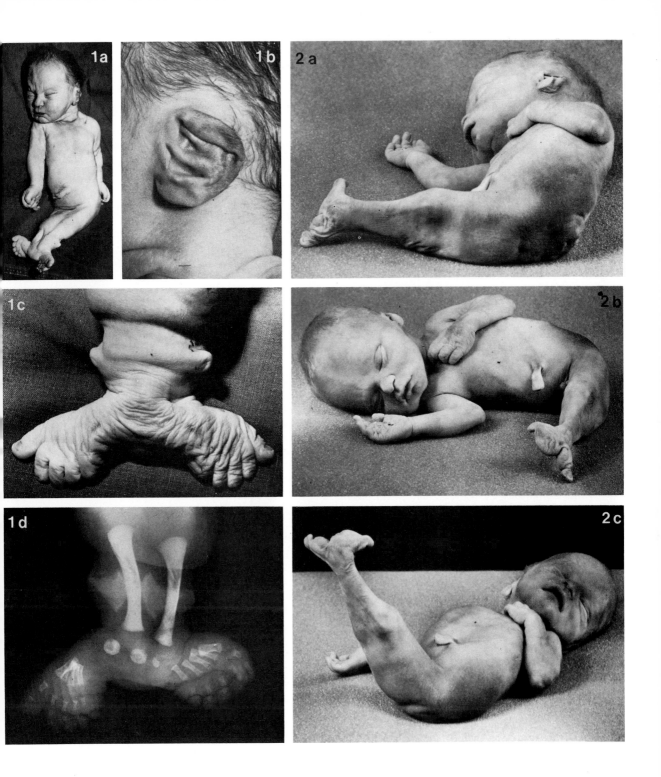

40. Meckel–Gruber Syndrome

(Dysencephalia Splanchnocystica, Gruber Syndrome)

An autosomal recessive syndrome with encephalocele, postaxial hexadactyly, and cystic changes of the kidney.

Main signs:
1. Encephalocele; microcephaly, anencephaly.
2. Postaxial hexadactyly of the hands and feet.
3. Cystic dysplasia of the kidneys and fibrotic and/or cystic changes of the liver.
4. Anomalies of the efferent urinary tract (absent renal pelvis, hypo- or aplasia of the ureters).
5. Oligohydramnios.

Supplementary findings: Facial dysmorphisms: cleft palate, cleft lip; microphthalmia or anophthalmia, hypertelorism; broad, round face with full cheeks, full lips; macrostomia; anomalies of the tongue; narrow chin. Low-set ears. Short neck.

Cardiac defects. Internal and/or external genital anomalies.

Unremarkable pregnancy, oligohydramnios, stillbirth or short survival.

Manifestation: At birth; prenatal diagnosis possible from the 18th week of pregnancy onwards, with modern diagnostic methods (ultrasonography). High alpha fetoprotein.

Etiology: Autosomal recessive defect.

Frequency: Great Britain 1:140,000; Ashkenazi Jews 1:50,000; Finland 1:8,500; Massachusetts 1:13,250; Belgium 1:3,000; Gujarati Indians 1:1,300.

Course, prognosis: About one-third stillborn; two-thirds of the infants survive a maximum of 2½ hours. Isolated reports of longer survival: 34 weeks, 13 months, 28 months, 3 years, 4 years.

Differential diagnosis: Due to the variability of the Meckel–Gruber syndrome, the following syndromes should be considered: Potter sequence, trisomy 13, hydrolethalus syndrome, Smith–Lemli–Opitz syndrome.

Treatment: Not relevant; genetic counseling.

Illustrations:
1–4 A newborn male infant: encephalocele; postaxial hexadactyly of the hands and feet; polycystic kidneys.

J.K.

References:

Fraser, F.C. and Lytwyn, A. Spectrum of anomalies in the Meckel syndrome, or: 'Maybe there is a malformation syndrome with at least one constant anomaly'. *Am. J. Med. Genet.*, 9, 67–73 (1981).

Seller, M.J. Phenotypic variation in Meckel syndrome. *Clin. Genet.*, 20, 74–77 (1981).

Rehder, H. and Labbé. Prenatal morphology in Meckel's syndrome. *Prenatal Diagnosis*, 1, 161–172 (1981).

Anderson, V.M. Meckel syndrome: morphologic consideration. *Birth Defects*, 18 (3B), 145–160 (1982).

Lowry, R.B.L., Hill, R.H., Tischler, B. Survival and spectrum of anomalies in the Meckel syndrome. *Am. J. Med. Genet.*, 14, 417–421 (1983).

The Meckel Symposium. *Am. J. Med. Genet.*, 18, 559–771 (1984).

Young, I.D., Rickett, A.B., Clarke, D.M. High incidence of Meckel Syndrome in Gujarati Indians. *J. Med. Genet.*, 22, 301–304 (1985).

Shen-Schwartz, S. and Dave, H. Meckel syndrome . . . review of the literature. *Am. J. Med. Genet.*, 31, 349–355 (1988).

Pachi, A., Giancotti, A., Torcia, F. et al. Meckel–Gruber syndrome: ultrasonic diagnosis at 13 weeks . . . *Prenatal Diagnosis*, 9, 187 (1989).

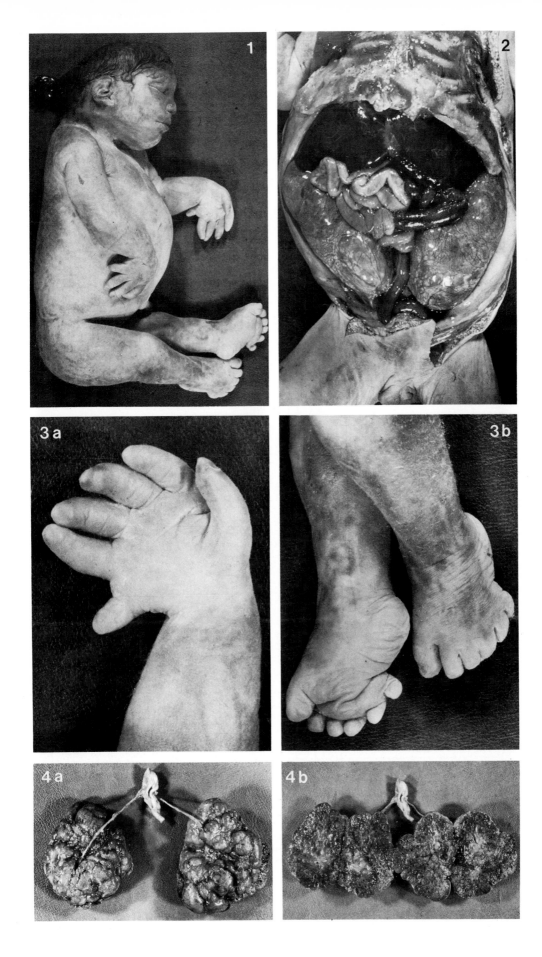

41. Lissencephaly

(Miller–Dieker Syndrome)

A characteristic syndrome with microcephaly, bitemporal depressions, long philtrum and thin upper lip, mild micrognathia, unusual dysplasia of the ears, anteverted nostrils, and lissencephaly (agyria).

Main signs:
1. Microcephaly.
2. Bitemporal depressions of the skull (due to failure of the frontal and temporal lobes to develop properly).
3. Long philtrum with thin upper lip.
4. Lissencephaly (CT), enlarged ventricles.

Supplementary findings: Mild micrognathia, dysplastic helices, anteverted nostrils, cardiac defects, cryptorchidism, corneal clouding, supernumerary fingers, seizures, abnormal muscle tone, severe mental retardation, postnatal growth retardation.

Manifestation: At birth.

Etiology: Chromosome 17 disorder in most cases—usually loss of part of the short arm, but ring chromosome 17 and translocation of chromosome 17 also possible. Autosomal recessive inheritance?

Frequency: Low: up to 1984, about 20 published cases.

Course, prognosis: Severe mental retardation, seizures, poor growth. About 50% of the children die before 6 months of age, the others in early childhood.

Differential diagnosis: Lissencephaly is also observed in a few very rare syndromes (Stratton et al., 1984; Dobyns et al., 1984, 1985), e.g., HARD + E syndrome.

Treatment: Symptomatic. Genetic counseling: with de novo chromosome mutation (high resolution banding) no increased risk of recurrence; with familial translocation, prenatal diagnosis: in the absence of chromosomal abnormality, recurrence risk 0–25% (?)

Illustrations:
1a A 24-day-old newborn girl with bilateral parietal depressions, high forehead, antimongoloid slant of the palpebral fissures, seizures.
1b Micrognathia, long prominent philtrum, anteverted nostrils, dysplastic rotated helices.
2 Cranial computed tomography: lissencephaly (agyria), enlargement of the lateral ventricles.

J.K.

References:
Jones, K.L., Gilbert, E.F., Kaveggia, E.G. et al. The Miller–Dieker syndrome. *Pediatrics*, 66, 277–281 (1980).
Dobyns, W.B., Stratton, R.F., Parke, J.T. et al. Miller–Dieker syndrome: lissencephaly and monosomy 17p. *J. Pediatr.*, 102, 552–558 (1983).
Stratton, R.F., Dobyns, W.B., Airhart, S.D. et al. New chromosomal syndrome: Miller–Dieker syndrome and monosomy 17p13. *Hum. Genet.*, 67, 193–200 (1984).
Dobyns, W.B., Stratton, R.F., Greenburg, F. Syndrome with lissencephaly. I: Miller–Dieker and Norman–Roberts syndromes and isolated lissencephaly. *Am. J. Med. Genet.*, 18, 509–526 (1984).
Dobyns, W.B., Kirkpatrick, J.B., Hittner, H.M. Syndromes with lissencephaly. II: Walker–Warburg and cerebro-oculo-muscular syndromes and a new syndrome with type II lissencephaly. *Am. J. Med. Genet.*, 22, 157–195 (1985).
Dobyns, W.B., Gilbert, E.F., Opitz, J.M. Further comments on the lissencephaly syndromes. *Am. J. Med. Genet.*, 22, 197–211 (1985).
Kotagal, P., Cruse, R.P., Estes, M.L. Norman–Roberts syndrome. *Am. J. Med. Genet.*, 29, 681–683 (1988).
Mielke, R., Lu, J.H. et al. Lissencephaly (Letter to the Editor). *Eur. J. Pediatr.*, 147, 487 (1988).
Warburg, M. and Prause, J.K. Reply to the letter. *Eur. J. Pediatr.*, 147, 487–488 (1988).

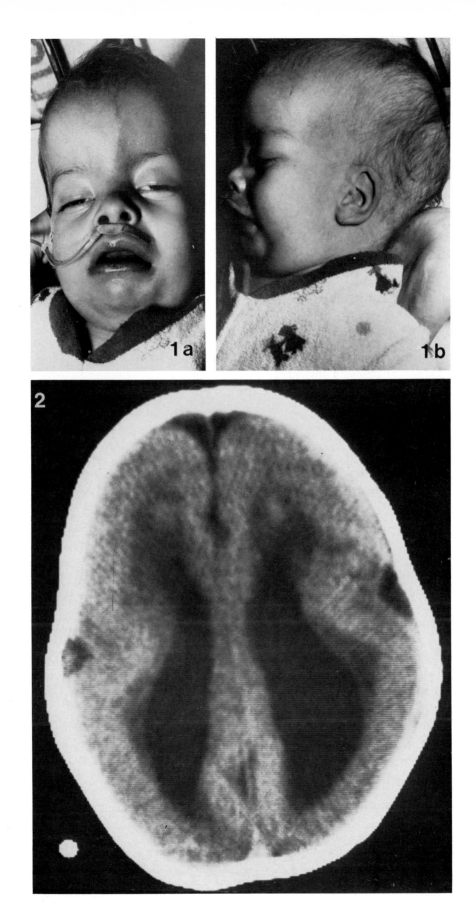

42. Trisomy 13

(D₁ Trisomy Syndrome, Pätau Syndrome, Anglo-American: Patau Syndrome)

A malformation syndrome with characteristic facies, hexadactyly, primordial growth deficiency, profound psychomotor retardation, and multiple other anomalies.

Main signs:
1. Typical facies with sloping forehead, hypo- or hypertelorism, mongoloid slant of the palpebral fissures, microphthalmia or anophthalmia, cleft lip and palate, and micrognathia (**1, 2, 5, 6**).
2. Microcephaly, profound psychomotor impairment, seizures, hypotonia, rarely hypertonia.
3. Postaxial hexadactyly, mainly of the upper extremities, hyperextensible thumbs; narrow, hyperconvex fingernails (**3**). Simian crease. Protruding calcaneus.
4. Localized skin defects in the occipital area (**7**). Capillary hemangiomas.
5. Cryptorchidism, partial fusion of the penis and scrotum, hypospadias.

Supplementary findings: Omphalocele.
   Cardiac defects of various types, especially ventricular septal defect and patent ductus arteriosus.
   Polycystic kidneys and anomalies of the urinary tract.
   Malformations of the brain as with holoprosencephaly (p.42), anomalies of the cerebellum.

Manifestation: At birth.

Etiology: Genetic imbalance due to trisomy of chromosome 13 or to a three-fold dose of the genetic material located on this chromosome. The extra chromosome almost always exists independently; very rarely, it is attached to another chromosome.

Frequency: About 1:10,000 live births.

Course, prognosis: Practically no psychomotor development. About 85% die before reaching 1 year of age.

Treatment: Symptomatic. Prenatal diagnosis after birth of an index case, especially in older mothers or in the case of a balanced translocation in one of the parents.

Differential diagnosis: Meckel syndrome, which usually shows encephalocele; polycystic kidneys. Normal chromosomes.

Illustrations:
1 Patient 1 on the first day of life. Birth measurements: 2230 g, length 48 cm, head circumference 26 cm. Death on the first day of life. Holoprosencephaly, microphthalmia, ventricular septal defect, renal cortical cysts, duplication of the renal pelvis and ureter bilaterally.
2–4 Patient 2 on the first day of life: the ninth child of a 40-year-old woman. Birth measurements within normal limits. Death at age 9 days. Omphalocele, coloboma of the iris, renal cortical cysts, duplication of the renal pelvis and ureter bilaterally, undescended testes, hypospadias, hypoplasia of the mitral and aortic valves.
5 and 6 Patient 3 at age 7 days. Death on the 19th day of life. Hexadactyly of the hands, microphthalmia, high-arched palate, bifid uvula, persistence of the left superior vena cava, ventricular septal defect, patent ductus arteriosus, horseshoe kidneys, bicornuate uterus.
7 and 8 Patient 4 at age 2 days. Birth measurements: 2000 g, length 44 cm, head circumference 31 cm. Death at age 2 days. Holoprosencephaly, hexadactyly of both hands, club feet, bilateral cleft lip and palate. Atresia of the pulmonary valve, ventricular septal defect, overriding aorta, patent ductus arteriosis, bicornate uterus.

H.-R.W.

References:
Hamerton, J.L. *Human Cytogenetics, vol 2.* Academic Press, New York and London, 1971.
Grouchy, J.de and Turleau, C. *Atlas des maladies chromosomiques*, 2. édit., Expansion scientifique française, Paris, 1982.

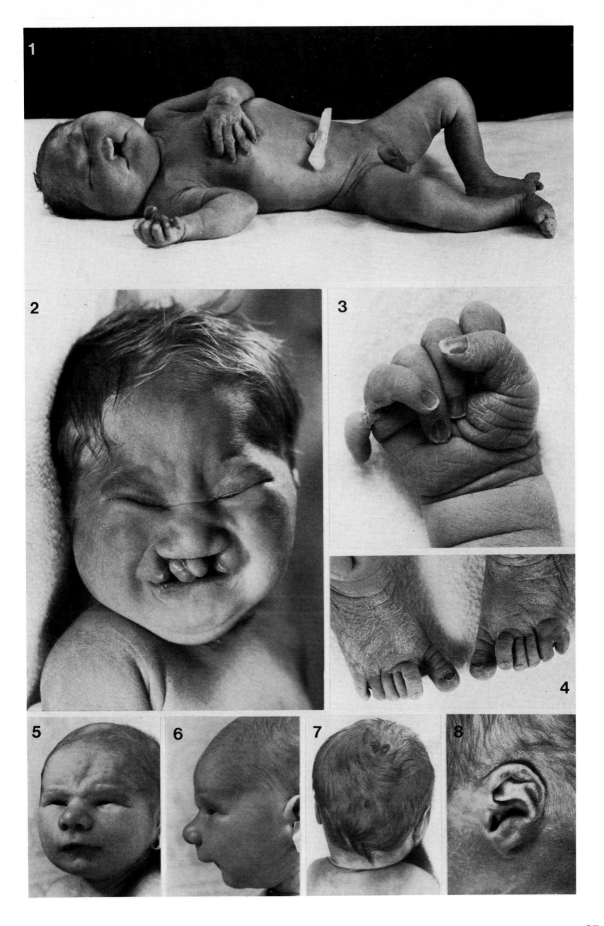

43. Trisomy 18

(Edwards' Syndrome)

A syndrome of primordial growth deficiency, typical facial dysmorphism, profound psychomotor retardation, and multiple other anomalies.

Main signs:
1. Characteristic facies, especially distinguished by protruding forehead, short—sometimes upward-slanting—palpebral fissures, micrognathia, microstomia, short philtrum, not infrequently cleft lip and palate or single components thereof. Narrow microcephalic skull with prominent occiput, dysplasia of the auricles of the ears (4–8).
2. Pronounced pre- and postnatal growth deficiency.
3. Profound psychomotor retardation, seizures; hypertonia after initial hypotonia (1).
4. Flexion contractures of the fingers with overlapping of the second and fifth over the third and fourth fingers respectively (2); hypoplastic nails, especially of the feet; usually partial syndactyly, short dorsiflexed big toes; protruding calcanei, 'rocker-bottom feet' (3).
5. Short sternum; small, relatively widely spaced nipples; umbilical and inguinal hernias; cutis laxa.

Supplementary findings: Aplasia of the radius, polydactyly.

Anomalies of the central nervous system such as hydrocephalus and myelomeningocele.

Cardiac defects, especially ventricular septal defect and patent ductus arteriosus.

Diaphragmatic hernia, omphalocele.

Hypospadias, cryptorchidism, bifid uterus, ovarian hypoplasia, renal anomalies (hydronephrosis, renal cysts, etc.).

Manifestation: At birth.

Etiology: Genetic imbalance due to trisomy of chromosome 18 or to a three-fold dose of the genetic material located on this chromosome. Almost without exception, the extra chromosome exists as an independent entity (and not translocated onto another chromosome).

Frequency: About 1:8,000 births. Predominantly females.

Course, prognosis: Practically no psychomotor development. In 90% of the cases, death occurs during the first year of life.

Treatment: Symptomatic. Prenatal diagnosis in mothers who have previously borne such a child, especially older mothers, or in the case of a balanced translocation in one of the parents.

Illustrations:
1–3 Patient 1. Birth measurements: 2220 g, length 45 cm, head circumference 31 cm. Death at age 4 weeks. Hypertrophy of the clitoris, stenosis of the aortic isthmus, patent ductus arteriosus, bicuspid pulmonary and aortic valves, ventricular septal defect with overriding aorta, tandem (fused) kidneys on the left with double renal pelvis.
4 and 5 Patient 2. Birth measurements: 2260 g, length 45 cm, head circumference 32 cm. Death at age 3 days. Partial syndactyly involving all fingers and toes, ventricular septal defect with overriding aorta, diaphragmatic hernia.
6–8 Patient 3. Birth measurements: 1690 g, length 40 cm, head circumference 31.5 cm. Death at age 8 weeks. Syndactyly, camptodactyly, hypoplastic labia majora, horseshoe kidney, Meckel's diverticulum, diaphragmatic hernia, atrial and ventricular septal defects, bicuspid aortic valve, hypoplasia of the left pulmonary veins.

H.-R.W.

References:

Hamerton, J.L. *Human Cytogenetics, vol II.* Academic Press, New York and London, 1971.
Schinzel, A. and Schmid, W. Trisomie 18 . . . *Helv. Pediatr. Acta*, 26, 673 (1971).
Grouchy, J. de and Turleau, C. *Atlas des maladies chromosomiques*, 2. édit., Expansion scientifique française, Paris, 1982.

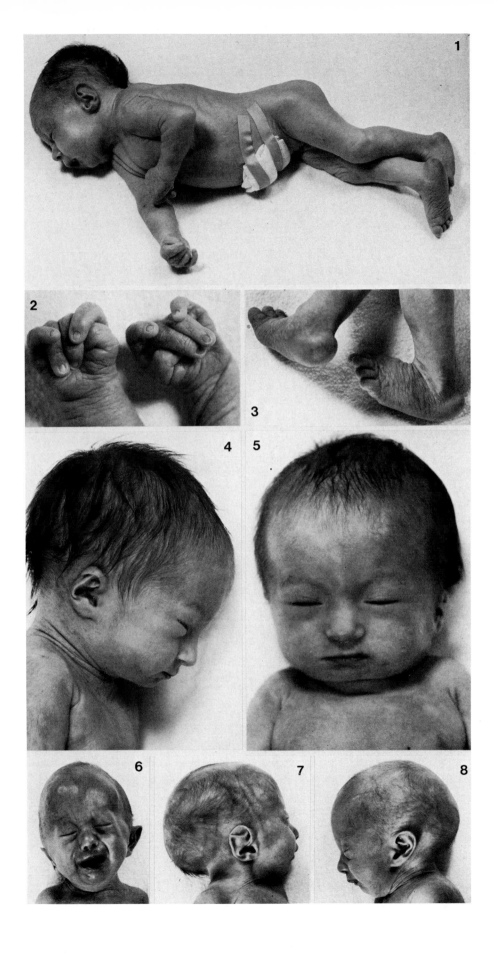

44. Down's Syndrome

(Trisomy 21 Syndrome, Mongolism, Mongoloidism)

A malformation syndrome with mental retardation and very characteristic physical appearance.

Main signs:
1. 'Flat face' with mongoloid slant of the palpebral fissures, epicanthus, low nasal root, small nose, and dysplastic external ears (**1–8, 12–14**) with short cranium and steeply sloping occiput (**14**). Macroglossia (frequently with fissured tongue); dysodontiasis.
2. Short-appearing neck with loose skin (more apparent in the young child). Relatively short stature. Short, stubby hands and fingers with frequent clinodactyly of the little fingers and simian crease of the palms (**15**); widely spaced big and second toes (**13, 16**).
3. Muscular hypotonia and generalized hypermobility of the joints with laxity of the ligaments (**9–11**).
4. Mental retardation, moderate to severe.

Supplementary findings: Cardiac defects in almost half of the cases (usually septal defects, e.g., AV canal).

Mild exophthalmos; strabismus, nystagmus; small white 'porcelain' (Brushfield) spots in the still pale-colored iris of the young infant; occasional cataracts.

Duodenal atresia or stenosis in 1–2% of cases.

Hypoplasia of the pelvis with flaring of the ilia and abnormally small angle between the ilium and the roof of the acetabulum on X-ray. Relatively small penis and frequent cryptorchidism (**10**).

Tendency to localized redness of the cheeks and nose (**6**), to dryness of the skin, to cutis marmorata, and to constipation; above-average frequency of thyroid dysfunction.

Manifestation: At birth.

Etiology: Frequently, increased maternal age. The syndrome is the expression of a chromosomal aberration, namely of trisomy 21, or the disturbance of genetic equilibrium caused by a three-fold dose of the genetic material located on this chromosome. In over 95% of cases the chromosome exists independently; infrequently (about 3%) it is attached to another chromosome (translocation).

Frequency: One case in about 650 births. More than 5% of all mentally retarded children have Down's syndrome.

Course, prognosis: Very dependent on the presence and severity of a cardiac defect. Distinctly increased susceptibility to respiratory tract ailments. Increased disposition to acute leukemia.

As infants, rather sluggish and apathetic, but from age 2 or 3 years, hyperactive behavior. Affected males are infertile.

Almost 80% of patients without a cardiac defect reach 30 years of age. From the fourth decade of life, Alzheimer's disease must be expected.

Treatment: Cardiac surgery may be indicated. Physiotherapy and aids for the handicapped. Genetic counseling for the parents and preventive measures in case of increased risk of recurrence.

Illustrations:
1–8 Facial appearance of, respectively, a 4-week-old, 7-month-old, 10-month-old, 1¼-year-old, 1¾-year-old, 2¾-, 6½-, and 15-year-old child.
9–11 Hypotonia and hyperextensibility in a 10-month-old and 1½-year-old child, respectively.
12–14 Typical flaccid stance of a 6½- and 9½-year-old child.
15 and 16 Simian crease and 'prehensile' foot in a 6-month- and a 1-month-old child respectively.

H.-R.W.

References:
Wiedemann, H.-R. Pathologie der Vererbung und Konstitutionspathologie. In: *Lehrbuch der Kinderheilkunde*, 24th edn. Joppich, G. and Schulte, F. (eds). G. Fischer, Stuttgart, 1980.
Burgio, G.R., Fraccaro, M., Tiepolo, L. (eds): *Trisomy 21*. Springer, Heidelberg, 1981.
Fort, P., Lifshitz, F. et al. Abnormalities of thyroid function in infants with Down syndrome. *J. Pediatr.*, 104, 545 (1984).
Pueschel, S. and Pezzullo, J.C. Thyroid dysfunction in Down syndrome. *Am. J. Dis. Child.*, 139, 636–639 (1985).
Koch, G., Neuhäuser, G. et al. Down syndrome. *Bibliographica Genetica Medica*, 21, (311 pp), Erlangen, 1986.
Baird, P.A. and Sadovnick, A.D. Life expectancy in Down syndrome. *J. Pediatr.*, 110, 849–854 (1987).

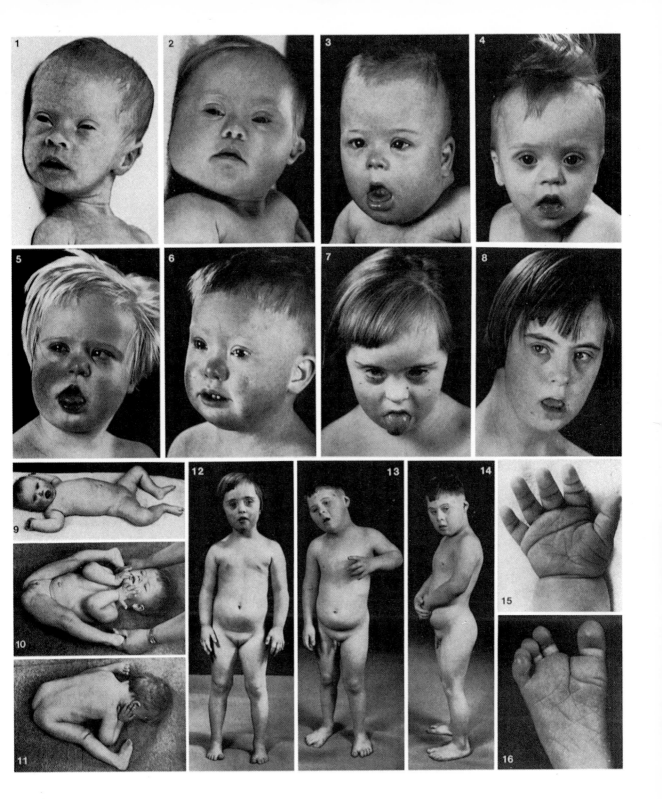

45. Cri Du Chat Syndrome

(Cat Cry Syndrome, Chromosome 5$_p$_ Syndrome)

A syndrome of typical facial dysmorphism, primordial growth deficiency, psychomotor retardation, and catlike cry in early infancy.

Main signs:
1. Face in infancy round and usually flat. Hypertelorism, epicanthal folds, usually antimongoloid slant of the palpebral fissures, strabismus, low broad nasal root, and micrognathia (1–3).
2. Primordial growth deficiency.
3. Microbrachycephaly and severe psychomotor retardation.
4. Catlike cry (unusually plaintive, high-toned, weak) as characteristic feature in early infancy.
5. Congenital stridor.

Supplementary findings: Frequently dysplasia or unusual configuration of the external ears (3). Short neck; scoliosis at a later age.

Malocclusion, high palate, bifid uvula.

Partial syndactyly, short metacarpal and metatarsal bones, simian crease.

Muscular hypotonia, inguinal hernia, diastasis recti abdominis.

Manifestation: At birth.

Etiology: Loss of the tip of the short arm of chromosome 5. As long as neither of the parents has a corresponding translocation, no increased risk of recurrence.

Frequency: Relatively low, about 1:50,000 newborns; up to 1980, about 400 had been reported.

Course, prognosis: Decreased life expectancy. The characteristic cry is lost during the first months of life.

Differential diagnosis: Wolf syndrome (deletion of the short arm of chromosome 4), which however includes 'fish mouth', cleft lip and palate, coloboma, cardiac defect, hypospadias.

Treatment: Symptomatic. Prenatal diagnosis in cases of increased recurrence risk.

Illustrations:
1, 2, and 3 Two affected girls, aged 2 and 6 months.

H.-R.W.

References:

Niebuhr, E. The cri du chat syndrome . . . *Hum. Genet.*, 44, 227 (1978).

Wilkins, L.E., Brown, J.A., Wolf, B. Psychomotor development in 65 home-reared children with cri-du-chat syndrome. *J. Pediatr.*, 97, 401 (1980).

Grouchy, J.de and Turleau, C. *Atlas des maladies chromosomiques*, 2. édit., Expansion scientifique française, Paris, 1982.

Wilkins, L.E., Brown, J.A. et al. Clinical heterogeneity in 80 home-reared children with cri du chat syndrome. *J. Pediatr.*, 102, 528–533 (1983).

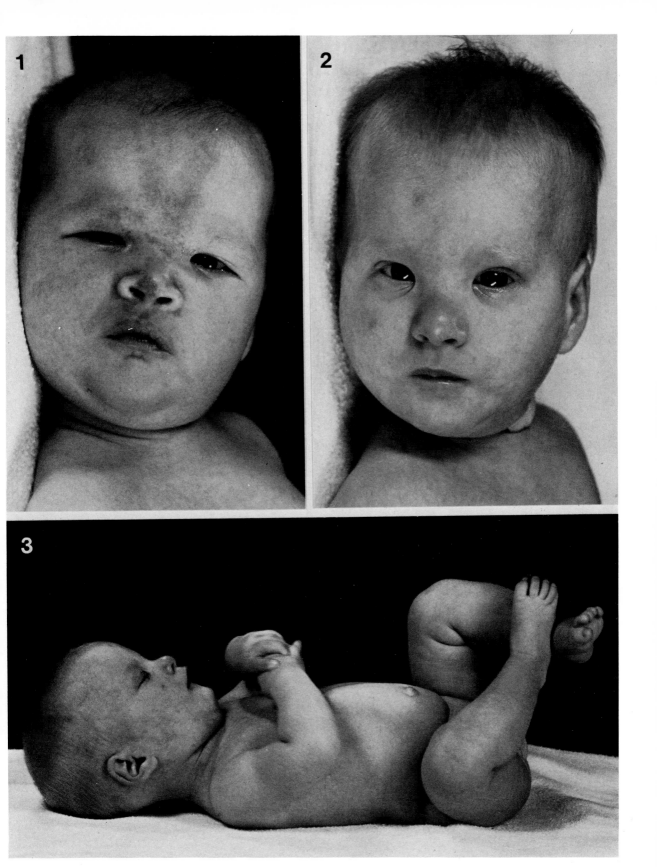

46. Wolf Syndrome

(Chromosome 4ₚ₋ Syndrome, Wolf–Hirschhorn Syndrome)

A characteristic chromosome deletion syndrome with microcephaly, abnormally formed cranium, hypertelorism, ptosis, coloboma of the iris, broad hooked aquiline nose, dysplasia of the external ears, and psychomotor retardation.

Main signs:
1. Intrauterine growth retardation: birth weight around 2000 g with normal period of gestation.
2. Microcephaly, cranial asymmetry, hemangiomata of the forehead, prominent glabella, ocular hypertelorism, divergent strabismus, ptosis of the eyelids, antimongoloid slant of the palpebral fissures, coloboma of the iris (30%).
3. Narrow external auditory canals, low-set dysplastic helices, preauricular tag and pits (50%), broad aquiline nose, short philtrum, 'carp mouth', frequent cleft lip or palate, micrognathia.
4. Cryptorchidism, hypospadias.

Supplementary findings: Stenosis or atresia of the nasolacrimal ducts, widely spaced hypoplastic nipples.

Hip dysplasia, club feet, long fingers, hypoplasia or duplication of the thumbs and halluces.

Scalp defects, hernias, diastasis recti.

Cardiac defects, hypoplasia of the cerebellum, agenesis of the corpus callosum, hypoplasia of the olfactory nerve.

Multicystic renal degeneration, hydronephrosis, unilateral renal agenesis, hypoplasia of the uterus, vaginal aplasia.

Manifestation: At birth.

Etiology: Loss of the tip of the short arm of chromosome 4. About 10% of patients can be explained by a balanced parental translocation. When the parental chromosomes are unremarkable, no increased risk of recurrence.

Frequency: Low; to date over 100 cases described.

Course, prognosis: Increased postnatal mortality (one-third of the patients die in the first year of life). Feeding problems, muscular hypotonia, seizures (80%), increased susceptibility to infections, severe psychomotor retardation, delayed dentition, kyphoscoliosis, delayed or precocious puberty. The oldest patient known to date is 24 years old. Two-thirds of the cases have been girls.

Differential diagnosis: Cri du chat syndrome (p.92).

Treatment: Symptomatic. Prenatal diagnosis in cases of parental translocation.

Illustrations:
1 and 2 Newborn girls.
1 Strabismus, hooked aquiline nose, microretrognathia, dysplastic helices.
2 Hypoplastic orbital boundaries, coloboma of the iris on the right, 'carp mouth'.

J.K.

Reference:
Schinzel, A. *Catalogue of unbalanced chromosome aberrations in man.* Walter de Gruyter, Berlin – New York, 1984.

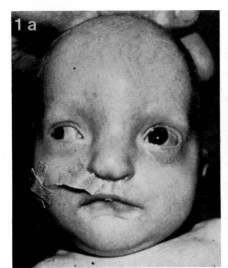

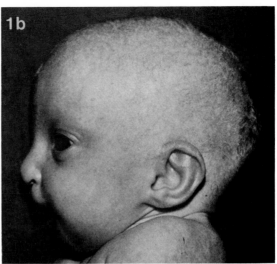

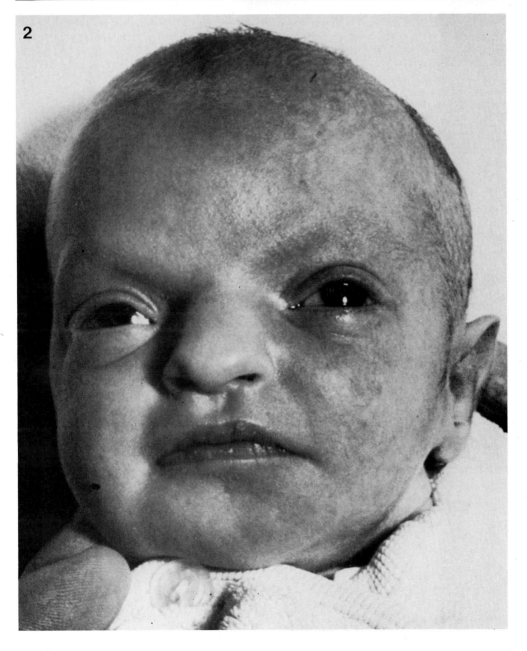

47. Happy Puppet Syndrome

(Angelman Syndrome)

Mental retardation, microcephaly, unusual facial features, unprovoked laughing spells, and ataxic jerky movements of the extremities characterize this syndrome.

Main signs:
1. Moderate to severe mental retardation; paroxysms of laughing ('happy'); no development of speech.
2. Microbrachycephaly (not in every case), occipital groove; hypoplasia of the midface, macrostomia, prognathism, protrusion of the tongue with laughter, widely spaced teeth; atrophy of the optic nerve and defective pigmentation of the choroid and iris.
3. Stiff gait, ataxic jerky ('puppet') movements of the extremities; muscular hypotonia; occasionally hyperreflexia; characteristically abnormal EEG with bilateral irregular spike and wave activity (24-hour EEG), occasionally clinical seizure disorder.

Manifestation: Prenatal onset? Diagnosis after about age 12 months. Laughing episodes after the first or second year of life. Onset of epilepsy between the 6th and 42nd months of life. The facial characteristics become more pronounced with time.

Etiology: Unknown. Various causes possible. Affected siblings have been reported repeatedly, males and females. Deletion in the proximal segment of chromosome 15 has been observed; there has been some evidence that in these cases the deleted chromosome is of maternal origin. (With paternal origin, the Prader–Willi phenotype seems to occur—imprinting? Cf. p.286.)

Frequency: Up to now, 69 patients have been described sporadically from all over the world, frequently from institutions for the handicapped. Six unequivocal sibling observations. Normal birth order and sex ratio.

Course, prognosis: No progression of the mental disorder. No development of speech. Decrease of epileptic disorder with age. The oldest known patient is 75 years old.

Treatment: Symptomatic treatment of epilepsy, if at all indicated.

Illustrations:
1a and 1b Patient 1, a mentally retarded, microcephalic boy, aged 8½ years. Hypoplasia of the midface, macrostomia, prognathism, dental prosthesis for severely malpositioned teeth.
2a and 2b Patient 2, a girl aged 3 years and 9 months. Microcephaly, hypoplasia of the midface, macrostomia, prognathism, widely spaced teeth. Mental retardation.
3a and 3b Patient 3, a similarly affected girl aged 8 years and 9 months.

J.K.

References:

Kuroki, Y., Matsui, I., Yamamoto, Y. et al. The 'happy puppet' syndrome in two siblings. *Hum. Genet.*, 56, 227–229 (1980).

Hersh, J.H., Bloom, A.S., Zimmerman, A.W. et al. Behavioral correlates in the happy puppet syndrome: a characteristic profile? *Develop. Med. Child. Neurol.*, 23, 792–800 (1981).

Dooley, J.M., Berg, J.M., Pakula, Z. et al. The puppet-like syndrome of Angelman. *Am. J. Dis. Child.*, 135, 621–624 (1981).

Pashayan, H.M., Singer, W., Bove, C. et al. The Angelman syndrome in two brothers. *Am. J. Med. Genet.*, 13, 295–298 (1982).

Williams, C.A. and Frias, J.L. The Angelman ('happy puppet') syndrome. *Am. J. Med. Genet.*, 11, 453–460 (1982).

Bjerre, I., Fagher, B., Ryding, E. et al. The Angelman or 'happy puppet' syndrome. *Acta Pediatr. Scand.*, 73, 398–402 (1984).

Barraitser, M., Patton, M., Lam, S.T.S. et al. The Angelman (happy puppet) syndrome: is it autosomal recessive? *Clin. Genet.*, 31, 323–330 (1987).

Fisher, J.A., Burn, J., Alexander, F.W. et al. Angelman (happy puppet) syndrome in a girl and her brother. *J. Med. Genet.*, 24, 294–298 (1987).

Willems, P.J., Dijkstra, I., Brouwer, O.F. et al. Recurrence risk in the Angelman ('happy puppet') syndrome. *Am. J. Med. Genet.*, 27, 773–780 (1987).

Magenis, R.E., Brown, M.G., Lacy, D.A. et al. Is Angelman syndrome an alternative result of del (15) (q11q13)? *Am. J. Med. Genet.*, 28, 829–838 (1987).

Dörries, A., Spohr, H.-L., Kunze, J. Angelman ('happy puppet') syndrome—8 new cases with documented cerebral computer tomography: review of the literature. *Eur. J. Pediatr.*, 148, 270–273 (1988).

Boyd, S.G., Harden, A. et al. The EEG in early diagnosis of the Angelman . . . syndrome. *Eur. J. Pediatr.*, 147, 508–513 (1988).

Knoll, J.H.M., Nicholls, R.D. et al. Angelman and Prader–Willi syndromes share a common chromosome 15 deletion but differ in parental origin of the deletion. *Am. J. Med. Genet.*, 32, 285–290 (1989).

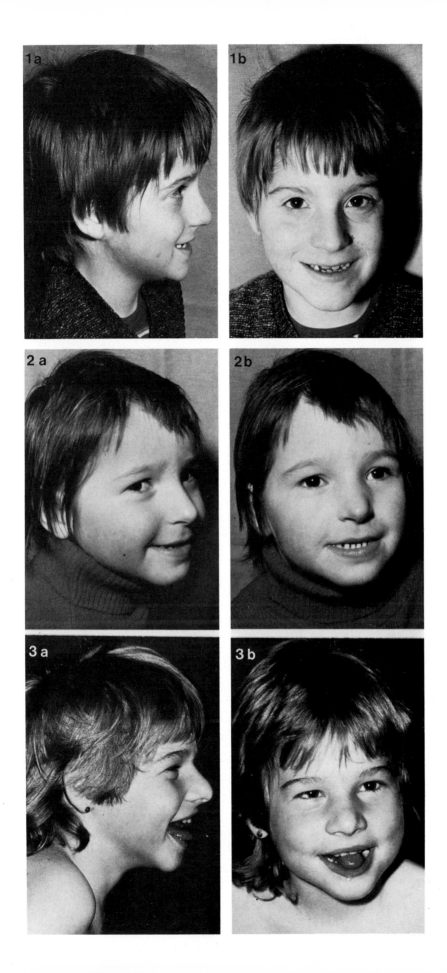

97

48. Rett Syndrome

A progressive syndrome exclusively of females, with cessation of development after the 9th to 18th month of life, rapid mental deterioration with autistic features, stereotype movements of the hands, tremors of the trunk, ataxia, microcephaly, paraspasm, and epilepsy.

Main signs:
1. After normal initial development, rapid onset of developmental retardation beginning between the 7th and 18th month of life. Loss of acquired speech, of target-specific grasping, of purposeful hand movements, of interest in the surroundings. Within a year, transition to moderate or severe mental retardation, autism, and sleep disorders.
2. Cessation of head growth, to microcephaly by the third year of life; ataxia of the trunk and extremities, anxiety, hyperventilation, aerophagia; vasomotor disturbances with sweating, red-blue discoloration of the feet; bizarre patterns of movement ('hand-wringing' in front of the chest or mouth, poor tone, irregular coordination), loss of ability to walk, spastic paraparesis, severe progressive kyphoscoliosis, joint contractures, confinement to a wheelchair, constipation. Epilepsy after the fourth year of life; autistic-ataxic dementia.

Supplementary findings:
1. Unremarkable maternal pregnancy, uncomplicated birth at term, no increased abortions, no stillbirths; length and head circumference of the child normal at birth.
2. No specific laboratory findings: CSF electrophoresis negative as a rule; in some patients decrease or absence of the τ-fraction. Blood ammonia slightly elevated in a few patients. Abnormal EEG after the third year of life. Nerve conduction velocity normal. Electromyography shows mild signs of denervation; computer tomography of the brain shows mild signs of cerebral atrophy; white matter normal. Nonspecific findings on electron microscopy of conjunctival and skin biopsies. Autopsy findings: micrencephaly, atrophy of the brain, decreased pigmentation of the substantia nigra, electron-optical increase of neuronal lipofuscin.

Manifestation: After the 7th–18th month of life. Diagnosis between the third and fifth years of life.

Etiology: Most likely X-linked dominant disorder with lethality in male hemizygote embryos. Always new mutations. Three reports of affected siblings: once in half sisters with the same mother, and in two sets of identical twins. No increase in tendency to abortions in the mothers of daughters affected with Rett syndrome. No patient with Rett syndrome has had children. Isolated 'forme fruste' observations or of atypical forms (Hagberg).

Frequency: Probably diagnosed too infrequently (according to one study about 1 case in 15,000 girls). To date more than 675 patients are known worldwide.

Course, prognosis: Progressive course, as described above, to spastic quadriparesis, dementia, autism, kyphoscoliosis. No exact data about life expectancy is known. The oldest patient to date is 34 years old.

Treatment: No specific therapy known. Symptomatic, anticonvulsive treatment in some cases. Physical therapy. Ketogenic diet?

Illustrations:
1a Female infant at 3 months, normal psychomotor development, neurologically unremarkable.
1b The same girl at age 12 years: autistic, ataxic dementia, microcephaly, characteristic 'hand-wringing' movements.
2a and 2b A 2¾-year-old girl with probable normal development in early infancy followed by decrease in performance, on to severe dementia; small cranium, variable muscle tone, constant stereotyped hand-washing movements, markedly abnormal EEG.

J.K.

References:
Hagberg, B., Aicardi, J., Dias, K. et al. A progressive syndrome of autism, dementia, ataxia, and loss of purposeful hand use in girls: Rett's syndrome. Report of 35 cases. *Ann. Neurol.*, 14, 471–479 (1983).
Hagberg, B., Goutières, F., Hanefeld, F. et al. Rett syndrome: criteria of inclusion and exclusion. *Brain Dev.*, 7, 372–373 (1985).
Hanefeld, F. The clinical pattern of Rett syndrome. *Brain Dev.*, 7, 320–325 (1985).
The Rett Syndrome. *Am. J. Med. Genet. Suppl.*, 1, Alan R. Liss Inc. (1986).
Bachmann, C., Schaub, J., Colombo, J.P. et al. Rett syndrome revisited: a patient with biotin dependency. *Eur. J. Pediatr.*, 144, 563–566 (1986).
Spiess, Y., Boltshauser, F., Hänggeli, Ch.A., et al. Rett-Syndrom: ein progredientes neurologisches Syndrom bei Mädchen. *Schweiz. Med. Wochenschr.*, 116, 458–463 (1986).
Tariverdian, G., Kantner, G., Vogel, F. A monozygotic twin pair with Rett syndrome. *Hum. Genet.*, 75, 88–90 (1987).
Papadimitriou, J.M., Hockey, A., Tan, N. et al. Rett syndrome: abnormal membrane-bound lamellated inclusions in neurons and oligodendroglia. *Am. J. Med. Genet.*, 29, 365–368 (1988).
Partington, M.W. Rett syndrome in monozygotic twins. *Am. J. Med. Genet.*, 29, 633–637 (1988).

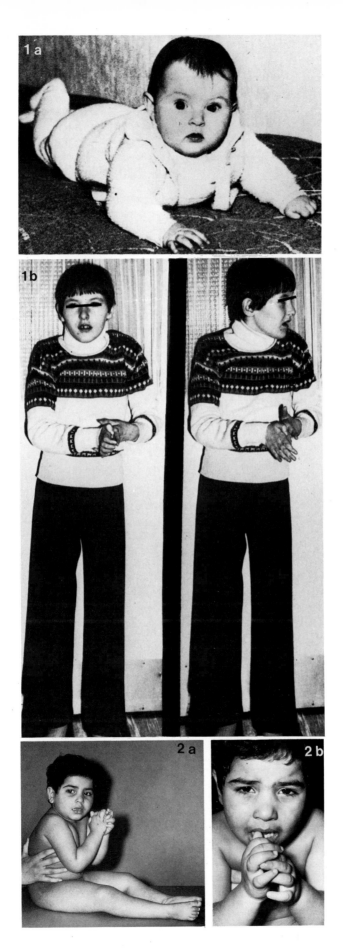

49. Fragile X Syndrome

(Marker X Syndrome; X-Linked Mental Retardation; Martin–Bell Syndrome)

A well-known syndrome (whose basic defect is still not sufficiently clarified) of mental retardation mainly in males, large ears, macroorchidism, and fragile X chromosome.

Main signs:
1. Mental retardation of varied severity (IQ below 50 in 25%).
2. Large ears.
3. Macroorchidism (30–75 ml).
4. Autism, occasionally.
5. Frequency of the fragile X in folic acid-deficient lymphocyte cultures from male probands varies between a few per cent and more than 50%.

Supplementary findings: Increased weight and head circumference above the 97th percentile at birth. Delayed psychomotor development: muscular hypotonia, thin legs, walking after 18 months, delayed speech (development after the third year). Shy as toddlers, with poor social contact. Increasingly hyperactive after age 3–4 years. In adolescence, distinct mental retardation, repetitive speech, echolalia. Occasional seizures. Tall stature, flat feet, hyperextensible joints, prolapse of the aortic and mitral valves, myopia as a result of mesenchymal weakness. The adult male after puberty shows the full clinical picture including typical facial features with long oval face and prognathism. Normal testosterone synthesis, normal testicular histology.

Women and 'Fra X':
1. 60% of heterozygous women are normal, but about 10% of these manifest psychoses.
2. 33% of heterozygous women are mentally retarded; of these, 20% become psychotic.
3. 50% of heterozygous women do not have a fragile X.
4. 20% of heterozygous women show the same characteristic facial features as affected men.
5. Fra X women show increased fertility (fourfold frequency of twin births).

Manifestation: Delayed psychomotor development after the fifth month of life; delayed speech (begins after the third year of life); full clinical picture after puberty.

Etiology: X-linked disorder with unusual segregation, with markedly varied penetrance in males and variable expression in females. Fragile X from folic acid or thymidine deficiency in lymphocyte cultures. Determination of the rate of new mutations is difficult. A preliminary estimate yielded a high rate of new mutations of 7.2×10^{-4} in males.

Frequency: 0.73 Fra X patients : 1,000 school boys (Tessa Webb 1986); 1 Fra X patient : 1,090 men (Opitz 1986); 1 Fra X patient : 1,500 school boys (Gustavson et al. 1986); fragile X in up to 7% of mildly mentally retarded school girls with IQs 55–75 (Turner et al. 1980).

Course, prognosis: At present there are no 'life tables'. The oldest known patient is 55 years old. Decreased life expectancy?

Differential diagnosis: Sotos syndrome.

Treatment: No definite results with folic acid therapy. Genetic counseling: In Fra X families, 20% of healthy brothers of Fra X patients have the affected gene. These brothers transmit the gene to their children with no risk of the disorder. However, their daughters will transmit the risk. If the female transmitter is retarded, 50% of her sons will be affected and 30–40% of her daughters. Prenatal cyto- and especially molecular genetic diagnosis is possible in informative families.

Illustrations:
1a–1c A characteristically affected 5-year-old boy.
2 A correspondingly affected 22-year-old man.

J.K.

References:

Schwinger, E. and Froster-Iskenius, U. *Das Marker-X-Syndrom. Klinik und Genetik*. Ferdinand Enke, Stuttgart, 1984.
International Workshop on the Fragile X and X-linked Mental Retardation. *Am. J. Med. Genet.*, 17, 5–385 (1984).
X-linked mental retardation. 2. *Am. J. Med. Genet.*, 23, 1–737 (1986).
Opitz, J.M., Neri, G. et al. X-linked mental retardation. 3. *Am. J. Med. Genet.*, 30, 1–702 (1988).
Sherman, S.L., Rogatko, A. et al. Recurrence risks for relatives in families with an isolated case of the fragile X syndrome. *Am. J. Med. Genet.*, 31, 735–765 (1988).

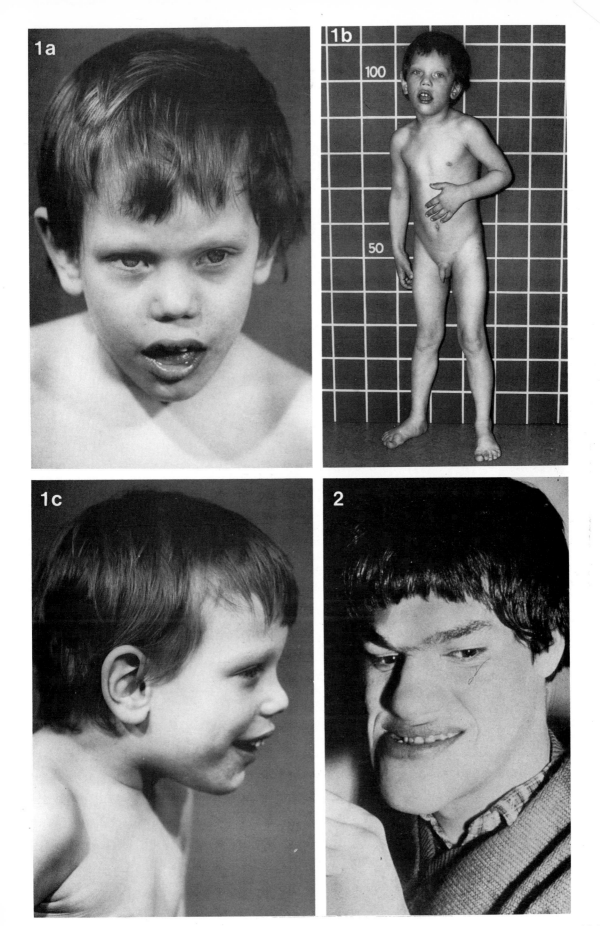

101

50. Infantile Cortical Hyperostosis

(Caffey Syndrome; Caffey–Silverman Syndrome)

A clinical picture occurring chiefly in young infants with firm, frequently asymmetric soft-tissue swellings, generally of the face or jaw and the extremities, with marked osseus swelling on the X-ray and usually eventual complete recovery.

Main signs:
1. Painful, firm often asymmetric soft-tissue swellings located on the face and/or the extremities and accompanied or heralded by fever and general irritability (**1, 3**).
2. X-rays show periosteal hyperostosis, often severe, usually affecting several areas of the skeleton, preferentially the mandible, clavicles, scapulae, ribs, and long bones (**2, 4, 5**).

Supplementary findings:
Occasionally pseudoparesis of part of an extremity during the acute swelling phase. Leukocytosis, elevated ESR, and possible thrombocytosis during the acute phase. Frequently moderately elevated serum alkaline phosphatase.

Manifestation:
Early infancy. (Prenatal onset has also been demonstrated on X-ray.) The hyperostosis is usually detectable within weeks of the onset of external swelling.

Etiology:
Numerous sporadic cases along with increased occurrence in some families, especially in siblings but also in successive generations, for which an autosomal dominant gene with incomplete penetrance and variable expression is thought to be responsible.

Frequency:
Relatively low, although about 500 cases have probably been reported.

Course, prognosis:
Course occasionally intermittent, with several phases or exacerbations. In isolated cases a more chronic course may lead to distinct bowing or to overgrowth of the long bones, and to marked delay of the gross motor development. Prognosis as a rule favorable. Usually complete clinical, followed after several months by radiological, recovery.

Differential diagnosis:
Trauma, accidental or abusive; inflammatory or toxic conditions; and (C-, D-) vitamin deficiency must be ruled out, and perhaps on occasion cherubism (p.106). Prolonged prostaglandin E_1 treatment can produce an identical radiological picture.

Treatment:
Symptomatic. Prevention of contractures. In severe cases, careful administration of corticosteroids may be indicated during the acute phase.

Illustrations:
1 A 9-week-old infant with asymmetric firm soft-tissue swellings on both lower legs and upper extremities.
3 Similarly affected 1-month-old child with anteriorly convex bowing of the tibia.
2 Hyperostosis of the lower edge of the body of the mandible in a 10-month-old infant.
4 and 5 Marked cortical hyperostosis of the tibia and arm bones of the infant in **1**.

H.-R.W.

References:

Spranger, J.W., Langer, L.O., Jr., Wiedemann, H.-R. *Bone Dysplasias. An Atlas of Constitutional Disorders of Skeletal Development.* G. Fischer and W.B. Saunders, Stuttgart and Philadelphia, 1974.

Finsterbusch, A. and Rang, M. Infantile cortical hyperostosis. Follow-up of 29 cases. *Acta Orthop. Scand.,* 46, 727 (1975).

Fried, K., Manor, A., Pajewski, M. et al. Autosomal dominant inheritance with incomplete penetrance of Caffey disease (infantile cortical hyperostosis). *Clin. Genet.,* 19, 271 (1981).

Gentry, R.R., Rust, R.S. et al. Infantile cortical hyperostosis . . . without mandibular involvement. *Pediatr. Radiol.,* 13, 236–238 (1983).

Maclachlan, A.K., Gerrard, J.W. et al. Familial infantile cortical hyperostosis in a large Canadian family. *Canad. Med. Assoc. J.,* 130, 1172–1174 (1984).

Langer, R. and Kaufmann, H.-J. Pränatale Diagnosestellung bei Caffey'scher Erkrankung . . . *Klin. Pädiatr.,* 197, 473–476 (1985).

Tabardel, Y., Seghaye, M.C. et al. Maladie de Caffey–Silverman néonatale avec thrombocytose . . . *Arch. Fr. Pediatr.,* 45, 263–265 (1988).

Töllner, U. and Alzen, G. Das Caffey–Silverman-Syndrom . . . *Pädiatr. Prax.,* 37, 309–314 (1988).

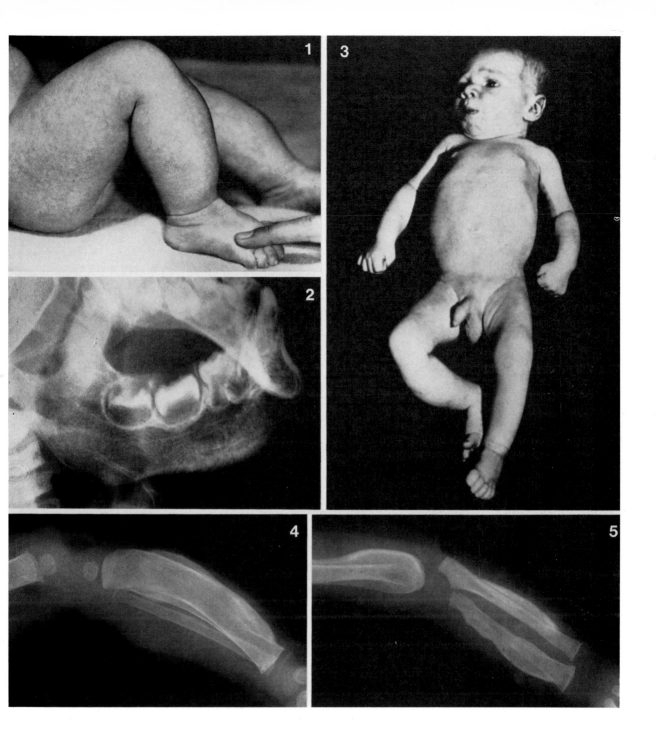

103

51. Craniometaphyseal Dysplasia

A hereditary systemic defect of ossification with widening of the metaphyses, thickening of the skull bones, and often impaired hearing.

Main signs: Hypertelorism (2) with paranasal bony ridges (1, 2) and bulging of the broad nasal root and the glabella (3) which, together with a large, occipito-frontally protruding cranium, produce a characteristic appearance. Narrowing of the nostrils with mouth breathing.

Supplementary findings: Compression of the auditory, optic, and facial nerves not unusual. Involvement of dentition possible.

On X-ray, frontal and occipital hyperostosis or sclerosis of the cranium (4); abnormally shaped long bones with club-shaped flaring of the metaphyses (5).

Increased alkaline phosphatase and other biochemical findings possible.

Manifestation: Variable. Possibly as early as the first year of life; more frequently, later in childhood.

Etiology: Monogenic hereditary disorder with variable expression. Heterogeneity. Autosomal dominant form more frequent than a perhaps more severe autosomal recessive type.

Frequency: Low.

Course, prognosis, treatment: Life expectancy normal as a rule. Good development of height. Symptomatic treatment of neural, dental, and other complications. Administration of human calcitonin or calcitriol (1,25 $(OH)_2-$ vitamin D_3) may have a favorable effect in isolated cases, as shown by recent reports.

Illustrations:

1–3 A 6-year-old boy, normally developed for his age but with defective hearing.

4–6 His X-rays, 6 shows typical mild changes.

H.-R.W.

References:

Spranger, J.W., Langer, L.O., Jr., Wiedemann, H.-R. *Bone Dysplasias. An Atlas of Constitutional Disorders of Skeletal Development.* G. Fischer and W.B. Saunders, Stuttgart and Philadelphia, 1974.

Beighton, P., Hamersma, H., Horan, F. Craniometaphyseal dysplasia—variability of expression within a large family. *Clin. Genet.*, 15, 252 (1979).

Penchaszadeh, V.B., Gutierrez, E.R., Figueroa, P. Autosomal recessive craniometaphyseal dysplasia. *Am. J. Med. Genet.*, 5, 43 (1980).

Carnevale, A., Grether, P. et al. Autosomal dominant craniometaphyseal dysplasia . . . *Clin. Genet.*, 23, 17–22 (1983).

Cole, D.E. and Cohen, M.M. A new look at craniometaphyseal dysplasia. *J. Pediatr.*, 112, 577–579 (1988).

Key, L.L., Volberg, F. et al. Treatment of craniometaphyseal dysplasia with calcitriol. *J. Pediatr.*, 112, 583–587 (1988).

Fanconi, S., Fischer, J.A. et al. Craniometaphyseal dysplasia . . . Therapeutic effect of calcitonin. *J. Pediatr.*, 112, 587–591 (1988).

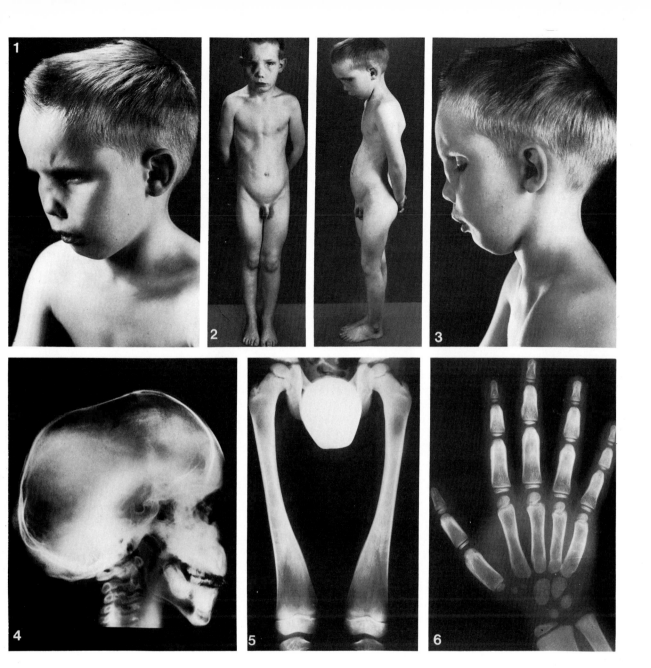

52. Cherubism

A condition almost exclusively involving the jaw bones, with typical facial dysmorphism.

Main signs:
1. Usually bilateral, symmetrical, indolent swelling of the submandibular or malar regions (1–4) due to fibrous replacement of the greater part of the jaw bones (upper and/or lower jaws; lower jaw especially). When the floor of the orbit is involved, the eye is cranially displaced and the sclera is visible below the rim of the iris (1, 3), the 'heavenward' glance and the 'cherubic' cheeks giving the syndrome its name.
2. Hypertelorism almost always present.
3. Severely affected primary dentition with many malpositioned or exfoliated teeth (2, 5); hypodontia of the secondary dentition.

Supplementary findings: During the stage of increasing swelling, possible enlargement of the regional lymph nodes and elevation of serum alkaline phosphatase.

X-ray examination of the rest of the skeleton may demonstrate mild cystic translucencies in other areas (e.g., bones of the hands).

Manifestation: The first years of life.

Etiology: Hereditary disorder with autosomal dominant transmission, variable expression, and incomplete penetrance in females.

Frequency: Low; apparently, up to 1980, more than 100 cases reported.

Course, prognosis: The tumorlike dysplasia affects tooth development, with corresponding results; it may impair nasal breathing and tongue function. After years of progression, the swelling ceases before, during, or soon after puberty, then gradually regresses. Thus, it is self-limited and benign. Complete healing, but with atrophy of the alveolar processes and reossification of the basal areas of the jaw.

Diagnosis: From appearance, X-rays (5), and in some cases histological findings on biopsy (proliferating loose fibrous tissue with spindle cells and multinucleated giant cells; little membranous bone formation).

Treatment: Curettage of tissue hindering nasal breathing or function of the tongue, may be indicated. X-ray therapy contraindicated. Timely application of prostheses. A modelling osteotomy may be indicated after adolescence.

Comment: An autosomal recessive hereditary syndrome comprising cherubism, gingival fibromatosis, hypertrichosis, small stature, mental retardation, and epilepsy is called Ramon syndrome.

Illustrations:
1–4 Physically and mentally normal 4-year-old boy with cherubism (mother and sister of the boy similarly affected—the former now in the healing stage). Broad, flat midface with very wide nasal root, slight hypertelorism, prominent zygomatic arches, small and flat nose with anteverted nares; eyeball rotated slightly 'heavenwards'. Distension of the lower half of the face. Marked protrusion of the upper dental plates; child unable to close his mouth because of distension of the alveolar processes; severe deficiency of teeth.
5 Vast multicystic distension of the upper and lower jaws with marked thinning of the cortex. Maxillary sinuses cannot be delineated with certainty; zygomatic arches displaced cranially; orbits narrowed; nasal bone almost horizontal; positional anomalies of the tooth buds.

H.-R.W.

References:
Hoppe, W., Spranger, J., Hansen, H.G. Cherubismus. *Arch. Kinderheilkd.*, 174, 310 (1966).
Khosla, V.M. and Korobkin, M. Cherubism. *Am. J. Dis. Child.*, 120, 458 (1970).
Peters, W.J.N. Cherubism: a study of twenty cases from one family. *Oral Surg., Oral Med., Oral Path.*, 47, 307 (1979).
Hoyer, P.F. and Neukam, F.-W. Cherubismus . . . *Klin. Pädiatr.*, 194, 128 (1982).
[Pina-Neto, J.M., Moreno, A.F.C. et al. Cherubism,, gingival fibromatosis, epilepsy, and mental deficiency . . . *Am. J. Med. Genet.*, 25, 433–441 (1986).]

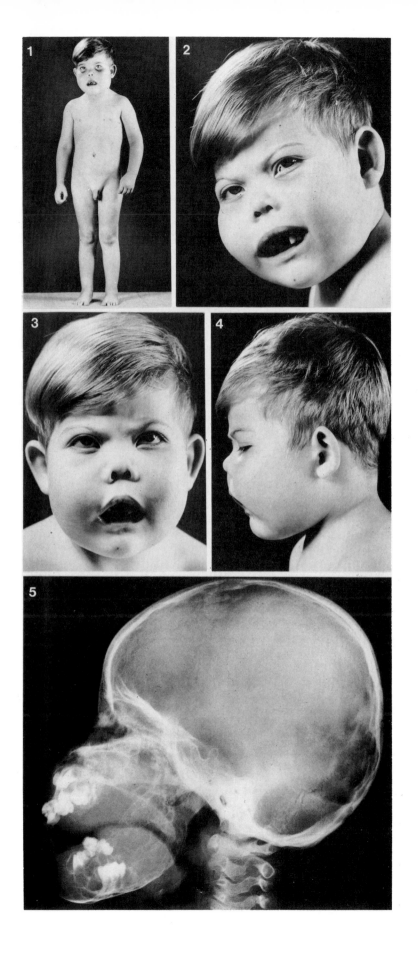

53. Menkes Syndrome

(Kinky Hair Syndrome, Menkes Disease, Steely Hair Syndrome, Trichopoliodystrophy)

A disease of copper metabolism in boys, with depigmented monilethrix, relatively typical facies, growth retardation, psychomotor retardation, seizures, and a poor prognosis.

Main signs:

1. Sparse, kinky, short, brittle hair, still pigmented during the first weeks of life, thereafter depigmented. Microscopically, twisting in the long axis, varying thickness of the shaft. Sparse eyebrows (**2, 3**).
2. Face puffy; characterized by full cheeks, 'carp mouth', micrognathia, low nasal root, and short philtrum (**1, 2**). High palate, broad alveolar ridges. Posteriorly rotated, poorly modeled ears.
3. Pale, doughy skin with seborrheic changes (**3**).
4. Psychomotor retardation; microcephaly. Seizures. Spasticity alternating with hypotonia.
5. Growth deficiency. Metaphyseal flaring, spurs, and increased density of the long bones, rosary. Pectus excavatum (**1**), possible club feet.

Supplementary findings: Not infrequently small size at birth; early failure to thrive, wasting.

Tendency to hypo-, less frequently hyperthermia. Increased infections.

Skeleton: wormian bones along the sagittal suture. After the second month of life, flaring of the metaphyses, which gradually regresses during the latter half of infancy (**4, 5**). Osteoporosis, periosteal bone formation. Vacuolated promyelocytes in the bone marrow.

On angiography, characteristic corkscrew twisting, elongation, and varying caliber of the cerebral, visceral, and soft tissue vessels. Subdural hemorrhages. Low levels of copper in serum and some tissues, but elevated levels in the mucosa of the small intestine and elsewhere (defect of copper distribution).

Manifestation: In the first months of life.

Etiology: X-linked recessive disorder, thus males affected. The exact pathogenesis is not clear.

Frequency: About 2 cases in 100,000 live-born males (between the first description, in 1962, and 1985 about 90 cases were recognized).

Course, prognosis: With the onset of seizures in the second to third month of life, arrest of psychomotor development and shortly thereafter loss of acquired abilities, on to coma. Death usually in the second year of life. However, deviations of the clinical course with different variants of the disease occur, including a less severe form with later manifestation and longer survival—into the second decade.

Treatment: Symptomatic. Neither oral nor parenteral copper administration has been shown to alter the course of disease with certainty; however, substitution therapy should always be tried initially. Genetic counseling. Prenatal diagnosis.

Illustrations:

1–5 Photographs and X-rays of an 8-month-old patient. Normal development up to the first seizure at age 2½ months, then arrest of development and shortly thereafter regression. Frequent infections, frequent hypothermia. Death at 12 months from meningitis.

H.-R.W.

References:

Heyne, K., Dörner, K., Graucob, E., Wiedemann, H.-R. Monophyle Vakuolisierung von Promyelozyten bei Menkes-Syndrom . . . *Klin. Pädiatr.*, 190, 576 (1978).

Grover, W.D., Johnson, W.C., Henkin, R.I. Clinical and biochemical aspects of trichopoliodystrophy. *Ann. Neurol.*, 5, 65 (1979).

Dobrescu, O., Larbrisseau, A., Dubé, L.-J. et al. Trichopoliodystrophie . . . *Can. Med. Assoc. J.*, 123, 490 (1980).

Taylor, C.J. and Green, S.H. Menkes' syndrome (trichopoliodystrophy): use of scanning electron microscope in diagnosis and carrier identification. *Develop. Med. Child. Neurol.*, 23, 361 (1981).

Moore, C.M. and Howell, R.R. Ectodermal manifestations in Menkes disease. *Clin. Genet.*, 28, 532–540 (1985).

Tønnesen, T., Horn, N. et al. Measurement of copper on chorionic villi for first-trimester diagnosis of Menkes' disease. *Lancet*, I, 1038–1039 (1985).

Wendler, H. and Mutz, I. Menkes-Syndrom mit exzessiven Skelettveränderungen. *Fortschr. Röntgenstr.*, 143, 351–355 (1985).

Kolb, H.-J. and Guthoff, T. Klinische Aspekte des Menkes-Syndroms. *Monatschr. Kinderheilkd.*, 135, 827–831 (1987).

Menkes, J.H. Kinky hair disease. In: *Neurocutaneous Diseases.* Gomez, M.R. (ed.) Butterworths, Boston, 1987, pp.284–292.

Baerlocher, K. and Nadal, D. Das Menkes-Syndrom. *Ergeb. Inn. Med. Kinderheilkd.*, 57, 77–144 (1988).

Gerdes, A.-M., Tønnesen, T. et al. Variability in clinical expression of Menkes syndrome. *Eur. J. Pediatr.*, 148, 132–135 (1988).

Nadal, D. and Baerlocher, K. Menkes' disease . . . *Eur. J. Pediatr.*, 147, 621–625 (1988).

Sander, C., Niederhoff, H. et al. Life span and Menkes kinky hair syndrome . . . *Clin. Genet.*, 33, 228–233 (1988).

Westman, J.A., Richardson, D.C. et al. Atypical Menkes steely hair disease. *Am. J. Med. Genet.*, 30, 853–858 (1988).

Tønnesen, T., Gerdes, A.-M., Damsgaard, E. et al. First trimester diagnosis of Menkes disease . . . *Prenatal Diagnosis*, 9, 159 (1989).

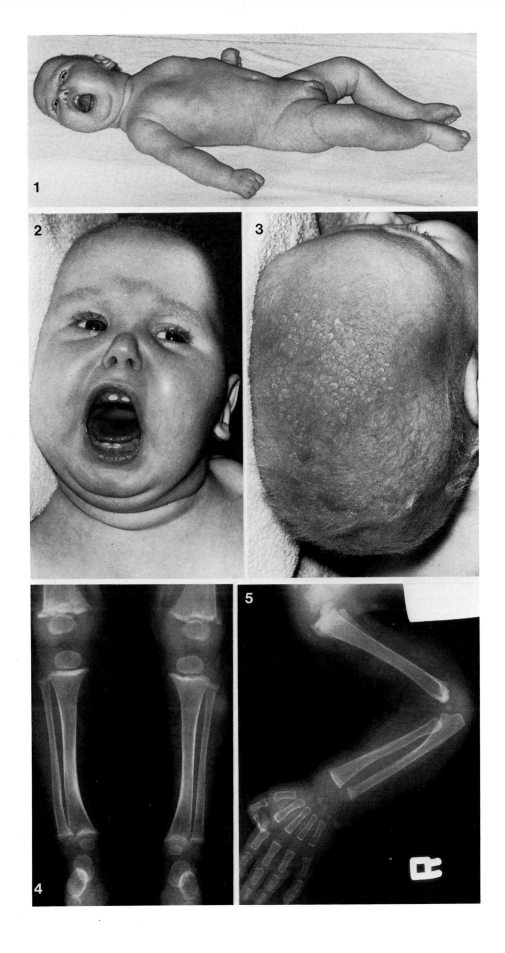

109

54. Glycogen Storage Disease Type I

(Formerly also referred to, erroneously, as von Gierke Syndrome)

A hereditary metabolic disease with—when treatment is inadequate or delayed—possible unusual facies, considerable growth deficiency, and markedly protuberant abdomen.

Main signs:
1. Unusual facies, best defined as a Rubens or doll face, in some cases (**1, 2, 4, 5**).
2. Small stature.
3. Protuberant abdomen as a result of liver enlargement (**3**). Hyperlordosis when standing.
4. Mental retardation as a result of hypoglycemia and hypoglycemic seizures.
5. Poorly developed hypotonic musculature (**3**).

Supplementary findings: Acidotic respiration.
Bleeding tendency.
Enlarged kidneys; hepatoma.
Osteoporosis.
Kidney stones, xanthomas, gouty tophi and arthritis.
Fasting hypoglycemia unresponsive to glucagon or adrenalin; elevated lactate, pyruvate, triglycerides, phospholipids, cholesterol and uric acid.

Manifestation: At birth. Growth retardation apparent in late infancy. Xanthomas, gouty tophi and arthritis usually not until adulthood.

Etiology: Autosomal recessive disease; glucose-6-phosphatase deficiency in the liver, kidneys, and mucosa of the small intestines.

Frequency: Low (about 1:400,000).

Course, prognosis: Average life expectancy somewhat reduced due to the metabolic state with lactic acidosis, later by gouty nephritis. Progression of liver enlargement probably limited to childhood.

Treatment: Frequent carbohydrate-rich meals; at night, constant gastric-tube feedings. Alkalization in stress situations during the first years of life; timely antibiotic treatment of bacterial infections; allopurinol to reduce uric acid levels. Liver transplantation?

Illustrations:
1–3 Patient 1 at age 18 months. Delayed development; height deficit 11 cm.
4 and 5 Patient 2 at age 18 months. Height deficit 9 cm. Hypoglycemic seizures up to the sixth year of life. Liver at the level of the umbilicus. Follow-up at age 10 years: no further relative liver enlargement. Height deficit now 13 cm.

H.-R.W.

References:
Stanbury, J.B., Wyngaarden, J.B., Fredrickson, D.S. *The Metabolic Basis of Inherited Disease.* McGraw-Hill Book Company, 5th edn. 1983, 141–167.
Malatack, J.J., Finegold, D.N. et al. Liver transplantation for type I glycogen storage disease. *Lancet,* I, 1073–1075 (1983).

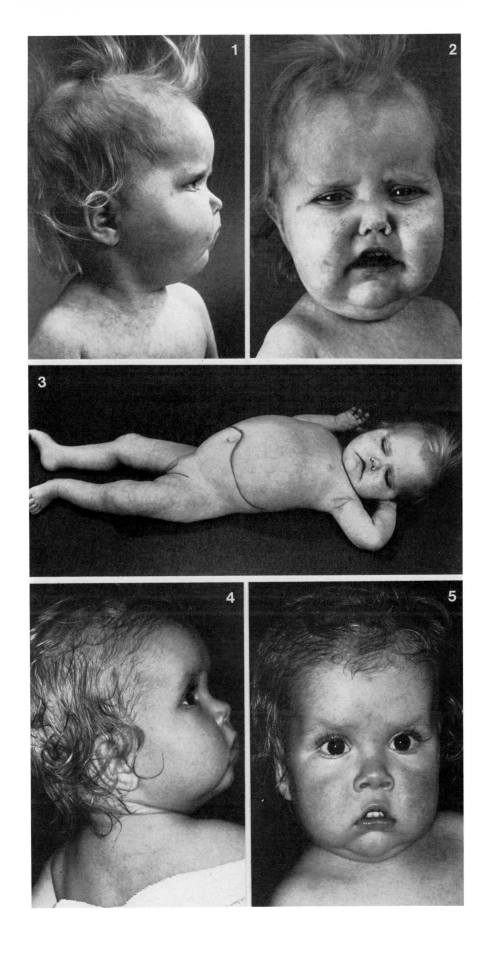

111

55. Niemann–Pick Disease

An autosomal recessive sphingolipidosis with different clinical forms, with protruding abdomen due to hepatosplenomegaly, neurological complications of variable severity, cherry-red spot of the retina, thin extremities, and growth deficiency characterizing the clinical picture.

Main signs:
Type A (acute form with neurological complications): large abdomen as a result of hepatosplenomegaly, feeding difficulties, progressive psychomotor decline within the first to second year of life, thin extremities, yellow-brown discoloration of the skin, cherry-red spot in the macula (50%), corneal clouding, muscular hypotonia. Storage cells in the bone marrow, spleen, adrenals, and lungs. *Type B* (chronic form without neurological complications): enlargement first of the spleen, then of the liver; normal intellect; growth deficiency; dyspnea; recurrent lung infections. *Type C* (chronic form with neurological complications): manifestation after the third year of life; then, regression of speech and intellect, ataxia, grand mal seizures, muscular hypotonia, hyperreflexia, cholestasis. *Type D* (Nova Scotia variant): similar to type C, progressive psychomotor deterioration between the second and fifth years, hepatosplenomegaly, impaired coordination, seizures. *Type E* (adult form without neurological complications): moderate hepatosplenomegaly (late-onset type C?). *Type F* ('sea-blue histiocytosis' = ophthalmoplegic neurolipidosis): hepatosplenomegaly, dementia, ataxia, supranuclear vertical ophthalmoplegia: partial to complete loss of voluntary vertical eye movement, especially downward, as well as vertical optokinetic nystagmus. Analogous limitation horizontally and of convergence. Intact: vestibular reflexes, fundus, and electroretinogram.

Supplementary findings: Spleen: mild hematological sequelae with microcytic anemia, thrombocytopenia. Liver: slight elevation of SGOT, SGPT, and alkaline phosphatase, especially in type B. Lymph nodes: enlarged in the mesentery, in the hilum of the spleen, liver, and lungs. Thymus and tonsils are infiltrated with storage cells. Bones: osteoporosis, coxa valga, dilated medullary spaces in the long bones and metacarpals. Heart: endocardial fibroelastosis. Lungs: diffuse reticular and finely nodular infiltrations. CNS: atrophy (types A and C up to 50–90% of the normal weight), disorganization of cortical structures, of the basal ganglia, of the brain stem, of the spinal cord, and of the spinal ganglia. Further organs: special storage cells in the bone marrow: with May–Grünwald–Giemsa stain numerous large, partly binucleated cells with light, vacuolated cytoplasm and frequently with one or more dark-colored dense inclusion bodies barely the size of erythrocytes. Less numerous, somewhat smaller storage cells with blue-green cytoplasmic granules ('sea-blue' cytoplasm), which although not specific, suggest type F disease.

Manifestation: Biochemically diagnosable in part prenatally, otherwise from birth on or after manifestation. Type A: organomegaly after the sixth month of life, retardation after 1 year. Type B: organomegaly somewhat later than in Type A. Type C: hepatomegaly and mental deterioration after the second year. Type D: organ and CNS involvement between the second and fourth years. Type E: adult form. Type F: in the first decade.

Etiology: Autosomal recessive inheritance. Intra- and intergenetic heterogeneity? Impaired sphingomyelinase activity in type A (10% of normal activity), activity in type B slightly higher than in type A; activity in type C 38–63%, in types D and E normal to elevated.

Frequency: Over 100 patients known; of these, 85% type A, in Ashkenazi Jews. Type D endemic in Nova Scotia. The ophthalmological neurolipidosis has been documented in 39 cases to date.

Course, prognosis: Type A: death before the fourth year from pneumonia. Type B: endangered by pneumonias. Type C and D: death between the 5th and 15th years. Type E: Unknown. Type F: death from pneumonia in 12 patients between the 5th and 29th years.

Treatment: No specific therapy. Splenectomy for cosmetic or mechanical indications or in case of hypersplenism. Genetic counseling. Prenatal diagnosis for types A and B only.

Illustrations:
1 A 3½-year-old patient with marked hepatosplenomegaly (fundi: 'red spot'). Mild expression of type A?
2 A younger sibling; **2a** caput medusae, lipid storage in the skin.
3 A mentally retarded patient, aged 6, with type F; **3a** paralysis of vertical eye movement.

J.K.

References:
Boltshauser, E., Hanefeld, F. et al. Ophthalmoplegische Neurolipidose. In: *Aktuelle Neuropädiatrie*, 2, 258–270 (1981).
Brady, R.O. Sphingomyelin lipidoses: Niemann–Pick disease. In: Stanbury, J.B., Wyngaarden, J.B., Fredrickson, D.S. *The Metabolic Basis of Inherited Disease.* McGraw-Hill Book Co., 5th edn., 831–841 (1983).
Pentchev, P.G. et al. A defect of cholesterol esterification in Niemann–Pick disease (type C) patients. *Proc. Natl. Acad. Sci.*, 82, 8247–8251 (1985).

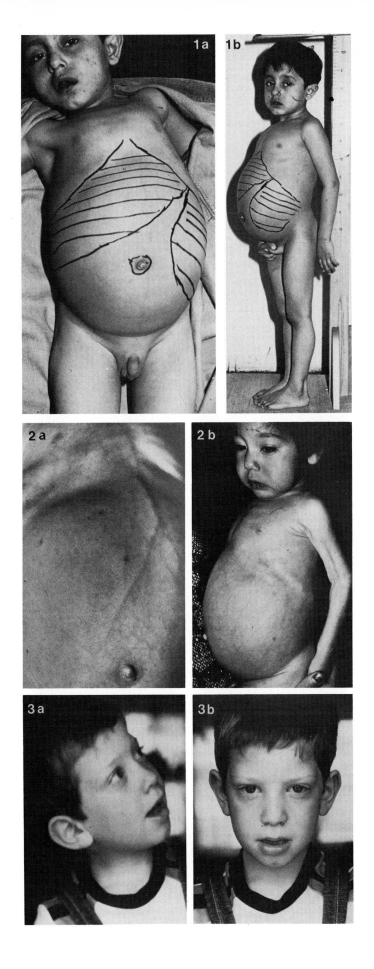

56. Gaucher's Disease, Types II, III, and Norrbottnian Type

Autosomal recessive glucosylceramide lipidoses of the infantile, juvenile, and Norrbottnian types.

Main signs:
Type II, Acute Neuropathic Form = Infantile Type: hepatosplenomegaly, about 6 months later neurological complications: cranial nerve and extrapyramidal signs. Trismus, strabismus, and retroflexion of the head form the typical triad. Feeding difficulties and problems with secretions due to uncoordinated movements of the oropharynx. Progressive spasticity, hyperreflexia, pathological reflexes. Rarely seizures. Eventual generalized muscular hypotonia and apathy. Recurrent pneumonias. *Type III, Subacute Neuropathic Form = Juvenile Type:* Hepatosplenomegaly, then spasticity, ophthalmoplegia, ataxia, retardation, seizures. *Type Norrbottnian:* Clinical course in five stages. Growth retardation after the first year of life (-1 to -5 SD), thoracic kyphosis, hip pain, fractures of the neck of the femur, other fractures of the bones, moderate to excessive splenomegaly, abdominal pain with episodes of unexplained fever, hepatomegaly, hyperplasia of the lymph nodes, dyspnea (due to enlarged spleen), irregular pigmentation of the areas of skin exposed to sun, intellectual retardation after the first year of life, disorder of fine and coarse movements, spastic paraparesis, seizures, oculomotor apraxia, mild hearing defect.

Supplementary findings: Foam cells with cytoplasm of 'wrinkled paper' appearance and eccentric nuclei of varied size, demonstrable in all organs: in the reticuloendothelial system, in the red splenic pulp, in the sinusoids of the liver and lymph nodes, in alveolar capillaries, in bone marrow, in the adventitia of arterioles, in veins and lymph vessels and capillaries; also in the pancreas, the thyroid, and the adrenals.

Type Norrbottnian: radiologically, decrease of the cortex of the Erlenmeyer-flask deformity distal femur, vertebral compression, acute cystic necrosis of the head of the femur, also of the trochanter. Shortly before death, fine granular pulmonary markings. Microcytic normochromic anemia, leukopenia, thrombocytopenia, epistaxis, petechiae, decreased factors V, VII–XII. Gaucher cells in bone marrow. Abnormal EEG.

Manifestation: Type II: 3rd–18th month; Type III: late infancy to adulthood; Norrbottnian Type: birth to 14th year of life.

Etiology: Autosomal recessive storage disease of glycolipid metabolism due to subnormal activities of glucocerebrosidase. Intragenetic heterogeneity. Interestingly, the Norrbottnian Type may run different courses within the same family.

Frequency: Type I (see p.304): 1:2,500 births among the Ashkenazis; Type II: less frequent than Type I, worldwide; Type III: less frequent than Type I, worldwide; Norrbottnian Type: North Sweden, 22 cases to date.

Course, prognosis: Type II: death during the first 3 years of life. Type III: death between the 6th and 12th years of life. Cause of death: recurrent infections, pneumonias.

Treatment: See Type I; but no splenectomy—unless prior to bone marrow transplantation.

Illustrations:
1 and 2 Barely 1-year-old child with hepatomegaly and Type II. Oculomotor apraxia, amimia.

J.K.

References:

Brady, R.O. and Barranger, J.A. Glucosylceramide lipidosis: Gaucher's disease. In: Stanbury, J.B., Wyngaarden, J.B., Fredrickson et al (eds.) *The Metabolic Basis of Inherited Disease*, 5th edn. McGraw-Hill Book Co., pp.842–856 (1983).

Dreborg, S., Erikson, A., Hagberg, B. Gaucher disease—Norrbottnian type. I. General clinical description. *Eur. J. Pediatr.*, 133, 107–118 (1980).

Blom, S. and Erikson, A. Gaucher disease—Norrbottnian type. Neurodevelopmental, neurological and neurophysiological aspects. *Eur. J. Pediatr.*, 140, 316–322 (1983).

Rappaport, J.M. and Ginns, E.I. Bone-marrow transplantation in severe Gaucher disease. *New Engl. J. Med.*, 311, 84–88 (1985).

Zlotogora, J. et al. Genetic heterogeneity in Gaucher disease. *J. Med. Genet.*, 23, 319–322 (1986).

Erikson, E. Gaucher disease—Norrbottnian type (III). *Acta Pediatr. Scand.* (suppl.), 326, 1–42 (1986).

Beaudet, A.L. Gaucher's disease. *N. Engl. J. Med.*, 316, 619–621 (1987).

Hobbs, J.R., Hugh Jones, K., Shaw, P.J. et al. Beneficial effects of pre-transplant splenectomy on displacement bone marrow transplantation for Gaucher's disease. *Lancet*, I, 1111–1115 (1987).

Tsuji, S., Choudary, P.V., Martin, B.M. et al. A mutation in the human glucocerebrosidase gene in neuronopathic Gaucher's disease. *N. Engl. J. Med.*, 316, 570–575 (1987).

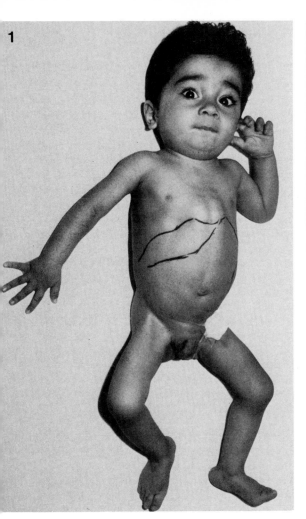

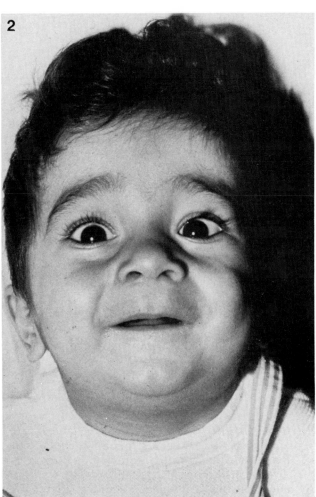

57. GM$_2$ Gangliosidoses: Tay–Sachs Disease and Sandhoff's Disease

Tay–Sachs disease and Sandhoff's disease are autosomal recessive GM$_2$ gangliosidoses with hexosaminidase defects, rapid psychomotor deterioration, hypotonia to generalized paralysis, and eventual spasticity, blindness, seizures, and cherry-red spot of the macula.

Main signs:
1. Increasing muscular weakness after the third month of life, startle reflex in response to noise, progressive psychomotor decline, loss of sitting and standing reflexes.
2. After 18 months of age in Tay–Sachs patients —or earlier in Sandhoff's patients—progressive deafness, blindness, seizures, pareses, spasticity.
3. Doll-like face with pale translucent skin, long eyelashes, fine hair, and unusual pink facial coloring.
4. Cherry-red spot in the macular region in over 95% of patients.
5. Mild hepatosplenomegaly in Sandhoff's disease patients.

Supplementary findings: Vomiting, starting in early infancy and increasing; recurrent pneumonias; progressive macrocephaly after the 16th month of life, as a result of cerebral gliosis (probably less as a result of ventricular enlargement). Lipidosis of the cortical, autonomic, and rectal mucosa neurons with ballooning of the cytoplasm and peripherally displaced nucleus. Central demyelinization, cortical gliosis. No pathological changes of the visceral organs in Tay–Sachs disease, slight hepatosplenomegaly in Sandhoff's disease.

Manifestation: Biomechanically, after birth. Clinically: earliest signs between the 3rd and 6th months of life.

Etiology: Tay–Sachs disease is an autosomal recessive disorder due to hexosaminidase A deficiency. Hexosaminidase A consists of two non-identical subunits, the alpha chain, coded by a locus on chromosome 15, and the beta chain, coded by a locus on chromosome 5. Mutations of the alpha locus on chromosome 15 lead to Tay–Sachs disease, or the juvenile or adult form of GM$_2$ gangliosidosis. Mutations of the beta locus on chromosome 5 lead to Sandhoff's disease. At present we are aware of 11 forms of GM$_2$ gangliosidosis (6 hexosaminidase A mutants, 3 hexosaminidase B mutants, and 2 activator mutants). The gene for Sandhoff's disease is located on the long arm of chromosome 5; for Tay–Sachs disease, on the long arm of chromosome 15.

Frequency: Tay–Sachs disease: thousands of patients known, especially among the Ashkenazi Jews, with a heterozygote frequency of 1:25. About 100 patients with Sandhoff's disease known.

Diagnosis: Demonstration of decreased activity of hexosaminidase A and/or B in serum, leukocytes, or fibroblast cultures. Demonstration of heterozygosity possible. Prenatal diagnosis.

Course, prognosis: As a rule, patients die by about the third year of life of pneumonia.

Treatment: Symptomatic. Genetic counseling, contraception, prenatal diagnosis. Screening programs to identify heterozygotes especially important for the Ashkenazi Jews.

Illustrations:
1 A 16-month-old child with Sandhoff's disease. Exaggerated startle response, especially for acoustic stimuli. Increasing spasticity of the flexors of the upper extremities and extensors of the lower extremities.
2a–2c A 1-year-old markedly retarded and hypotonic girl with Tay–Sachs disease. 'Doll' face; long eyelashes. Hyperacusis. Red spot.

J.K.

References:

O'Brien, J.S. The gangliosidoses. In: Stanbury, J.B., Wyngaarden, J.B., Fredrickson et al (eds.). *The Metabolic Basis of Inherited Disease*, 5th edn. McGraw-Hill Book Co., pp. 945–969 (1983).

Schulte, F.J. Clinical course of GM$_2$ gangliosidoses. A correlative attempt. *Neuropediatrics*, 15 (suppl.) 66–70 (1984).

Pampiglione, G. and Harden, A. Neurophysiological investigations in GM$_1$ and GM$_2$ gangliosidoses. *Neuropediatrics*, 15 (suppl.) 74–84 (1984).

Sandhoff, K. and Conzelmann, E. The biochemical basis of gangliosidoses. *Neuropediatrics*, 15 (suppl.) 85–92 (1984).

Grebner, E.E. and Jackson, L.G. Prenatal diagnosis for Tay–Sachs disease using chorionic villus sampling. *Prenatal Diagnosis*, 5, 305–321 (1985).

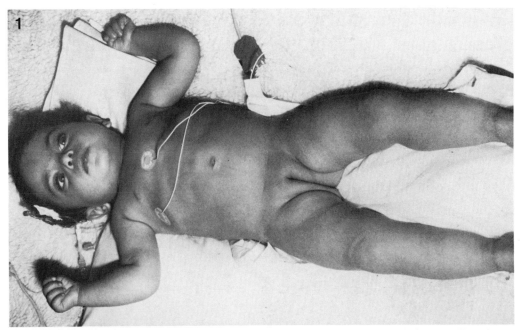

1

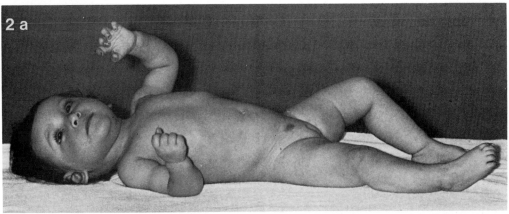

2 a

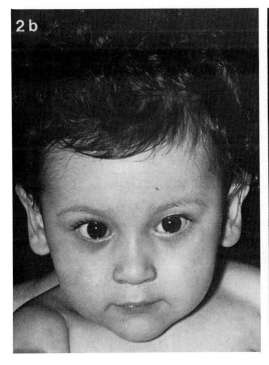

2 b

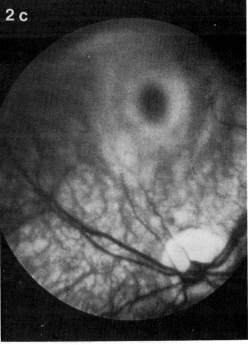

2 c

58. Mucopolysaccharidosis Type I-H

(Hurler's Syndrome, Pfaundler–Hurler Disease)

An autosomal recessive mucopolysaccharide storage disease, which leads to the development of typical facial dysmorphism, stunted growth, dementia, corneal clouding, and hepatosplenomegaly.

Main signs:
1. Characteristic facies with low, flat nasal root; broad tip of the nose; large nares; hypertelorism; exophthalmos; corneal clouding; thick, pouting lips (1–4); large tongue; widely spaced teeth; hypertrophy of the alveolar processes and gums (8). Macrocephaly (6). Abundant, thick scalp hair (1, 2). Increasing dementia.
2. Growth deficiency after initial normal growth in early infancy; short neck; gibbus (4, 6).
3. Joint contractures (3), claw hands (7), broad stubby feet. Indurations of the skin and cartilage.
4. Protruding abdomen, diastasis recti, hernias.

Supplementary findings: Chronic purulent rhinitis. Abundant lanugo-like body hair.

Heart: Valvular defects, enlargement, failure.

Progressive changes of bony structure and form as in a dysostosis multiplex: osteoporosis with coarse trabeculations, thickened skull, broad ribs and clavicles, crudely formed scapulae, oval and partly hook-shaped vertebral bodies; broadening and shortening of the long bones (5). Dysplasia of the pelvis.

Intracranial pressure frequently increased due to interference with circulation of the cerebrospinal fluid as a result of mucopolysaccharide deposits in the meninges. Increased levels of chondroitin sulfate B and heparan sulfate in the urine; alpha-L-iduronidase in the tissues decreased or not demonstrable.

Manifestation: Biochemically, from birth on; radiologically, the first months of life; clinically, from six months onwards.

Etiology: Autosomal recessive disease. The above-mentioned mucopolysaccharides are not degraded due to absence of alpha-iduronidase, but are stored in various organs, which leads to functional and morphological anomalies of these organs.

Frequency: About 1:100,000.

Course, prognosis: Progression until death in the second decade of life. (Infection, heart failure or aspiration.)

Differential diagnosis: The Hunter's syndrome (mucopolysaccharidosis type II) affects only males. It is clinically similar, but more slowly manifest and milder (however with relatively early hearing impairment), usually runs a more prolonged course, and as a rule, shows no corneal clouding.

Treatment: Symptomatic. Prevention by means of prenatal diagnosis.

Comment: Alpha-L-iduronidase deficiency can, in addition to the above-described classic Hurler phenotype (mucopolysaccharisosis I-H), also lead to Scheie disease (MPS I-S), to Hurler/Scheie variant (MPS I-H/S), and to further phenotypes, which are—all?—presumably due to allelic mutations of the same gene. Patients with Scheie disease are of normal height and mental development; they first come to attention in the second decade of life due to joint contractures, impaired vision, and corneal clouding. The Hurler/Scheie variant shows an intermediate phenotype.

Illustrations:
1–5 Patient 1 at age 5 years. Height 93 cm (50th percentile for a 2½-year-old girl), marked dementia, pronounced hepatomegaly.
6 Patient 2 at age 1¼ years. Height 85 cm (97th percentile), head circumference 52.5 cm (50th percentile for a 10-year-old boy). Hepatomegaly. Bilateral inguinal hernia.
7 and 8 Patient 3. Hand and oral cavity at age 2½ years.

H.-R.W./J.K.

References:
Spranger, J. Mucopolysaccharidosen. *Hdb. Inn. Med.*, bd. VII/1, 209. Springer, Berlin Heidelberg New York, 1974.
Spranger, J.W., Langer, L.O., Jr., Wiedemann, H.-R. *Bone Dysplasias. An Atlas of Constitutional Disorders of Skeletal Development.* G. Fischer and W.B. Saunders, Stuttgart and Philadelphia, 1974.
McKusick, V.A. *Heritable Disorders of Connective Tissue.* Mosby, Saint Louis, 1979.
Mueller, O.T., Shows, T.B. et al. Apparent allelism of the Hurler, Scheie, and Hurler/Scheie syndromes. *Am. J. Med. Genet.*, 18, 547–556 (1984).
Roubicek, M., Gehler, J. et al. The clinical spectrum of alpha-L-iduronidase deficiency. *Am. J. Med. Genet.*, 20, 471–481 (1985).
Whitley, C.B., Gorlin, R.J. et al. A non-pathologic allele (I^W) for low alpha-L-iduronidase enzyme activity vis-à-vis prenatal diagnosis of Hurler syndrome. *Am. J. Med. Genet.*, 28, 233–243 (1987).
Spranger, J. Mini review: inborn errors of complex carbohydrate metabolism. *Am. J. Med. Genet.*, 28, 489–499 (1987).

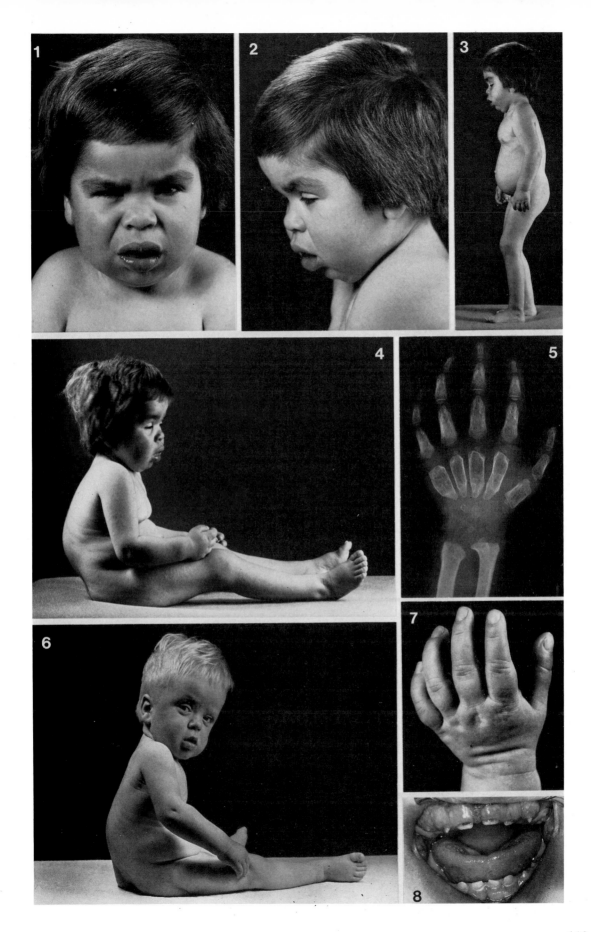

59. Mucopolysaccharidosis Type II

(Hunter's Disease)

A mucopolysaccharide storage disease exclusively in males and leading to relatively typical facial dysmorphism, early hearing impairment, hepatosplenomegaly, small stature, and generally severe mental retardation.

Main signs:
1. Coarse facial features—similar to, but not as pronounced as in Hurler's disease—with broad low nose, hypertelorism, 'full' cheeks, thick lips, large tongue, widely spaced teeth, and macrocephaly (**4, 5**). Impaired hearing beginning in early childhood. Usually no corneal clouding. Irritability, mental retardation or dementia (not with type B; see below).
2. Small stature after transiently normal growth in the first year or two of life; short neck.
3. Joint contractures (**1, 2**), claw hands (**3**). Induration, usually nodular, of skin and cartilage.
4. Pes cavus, hernias (**1, 2**), diastasis recti. Protuberant abdomen (**2**).

Supplementary findings: Chronic suppurative rhinitis. Hepatosplenomegaly.

Heart: valvular defects, enlargement, cardiac failure.

Changes of bony form and structure as in Hurler's syndrome; however, less severe at a given age. Pseudoarthrosis of the femoral head (type B). Increased intracranial pressure from impaired circulation of the cerebrospinal fluid, seldom progressive.

Increased heparan sulfate and chondroitin sulfate B in the urine.

Manifestation: Biochemically, from birth; clinically, after the end of the first year of life.

Etiology: X-linked recessive disease. Gene localized to the long arm of the X chromosome (Xq 26). Decreased activity of the enzyme iduronate sulfatase results in storage of mucopolysaccharides in the cells of various organs and thus to anomalies of their functions and morphologies.

Frequency: About 1:50,000.

Course, prognosis: Slowly progressive in the first years of life. After the fourth or fifth year of life, two forms can be distinguished by their different courses: type A, rapidly progressive with death before the 15th year of life; type B, slowly progressive and with only slight or no noticeable mental impairment, and death—usually from cardiac failure—in adulthood. The oldest-known patient lived to be 60 years old.

Differential diagnosis: Mucopolysaccharidosis type I-H (q.v.).

Treatment: Symptomatic. Genetic counseling. Biochemical identification of the female carriers and prenatal diagnosis possible.

Illustrations:
1–5 Patient (type A) at age 5 years (**1, 2, 4**) and 4 years (**3, 5**). Psychomotor development normal up to 18 months of age; thereafter, developmental standstill. At 111 cm, height still normal. Liver four fingerbreadths below the costal margin. At 5¾ years, a shunt operation for increased intracranial pressure.

H.-R.W.

References:

Spranger, J. Mucopolysaccharidosen. *Hdb. Inn. Med.*, bd. VII/1, 209. Springer, Berlin Heidelberg New York, 1974.
Spranger, J.W., Langer, L.O., Jr., Wiedemann, H.-R. *Bone Dysplasias. An Atlas of Constitutional Disorders of Skeletal Development.* G. Fischer and W.B. Saunders, Stuttgart and Philadelphia, 1974.
McKusick, V.A. *Heritable Disorders of Connective Tissue.* C.V. Mosby, Saint Louis, 1979.
Young, J.D., Harper, P.S. et al. A clinical and genetic study of Hunter's syndrome. 1. Heterogeneity. *J. Med. Genet.*, 19, 401–407 (1982).
Archer, I.M., Young, I.D. et al. Carrier detection in Hunter's syndrome. *Am. J. Med. Genet.*, 16, 61–69 (1983).
Lykkelund, C., Søndergaard, F. et al. Feasibility of first trimester prenatal diagnosis of Hunter syndrome . . . *Lancet,* II, 1147 (1983).
Kleijer, W.J., Diggelen, O.P. van et al. First trimester diagnosis of Hunter Syndrome . . . *Lancet,* II, 472 (1984).
Zlotogora, J. and Bach, G. Heterozygote detection in Hunter syndrome. *Am. J. Med. Genet.*, 17, 661–665 (1984).
Upadhyaya, M., Sarfarazi, M., et al. Localization of the gene for Hunter syndrome . . . *Hum. Genet.*, 74, 391–398 (1986).

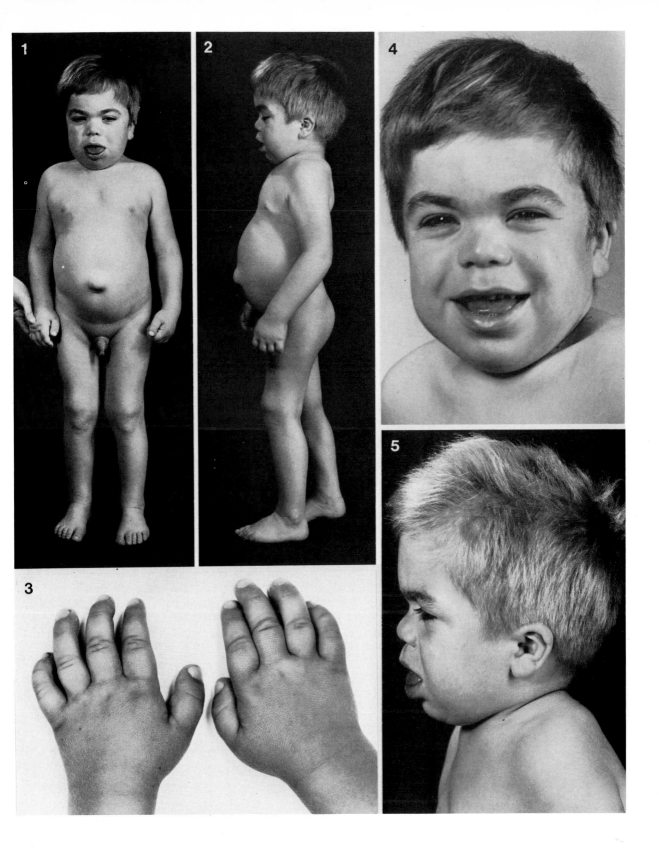

60. Mucopolysaccharidosis Type III

(Sanfilippo's Syndrome)

An autosomal recessive mucopolysaccharide storage disease, which leads to coarsening of the facial features, to behavioral disturbances and dementia, and to hepatomegaly.

Main signs:
1. Flat nasal root; full pouting lips; enlarged tongue; generally coarsened facial features, which in older children are reminiscent of those in Hurler's syndrome. Abundant coarse scalp hair; thick bushy eyebrows, sometimes with synophrys (1–5).
2. Increasing irritability, aggressiveness, dementia.
3. Up to the tenth year of life, above-average height; thereafter, slowing of growth.
4. No corneal clouding.

Supplementary findings: Hepatosplenomegaly. Broad dental laminae. Occasionally umbilical or inguinal hernias, decreased joint mobility. Increased susceptibility to infections.

Sleep disorders. Optic atrophy in isolated cases.

Changes of bony structure and form similar to those of mucopolysaccharidosis I-H, but much less severe.

Increased excretion of the mucopolysaccharide heparan sulfate in the urine.

Manifestation: Biochemically, from birth; clinically, by behavioral disturbance and mental retardation, usually after the third year and by somatic signs, after about the fourth or fifth year of life.

Etiology: Autosomal recessive disease. Heterogeneity. The vastly uniform clinical picture is based on the absence of one of the following enzymes: heparan sulfate sulfatase (Sanfilippo's syndrome type A), alpha-N-acetylglucosaminidase (type B), acetyl CoA: alpha-glucosaminide-N-acetyltransferase (type C), or N-acetyl-glucosaminide-6-sulfatase (type D). Patients with type A disease are somewhat more severely affected than those with type B (earlier manifestation, more rapid progression); those with type C appear to take an intermediate course.

Frequency: About 1:30,000.

Course, prognosis: Characterized by rapid loss of mental and motor abilities, so that meaningful communication becomes impossible by 6 to 10 years of age. Spastic tetraplegia with dysphagia in the terminal phase. Death, usually as the result of pneumonia, in the second decade of life.

Treatment: Symptomatic. Genetic counseling. Prenatal diagnosis possible.

Illustrations:

1 and 2 Patient 1, aged 7 years: macrocephaly (head circumference 55.5 cm). Height 138 cm (average height of a 10-year-old girl). IQ 38 (Kramer–Binet). Mild joint contractures.

3–5 Patient 2 at age 3 years. Head circumference, height, and psychomotor development still within normal limits. Hepatomegaly. Biochemically type B. Note that the facial features of the younger patient more closely resemble those of Hurler's syndrome than do those of patient 1.

H.-R.W.

References:

Spranger, J. Mucopolysaccharidosen. *Hdb. Inn. Med.*, bd. VII/1, 209. Springer, Berlin Heidelberg New York, 1974.
Spranger, J.W., Langer, L.O., Jr., Wiedemann, H.-R. *Bone Dysplasias. An Atlas of Constitutional Disorders of Skeletal Development.* G. Fischer and W.B. Saunders, Stuttgart and Philadelphia, 1974.
McKusick, V.A. *Heritable Disorders of Connective Tissue.* C.V. Mosby, Saint Louis, 1979.
Kleijer, W.J., Janse, H.C. et al. First-trimester diagnosis of mucopolysaccharidosis III A . . . *N. Engl. J. Med.*, 314, 185–186 (1986).
Kaplan, P. and Wolfe, L.S. Sanfilippo syndrome type D. *J. Pediatr.*, 110, 267–271 (1987).
Spranger, J. Mini review: inborn errors of complex carbohydrate metabolism. *Am. J. Med. Genet.*, 28, 489–499 (1987).
Toone, J.R. and Applegarth, D.A. Carrier detection in Sanfilippo A syndrome. *Clin. Genet.*, 33, 401–403 (1988).
Sewell, A.C., Pontz, B.F. et al. Mucopolysaccharidosis type IIIC (Sanfilippo) . . . *Clin. Genet.*, 34, 116–121 (1988).
Turki, I., Kresse, H., Scotto, J. et al. Sanfilippo disease, type C . . . *Neuropediatrics*, 20, 90–92 (1989).

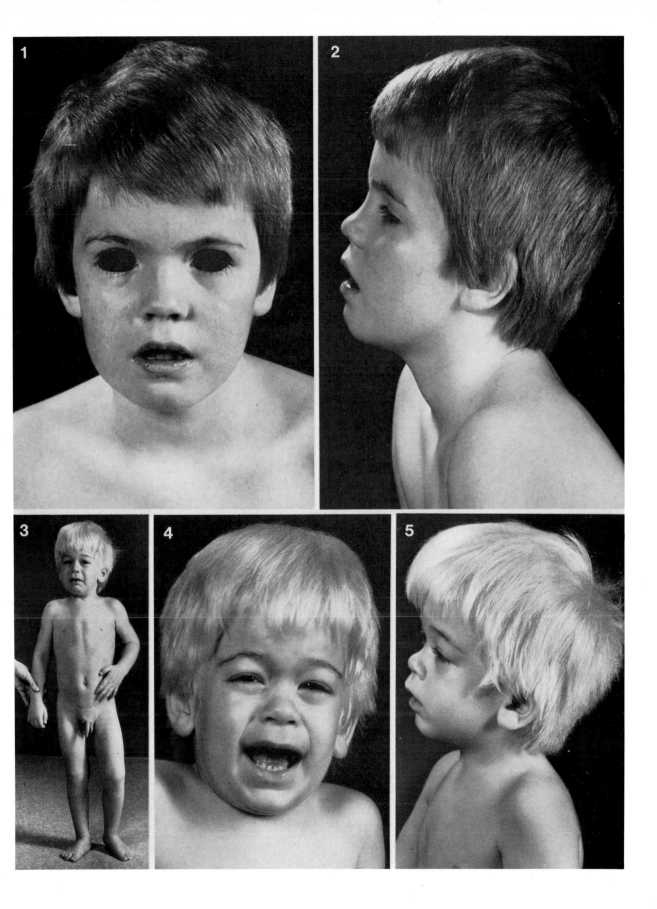

123

61. Mucopolysaccharidosis Type IV

(Morquio–Brailsford Syndrome, Morquio's Syndrome)

A mucopolysaccharide storage disease, which—in its classic form—leads to relatively typical facial dysmorphism, marked disproportionate growth retardation, joint dysplasia, corneal clouding, and all in all a characteristic clinical picture.

Main signs:

1. Moderately coarse facial features with macrostomia, short nose, and prominent jaw (**1, 2**). Corneal clouding, dental caries, grey-blue discoloration of the teeth as a result of enamel hypoplasia.

2. Usually severe growth deficiency, especially of the trunk, with a very short neck (**1, 2**). Head held in dorsiflexion. Pectus carinatum, flaring of the lower rib cage, kyphoscoliosis.

3. Swelling and limitation of movement at the joints with malpositioning (e.g., ulnar deviation of the hands, pronounced knock-knees), hyperextensibility of the finger joints, and instability of the vertebral ligaments. Hands and feet short and stubby.

Supplementary findings: Normal intelligence. Inguinal hernias. Inelastic, indurated skin.

Progressive hearing impairment starting in the first decade of life or thereafter.

Aortic regurgitation.

Changes in bony form and structure similar to those of Hurler's syndrome, but with more marked changes in the epiphyses and more severe generalized platyspondyly. Hypo- or aplasia of the odontoids.

Increased urinary excretion of the mucopolysaccharides keratin sulfate and chondroitin-4-sulfate; a tendency to normalization with increasing age in this respect.

Manifestation: Biochemically, from birth; radiologically, in mid-infancy; clinically, from the second to third year of life. Corneal clouding not recognizable without a slit lamp before age 10 years.

Etiology: Autosomal recessive disorder. Heterogeneity. Deficiency of galactosamine-6-sulfate sulfatase (type A) or beta-galactosidase (type B).

Frequency: Estimated at about 1:100,000.

Course, prognosis: Progression of signs and symptoms. Attainable adult height usually not greater than 1.20 m. Average life expectancy shortened by heart failure and especially as a result of compression of the medulla oblongata and the spinal cord. Life expectancy, which in the past was about 20 years, has been definitely prolonged since the introduction of therapy.

Differential diagnosis: Includes the other mucopolysaccharidoses, especially Hurler's syndrome (p.118), which, however, shows mental retardation or dementia, early corneal clouding, a different pattern of MPS excretion in the urine, etc.

Also, differentiation from the skeletal dysplasias especially with severe involvement of the vertebral column (see spondyloepiphyseal dysplasia congenita, p.246; metatrophic dysplasia, p.240; osteodysplasia type Kniest, p.250).

Treatment: No specific therapy known. Fusion of the upper cervical vertebrae no later than the fifth year of life. Orthopedic measures. Replacement of the aortic valve may be considered. Hearing aids may be indicated. Psychological care and guidance.

Illustrations:

1 and 2 A 14-year-old patient. Increased excretion of keratan sulfate.

H.-R.W.

References:

Spranger, J.W., Langer, L.O., Jr., Wiedemann, H.-R. *Bone Dysplasias. An Atlas of Constitutional Disorders of Skeletal Development.* G. Fischer and W.B. Saunders, Stuttgart and Philadelphia, 1974.

McKusick, V.A. *Heritable Disorders of Connective Tissue.* Mosby, Saint Louis, 1979.

Holzgreve, W., Gröbe, H., Figura, K.v. et al. Morquio syndrome: clinical findings in 11 patients with MPS IV A and 2 patients with MPS IV B. *Hum. Genet.*, 57, 360 (1981).

Fujimoto, A. and Horwitz, A.L. Biochemical defect of non-keratan-sulfate-excreting Morquio syndrome. *Am. J. Med. Genet.*, 15, 265–273 (1983).

Hecht, J.T., Scott, C.I., Jr. et al. Mild manifestations of the Morquio syndrome *Am. J. Med. Genet.*, 18, 369–371 (1984).

Beck, M., Glössl, J. et al. Heterogeneity of Morquio disease. *Clin. Genet.*, 29, 325–331 (1986).

Spranger, J. Mini review: inborn errors of complex carbohydrate metabolism. *Am. J. Med. Genet.*, 28, 489–499 (1987).

Nelson, J. et al. Clinical findings in 12 patients with MPS IV A . . . *Clin. Genet.*, 33, 111–130 (1988).

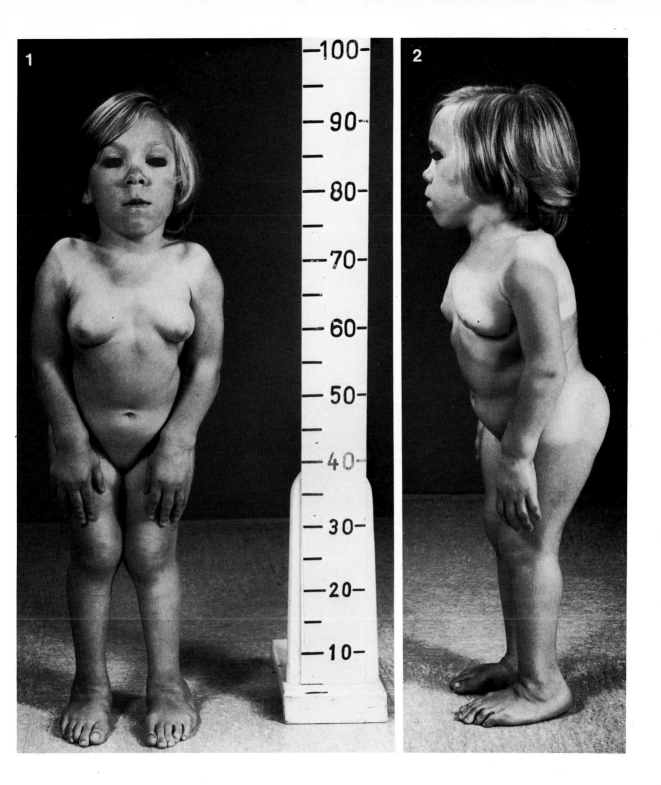

62. Maroteaux–Lamy Syndrome

(Polydystrophic Dysplasia, Mucopolysaccharidosis Type VI)

An autosomal recessive mucopolysaccharide storage disease distinguished by characteristic facial changes, corneal clouding, small stature, and hearing impairment with normal intelligence.

Main signs:
1. Hurler-like facial dysmorphism with large nose; thick lips, low nasal bridge; corneal clouding; macroglossia; widely spaced, late erupting teeth; macroencephaly. Normal intelligence.
2. Growth deficiency with increasing curvature of the spine; prominent sternum.
3. Mild joint contractures (claw hands).
4. Hearing defects of various degrees of severity.
5. Large abdomen with hepatosplenomegaly; hernias.
   The complete picture resembles that of mucopolysaccharidosis Type I.

Supplementary findings: Recurrent infections of the respiratory tract, diarrhea, cardiac complications.

Manifestation: The severe form, type A, can be recognized at the end of the first year of life (humpback when sitting). The milder form, type B, is usually diagnosed between the sixth and tenth years of life on the basis of growth retardation.

Etiology: Autosomal recessive disorder with arylsulfatase B deficiency. Intragenetic heterogeneity. Gene localized to the long arm of chromosome 5.

Frequency: Less than 1 in 100,000 births.

Course, prognosis: Patients with the mild form (type B) survive into the third decade of life and longer. They frequently die of cardiac complications. Patients with the more severe form (type A) begin to deteriorate in late infancy, and have severe deformities by 3–6 years of age. Exact data on the course after the tenth year of life are poorly documented.

Differential diagnosis: In the late phase, especially mucopolysaccharidosis I (Hurler), but also the other mucopolysaccharidoses.

Treatment: Symptomatic corrective measures. Treatment of respiratory infections. Prenatal diagnosis and genetic counseling.

Illustrations:
1a and b Patient 1 at age 11 months. Type A form clinically diagnosed from the kyphosis apparent when the child was sitting. Facial features not yet remarkable.
2a Patient 2 at age 15 years with hyperlordosis and curvature of the thoracic spine.
2b Hurler-like facies, normal intelligence.
2c Small stature.

J.K.

References:

Gehler, J. Phänotyp bei Heteroglykanosen und Sphingolipidosen. *Monatschr. Kinderheilkd.*, 129, 610–620 (1981).
Kresse, H., Cantz, M., Figura, K.von et al. The mucopolysaccharidoses: biochemistry and clinical symptoms. *Klin. Wochenschr.*, 59, 867–876 (1981).
Pilz, H., Figura, K.von, Goebel, H.H. Deficiency of araylsulfatase B in two brothers aged 40 and 38 years (Maroteaux–Lamy syndrome, type B). *Ann. Neurol.*, 6, 315–325 (1979).
Black, S.H., Pelias, M.Z. et al. Maroteaux-Lamy syndrome in a large consanguineous kindred. *Am. J. Med. Genet.*, 25, 273–279 (1986).
Spranger, J. Mini review: inborn errors of complex carbohydrate metabolism. *Am. J. Med. Genet.*, 28, 489–499 (1987).

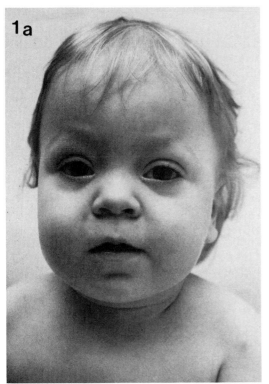

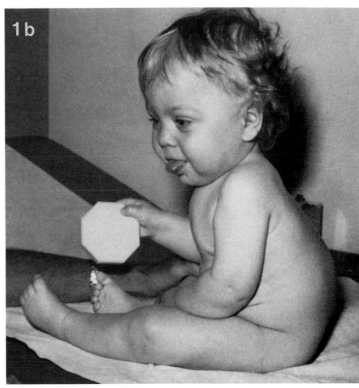

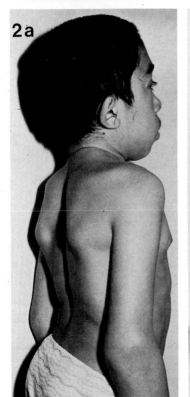

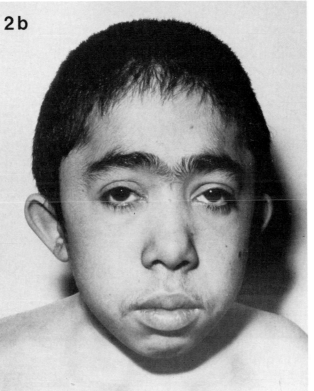

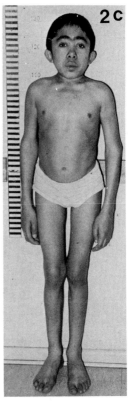

63. Fucosidosis

An autosomal recessive oligosaccharidosis with Hurler-like facial dysmorphism, spasticity, hepatomegaly, angiokeratoma corporis diffusum, and severe progressive psychomotor retardation and neurological deterioration.

Main signs:
1. Macrocephaly, brachycephaly, facial dysmorphism with prominence of the forehead and supraorbital region, depressed nasal root, hypertelorism, exophthalmos, thick growth of scalp hair and eyebrows, thick pouting lips, large tongue, gingival hypertrophy, seizures, spastic tetraplegia. Progressive dementia.
2. Growth deficiency, short neck, thoracolumbar gibbus.
3. Joint contractures. Claw hands, broad hands and feet with hourglass nails, thick skin, elevated salt content of sweat (type I only), an- or hypohydrosis, angiokeratoma corporis diffusum (type II only) over the thorax and inner surfaces of the hands and feet.
4. Large abdomen, hepatomegaly and cardiomegaly (type I only).

Supplementary findings: Tortuous conjunctival vessels, pigmented retinopathy; mild corneal clouding can occur. Dysfunction of the gall bladder. X-ray: progressive thickening of the diploic spaces, early frontal and supraorbital synostosis, absent or poorly developed paranasal sinuses. Short odontoid process, cervical platyspondyly, thoracolumbar kyphosis, short sacrum, absent or rudimentary coccyx. Sclerosis and irregularly serrated form and thickening of the roof of the acetabulum, flattening and irregularities of the head of the femur, coxae valgae, broadening of the shafts of the long tubular bones.

Manifestation: Biochemically, prenatally and after birth. Clinically: type I (infantile type) between the 3rd and 18th months (60% of all patients); type II (late infantile–juvenile form) from the first to second year of life; type III (adult form) later.

Etiology: Autosomal recessive disorder. Absence or diminished activity of alpha-L-fucosidase in the liver, lungs, kidneys, brain, skin, lymphocytes, and serum. Intragenetic heterogeneity. Further sub-types possible. The gene for fucosidosis has been localized to chromosome 1.

Frequency: About 50 patients known; about 60% of them are of the infantile type.

Course, prognosis: Type I (infantile type): death around the fifth year of life. Type II (juvenile type): death after the 20th year. Type III (adult type): too few patients known.

Differential diagnosis: The phenotype is comparable to that of mucopolysaccharidosis I (Hurler). Angiokeratoma corporis diffusum also occurs with Fabry's disease and aspartyl glucosaminuria.

Treatment: Symptomatic. Prevention through prenatal diagnosis.

Illustrations:
1 A 10-year-old fucosidosis patient and his 5-year-old healthy sibling.
2a A 19-year-old patient, brother of the children in 1: thick scalp hair and heavy eyebrows; prominent forehead and supraorbital ridges; exophthalmos; depressed nasal root and broad tip of the nose; thick lips; macroglossia—all in all coarse facies. Angiokeratoma corporis diffusum on the thorax. Type II fucosidosis.
2b–2d Angiokeratoma on the trunk, palms, and soles (patient showed broad, somewhat plump feet and broad hourglass nails).

J.K.

References:
Beaudet, A.L. Disorders of glycoprotein degradation: mannosidosis, fucosidosis, sialidosis, aspartylglucosaminuria. In: *The Metabolic Basis of Inherited Disease*, 5th edn. Stanbury, J.B., Wyngaarden, J.B., Fredrickson, D.S. et al (eds.) McGraw-Hill, 1983.
Lee, F.A., Donnell, G.N., Gwinn, J.L. Radiographic features of fucosidosis. *Pediatr. Radiol.*, 5, 204–208 (1977).
Christomanou, H. and Beyer, D. Absence of alphafucosidase activity in two sisters showing a different phenotype. *Eur. J. Pediatr.*, 140, 27–29 (1983).
Jackson, K. and Dawson, G. Molecular defect in processing alpha-fucosidase in fucosidosis. *Biochem. Biophys. Res. Commun.*, 133, 90–97 (1985).
Spranger, J. Mini review: inborn errors of complex carbohydrate metabolism. *Am. J. Med. Genet.*, 28, 489–499 (1987).
Fritsch, G. and Paschke E. Fukosidose. *Pediatr. Prax.*, 37, 469–476 (1988).
Willems, P.J., Garcia, C.A. et al. Intrafamilial variability in fucosidosis. *Clin. Genet.*, 34, 7–14 (1988).

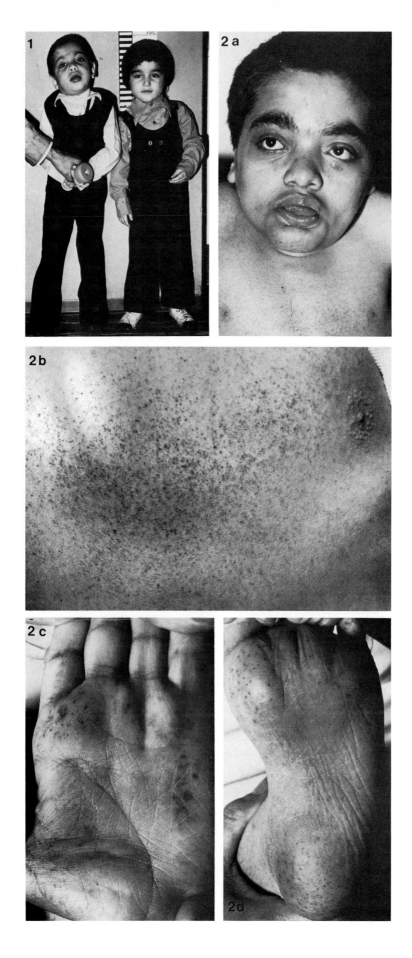

64. Mannosidosis

An autosomal recessive oligosaccharidosis with an alpha-mannosidase defect, psychomotor retardation or deterioration, macrocephaly, hearing defect, hepatomegaly, and 'dysostosis multiplex'.

Main signs: Clinical heterogeneity. Type I refers to a severe infantile form and type II, a milder late infantile–juvenile to adult form.
1. Psychomotor retardation. Developmental stand-still by about the end of the second year of life; coarse facial features; hearing defect.
2. Hepatomegaly; hernias.
3. Lens opacities and corneal clouding (typical retro-lental opacity in the form of a wheel-spoke pattern).
4. Thickening of the calvarium; ovoid configuration of the vertebral bodies, which appear flattened and beaked; occasional gibbus.
5. Recurrent bacterial infections.

Type I: rapid mental deterioration; marked hepato-splenomegaly; severe dysostosis multiplex; hearing defect.

Type II: mental retardation noted in the school-age child; especially severe hearing impairment; milder skeletal involvement.

Supplementary findings: Vacuolated lymphocytes in most cases; absent mucopolysacchariduria; low IgG level; increased PR interval on ECG.

Manifestation: Biochemically, from birth. Clinically: type I, onset between the 3rd and 12th months; type II, onset between the first and fourth years of life.

Etiology: Autosomal recessive alpha-mannosidase deficiency, intragenetic heterogeneity. Localization of the gene on chromosome 19. The enzyme activities can be subdivided into two acidic forms, A and B, and a neutral form, C. In mannosidosis, types A and B are deficient.

Frequency: Low; about 60 patients have been described up to now.

Course, prognosis: Type I: Death between the third and tenth years of life from recurrent bacterial infections. Type II: Survival into adulthood possible.

Differential diagnosis: The clinical picture resembles those of the mild forms of mucopolysaccharidosis. Biochemical elucidation.

Treatment: Symptomatic; antibiotics for bacterial infections. Prenatal diagnosis possible.

Illustrations:
1a–1c Patient 1, an 18-month-old girl, type II. Early stage of coarsening of facial features, macroglossia, claw hands, 'dysostosis multiplex', retardation.
2a–2c Patient 2, likewise type II, 2½ years old; coarse facial features with flat profile, depressed nasal root, protruding lips; prominent forehead and macrocephaly (above the 97th percentile).
3a–3c Patient 3 at 7 (**a, b**) and 12 (**c**) years; small stature, short neck, coarse facial features, retardation; also type II.

J.K.

References:
Beaudet, A.L. Disorders of glycoprotein degradation: mannosidosis, fucosidosis, sialidosis, and aspartylglucosaminuria. In: Stanbury, J.B., Wyngaarden, J.B., Fredrickson, D.S. et al (eds.) *The Metabolic Basis of Inherited Disease*, 5th edn. McGraw-Hill Book Co., pp.788–802 (1983).
Poenaru, L. et al. Antenatal diagnosis in three pregnancies at risk for mannosidosis. *Clin. Genet.*, 16, 428–432 (1979).
Spranger, J. Mini review: inborn errors of complex carbohydrate metabolism. *Am. J. Med. Genet.*, 28, 489–499 (1987).

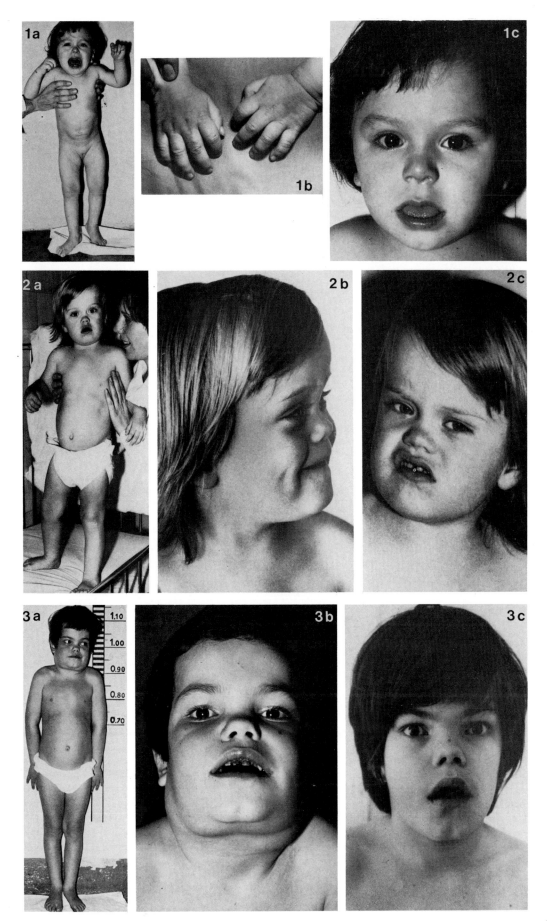

131

65. GM₁-Gangliosidosis

An autosomal recessive storage disease with defective ß-galactosidase and very variable phenotype: depending on the form, either an acute infantile onset with rapid neurological deterioration and severe bone deformities, or normal intelligence and survival into adulthood.

Main signs: Infantile form: shortly after birth, generalized edema of the extremities, poor appetite, vomiting. Subsequently, no sitting or crawling. Mentally dull, irregular respirations, recurrent pneumonias, seizures. Initial muscular hypotonia, followed by spastic paresis in the second year. Blindness, deafness. Prominent forehead, depressed nasal root, large low-set ears, coarse facies, gingival hypertrophy, macroglossia, macrocephaly, cherry-red spot of the fundus (50%), dorsolumbar kyphosis.

Juvenile form: later onset. During the first year, unremarkable psychomotor behavior, good appetite and weight gain. Ataxia after the first year of life as the first sign. Internal strabismus, nystagmus, impaired coordination, loss of speech, generalized muscular hypotonia, progressive psychomotor retardation, lethargy, followed by spasticity of the upper and lower extremities. Seizures after the 16th month of life. Recurrent pneumonias. Relatively late development of mild facial dysmorphism.

Adult form: onset in the school-child of progressive cerebellar dysarthria, spasticity, and ataxia. Mild intellectual decline. Neurological complications ten years after the first symptoms, at about age 20 years.

Supplementary findings: Infantile form: deformity of the vertebral bodies with anterior beaking, periosteal new-bone formation in the long bones, broadening of the ribs, deformity of the pelvis and bones of the hands and feet. Hepatosplenomegaly.

Juvenile form: eventual blindness, only mild radiological signs.

Adult form: no seizures, no impairment of sight.

Manifestation: Biochemically, from birth; clinically, varied: Infantile form: shortly after birth, rapidly progressive. Juvenile form: in the second year of life, slow progression. Adult form: after the 20th year of life.

Etiology: Deficiency of ß-galactosidase. The fact that the progression of the different forms is constant within families is explained by intragenetic heterogeneity. Autosomal recessive disorder. Further phenotypic variants are possible. The gene for ß-galactosidase is located on the short arm of chromosome 3.

Frequency: Of the infantile form, presently about 100 patients known; of the juvenile form, 20; and of the adult form, 10.

Course, prognosis: Infantile form: death about the second year as a result of recurrent pneumonias. Juvenile form: Death between the third and tenth years of life, or shortly after. Adult form: all known patients have survived to date.

Differential diagnosis: Mucolipidosis Type II (I-cell disease).

Treatment: Symptomatic. Genetic counseling. Prenatal diagnosis possible.

Illustrations:

3 An 11-year-old boy with the juvenile form. Macrocephaly, moderately coarse facial features with bushy eyebrows, depressed nasal root and macroglossia; short trunk with barrel-shaped chest and pigeon breast. Impairment of voluntary motor coordination.

1 and 2 The child in 3 with his 6½-year-old brother. The phenotype of the latter is, in comparison, still unremarkable with some mental deterioration and loss of speech; kyphosis when sitting, awkward gait.

J.K.

References:

O'Brien, J.S. The gangliosidoses. In: *The Metabolic Basis of Inherited Disease*. Stanbury, J.S., Wyngaarden, J.B., Fredrickson, D.S. et al (eds.), 5th edn. McGraw-Hill Book Co, pp.945–969 (1983).

Kohlschütter, A. Clinical course of GM₁ gangliosidoses. *Neuropediatrics*, 15 (suppl.), 71–73 (1984).

Pampiglione, G. and Harden, A. Neurophysiological investigations in GM₁ and GM₂ gangliosidoses. *Neuropediatrics*, 15 (suppl.), 74–84 (1984).

Sandhoff, K. and Conzelmann, E. The biochemical basis of gangliosidoses. *Neuropediatrics*, 15 (suppl.), 85–92 (1984).

Giugliani, R., Dutra, J.C., Pereira, M.L.S. et al. GM₁ gangliosidosis: clinical and laboratory findings in eight families. *Hum. Genet.*, 70, 347–354 (1985).

Spranger, J. Mini review: inborn errors of complex carbohydrate metabolism. *Am. J. Med. Genet.*, 28, 489–499 (1987).

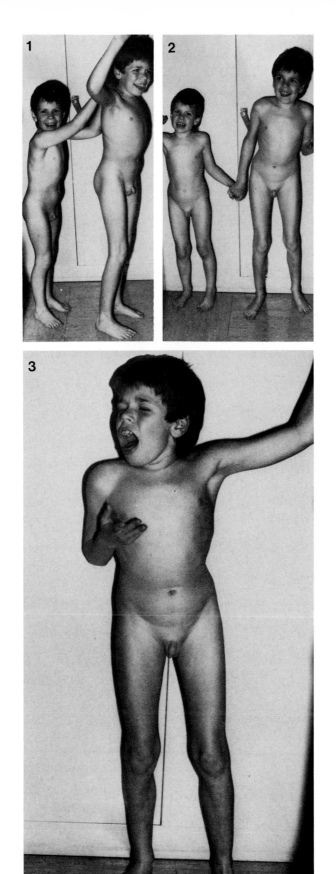

66. Mucolipidosis

An autosomal recessive disorder with elevation of several lysosomal enzymes and Hurler-like signs with variable expressivity (type II = I-cell disease = Leroy syndrome; type III = pseudo-Hurler polydystrophy; type IV).

Main signs:

Type II: 1. Intrauterine growth retardation, early coarsening of the facial features, exophthalmos, mouth held open, gingival hyperplasia, thick hair, prominent forehead, scaphocephaly (premature closure of the sagittal suture), depressed nasal root.
2. Kyphoscoliosis, lumbar gibbus, luxation of the hip, club feet, joint contractures, hernias. Beaking and wedging of the vertebral bodies, broadening of the ribs, proximal tapering of the metacarpals. Circular periosteal new-bone formation, around the shaft of the humerus and other long bones.
3. Thick firm skin especially over the finger joints, short fingers, paw-like claw hands.
4. Puffy eyelids, corneal clouding, increase of corneal diameter.
5. Hepatosplenomegaly, cardiomegaly, cardiac defects.
6. Disproportionate growth deficiency, severe developmental retardation, recurrent lung infections.

Type III: Three different, severe forms:
1. Marked limitation of movement in all joints, progressive until puberty. Firm thick skin, paw-like hands, disproportionate growth deficiency, coarsening of the facial features between the sixth and tenth years of life. By the end of the first decade of life, corneal clouding, carpal tunnel syndrome. Intelligence varied: normal to rapidly deteriorating, depending on the form.
2. Severe anomalies of the pelvis and spine. Hyperlordosis, hip dysplasia, short neck, final height 130–140 cm.
3. No mucopolysacchariduria.

Type IV: 1. Slow neurological decline with increased knee and ankle jerks, hypotonia, dystonia, moderate to severe psychomotor deterioration, mild coarsening of facial features.
2. Strabismus, corneal clouding.
3. No mucopolysacchariduria, no organomegaly, skeleton normal.

Supplementary findings: Type II: Numerous cytoplasmic inclusion bodies (I-form) in skin fibroblasts. Type III: Inclusion bodies as in type II. Type IV: Cytoplasmic granular inclusions and lamellar structures in skin cells.

Manifestation: Type II: first months of life. Type III: age 4–5 years. Type IV: in the first decade of life.

Etiology: Autosomal recessive disorder with decreased intracellular and increased extracellular activities of lysosomal acid hydrolases (10- to 20-fold increase of ß-hexosaminidase, iduronate sulfatase, arylsulfatase A in serum). Intragenetic and intergenetic heterogeneity.

Frequency: Low. Type II: about 50 patients. Type III: fewer than 50 patients known. Type IV: 15 patients.

Course, prognosis: Type II: death before the fifth year of life. Type III: the oldest patient is over 30 years old. Type IV: the oldest patient is over 23 years old.

Differential diagnosis: Type II: Hurler disease. Type III: MPS VI (Maroteaux–Lamy). Classification within type III depends on the diagnostic center. Type IV: mucolipidoses II and III. Biochemical elucidation.

Treatment: Symptomatic. Prenatal diagnosis identifies only the homozygotes of type II. Apparently type III can be diagnosed prenatally. Type IV: still not diagnosable with certainty (electron microscopic search for inclusion bodies?).

Illustrations:

1a and 1b 7-month-old, growth deficiency, coarsening of facial features, thick scalp hair. Prominent forehead, exophthalmos, appears similar to mucopolysaccharidosis (mucolipidosis II).
2a 16-year-old, growth deficiency, lordosis with large protruding abdomen, joint contractures (mucolipidosis III). **2b** Hurler appearance, coarsened facies, thick scalp hair, exophthalmos, synophrys, thick lips, depressed nasal root. Intelligence normal. **2c and 2d** Joint contractures, short fingers, paw-like claw hands.

J.K.

References:

Neufeld, E.F. and McKusick, V.A. Disorders of lysosomal enzyme synthesis and localization: I-cell disease and pseudo-Hurler polydystrophy. In: Stanbury, J.S., Wyngaarden, J.B., Fredrickson, D.S. et al (eds.) *The Metabolic Basis of Inherited Disease*, 5th edn. McGraw-Hill Book Co., pp.778–787 (1983).

Okada, S. et al. I-cell disease: clinical studies of 21 Japanese cases. *Clin. Genet.*, 28, 207–215 (1985).

Ornoy, A. et al. Letter to the editor: Early prenatal diagnosis of mucolipidosis IV. *Am. J. Med. Genet.*, 27, 983–985 (1987).

Spranger, J. Mini review: Inborn errors of complex carbohydrate metabolism. *Am. J. Med. Genet.*, 28, 489–499 (1987).

Pazzaglia, U.E., Beluffi, G. et al. Study of bone pathology in early mucolipidosis II . . . *Eur. J. Pediatr.*, 148, 553–557 (1989).

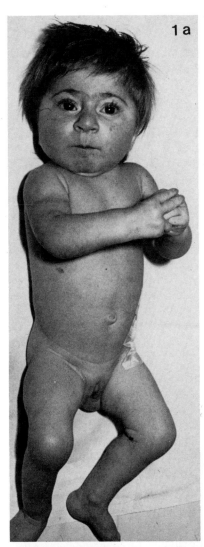

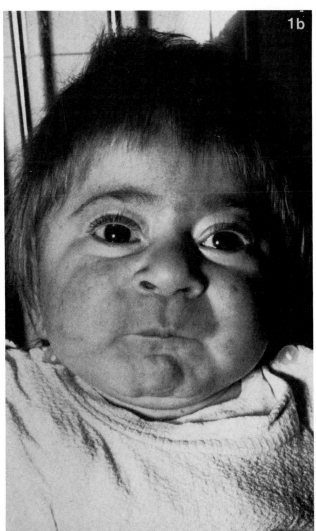

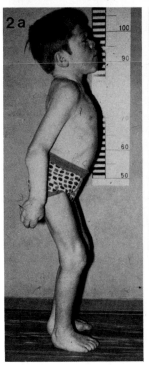

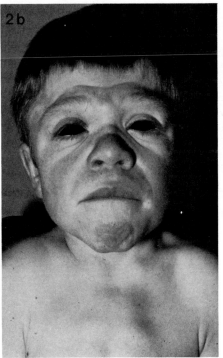

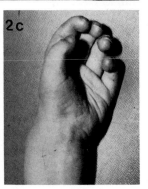

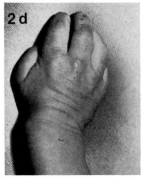

135

67. Exomphalos–Macroglossia–Gigantism Syndrome

(EMG Syndrome, Wiedemann–Beckwith Syndrome)

A congenital, relatively frequent, and very characteristic metabolic dysplasia syndrome of practical importance with peculiar facies, 'grooved' ears, congenital and/or postnatal generalized 'gigantism', sometimes with umbilical hernia, muscular macroglossia, and other organomegaly in addition to possible post-natal hypoglycemia.

Main signs:
1. Frequent mild exophthalmos often associated with a relatively small head with protruding occiput (**2, 4–6**) and telangiectatic nevi of the upper half of the face in infancy. Hypoplasia of the midface, possible soft-tissue folds under the eyes (**5, 9, 10**). Variously developed slit- or notch-like indentations of the external ears (**12–14**) and/or a groove on the dorsal edge of the helix in the great majority of cases. Congenital macroglossia, often with macrostomia, prognathism. Omphalocele (**1**); or simply a large umbilical hernia (**2**). Congenital nephromegaly (ultrasonography imperative), hepato-, pancreato-, and in some cases cardiomegaly. Congenital macrosomia and/or postnatal 'gigantism', whereby height, weight, and skeletal and dental maturity may be above the norm for years.
2. Possible severe prolonged therapy-resistant hypoglycemia in the newborn period and infancy.

Supplementary findings: Not infrequently the presence or development of fairly distinct hemihypertrophy (of a lower extremity alone or of the whole half of the body).

Infrequent hypertrophy of the clitoris and/or labia, or penis.

Substantially increased tendency to neoplasia (especially Wilms tumors and carcinoma of the adrenal cortex), especially in children with distinct hemihypertrophy.

Mental development usually normal (in the absence of severe hypoglycemic damage).

Manifestation: At birth and thereafter (macrosomia).

Etiology: An autosomal dominant gene with extremely variable expression and incomplete penetrance has been assumed. In apparently sporadic cases (i.e., thorough investigation for possible carriers negative), new mutation possible, low risk of recurrence; with familial occurrence, risk of recurrence up to 50%. In atypical cases chromosome analysis is indicated.

Frequency: Relatively high; many hundreds of cases have been recognized.

Course, prognosis: After possible postpartum adaptive difficulties (e.g., polycythemia, hypoglycemia, feeding and respiratory difficulties, etc.), usually good. Regression of visceromegaly; gradual slowing of growth, often with eventual normal height; unremarkable sexual maturation; tendency to attain normal proportions, including those of the facial features, and better tongue-to-mouth proportions.

Regular close follow-up, especially of the abdomen for possible tumor development, and with routine ultrasonography, is mandatory in the first years of life.

Differential diagnosis: Infant of diabetic mother, which does not include macroglossia, ear grooves, umbilical hernia, etc. Hypothyroidism, which is unlikely with accelerated growth and absence of constipation, etc., blood tests.

Treatment: Initially, blood sugar determinations at regular intervals; in some cases prednisolone or diazoxide. Repair of omphalocele. Partial glossectomy may be indicated, possibly at a young age. Orthodontic care. Orthopedic treatment for hemihypertrophy. Genetic counseling. Ultrasonographic prenatal diagnosis in some cases.

Illustrations:
1 Premature infant; exomphalos, macroglossia; brother of the patient in **10**.
2 A 6-month-old child; typical facies (ear shown in **12**), large umbilical hernia; probably frequent early hypoglycemic seizures; persisting tendency to hypoglycemia.
3, 7, and 11 Young children, *post partum* surgery for exomphalos, accelerated growth, mentally normal.
4–6 and 8–10 Typical facies at various ages.
13 Ear of patient in **3**.
14 Ear of patient in **5**.

H.-R.W.

References:

Lemke, J., Meinecke, P. et al. Das Wiedemann–Beckwith-Syndrom. *Monatschr. Kinderheilkd.*, 134, 554–557 (1986).
Pettenati, M.J., Haines, J.L. et al. Wiedemann–Beckwith syndrome . . . review of the literature. *Hum. Genet.*, 74, 143–154 (1986).
Engström, W., Lindham, S. et al. Wiedemann–Beckwith syndrome (review). *Eur. J. Pediatr.*, 147, 450–457 (1988).
Litz, C.E., Kaylor, K.A. et al. Absence of detectable chromosomal and molecular abnormalities in monozygotic twins discordant for the Wiedemann–Beckwith syndrome. *Am. J. Med. Genet.*, 30, 821–833 (1988).

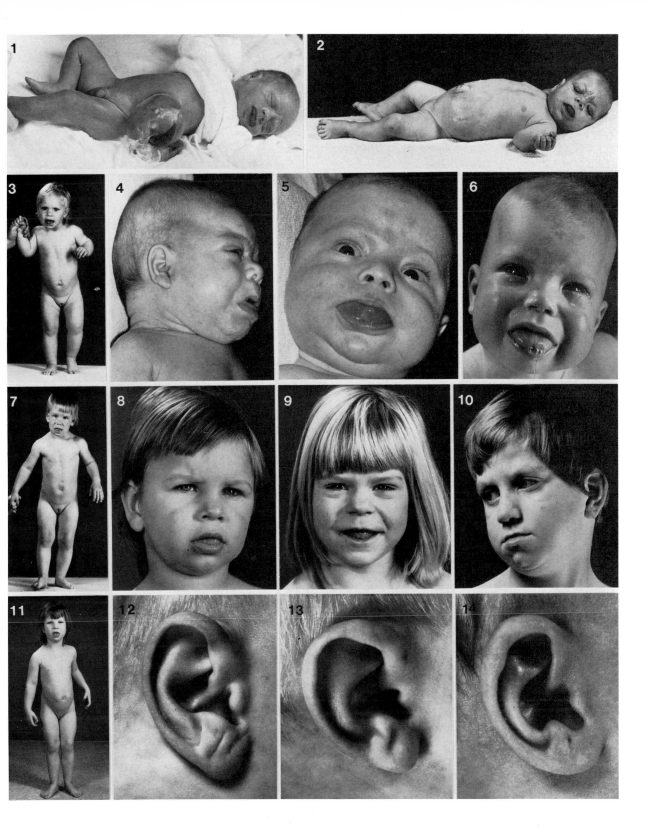

68. Sotos Syndrome

(Sotos Sequence, Cerebral Gigantism Type Sotos)

A syndrome of childhood gigantism, usually with above-normal size at birth, unusual facies, acromegalic changes, and signs of non-progressive cerebral involvement.

Main signs:

1. Congenital macrosomia and/or postnatal somatic 'gigantism' (**3, 4**) with discordant acceleration of bone age and dentition (phalanges and metacarpals > carpals).
2. Macrocephaly and abnormally large hands and feet.
3. Unusual physiognomy (prominent forehead with high or 'receding' hairline (**1**); hypertelorism; slight antimongoloid slant of the palpebral fissures).
4. Congenital nonprogressive cerebral impairment with psychomotor retardation, impairment of fine motor activity.

Supplementary findings: Usually dolicocephaly, large ears, prognathism, high palate, and unusually long arms. Not infrequently development of kyphoscoliosis. Cranial ultrasound or CT shows slight to moderate enlargement of the cerebral ventricles, especially the IIIrd (no increased intracranial pressure). EEG frequently abnormal.

Congenital cardiac defect relatively frequent.

No evidence of a constant endocrinological or biochemical abnormality.

Manifestation: At birth and during infancy.

Etiology: Genetically determined syndrome. Usually sporadic occurrence. Evidence for dominant as well as possible recessive transmission. Thus probable heterogeneity.

Frequency: Not particularly rare (several hundred case reports in the literature).

Course, prognosis: Self-limitation of the accelerated growth by the end of the first, or at least the beginning of the second decade of life. Onset of puberty at the usual age or somewhat earlier. Adult height within the normal range. The degree of mental retardation is of considerable importance. Apparently increased tendency to develop malignant tumors.

Differential diagnosis: Other primordial overgrowth syndromes, including the fragile X syndrome (e.g., p.136, p.140).

Treatment: Follow-up examinations at regular intervals. All appropriate measures to educate children with developmental or psychomotor retardation. Precautionary measures against, or early treatment of, scoliosis. Genetic counseling.

Illustrations:

1–4 A child with Sotos syndrome. Length at birth 60 cm. At age 14 months (**1, 3, 4**), average height of a 2¼-year-old; head circumference corresponding to that of an 8-year-old. Hand length of a 5-year-old, early eruptions of teeth, bone age 3 years. Prominent forehead with frontal baldness, appearance of a child older than his age; large, somewhat low-set ears; large genitalia; very large feet. Gross motor retardation, clumsy motor performance; clearly enlarged IIIrd ventricle. At 2 years 4 months, height of a 4-year-old; enormous feet. At 3 years 11 months (**2**), average height of a 6¼-year-old. 'Too old' appearance. Clumsy, restless, mentally subnormal behavior.

H.-R.W.

References:

Jaeken, J., Schueren-Lodeweyck, M. van der and Eeckels, R. Cerebral gigantism syndrome. A report of 4 cases and review of the literature. *Z. Kinderheilkd.*, 112, 332 (1972).
Wiedemann, H.-R. Diencephale Syndrome des Kindesalters. *Pädiat. Prax.*, 11, 95 (1972).
Sotos, J.F., Cutler, E.A., Dodge, P. Cerebral gigantism. *Am. J. Dis. Child.*, 131, 625 (1977).
Beman, H. and Nilsson, D. Sotos syndrome in two brothers. *Clin. Genet.*, 18, 421 (1980).
Smith, A., Farrar, J.R., Silink, M. et al. Dominant Sotos syndrome. *Arch. Dis. Child.*, 55, 579 (1980).
Dodge, P.R., Holmes, S.J. et al. Cerebral gigantism. *Develop. Med. Child. Neurol.*, 25, 248–252 (1983).
Bale, A.E., Drum, M.A. et al. Familial Sotos syndrome . . . *Am. J. Med. Genet.*, 20, 613–624 (1985).
Wit, J.M., Beemer, F.A. et al. Cerebral gigantism . . . *Eur. J. Pediatr.*, 144, 131–140 (1985).
Kaneko, H., Tsukahara, M. et al. Congenital heart defects in Sotos sequence. *Am. J. Med. Genet.*, 26, 569–576 (1987).
Verloes, A., Sacré, J.-P. et al. Sotos syndrome and fragile X chromosomes. *Lancet*, II, 329 (1987).
Goldstein, D.J., Ward, R.E. et al. Overgrowth, congenital hypotonia, nystagmus, stabismus, and mental retardation: variant of dominantly inherited Sotos sequence? *Am. J. Med. Genet.*, 29, 783–792 (1988).
Blackett, P.R., Coffman, M.A. et al. Dominantly inherited childhood gigantism resembling Sotos' syndrome. *Am. J. Med. Sci.*, 296, 181–185 (1989).

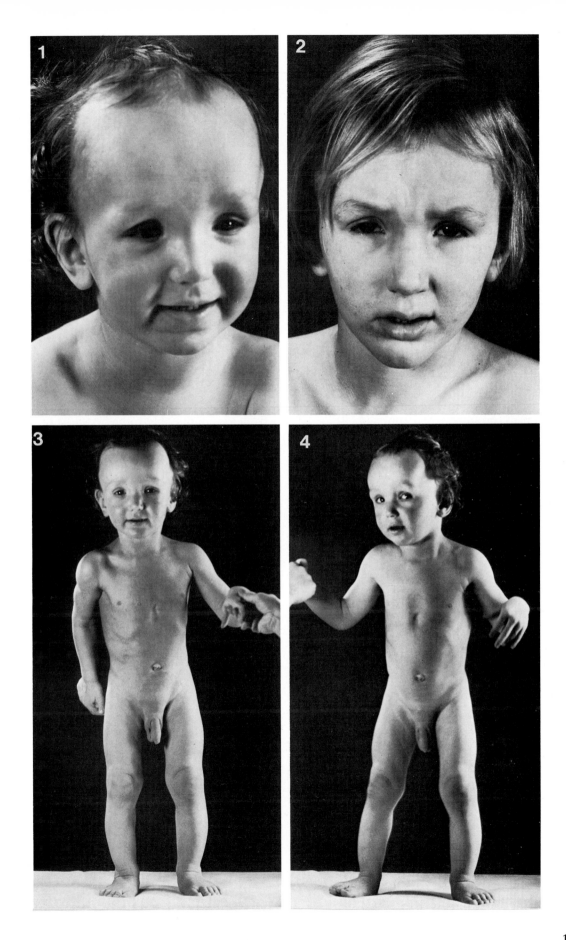

139

69. Weaver Syndrome

A further syndrome of childhood 'gigantism', usually with congenital macrosomia, macrocephaly, distinctive facies, psychomotor retardation, unusual voice, increased muscle tone, and additional anomalies.

Main signs:
1. Congenital macrosomia and/or postnatal somatic 'gigantism' (**1**).
2. Marked macrocephaly (without signs of increased intracranial pressure) with broad, protruding forehead (**2**).
3. Distinctive appearance: marked hypertelorism or telecanthus; broad, low nasal root; prominent or long philtrum; receding chin; and large ears (**1, 2**).
4. Developmental retardation a regular feature. Deep, hoarse voice. Muscular hypertonia (less frequently hypotonia).

Supplementary findings: Possible early limitation of motion of the elbows and knees. Club feet. Camptodactyly of the fingers, clinodactyly of the toes, broad thumbs, simian creases in some cases. Thin, deeply inserted nails; prominent fingertip pads.

Loose nuchal skin; inguinal and/or umbilical hernias.

X-rays: Discordant acceleration of bone age (carpals > phalanges and metacarpals); low broad iliac wings; widening of the distal ends of the long bones, especially the femora (**3**).

Manifestation: At birth and thereafter.

Etiology: Undetermined; genetic factors probably play a role, although a definite mode of inheritance has not yet been established.

Frequency: Low (about 25 cases have been reported since 1974).

Course, prognosis: To date hardly any long-term observations; apparently normal, decreased, or excessive final height may result. In each case the mental development is key to the prognosis.

Differential diagnosis: Other primordial 'gigantism' syndromes (see, e.g., p.136, p.138).

Treatment: Symptomatic. Any measures to promote psychomotor development. Early measures to prevent obesity.

Illustrations:
1–3 A 15-month-old boy, the first child of healthy, young, nonconsanguineous parents. Birth at term after an unremarkable pregnancy: 57 cm, 4970 g, and head circumference 36 cm; club feet. At 15 months 93 cm (like a 2½-year-old), about 17 kg, and head circumference 52 cm (both those of a 4-year-old).

H.-R.W.

References:

Weaver, D.D., Graham, C.B., Thomas, I.T., et al. A new overgrowth syndrome with accelerated skeletal maturation, unusual facies, and camptodactyly. *J. Pediatr.*, 84, 547 (1974).
Fitch, N. The syndromes of Marshall and Weaver. *J. Med. Genet.*, 17, 174 (1980).
Majewski, F., Ranke, M., Kemperdick, H. et al. The Weaver syndrome: a rare type of primordial overgrowth. *Eur. J. Pediatr.*, 137, 277 (1981).
Meinicke, P., Schaefer, E. et al. The Weaver syndrome in a girl. *Eur. J. Pediatr.*, 141, 58–59 (1983).
Farrell, S.A. and Hughes, H.E. Weaver syndrome with pes cavus. *Am. J. Med. Genet.*, 21, 737–739 (1985).
Ardinger, H.H., Hanson, J.W. et al. Further delineation of Weaver syndrome. *J. Pediatr.*, 108, 228–235 (1986).
Thompson, E.M., Hill, S. et al. A girl with Weaver syndrome. *J. Med. Genet.*, 24, 232–234 (1987).

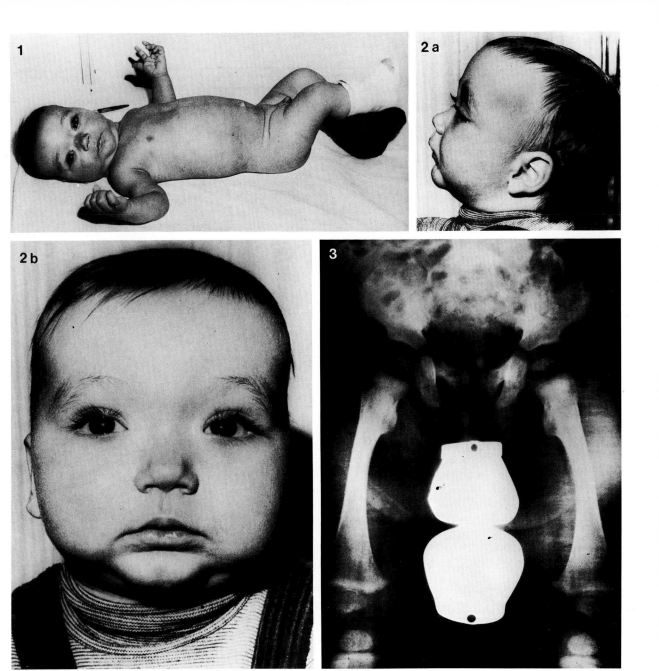

70. Marfan Syndrome

(Arachnodactyly)

A characteristic hereditary disorder with disproportionate tall stature, defects of the eyes, and tendency to develop aortic aneurysms.

Main signs:
1. Tall stature, mainly due to excessively long extremities, particularly the distal portions, resulting in eunuchoid body proportions and arachnodactyly (**1, 2**).
2. Marked deficit of fatty tissue. Muscular hypoplasia and hypotonia (**1, 4, 6**).
3. Long, narrow face with high palate (**1, 4**) and narrowly spaced teeth; dolichocephaly.
4. Signs of connective tissue weakness; hernias, hyperextensible joints, dislocation of the joints, kyphoscoliosis, pes planus, striae, and others; pectus carinatum or excavatum (**1, 4, 7**).

Supplementary findings: Dislocation of the lenses in about 75% of cases, usually upwards; when less pronounced, recognizable on slit-lamp examination; danger of glaucoma. Usually marked myopia. Retinal detachment. Round lenses. Blue sclera.

General dilatation of the aorta (aortic valve incompetence), dissecting aneurysm. Less frequently similar involvement of the pulmonary artery or the mitral and tricuspid valves (prolapse of the mitral valve).

Manifestation: In infancy. However usually not diagnosed until childhood or later.

Etiology: Autosomal dominant disorder with variable expression; new mutations may be assumed for about 15% of the cases, often associated with increased paternal age. A fundamental connective tissue disorder is likely, although the exact defect has yet to be determined.

Frequency: Varied estimates between 1:66,000 and 1.5:100,000 of the general population.

Course, prognosis: Death as a result of cardiovascular complications possible at any age, especially after puberty. On the average, patients attain 30–50 years. If valvular endocarditis develops, the prognosis is very poor. Danger of going blind.

Differential diagnosis: Homocystinuria must be ruled out in every case since it is basically amenable to therapy. Stickler syndrome. Contractural arachnodactyly.

Treatment: Limitation of growth by means of hormone therapy at the appropriate time, also as an attempt to prevent severe scoliosis. Propranolol seems to slow the development of aneurysms. Vascular or cardiac surgery may be indicated. Avoidance of marked physical exertion. Genetic counseling.

Illustrations:
1–3 Patient 1 at age 14 years: height 174 cm, weight 48 kg (normal weight of a girl 159 cm tall). Both second toes shortened operatively, as they were 1.5 cm longer than the halluces. No evidence of cardiac defect at present. Myopia.
4 Patient 2 at age 9 years. No definite evidence of a cardiac defect. Myopia on the right, astigmatism on the left, round lenses. *No* dislocation of the lenses. Height at 13 years, 196.5 cm.
5 and 6 Patient 3 (sister of patient 2) at age 6 years. Suspected to have ballooning of the mitral valve. Round lenses, *no* dislocation. Normal amino acid chromatogram. Height at age 10 years, 174.5 cm.
7 The Marfan thumb sign (the thumb folded across the palm distinctly extends beyond the ulnar edge of the hand).

H.-R.W.

References:

Pyeritz, R.E. and McKusick, V.A. The Marfan syndrome: diagnosis and management. *N. Engl. J. Med.*, 772, (1979).
Donaldson, R.M., Emanuel, E.W., Olsen, E.G.J. et al. Management of cardiovascular complications in Marfan syndrome. *Lancet*, II, 1178 (1980).
Boucek, R.J., Noble, N.L., Gunja-Smith, Z. et al. The Marfan syndrome. A deficiency in chemically stable collagen cross-links. *N. Engl. J. Med.*, 988, (1981).
Chemke, J., Nisani, R., Feigl, A. et al. Homozygosity for autosomal dominant Marfan syndrome. *J. Med. Genet.*, 21, 173–177 (1984).
Pyeritz, R.E. The diagnosis and management of the Marfan syndrome. *Am. Fam. Physician*, 34, 83–94 (1986).
Burgio, R.G., Martin, A. et al. Asymmetric Marfan syndrome. *Am. J. Med. Genet.*, 30, 905–909 (1988).
Hofman, K.J., Bernhardt, B.A. et al. Marfan syndrome: neuropsychological aspects. *Am. J. Med. Genet.*, 31, 331–338 (1988).
Conference report: First international symposium on the Marfan syndrome. *Am. J. Med. Genet.*, 32, 233–238 (1989).

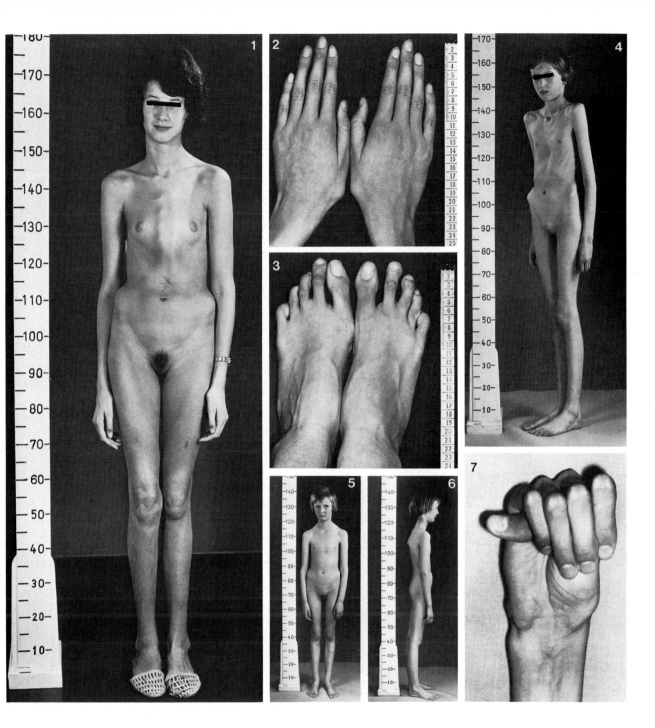

143

71. Contractural Arachnodactyly

(Beals–Hecht Syndrome, CCA Syndrome)

A syndrome of arachnodactyly with multiple congenital contractures of the limbs and characteristic changes of the external ear.

Main signs:
1. Multiple, mostly symmetrical, congenital contractures of the finger, knee, ankle, elbow, and (usually mildly involved) hip joints. Long, thin extremities, including hands and fingers, feet and toes, the proximal phalanges being especially long. Flexion contractures of the fingers at the proximal interphalangeal joints, often with ulnar deviation; thumbs often adducted; toes may be slightly incurved. Pes equinovarus or calcaneo valgus (1, 3).
2. Height normal or above average. Pectus excavatum or carinatum. Frequent development of kyphoscoliosis (1). Asthenic, Marfanoid habitus. Hypotonia.
3. Eyes somewhat deep-set in some cases; external ears may be posteriorly rotated with anomalies of the helix or antihelix and concha, giving the appearance of crumpled ears; high palate, retrognathia (2). Short nucha (1c).

Supplementary findings: No dislocation of the lens or iridodonesis as seen in Marfan syndrome (p.142) and homocystinuria (p.146); however, ocular anomalies may occur.

Cardiovascular disorders (as in Marfan syndrome) are much less frequent, but may occur, e.g., prolapse of the mitral valve.

Manifestation: At birth.

Etiology: Autosomal dominant disorder with variable expression.

Frequency: Low (to date about 90 cases in the literature).

Course, prognosis: Initially, motor retardation possible, especially as a result of knee and ankle contractures. Normal life expectancy (unless, as an exception, a serious cardiac defect is present). The contractures tend to improve; while the kyphoscoliosis, when present, tends to progress.

Differential diagnosis: Arthrogryposis (p.402); differentiation possible from the complete clinical picture. In the rare case of mental subnormality and rib and vertebral anomalies (supernumerary), a chromosomal aberration (trisomy 8) must be ruled out.

Treatment: Symptomatic, with intensive physiotherapy; surgical correction of malpositioned fingers, if necessary. Genetic counseling.

Illustrations:
1–3 A 3½-year-old mentally normal boy, the second child of healthy parents, after the birth of a healthy girl. Birth length 57 cm; subsequent height measurements above the 97th percentile. Congenital flexion contractures of the fingers and bilateral clinodactyly of the fifth finger; long narrow feet, initially in slight club-foot position (later valgus deformity and pes planus). Large cranium; hypertelorism; high, narrow palate with bifid uvula, slight micrognathia; large ears, posteriorly rotated on the right. Bluish sclera; eyes otherwise negative at repeat follow-up examinations. Winged scapulae; pigeon chest deformity of the thorax; pronounced muscular hypotonia; inguinal hernias. Kidneys normal. Chromosome analysis with banding negative. Low excretion of 5-hydroxyproline. Persistent ductus arteriosis (ligation at age 3 years). Persistence of the left superior vena cava; surgical repair of severe aortic dilatation and aortic valve replacement at age 5 years. Death due to heart failure at 5 years and 8 months.

H.-R.W.

References:

Beals, R.K. and Hecht, F. Congenital contractural arachnodactyly. *J. Bone Jt. Surg.*, 53-A, 987 (1971).
Bjerkreim, I., Skogland, L.B., Trystad, O. Congenital contractural arachnodactyly. *Acta Orthop. Scand.*, 47, 250 (1976).
Meinecke, P., Schaefer, E. et al. Congenitale kontrakturelle Arachnodactylie . . . *Klin. Pädiatr.*, 185, 64–70 (1983).
Anderson, R.A., Koch, S. et al. Cardiovascular findings in congenital contractural arachnodactyly . . . *Am. J. Med. Genet.*, 18, 265–271 (1984).
Arroyo, M.A.R., Weaver, D.D. et al. Congenital contractural arachnodactyly . . . review . . . *Clin. Genet.*, 27, 570–581 (1985).
Tamminga, P., Jennekens, F.G.J. et al. An infant with Marfanoid phenotype and congenital contractures . . . *Eur. J. Pediatr.*, 143, 228–231 (1985).
Currarino, G. and Friedman, J.M. A severe form of congenital contractural arachnodactyly . . . *Am. J. Med. Genet.*, 25, 763–773 (1986).

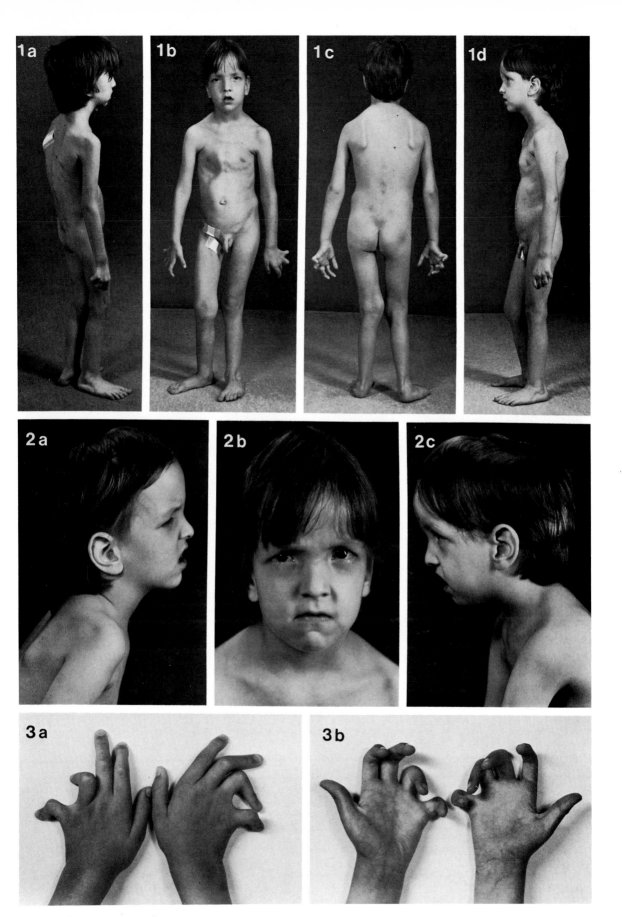

72. Homocystinuria

A metabolic disorder leading to tall stature, visual disorders, and frequently also mental retardation.

Main signs:
1. A clinical picture similar to Marfan syndrome, with age dependent progressive changes: tall stature with often eunuchoid body proportions, conspicuous in childhood and increasing until puberty; arachnodactyly; deficient subcutaneous fat. Long, narrow face (see especially patient 1, 1–3); high palate.
2. Pectus carinatum or excavatum (**2, 6**), scoliosis or kyphoscoliosis, knock-knees (**2**), hernias (**2**, postoperative), ankylosis, 'waddling' gait.
3. Thin, sparse, dry, blond hair; strikingly reddened cheeks, translucent skin. Tendency to eczema.
4. In a half to two-thirds of all cases, mental retardation of various grades of severity. Behavioral disturbances with decreased ability to concentrate, irritability, limited social contact, etc. Possible microcephaly.

Supplementary findings: Dislocation of the lens, usually inferiorly, occurring no later than the second decade of life; myopia; possible cataracts, secondary glaucoma, retinal detachment.

Tendency to form thromboemboli, even in early childhood and in every region of the body; severe premature arteriosclerosis due to homocystinemic damage to the endothelium.

Seizures in some cases.

Hepatomegaly.

Osteoporosis, punctate calcifications of the distal radial and ulnar epiphyses; shortened metacarpal IV in some patients.

Homocystine in the urine or hypermethioninemia demonstrable.

Manifestation: Biochemically, in the first weeks of life; clinically, in childhood or later.

Etiology: Autosomal recessive disorder with absence of the enzyme cystathionine synthetase (gene located on the long arm of chromosome 21 [21q21]). Subdivided into type A and type B according to whether responsive or nonresponsive to vitamin B_6 therapy. In addition there are further biochemically defined types of homocystinuria which, however, do not show the clinical picture described here.

Frequency: About 1:50,000 to 1:150,000 of the population.

Course, prognosis: Life expectancy of untreated patients substantially shortened due to thromboembolic complications.

Diagnosis: By means of special urinary tests and subsequent quantitative determination of homocystine in the blood plasma and urine. With thromboembolism of unknown origin in childhood, homocystinuria must always be considered.

Differential diagnosis: Marfan syndrome, in which, however, luxation of the lens is usually congenital and *upwards*, cheeks are not flushed, hair is unremarkable, joints are hyperextensible. Furthermore, no mental retardation, no analogous tendency to thromboembolism, no progression of signs, and usually a family history of similarly affected persons.

Treatment: About half of the cases respond to high doses of vitamin B_6 (with simultaneous folic acid substitution)—type A. Life-long treatment is required. Type B can be favorably influenced by a methionine-deficient and L-cystine-enriched diet on a long-term basis. Great restraint is needed with operative procedures, especially all avoidable procedures involving the vascular system (venepuncture, etc.) because of the danger of triggering thromboembolism. Genetic counseling. In some cases utilization of prenatal diagnostic possibilities.

Illustrations:
1–4 Patient 1 at age 5½ years. Height 129 cm (average height of a 7-year-old boy). Moderate mental retardation. Blond hair, reddened cheeks. Subluxation of the lenses and myopia diagnosed at age 2 years.
5–7 Patient 2 at age 3¾ years. Height 109 cm (average height of a 5-year-old). No mental retardation. Blond hair. Flushed cheeks, eczema. At age 2½ years slight myopia. No osteoporosis. Neither patient responded to treatment with pharmacological doses of vitamin B_6.

H.-R.W.

References:

Pullon, D.H.H. Homocystinuria and other methioninemias. In: *Neonatal screening for inborn errors of metabolism.* Bickel, H. et al (eds.). Springer, Berlin-Heidelberg-New York, 1980.

Fowler, B. and Børresen, A.L. Prenatal diagnosis of homocystinuria. *Lancet,* II, 875 (1982).

Munnich, A., Saudubray, J.-M. et al. Diet-responsive proconvertin (factor VII) deficiency in homocystinuria. *J. Pediatr.,* 102, 730–734 (1983).

Wilcken, D.E.L., Wilcken, B. et al. Homocystinuria—the effects of betaine . . . *N. Engl. J. Med.,* 309, 448–453 (1983).

Boers, G.H.J., Fowler, B. et al. Improved identification of heterozygotes for homocystinuria . . . *Hum. Genet.,* 69, 164–169 (1985).

Skovby, Fl. Homocystinuria. *Acta Pediatr. Scand.* (Suppl.), 321 (1985).

Amram, S., Palcoux, J.B. et al. Homocystinurie pyridoxino-résistante. *Arch. Fr. Pédiatr.,* 43, 715–717 (1986).

Abbott, M.H., Folstein, S.E. et al. Psychiatric manifestations of homocystinuria . . . *Am. J. Med. Genet.,* 26, 959–969 (1987).

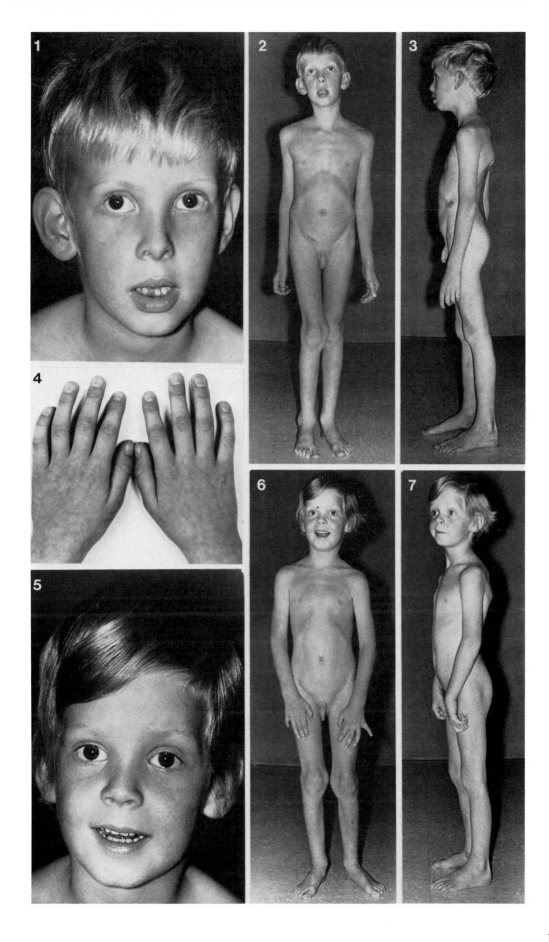

73. XYY Syndrome

A tall-stature syndrome in males, with frequent behavioral disorders and an extra Y chromosome.

Main signs:
1. Tall stature (> 180 cm).
2. Behavioral disorders in 50%.
3. Delayed speech development.

Supplementary findings: Average intelligence. Psyche frequently labile; patients may be unstable, easily led astray, and have a history of deviant behavior.

Increased occurrence of minor anomalies: relatively large head, asymmetrical cranium, dysplastic helices, epicanthus, strabismus, micrognathia; clinodactyly, single-crease fifth finger, simian crease; pectus carinatum, inguinal hernias. Tendency to acne and early varicosities of the lower leg and leg ulcers.

Double 'Y-chromosomal sex chromatin' demonstrable in a simple screening test; confirmation of the abnormal sex chromosome constitution by chromosomal analysis.

Manifestation: Tall stature beginning in puberty, severe acne.

Etiology: The syndrome, expressing the chromosomal aberration of a supernumerary Y chromosome, is caused by faulty separation of the chromosomes during spermatogenesis.

Frequency: About 1:1,000 newborn boys.

Course, prognosis: Average final height of about 1.85 m; occasionally, patients may be much taller. Extreme tallness is a marked psychological handicap, impairing the patient's ability to cope. Possible infertility.

Differential diagnosis: Other tall-stature syndromes, especially Marfan syndrome (p.142).

Treatment: Hormonal therapy if excessive growth is anticipated. Psychological guidance; psychotherapy may be indicated.

Illustrations:
1 A patient at age 14 years (1.82 m).
2 The same patient at 18 years (2.02 m).

H.-R.W./J.K.

References:

Any comprehensive pediatric or internal-medicine textbook.

Robinson, A., Lubs, H.A. et al. Summary of clinical findings: profiles of children with . . . 47, XYY karyotypes. *Birth Defects,* XV, no. 1, 261–266 (1979).

Grass, F., McCombs, J. et al. Reproduction in XYY males . . . implications for genetic counseling. *Am. J. Med. Genet.,* 19, 553–560 (1984).

Netley, C.T. Summary overview of behavioural development in individuals with neonatally identified X and Y aneuploidy. *Birth Defects,* XXII, no. 3, 293–306 (1986).

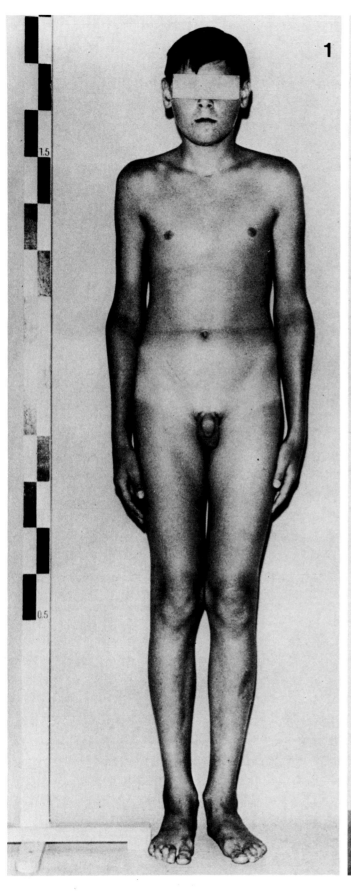

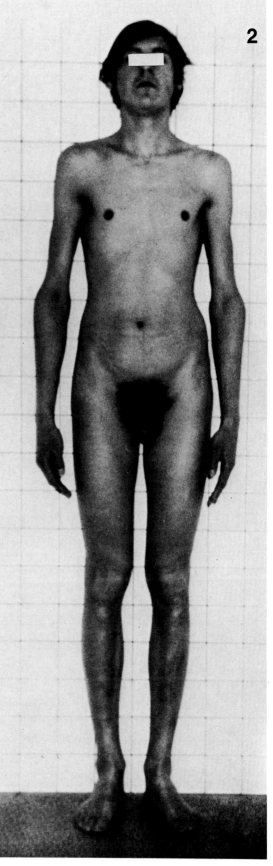

74. Malformation–Retardation Syndrome Due to Incomplete Triploidy

A syndrome of primary subnormality, frequent asymmetry, genital anomalies, and psychomotor retardation with mosaic triploidy.

Main signs:
1. Pre- and postnatal growth deficiency with relatively large, elongated cranium, micrognathia and sometimes low-set poorly formed ears (**1**).
2. Asymmetry of the body due to underdevelopment of one half of the face and/or one extremity (**2a, 2b, 3a**).
3. Hypogenitalism in males (micropenis, cryptorchidism, sometimes hypospadias or intersex features) (**2a, 3a**).
4. Mental retardation; possible seizure disorder.
5. Chromosomally: mosaic triploidy (2N/3N).

Supplementary findings: Average birth weight about 2200 g. Diverse anomalies of the hands and feet: club foot, syndactyly, camptodactyly, clinodactyly, and others (**3b, 3c**). Pigmentation anomalies in some cases.

Manifestation: At birth.

Etiology: The presence of (in the case of the patient in 1–3, 4%) triploid cells (in the given case, 69 XXY) as a mosaic (2N/3N).

Frequency: Low; to date somewhat over 20 cases reported.

Course, prognosis: Not infrequently, initial failure to thrive. Otherwise the prognosis is mainly dependent on the degree of psychomotor or mental retardation.

Diagnosis, differential diagnosis: Silver–Russell syndrome; however, psychomotor retardation and comparatively good body weight should facilitate the clinical differentiation. In case of doubt, chromosomal analysis of cultured skin fibroblasts.

Treatment: Symptomatic. Appropriate handicap aids.

Illustrations:
1–3 The same patient, the second child of healthy, young, nonconsanguineous parents, after a healthy brother.
1 Somewhat small neonate (47 cm; 2400 g; 34 cm head circumference) with relatively large cranium, micrognathia, radial abduction of both hands.
2 The patient at 3 years.
3 At 4½ years. Hypoplasia of the left side of the face and the left upper extremity. At both ages height corresponded to the 10th percentile, head circumference 50th–75th percentile. Genu valgus. Micropenis and bilateral undescended testes. Obvious mental retardation.
3b and 3c Proximally displaced thumbs; cutaneous syndactyly of fingers III/IV, of toes II–IV; clinocamptodactyly of fifth fingers bilaterally, hypoplasia of the fifth toes; widely spaced big and second toes. For a long time the patient was assumed to suffer from the Silver–Russell syndrome. Internal organs: horseshoe kidneys.

H.-R.W.

References:

Graham, J.M., Hoehn, H., Lin, M.S. et al. Diploid-triploid mixoploidy: clinical and cytogenetic aspects. *Pediatrics*, 68, 23–28 (1981).

Tharapel, A.T., Wilroy, R.S., Martens, P.R. et al. Diploid-triploid mosaicism: delineation of the syndrome. *Ann. Génét.*, 26, 229–233 (1983).

Meinecke, P. and Engelbrecht, R. Fehlbildungs-Retardierungssyndrom infolge inkompletter Triploidie. *Monatschr. Kinderheilkd.*, 136, 206–208 (1988).

Küster, W., Beckmann, H., Gebauer, H.J. et al. Triploidie bei Neugeborenen. *Monatschr. Kinderheilkd.* 136, 210–213 (1988).

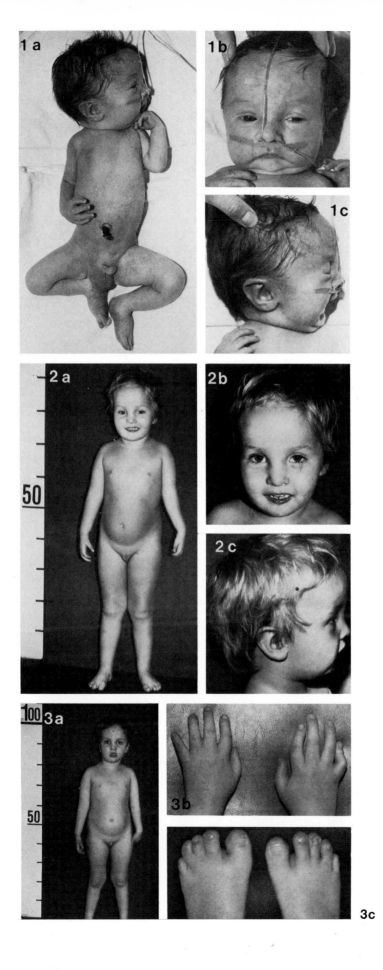

75. Silver–Russell Syndrome

(Russell–Silver Syndrome)

A syndrome of pre- and postnatal slender, small stature, relatively very large cranium with correspondingly small triangular face and micrognathia, fairly marked asymmetry of the body, and clinobrachydactyly of the little fingers.

Main signs:
1. Congenital small size (length and weight) with birth at term. Disproportionately large cranium (**1** p. 155) with prominent forehead, high hair line and frequently very late closure of the anterior fontanelle—however, normal head circumference at birth and normal further development: 'pseudohydrocephalus'. Small triangular face, often with fine, small nose, short philtrum, and large thin-lipped mouth with down-turned corners. Micrognathia (**3** p. 155).
2. Postnatal continuation of slow growth in height and especially weight (under or about the third percentile; final height about 150 cm). Not infrequently distinct asymmetry due to underdevelopment of one side of the body or a part thereof. The upper extremities may be relatively short (**2a** p. 155), and the lower extremities long. Slender build, also with narrow thorax and insufficiently developed musculature (**2** p. 155).
3. Clino- or clinobrachydactyly of the little fingers. Delayed bone age (**4** p. 155).

Supplementary findings: High squeaky voice persisting for years. Marked tendency to heavy sweating. Café au lait spots of the skin in some patients. Hip or other skeletal dysplasias. Malformations of the urogenital system. With marked asymmetry of the lower extremities, tilting of the pelvis and secondary scoliosis.

Possible signs of dissociated precocious puberty: most frequently, early elevation of gonadotropin in the urine.

Gross motor development may be delayed. Exceptionally, mental retardation (about 15% of cases).

Manifestation: Pre- and postnatally.

Etiology: Usually sporadic occurrence. Cases suggesting autosomal dominant or autosomal recessive inheritance are the exception. Considerable phenotypic variability.

Frequency: Moderately low; but over 200 publications.

Course, prognosis: Usually relatively favorable (apart from the small adult height); in the individual cases dependent on the degree of expression of the clinical picture and on the significance of possible additional malformations and handicaps.

Treatment: Physiotherapy or orthopedic, nephrourological, or psychological care may be needed. Growth hormone deficiency and response to high doses of HGH may occur.

Illustrations:
1–3 A 2-year-old girl of normal psychomotor development (birth at term, 1800 g and 49 cm). Height age, 18 months (i.e., below the 10th percentile); weight age, 9 months (i.e., below the 3rd percentile). Congenital hemiatrophy of the whole right side of the body including the ear and nose (osseus atrophy shown in **3a**); secondary tilting of the pelvis and mild secondary scoliosis. Relatively large, but normal-for-age, cranium (46.5 cm). Prominent, slightly bulging forehead. Small face; microretrognathia. Clinobrachydactyly of the fifth fingers; zygodactyly on the right. Rather unusually tall lumbar vertebral bodies. Ectopic ureterocele with megaureter and hydronephrosis on the left and with left quiescent accessory kidney and ureter. Markedly elevated gonadotropins in the urine.

H.-R.W./J.K.

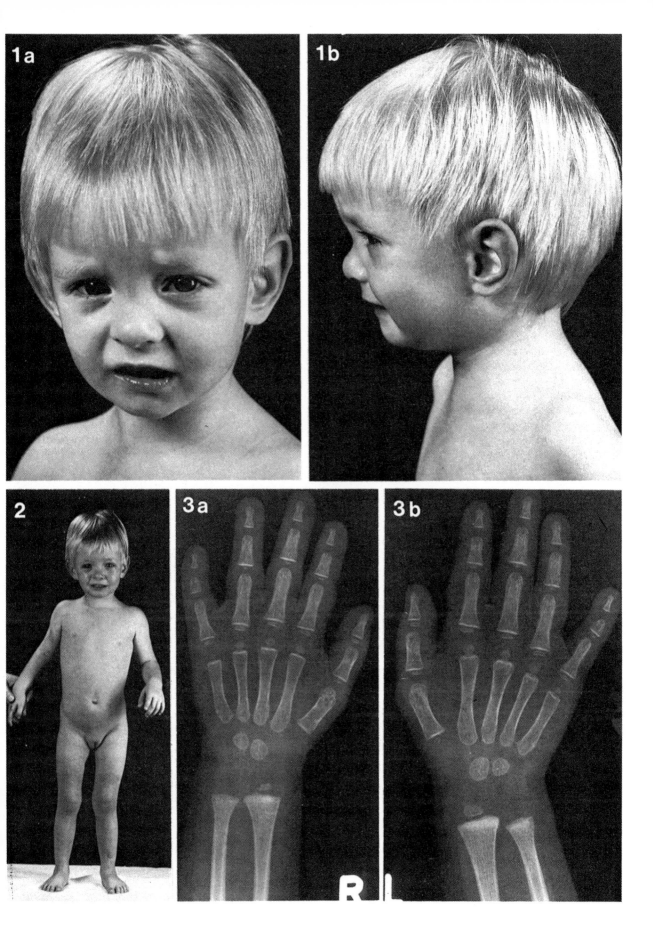

76. Silver–Russell Syndrome (cont.)

(Russell-Silver Syndrome)

Illustrations:
1–5 A child born at term with birth weight 1750 g; mental development within normal limits. Shown at 4½ months (52 cm, 3320 g), at 3 years 4 months (75 cm, 5500 g), and 12 years 5 months (126.5 cm, 14.8 kg, each far below the third percentile). Extremely slender build. Long cranium with large protruding forehead, and high and initially thin hairline, head circumference normal for age. Right half of the face somewhat fuller than the left. Slightly low-set ears. Congenital ptosis of the left upper eyelid. Relatively large thin-lipped mouth with slightly down-turned corners. Microretrognathia. Overbite, narrowly spaced teeth, especially in the lower jaw. Caries. Squeaky voice. Short upper extremities. Slight clinobrachydactyly of the little fingers; bilateral zygodactyly with a double nail on the left second toe. Extremely narrow, slim hand with markedly delayed bone age. Pseudoepiphyses of metacarpals I and II proximally and hypoplastic middle phalanx of fifth finger. Possible ventricular septal defect. Slightly dilated right renal pelvis on pyelography; hypospadias. Profuse sweating.

H.-R.W.

References:

Silver, H.K., Kiyasu, W., George, J. et al. Syndrome of congenital hemihypertrophy, shortness of stature, and elevated urinary gonadotropins. *Pediatrics*, 12, 368–375 (1953).

Russell, A. A syndrome of 'intra-uterine' dwarfism recognizable at birth with cranio-facial dysostosis, disproportionately short arms, and other anomalies (5 examples). *Proc. Roy. Soc. Med.*, 47, 1040 (1954).

Tanner, J.M., Lejarraga, H., Cameron, N. The natural history of the Silver–Russell syndrome: A longitudinal study of thirty-nine cases. *Pediatr. Res.*, 9, 611–623 (1975).

Angehrn, V., Zachmann, M., Prader, A. Silver–Russell syndrome. Observations in 20 patients. *Helv. Paed. Acta, 34, 297–308 (1979).*

Saal, H.M., Ragon, R.A., Pepin, M.G. Reevaluation of Russell–Silver syndrome. J. Pediatr., 107, 733–737 (1985).

Partsch, C.-J., Hermanussen, M., Sippell, W.G. Treatment of Silver–Russell type dwarfism with human growth hormone . . . *Acta Endocrinol. Suppl.*, 279, 139–146 (1986).

Davies, P.S., Valley, R., Preece, M.A. Adolescent growth and pubertal progression in the Silver–Russell syndrome. *Arch. Dis. Childh.*, 63, 130–135 (1988).

Patton, M.A. Russell–Silver Syndrome. *J. Med. Genet.*, 25, 557–560 (1988).

Chitayat, D., Friedman, J.M. et al. Hepatocellular carcinoma in a child with familial Russell–Silver syndrome. *Am. J. Med. Genet.*, 31, 909–914 (1988).

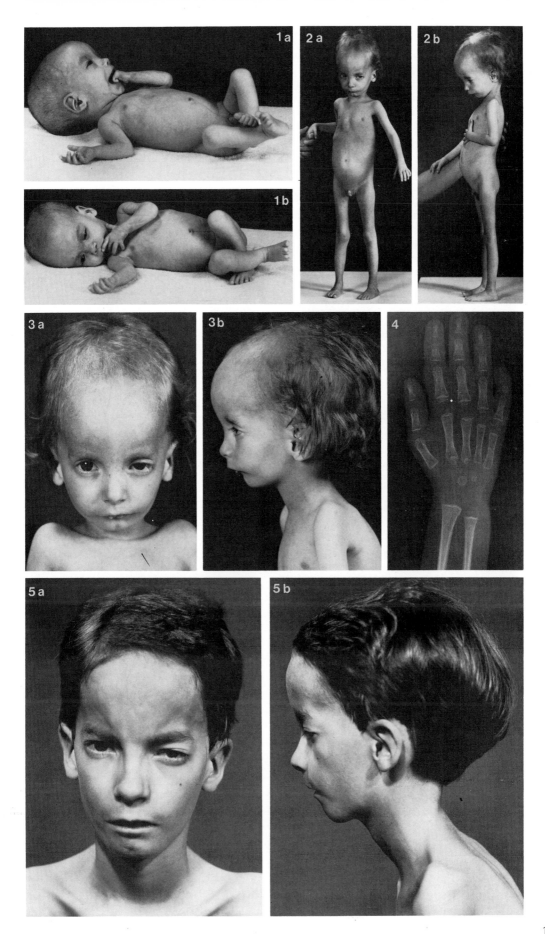

77. Blepharophimosis Syndrome

A genetically distinct syndrome with epicanthus medialis inversus, lateral displacement of the inner canthi, ptosis, and blepharophimosis in addition to female infertility in type I.

Main signs:
1. Epicanthus medialis inversus between the upper and lower lids, short palpebral fissure with displacement of the inner corner of the eye (telecanthus). Ptosis, flat nasal root, anteverted nares, and strabismus.
2. Dysplastic helices in some cases.
3. Primary hypogonadism with sterility in female type I patients.
4. Muscular hypotonia in early infancy.

Supplementary findings: Cardiac defects, occasionally mental retardation. Microphthalmia, anophthalmia, microcornea, hyperopia (hypermetropia), strabismus, nystagmus, amblyopia.

Manifestation: At birth.

Etiology: Infertility in type I patients, affecting females only, is transmitted as an autosomal dominant sex-linked characteristic. Penetrance is complete; the sex ratio of affected persons in an affected family is shifted to an excess of males.

Type II is inherited from both males and females by autosomal dominant transmission with incomplete penetrance. Among the children of affected males, predominately females are affected, and among the children of affected women, predominately males. The sex ratio of affected persons within the family is normal.

Frequency: Type I is more frequent than type II. This is of significance in genetic counseling with respect to the infertile women.

Course, prognosis: Cardiac defects and mental retardation will prevent some patients from living a full life.

Differential diagnosis: Blepharophimosis associated with malformations as part of other syndromes.

Treatment: Ophthalmological and surgical care. Definition and hormonal substitution treatment of the ovarian insufficiency.

Illustrations:
1 and 2 A 5-month-old female with epicanthus medialis inversus, telecanthus, ptosis, blepharophimosis, flat nasal root, and anteverted nares.

J.K.

References:

Callahan, A. Surgical correction of the blepharophimosis syndrome. *Trans. Amer. Acad. Ophthal. Otolaryng.*, 77, 687–695 (1973).

Pueschel, S.M. and Barsel-Bowers, G. A dominantly inherited congenital anomaly syndrome with blepharophimosis. *J. Pediatr.*, 95, 1010–1012 (1979).

Zlotogora, J., Sagi, M., Cohen, T. The blepharophimosis, ptosis, and epicanthus inversus syndrome: delineation of two types. *Am. J. Hum. Genet.*, 35, 1020–1027 (1983).

Oley, C. and Baraitser, M. Blepharophimosis, ptosis, epicanthus inversus syndrome (BPES syndrome). Syndrome of the month. *J. Med. Genet.*, 25, 47–51 (1988).

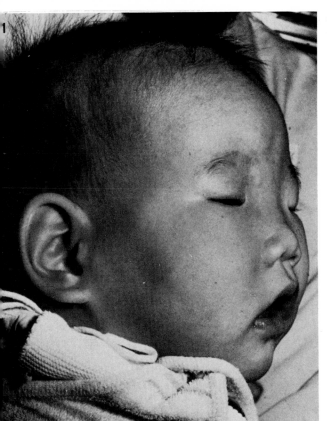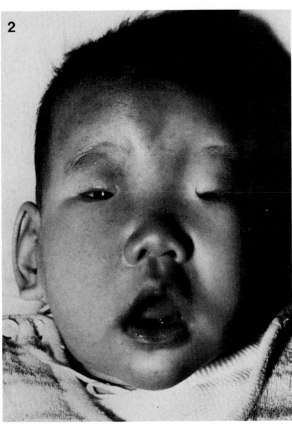

78. Primordial Small Stature with Relative Macrocrania, Peculiar Physiognomy, Further Minor Malformations, and Normal Psychomotor Development

A syndrome of primordial small stature, unusual facies with blepharophimosis, large dolichocephalic head, and normal mental development.

Main signs:
1. Primordial, for the most part proportional, slender short stature, well under the third percentile. Relative macrocephaly with dolichocephaly (1–3).
2. Facies: short, narrow palpebral fissures with slight antimongoloid slant under relatively thick eyebrows. Suggestion of epicanthus bilaterally. Low-set ears. Prominent nose. Small, thin-lipped, narrow mouth, which appears pinched (1, 4). Open bite. Massive caries (? secondary to difficulty in caring for the teeth because of the small opening of the mouth).
3. Hypogonadism, bilateral cryptorchidism. Simian crease left, suggested on the right; hypoplastic-appearing distal phalanges of the fingers; clinodactyly of the fifth fingers (5).

Supplementary findings: Slumped posture, winged scapulae; dorsal kyphosis, which could be compensated (2, 3).

Psychomotor development normal for age.

X-rays: Dysplasia of the first rib on the left. Discordant development of the ossification centers on the wrist X-ray and profoundly retarded bone age (by about 3½ years) (5).

Manifestation: At birth.

Etiology: Undetermined.

Course, prognosis: Apart from short stature expected to be favorable.

Differential diagnosis: Other syndromes with short stature and blepharophimosis.

Treatment: Symptomatic.

Illustrations:
1–5 A 7-year-old boy, the first child of healthy, young nonconsanguineous parents of normal height. A healthy younger brother. Birth of the proband shortly before term with 2250 g and 44 cm. At 7 years 2 months, 104 cm; head circumference at 6 years 10 months, 52.3 cm. No abnormality of internal organs; thorough endocrinological examination negative; chromosome analysis negative.

H.-R.W.

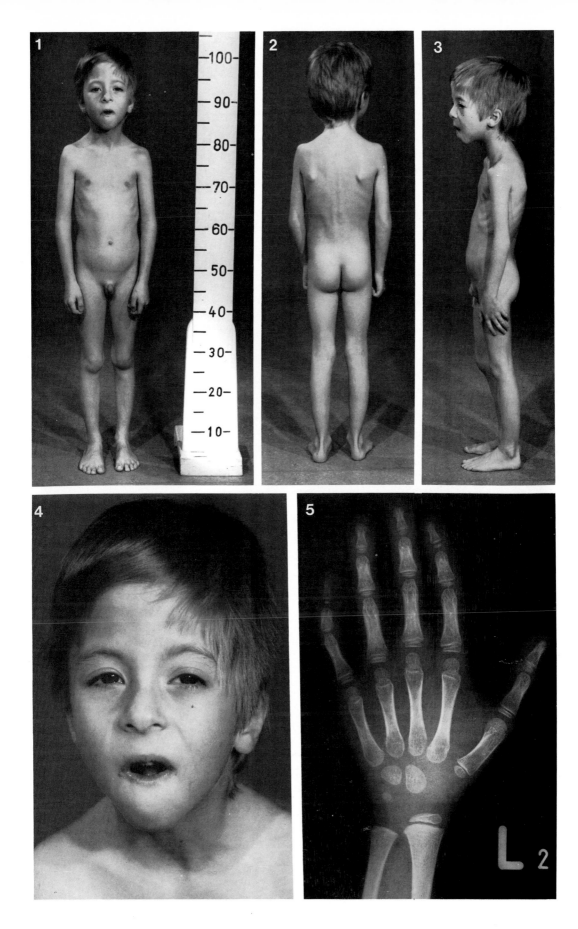

159

79. Syndrome of Blepharophimosis, Camptodactyly, Small Stature, Mental Retardation, and Sensorineural Hearing Impairment

A syndrome of unusual features of the face, hands, and feet combined with growth disorder, mental retardation, and impaired hearing.

Main signs:

1. Facies: High forehead, short narrow palpebral fissures, thick eyebrows and mild synophrys; low-set simple auricles; low nasal root, and small mouth (with diastema, high palate, bifid uvula) (1–3).
2. Camptodactyly of fingers II–V along with clinodactyly of the little fingers (6). Bilateral hallux-valgus deviation and dysplasia of the little toes with rudimentary or absent nails.
3. Small stature (under the third percentile at 5 and at 13½ years with somewhat short lower extremities (4, 5).
4. Primary mental retardation (IQ 44 at 13½ years).
5. Primary bilateral sensorineural hearing impairment.

Supplementary findings: Long narrow thorax with mild funnel chest.

Strabismus (operated); ocular fundi normal.

X-rays: Cone-shaped epiphyses of the proximal phalanges of toes II–V bilaterally.

Manifestation: At birth (hearing impairment recognized in infancy).

Etiology: Unknown.

Course, prognosis: Affected especially by the severe degree of mental retardation.

Differential diagnosis: Other small stature and blepharophimosis syndromes.

Treatment: Symptomatic.

Illustrations:

1–6 The proband at age 5 years (1, 2, 6) and 13½ years (3–5). First child of healthy young nonconsanguineous parents; premature birth; no serious problems in the first year of life. Several seizures between the third and fifth years of life; neurological examination negative. EEG negative, electromyogram unremarkable. Clinical and laboratory examinations negative. Chromosome analysis negative.

H.-R.W.

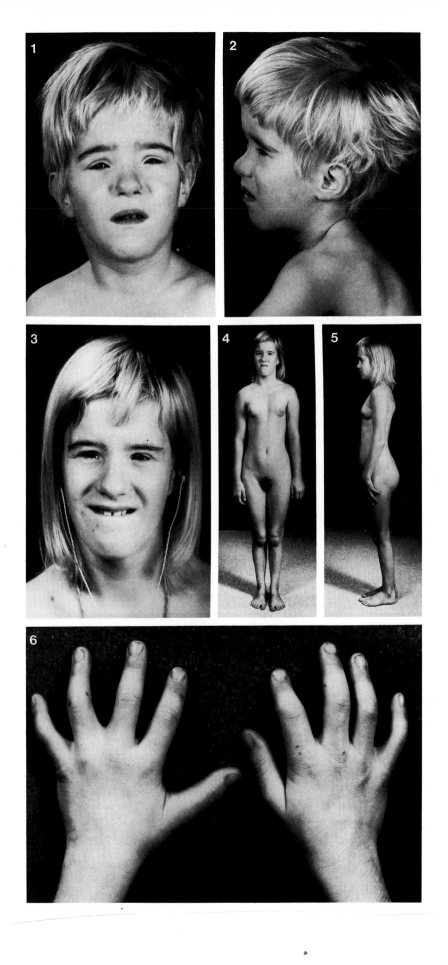

80. Rubinstein–Taybi Syndrome

(Broad Thumb–Broad Hallux Syndrome)

A syndrome of characteristic facies, microcephalic psychomotor retardation, small stature, and anomalies of the hands and feet with broad distal phalanges, especially of the thumbs and halluces.

Main signs:

1. Cranium and facies: microcephaly of varied grades of severity, frequently with prominent forehead and large anterior fontanelle. Antimongoloid slant of the palpebral fissures, broad nasal root, epicanthic folds, frequent strabismus, prominent eyebrows and eyelids, possible ptosis, and mild anomalies of the external ears (**1, 2, 6**). Beak-shaped nose, aquiline or straight, with anterior prolongation of the nasal septum (**2**). High palate, slightly receding chin.

2. Broad distal phalanges of the thumbs and halluces, also often of other rays (**3–7**). Thumbs not infrequently radially deviated at the interphalangeal joint ('hitchhiker thumb', **6, 7**). Possible clinodactyly and overlapping toes.

3. Psychomotor retardation (IQ usually under 50); frequent EEG anomalies.

4. Short stature (usually about or below the third percentile).

Supplementary findings: Frequently undescended testicles. Frequent hirsutism. Development of kyphoscoliosis. Heart and kidney defects possible.

X-rays may show deformity of the proximal phalanges in cases with abnormal angulation of the thumbs and/or halluces; sometimes duplication of the big-toe region. Generalized delay of ossification. Possible anomalies of the pelvis, vertebral column and/or thorax.

Manifestation: At birth and thereafter.

Etiology: Unknown; since there has been concordance in monozygotic twins, genetic factors must be assumed. No increased risk of recurrence in further children of parents with an affected child.

Frequency: Among the mentally retarded, up to 1 in 500 and higher.

Course, prognosis: For the most part dependent on the degree of mental retardation and the quality of support and education of the child. Average life expectancy probably shortened.

Differential diagnosis: The Cornelia de Lange syndrome should not be difficult to exclude.

Treatment: Symptomatic. Any appropriate handicap aids.

Illustrations:

1–5 A 6½-year-old girl, the second child of healthy nonconsanguineous parents after a healthy sibling. Head circumference at birth (with otherwise normal measurements), 32.5 cm; presently 47.6 cm (below the second percentile). Height and weight around the tenth percentile. General developmental retardation. Hirsutism. On X-ray, distinct asymmetry of the facial bones and skull; retarded bone age. Chromosomal analysis negative.

6 and 7 A characteristically affected 4-month-old infant.

H.-R.W.

References:

Thiele, U., Draf, U., Heldt, J.P. Das Rubinstein–Taybi-Syndrom. *Dtsch. Med. Wochenschr.*, 1505, 1978.

Baraitser, M. and Preece, M.A. The Rubinstein–Taybi syndrome: occurrence in two sets of identical twins. *Clin. Genet.*, 23, 318–320 (1983).

Gillies, D.R.N. and Roussounis, S.H. Rubinstein–Taybi syndrome: further evidence of a genetic aetiology. *Develop. Med. Child. Neurol.*, 27, 751–755 (1985).

Berry, C. Rubinstein–Taybi syndrome. *J. Med. Genet.*, 24, 562–566 (1987).

Hennekam, R.C.M., Lommen, E.J.P., Strengers, J.L.M. et al. Rubinstein-Taybi syndrome in a mother and son. *Eur. J. Pediatr.*, 148, 439 (1989).

Bonioli, E. and Bellini, C. Inheritance of Rubinstein–Taybi syndrome. *Am. J. Med. Genet.*, 32, 559 (1989).

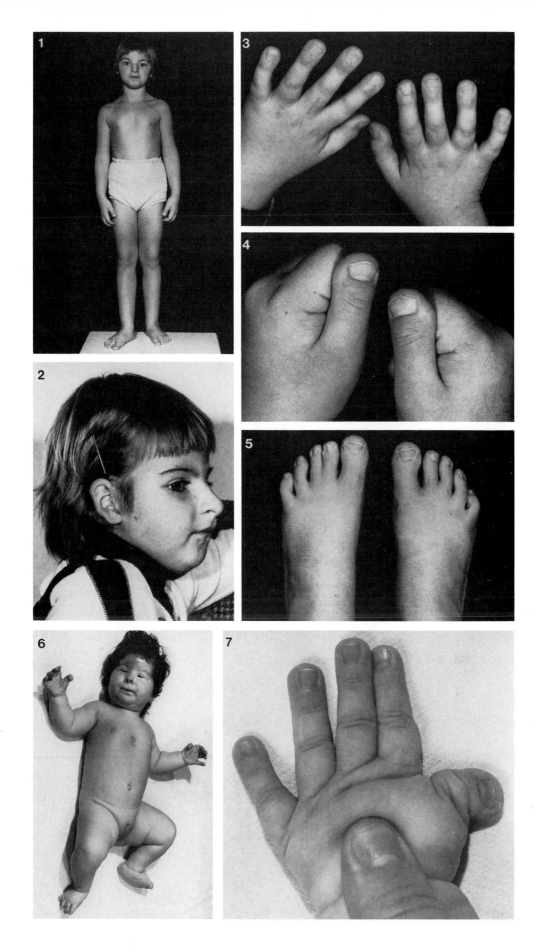

163

81. Syndrome of Dyscrania or Microcephaly, Psychomotor Retardation, and Short Stature with Anomalies of the Hands and Feet

A familial dyscrania-microcephaly-retardation syndrome with small stature and broad, short thumbs and halluces.

Main signs:
1. Dyscrania with high forehead, sloping occiput (1–3, 1a–3a); microcephaly.
2. Facies: slight antimongoloid slant of the palpebral fissures, low-set ears, slightly receding chin (1–3, 1a–3a).
3. Psychomotor retardation of variable severity.
4. Short stature (below the third percentile).
5. Short hands and feet with stubby, broad thumbs and halluces (1b–3b, 4, 5).

Supplementary findings: Unilateral undescended testes in both the boys illustrated, as well as inguinal hernias. Micropenis and marked scrotal hypoplasia in the child in 3.

Manifestation: At birth and thereafter.

Etiology: Genetically determined syndrome.

Course, prognosis: Essentially dependent on the degree of mental retardation.

Treatment: Symptomatic.

Illustrations:
1, 1a, and 1b A 9-month-old infant, the first child of young nonconsanguineous parents. Normal birth measurements. Head circumference at 9 months about the second percentile, at 2 years well under the second percentile. Initially, telangiectatic nevi spread over the face. Delayed closure of a very large anterior fontanelle. No psychomotor development (CT scan: dilated ventricles; EEG: increased seizure activity). Small size, on and below the third percentile. Short, stubby thumbs, contracted in the physiological position (1b), as are also the halluces. High arched palate, pectus carinatum, club feet, cardiac defect (VSD). Optic fundi negative; detailed clinical, laboratory, and enzymatic investigations negative. Chromosomal analysis negative.

2, 2a, 2b, 4 and 5 The 26-year-old mother of the proband: craniofacial dysmorphism, retardation, abnormal thumbs and big toes (also present in the mother's father and her two sisters). Extensive similarities of the mother's and son's palmar ridge patterns.

3, 3a, and 3b The 13-month-old son of one of the sisters of the proband's mother. The first child of young nonconsanguineous parents. Birth 3 weeks before term with 2300 g, 44 cm, and 32 cm head circumference. At 14 months microcephaly; premature closure of the cranial sutures; CT scan: partial dilatation of the cerebral ventricles. Psychomotor retardation. Small size (at 14 months around the third percentile). Plump paw-like hands and plumpish feet, broad thumbs and big toes. Fundi normal. Chromosomes normal (also in banded preparations).

H.-R.W.

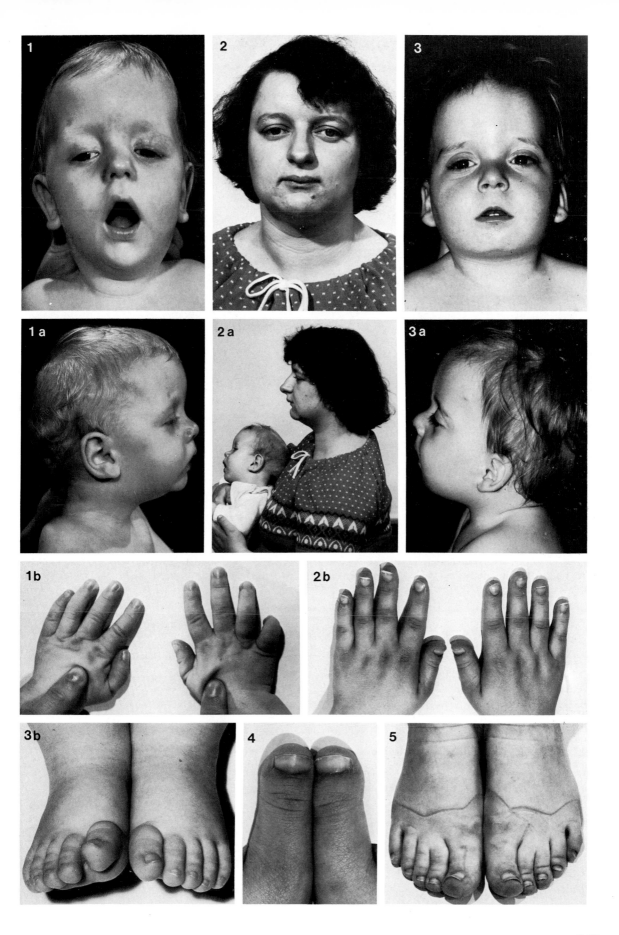

82. Cockayne Syndrome

A disorder manifesting, as a rule, from the second year of life onwards, and leading to severe growth retardation with typical facies, microcephaly, mental deficiency, neurological and ocular defects, and other anomalies.

Main signs:
1. Severe growth deficiency, disproportionate due to excessive length of the extremities and oversized hands and feet (1).
2. Typical facies, narrow, 'sunken in' and 'too old', with deep-set eyes, thin nose, prognathism (1–3).
3. Increasingly apparent microcephaly.
4. Progressive neurological defects (ataxia, sometimes tremor; hearing impairment, which may progress to deafness, and decreased visual acuity—see below) as well as mental retardation (due to a special form of orthochromatic leukodystrophy).

Supplementary findings: Development of ocular and visual defects, eventually blindness; retinitis pigmentosa; optic atrophy, cataracts (in about one-third of cases); possible corneal clouding.

Hypersensitivity to UV light with exanthemata and subsequent pigment changes and scarring.

Progressive development of flexion contractures of the large joints and increasing dorsal kyphosis.

Cryptorchidism in some patients; impaired sweating, disorder of water–salt metabolism, decreased resistance to infection.

Radiologically, calcifications of the basal ganglia, thickening of the calvaria, and other findings.

No evidence of a consistent endocrinological or biochemical abnormality.

Manifestation: Starting in the second year of life (after initial normal development for the greater part of the first year of life); however, a congenital form ('type 2') also occurs.

Etiology: Autosomal recessive disorder. Basic defect unknown. Cells are UV sensitive; defective DNA repair.

Frequency: Very low; about 100 cases have been described.

Course, prognosis: Progressive, leading eventually to complete dependence. Decreased life expectancy.

Differential diagnosis: 'Seckel syndrome' (p.168), Dubowitz syndrome (p.176), progeria (p.270), de Barsy syndrome (p.276), and Bloom syndrome (p.360) are readily excluded.

Treatment: Symptomatic. Avoidance of exposure to sunlight. Cataract operation, hearing aids may be indicated. Genetic counseling of the parents. Prenatal diagnosis.

Illustrations:
1–3 An 18-year-old, the only child of healthy parents. Birth measurements 3875 g and 55 cm. Quite unremarkable development until the second year of life; thereafter, marked, progressive, slowing of physical and mental development. Presently, typical senile facial appearance, microcephaly (43.5 cm), severe growth deficiency (97.5 cm) with long extremities and large hands and feet. Ataxia, tremor, mental retardation, photosensitivity. Visual and hearing impairments.

H.-R.W.

References:

Schönenfeld, H. and Frohn, K. Das Cockayne-Syndrom. *Monatschr. Kinderheilkd.*, 117, 103 (1969).
Bensmann, A., Brauner, M., Teboul-Faure, et al. Le syndrome de Cockayne. *J. Radiol. Electrol.*, 59, 375 (1978).
Soffer, D., Grotzky, H.W., Rapin, I. et al. Cockayne syndrome: unusual neuropathologic findings and review of the literature. *Ann. Neurol.*, 6, 340 (1979).
Houstin, C.S., Zaleski, W.A. et al. Identical male twins and brother with Cockayne syndrome. *Am. J. Med. Genet.*, 13, 211–223 (1982).
Smits, M.G., Gabreels, F.J.M. et al. Peripheral and central myelinopathy in Cockayne's syndrome ... *Neuropediatrics*, 13, 161–167 (1982).
Grunnet, M.L., Zimmerman, A.W. et al. Ultrastructure and electrodiagnosis of peripheral neuropathy in Cockayne's syndrome. *Neurology*, 33, 1606–1609 (1983).
Ohta, S., Shima, A. et al. Ultraviolet sensitivity of Cockayne syndrome ... *Cong. Anom.*, 23, 399–403 (1983).
Lehmann, A.R., Francis, A.J. et al. Prenatal diagnosis of Cockayne's syndrome. *Lancet*, I, 486–488 (1985).
Silengo, M.C., Franceschini, P. et al. Distinctive skeletal dysplasia in Cockayne syndrome. *Pediatr. Radiol.*, 16, 264–266 (1986).
Somer, M., Rossi, L. et al. Cockayne syndrome, early-onset type ... *Clin. Genet.*, 29, 473–474 (1986).
Sugita, K., Suzuki, N. et al. Cockayne syndrome with delayed recovery of RNA synthesis after ultraviolet irradiation but normal ultraviolet survival. *Pediatr. Res.*, 21, 34–37 (1986).
Patton, M.A., Giannelli, F., Frances, A.J. et al. Early onset of Cockayne's syndrome ... *J. Med. Genet.*, 26, 154 (1989).

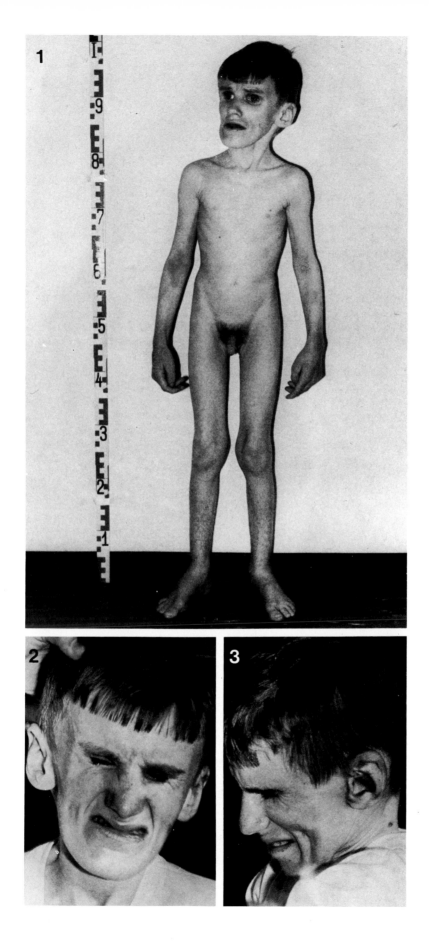

83. Seckel Syndrome

('Bird-headed Dwarfism')

A rare, autosomal recessive syndrome with intrauterine growth retardation, postnatal growth deficiency, mental retardation, microcephaly, prominent nose, and micrognathia ('bird-head appearance').

Main signs:
1. Intrauterine growth retardation. Birth weight about 1500 g.
2. Postnatal continuation of growth deficiency with SD of −5 to −11.
3. Microcephaly (−4 to −14 SD), premature closure of the cranial sutures. Mental retardation (IQ below 50–80).
4. Prominent aquiline nose, large eyes, antimongoloid slant of the palpebral fissures, micrognathia, dysplastic helices.

Supplementary findings: High palate, hypoplasia of the dental enamel, retarded bone age, hirsutism, fifth finger clinodactyly, hip dysplasia, cryptorchidism, clitoral hyperplasia. Further possible malformations of all kinds have been noted.

Manifestation: Prenatally; at birth.

Etiology: Autosomal recessive inheritance.

Frequency: Low; up to 1985 about 20 cases were observed.

Course, prognosis: A 13-year-old patient attained a height of 124 cm; the oldest known patient was 104 cm at 22 years. In one-third of all patients the IQ is below 50; in isolated cases IQs of 74 and 79 have been recorded.

Differential diagnosis: Mainly the osteodysplastic primordial growth deficiency types I–III. The microcephalic growth deficiency syndrome of Dubowitz, alcohol embryopathy, the Cornelia de Lange syndrome, trisomy 18, and Bloom syndrome can be well differentiated by phenotype.

Treatment: Symptomatic. Genetic counseling. Ultrasonographic diagnosis during pregnancy.

Illustrations:
1–3 A characteristically affected newborn.

J.K./H.-R.W.

References:

Majewski, F. and Goecke, T. Studies of microcephalic primordial dwarfism I: approach to a delineation of the Seckel syndrome. *Am. J. Med. Genet.*, 12, 7–21 (1982).

Thompson, E. and Pembrey, M. Seckel syndrome: an overdiagnosed syndrome. *J. Med. Genet.*, 22, 192–201 (1985).

Butler, M.G., Hall, B.D., Maclean, R.N. et al. Do some patients with Seckel syndrome have hematological problems and/or chromosome breakage? *Am. J. Med. Genet.*, 27, 645–649 (1987).

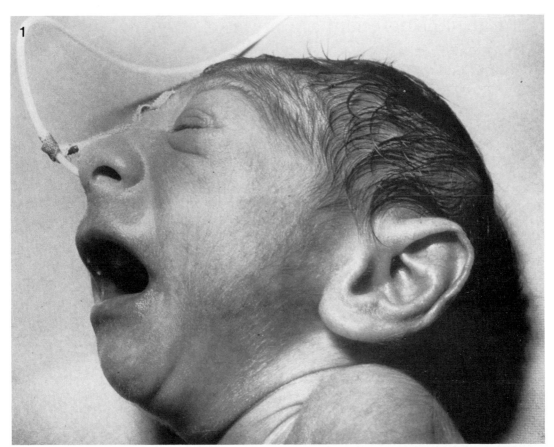

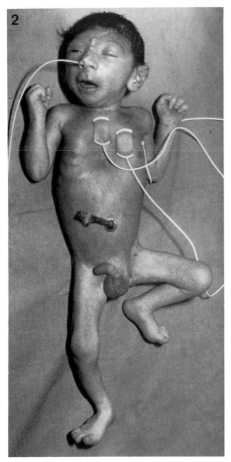

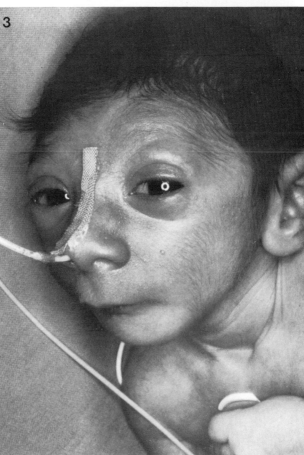

169

84. Primordial Microcephalic and Osteodysplastic Dwarfism

(Bird-headed Seckel-like Type with Osteodysplasia)

A clinical picture with very marked pre- and post-natal growth retardation, microcephaly, 'bird face', mental retardation, osteodysplasia, and further anomalies.

Main signs:
1. Marked intrauterine growth retardation.
2. Postnatal continuation of marked growth deficiency.
3. Microcephaly (low and receding forehead; prematurely closed, prominent cranial sutures; prominent occiput); psychomotor retardation.
4. 'Bird face' as a result of receding forehead, relatively large eyes, prominent aquiline nose, receding chin.
5. Osteodysplasias: S-shaped, long, narrow clavicles; atypical narrowing of the long bones (ventrolateral curving of the femora); abnormally shaped pelvis (ventral prolongation of the iliac crests, absent acetabular angle, elongated pubic and ischial bones, unusual narrowness of the hip joint space on X-ray) and marked disturbance of metaphyseal growth. Joints very poorly formed, causing an increase in mobility in some and marked limitation in others.

Supplementary findings: Marked hypotrichosis and dry, finely scaled skin. Urogenital anomalies. Fifth finger clinodactyly.

Manifestation: Intrauterine; at birth.

Etiology: Several types of 'Seckel-like' osteodysplastic primordial dwarfism occur. Heterogeneity? Autosomal recessive inheritance seems to be the most likely.

Frequency: Low. Similarity of the present case with the type 3 of Majewski et al. and especially with the observation of Winter et al.

Course, prognosis: Poor, with respect to mental development.

Differential diagnosis: other types of primordial microcephalic osteodysplastic dwarfism.

Treatment: Symptomatic. Genetic counseling. Ultrasonographic prenatal diagnosis possible in future pregnancies.

Illustrations:
1–9 The second child of young, healthy, nonconsanguineous parents after a healthy girl. (1–3, during the newborn period; 4–6, at 6 months; 7–9 at 18 months). Spontaneous birth 9 days after term with birth weight 1200 g, 36 cm length, 27 cm head circumference. Facial asymmetry; strabismus. Hypotrichosis; dry, scaly skin. Hypermobile knees, limitation of movement of the other large joints; rocker-bottom feet. Distally tapering fingers, fifth finger clinodactyly, bilateral simian crease. Bilateral cryptorchidism. Right hydronephrosis with ureteral stenosis. Measurements at 6 months: 3550 g, 52 cm length, 31 cm head circumference. At 3½ years length, 69 cm, head circumference 34 cm (all measurements well below the second percentile). CT scan: Hydrocephalus *int. et ext. e vacuo;* possible bilateral hypoplasia of the frontal lobes. Severely impaired mental and motor development. Chromosome analysis of cultured lymphocytes and fibroblasts (including banded preparations) negative.
7–9 Extremely delayed osseus development; horizontal acetabular roofs; short, relatively wide femoral necks; and narrow joint cavities.

H.-R.W.

References:

Majewski, F., Stoeckenius, M., Kemperdick, H. Studies of microcephalic primordial dwarfism III: an intrauterine dwarf with platyspondyly and anomalies of pelvis and clavicles—osteodysplastic primordial dwarfism Type III. *Am. J. Med. Genet.,* 12, 37–42 (1982).

Winter, R.M., Wigglesworth, J., Harding, B.N. Osteodysplastic primordial dwarfism: report of a further patient with manifestations similar to those seen in patients with types I and III. *Am. J. Med. Genet.,* 21, 569–574 (1985).

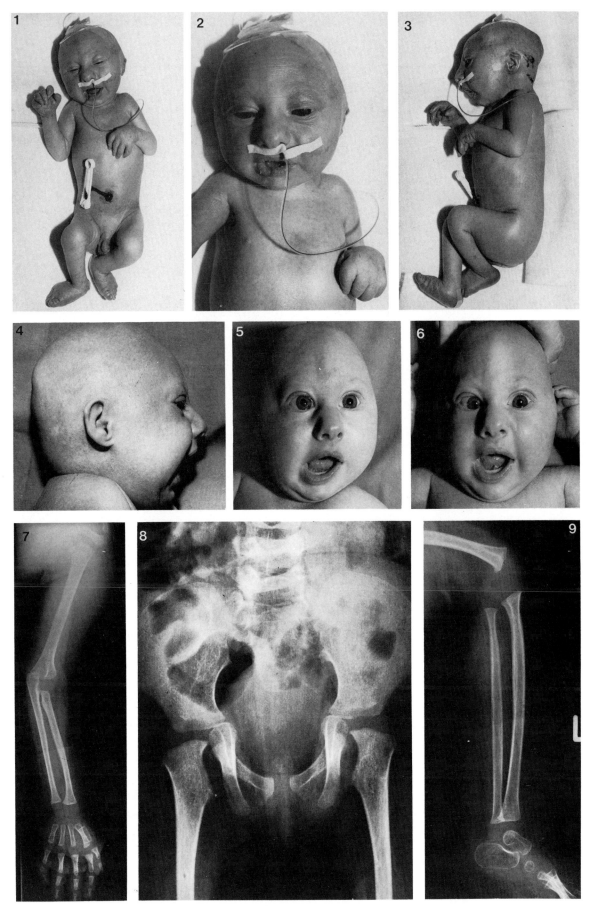

171

85. A Further Microcephaly–Growth Deficiency–Retardation Syndrome

An unknown syndrome with unusual facies, microcephaly and mental retardation, short stature, cardiac defects, and other anomalies.

Main signs:
1. Facies: Hypertelorism, epicanthic folds, blepharophimosis, prominent eyebrows, stenosis of the lacrimal duct, convergent strabismus; short, broad nose; gothic palate, retrognathia (1, 2).
2. Microcephaly (below the third percentile) with psychomotor retardation.
3. Short stature (below the third percentile).
4. VSD; persistent ductus arteriosis (operated); patent foramen ovale.
5. Complete cutaneous syndactyly of the third and fourth fingers bilaterally (3); mild syndactyly of the first and second toes bilaterally.

Supplementary findings: Hypotonia. Hip dysplasia and pes valgus. Unusual cry. Hypoplastic optic papillae, irregular pigmentation of the fundi.

Manifestation: At birth.

Etiology: Uncertain. Chromosomal analysis unremarkable (high-resolution technique).

Course, prognosis: Poor, in view of the mental impairment.

Diagnosis, differential diagnosis: Other microcephaly–growth deficiency syndromes.

Treatment: Cardiac care. Appropriate handicap aids.

Illustrations:
1–3 The second child of healthy parents; sibling healthy. At birth (in the 38th week of pregnancy), obvious intrauterine growth retardation, with birth weight 1900 g, length 42 cm and head circumference 30.5 cm. Oligohydramnios, small placenta.

H.-R.W.

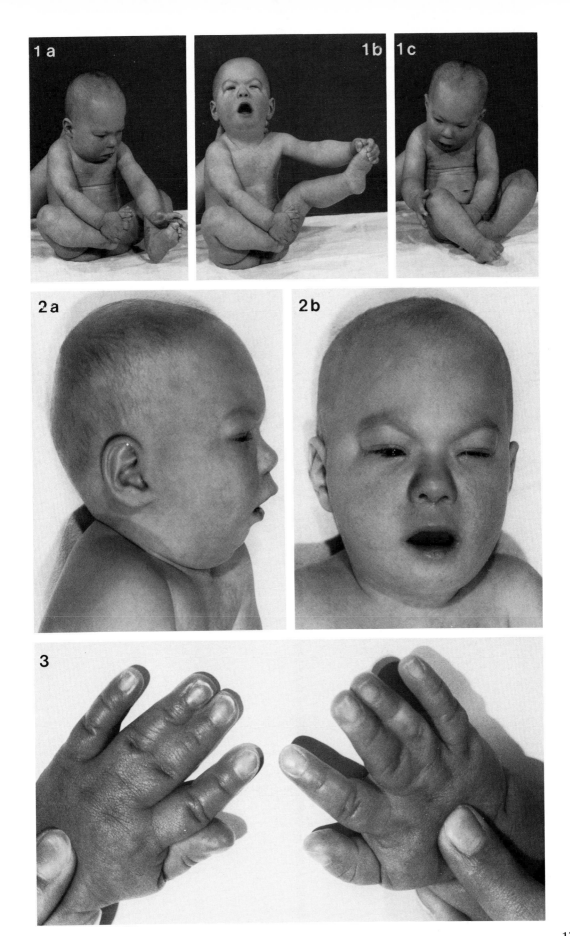

173

86. Coffin–Siris Syndrome

A characteristic syndrome of growth deficiency, microcephaly, psychomotor retardation, unusual facies, abnormalities of the hair, and aplasia of the terminal phalanges of the fifth fingers and toes.

Main signs:
1. Growth retardation of postnatal onset with delayed skeletal development. Microcephaly.
2. Marked psychomotor retardation.
3. Coarse facies with low nasal root, possible macrostomia and thick lips.
4. Quite sparse growth of scalp hair with hypertrichosis of the face and body.
5. Small hands and feet with aplasia of the distal phalanges of the fifth ray and hypoplasia of further distal phalanges including the nails on the hands and feet.

Supplementary findings:
1. Neurological signs in some cases (which may be due to a variety of cranial malformations).
2. Further skeletal anomalies of the spine, pelvis, or other areas.
3. Anomalies of the internal genitalia may occur in females.
4. Normal karyotype.

Manifestation: At birth and thereafter.

Etiology: Not yet clear. Several observations in siblings could suggest autosomal recessive inheritance.

Frequency: Low; to date, about 20 cases reported in detail.

Course, prognosis: Clouded by the mental retardation.

Diagnosis, differential diagnosis: Hydantoin embryopathy can be ruled out by the history, and trisomy 9p, by chromsomal analysis.

Treatment: Only symptomatic measures are possible. Appropriate handicap aids.

Illustrations:
1 and 2 A 5½-year-old girl, normal birth length, microcephalic, mentally retarded, with marked growth retardation (first child of healthy, young, nonconsanguineous parents) with all the characteristic findings. Typical facies, scanty scalp hair—through which the skin of the scalp is visible—and increased facial hair (**1**). Hypo- to aplasia of the distal phalanges and nails (**2**). Delayed ossification and hypoplasia or aplasia of the distal phalanx of the fifth ray of the same child at 7¾ years (**3**). The patient showed a hypertonic-hypotonic-ataxic disorder. Normal karyotype.

H.-R.W.

References:

Coffin, G.S. and Siris, E. Mental retardation with absent fifth fingernail and terminal phalanx. *Am. J. Dis. Child.*, 119, 433–439 (1970).
Haspeslagh, M., Fryns, J.P., Berghe, H. van den. The Coffin–Siris syndrome: report of a family and further delineation. *Clin. Genet.*, 26, 374–378 (1984).
Coffin, G.S. and Siris, E. The Coffin–Siris syndrome. *Am. J. Dis. Child.*, 139, 12 (1985).
Franceschini, P., Silengo, M.C., Bianco, R. et al. The Coffin–Siris syndrome in two siblings. *Pediatr. Radiol.*, 16, 330–333 (1986).
Meinecke, P., Engelbrecht, R., Schaefer, E. Coffin–Siris-Syndrom bei einem 5jährigen Mädchen. *Monatschr. Kinderheilkd.*, 134, 692–695 (1986).
Bassio, W.A. de. Coffin–Siris syndrome. Chapter 34 in: *Neurocutaneous Diseases*. Gomez, M.R. (ed.). Butterworths, Boston 1987 (pp.307–310).

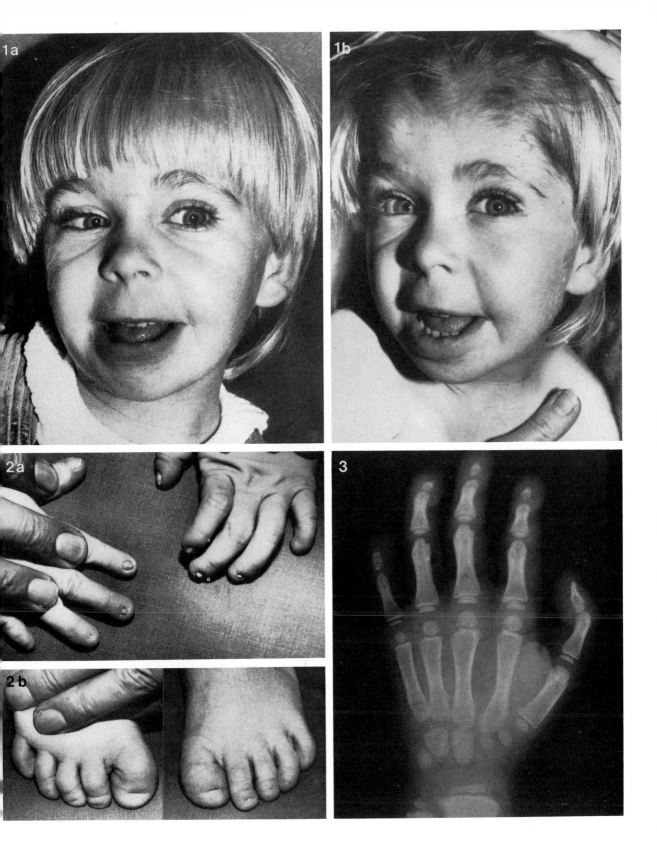

87. Dubowitz Syndrome

A malformation–retardation syndrome with primordial short stature, unusual facies, marked microcephaly, moderate mental retardation, hyperactivity, and eczema.

Main signs:
1. Typical facial dysmorphism, especially characterized by upper epicanthic folds, hypertelorism, relatively short palpebral fissures, ptosis, low nasal bridge (most noticeable in the young preschooler). Thin hair, hypoplasia of the lateral eyebrows; dysplasia of the external ears, micrognathia (1, 2).
2. Pre- and postnatal growth retardation. Marked microcephaly with comparatively mild—and not obligatory—mental retardation. Hyperactivity. Muscular hypotonia. High voice.
3. Decreased subcutaneous fatty tissue. Eczematous skin changes, especially after exposure to sunlight (1–4).

Supplementary findings: Syndactyly of the second and third toes (6).
Pes planus, pes planovalgus. Short radially deviated fifth fingers (5).
Tendency to inguinal hernias.
Cryptorchidism.
Vomiting and diarrhea in infancy.
Increased infections. Anemia.

Manifestation: At birth.

Etiology: Autosomal recessive disease. An autosomal dominant form was recently observed for the first time; thus, heterogeneity is likely.

Frequency: Between the first description, in 1971, and 1988 about 50 cases were described.

Prognosis: Occasional good catch-up of growth. Improvement of the eczema after about the third year of life. Statements about further development are not possible since almost all of the known patients are still in the pediatric age group. Apparently there is an increased tendency to aplastic anemia and the development of malignancies.

Differential diagnosis: Silver–Russell syndrome (p.152). Bloom syndrome (p.360): here, no mental retardation; skin manifestation is not eczema, but rather telangiectatic erythema; typical chromosomal changes. Fetal alcohol syndrome (p.480): here, corresponding maternal history, cardiac defect of the child.

Treatment: Symptomatic. Genetic counseling; in case of further pregnancy, prenatal diagnosis by means of ultrasonography.

Illustrations:
1–6 A patient at age 8 years. Birth weight 2750 g. Eczema and vomiting in infancy. Intelligence quotient 62, hyperactivity. Retractable testes. Measurements at age 8 years: Height 106 cm (corresponding to that of a 4½-year-old boy); weight 12 kg (corresponding to that of a 1¾-year-old boy); head circumference 48 cm (corresponding to that of an 18-month-old boy).

H.-R.W.

References:
Grosse, R., Gorlin, J., Opitz, J.M. The Dubowitz syndrome. *Z. Kinderheilkd.*, 110, 175 (1971).
Majewski, F., Michaelis, R., Moosmann, K., Bierich, J.R. A rare type of low birthweight dwarfism: the Dubowitz syndrome. *Z. Kinderheilkd.*, 120, 238 (1975).
Orrison, W.W., Schnitzler, E.R., Chun, R.W.M. The Dubowitz syndrome: further observations. *Am. J. Med. Genet.*, 7, 155 (1980).
Küster, W. and Majewski, F. The Dubowitz syndrome. *Eur. J. Pediatr.*, 144, 574–578 (1986).
Shuper, A., Merlob, P. et al. The diagnosis of Dubowitz syndrome in the neonatal period . . . *Eur. J. Pediatr.*, 145, 151–152 (1986).
Wilhelm, O.L. and Méhes, K. Dubowitz syndrome. *Acta Pediatr. Hung.*, 27, 67–75 (1986).
Winter, R.H. Dubowitz syndrome. *J. Med. Genet.*, 23, 11–13 (1986).
Berthold, F., Fuhrmann, W. et al. Fatal aplastic anemia in a child with features of Dubowitz syndrome. *Eur. J. Pediatr.*, 146, 605–607 (1987).
Kondo, I., Takeda, K. et al. A Japanese patient with the Dubowitz syndrome. *Clin. Genet.*, 31, 389–392 (1987).
Méhes, K. Personal communication 1987.
Belohradsky, B.H., Egger, J. et al. Das Dubowitz-Syndrom. *Erg. Inn. Med. Kinderheilkd.*, 57, 145–184 (1988).

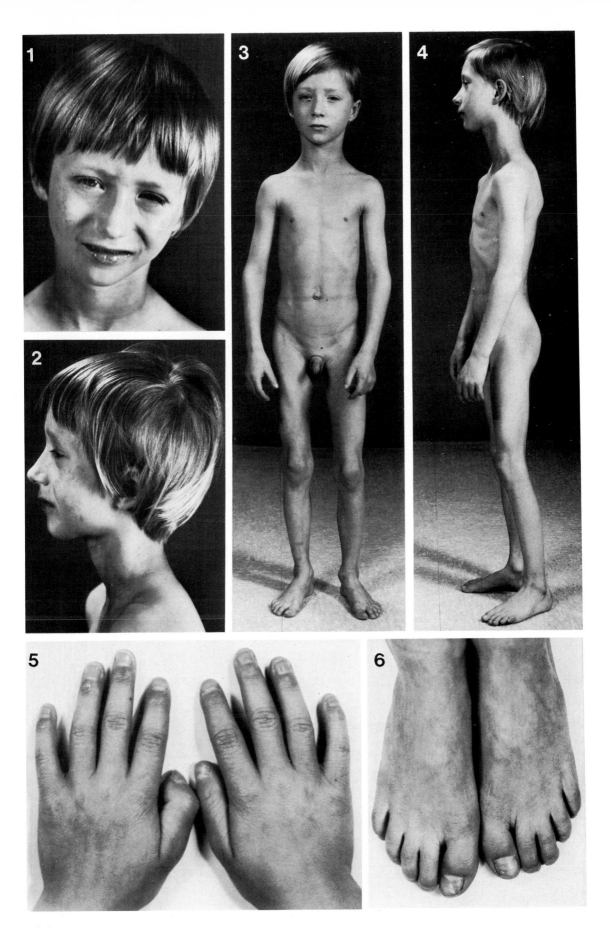

88. A Further Microcephaly–Small Stature–Retardation Syndrome

An unknown syndrome with peculiar facies, microcephaly and mental retardation, small stature, anal atresia, and other anomalies.

Main signs:
1. Facies: Antimongoloid slant of the palpebral fissures, bilateral ptosis (left more marked than right; possible IIIrd and XIIth nerve paralysis); broad nasal bridge; low-set, prominent, dysplastic ears; thin upper lip; and receding chin (1–8).
2. Microcephaly (around the second percentile) with psychomotor retardation.
3. Small stature (between the third and tenth percentiles).
4. Anal atresia.

Supplementary findings: High palate, dysodontiasis, bifid uvula, patent ductus arteriosus. Synostosis of the first ribs bilaterally; abnormally shaped scapulae and clavicles. Narrow hands; pillar-like legs, lacking contour (6, 9).

Manifestation: At birth.

Etiology: Unknown.

Course, prognosis: In view of the mental retardation, poor.

Differential diagnosis: Other microcephaly–growth deficiency syndromes.

Treatment: Appropriate handicap aids.

Illustrations:
1–9 The third child of healthy parents; numerous healthy siblings. Birth measurements 3100 g, 49 cm, and 33.5 cm (head circumference). No maternal alcoholism. Chromosome analysis normal.

H.-R.W.

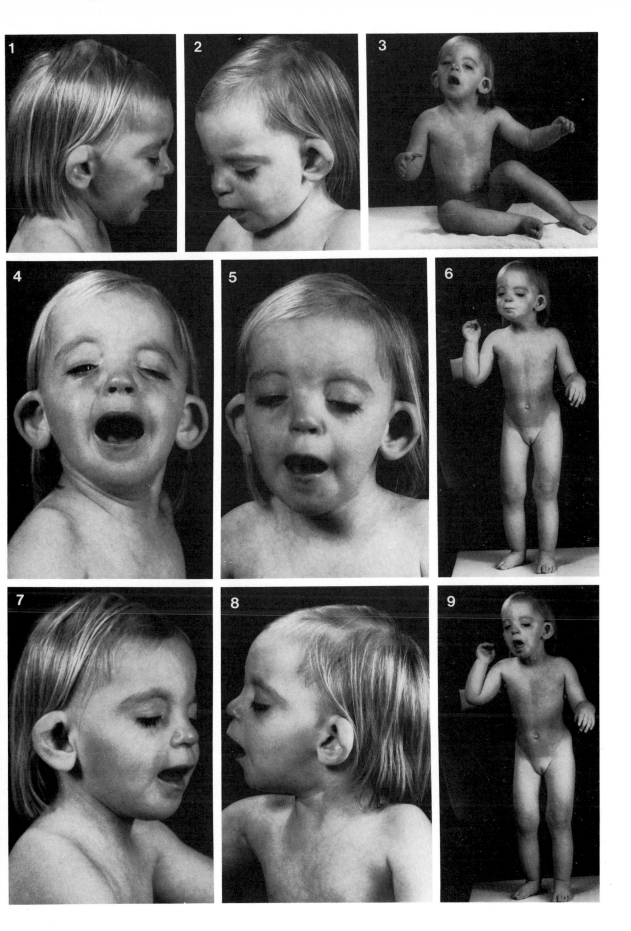

179

89. Mietens Syndrome

A malformation–retardation syndrome with small stature, short forearms held in flexion, unusual facies, corneal clouding, and moderate mental retardation.

Main signs:

1. Flexion contractures of the elbows with dislocation of the head of the radius and abnormally short forearms (**1–4**).
2. Small stature and mental retardation (IQ about 70–80).
3. Unusual facies with bilateral corneal clouding, nystagmus, strabismus, and narrow, pointed nose with hypoplastic alae nasi (**1, 2**).

Supplementary findings: Pes planus and valgus, moderately severe flexion contractures of the knees (**2**), hip dysplasia, pectus excavatum, and clinodactyly may also be present.

Manifestation: Pre- and postnatally.

Etiology: Genetically determined syndrome. Mode of inheritance not known, most likely autosomal recessive.

Frequency: Very rare.

Course, prognosis: Intelligence may be difficult to evaluate due to defective vision and limited arm motion. *If* vascular anomalies prove to be part of the syndrome (see below, text of Illustrations), the prognosis must be guarded.

Treatment: Ophthalmological and orthopedic care. All measures to promote the developmentally retarded child.

Illustrations:

1 and 2 Two of four affected siblings. Small stature; mental retardation. Corneal clouding; strabismus. Narrow nose with hypoplastic alae nasi. Abnormally short forearms with flexion contractures of the dislocated elbows. Flexion contractures of the knees; pes planus and valgus. The girl has a history of a ruptured aneurysm of the right anterior cerebral artery.

3 X-ray of a 5-month-old sibling.

4 X-ray of the boy shown in **1**.

H.-R.W.

References:

Mietens, C. and Weber, H. A syndrome characterized by corneal opacity, nystagmus, flexion of the elbows, growth failure, and mental retardation. *J. Pediatr.*, 62, 624 (1966).

Warring III, G.O. and Rodrigues, M.M. Ultrastructure and successful keratoplasty of sclerocornea in Mieten's syndrome. *Am. J. Ophthalmol.*, 90, 469 (1980).

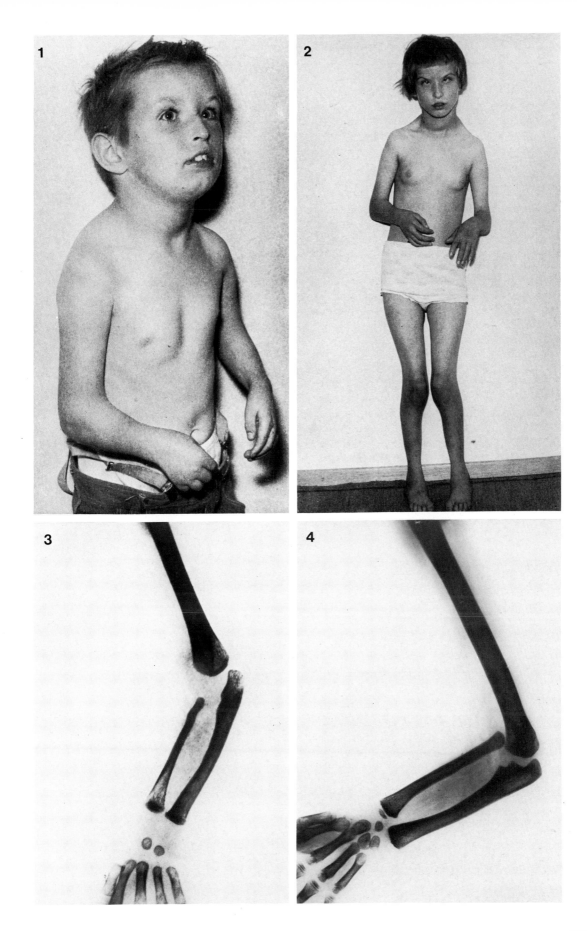

90. Brachmann–de Lange Syndrome

(Cornelia de Lange Syndrome, 'Typus degenerativus amstelodamensis')

A malformation–retardation syndrome of unknown etiology with characteristic facial dysmorphism, primordial short stature, and marked reduction anomalies of the extremities.

Main signs:

1. Pathognomonic facies with bushy eyebrows which meet over the root of the nose, hypertelorism, antimongoloid slant of the palpebral fissures; anteverted nares, long or prominent philtrum, narrow lips and down-turned corners of the mouth. Low anterior and posterior hairlines. Microbrachycephaly. Low, hoarse, expressionless voice.
2. Considerable mental retardation in most cases. Initial muscular hypertonia, which may interfere with feeding.
3. Hirsutism.
4. Short stature.
5. Short hands and feet, proximally displaced thumbs, short fifth finger, simian crease. With marked reduction, retrogression of the rays from the ulnar side with monodactyly and arm stumps in extreme cases; lower extremities generally not as severely affected.

Supplementary findings: Cylindrical trunk, small nipples. Cutis marmorata. Myopia, nystagmus, strabismus. Cardiac defects. Undescended testes, hypoplastic genitalia, and many more anomalies.

Manifestation: At birth.

Etiology: Unknown. The vast majority of cases are sporadic. However, there have been observations that would seem to support autosomal dominant inheritance as well as some that point to autosomal recessive. Heterogeneity cannot be excluded. The spectrum of phenotypic variation is very broad. The nonuniform chromosome anomalies occasionally reported are considered concomitant findings.

Frequency: Not rare; about 250 cases were published by 1971; recent estimate: 1:10,000 to 1:30,000.

Course, prognosis: No progression. Infections pose a threat to severely retarded or markedly hypertonic children, especially in infancy. Probably generally decreased life expectancy. Low risk of recurrence.

Treatment: Symptomatic.

Illustrations:

1–4 Patient 1 at age 10½ years. Birth weight 2450 g; length 39 cm. Subsequent linear growth just below the third percentile. Frequent infections in infancy. At 12 years, onset of grand mal epilepsy. Mental retardation. Head circumference, 49 cm, corresponds to that of a 3-year-old girl.

5 Patient 2 as a neonate with a severe right-sided reduction anomaly (monodactyly).

6 and 7 Patient 3 at age 7 months; weight 5000 g; length 58 cm; head circumference 36.5 cm (birth: weight 1770 g; length 41 cm; head circumference 28.5 cm). Marked muscular hypertonia and severe psychomotor retardation; feeding possible only with a stomach tube; seizures.

H.-R.W.

References:

Beck, B. and Fenger, K. Mortality, pathological findings and causes of death in the de Lange syndrome. *Acta Pediatr. Scand., 74,* 765–769 (1985).

Hawley, P.P., Jackson, L.G., Kurnit, D.M. Sixty-four patients with Brachmann–de Lange syndrome: a survey. *Am. J. Med. Genet., 20,* 453–459 (1985).

Opitz, J.M. Editorial comment: the Brachmann–de Lange syndrome. *Am. J. Med. Genet., 22,* 89–102 (1985).

Mosher, G.A., Schulte, R.L., Kaplan, P.A. et al. Brief clinical report: pregnancy in a woman with Brachmann–de Lange syndrome. *Am. J. Med. Genet., 22,* 103–107 (1985).

Robinson, L.K., Wolfsberg, E., Jones, K.L. Brachmann–de Lange syndrome: evidence for autosomal dominant inheritance. *Am. J. Med. Genet., 22,* 109–115 (1985).

Fryns, J.P., Dereymaeker, A.M. et al. The Brachmann–de Lange syndrome in two siblings of normal parents. *Clin. Genet., 31,* 413–415 (1987).

Bonorden, S.W. and Reinken, L. Ein interdisziplinär koordiniertes Therapiekonzept am Beispiel des Cornelia de Lange-Syndroms. *Klin. Pädiatr., 200,* 457–462 (1988).

Greenberg, F. and Robinson, L.K. Mild Brachmann–de Lange syndrome. *Am. J. Med. Genet., 32,* 90 (1989).

Filippi, G. The de Lange syndrome ... 15 cases. *Clin. Genet., 35,* 343–363 (1989).

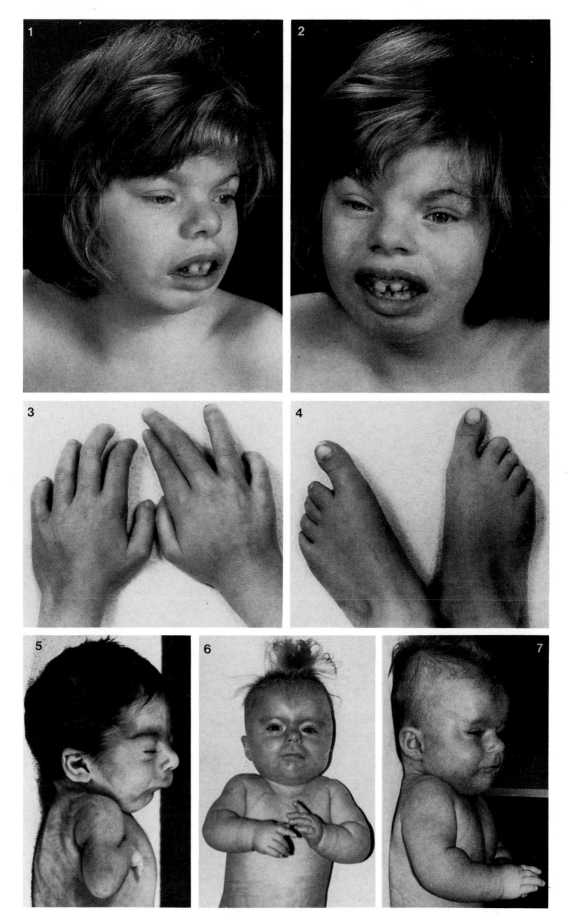

183

91. Oligosymptomatic Hypothyroidism

A form of hypothyroidism of delayed onset and mainly skeletal manifestations, with short stature as the principal sign.

Main signs:
1. Variably severe, for the most part proportional, short stature with thick-set appearance; thorax often broad and bell-shaped; frequent dorsal kyphosis and lumbar lordosis and quite pronounced muscle contours, especially of the thighs (1, 3, 4).
2. Often, distinctly waddling gait.
3. Radiologically, general delay of ossification and epiphyseal dysgenesis, the latter most pronounced in the hip joints as a multicentric crumbly appearance of the capital femoral epiphysis. Also flattening of the vertebral bodies. All in all a picture that most resembles that of polyepiphyseal dysplasia (5–7). Sella turcica frequently enlarged.
4. Mental development may seem normal; skin and hair may be quite unremarkable; obesity, constipation, etc. may be completely absent; and the conventional diagnostic laboratory tests (e.g., thyroxine (T_4) levels) may not yield clearly abnormal results.

Supplementary findings: Delayed dentition.

Unequivocal clarification by means of thyroid-stimulating hormone (TSH) determination (including thyroxine-releasing hormone (TRH) test). Ectopic thyroid tissue frequently demonstrable.

Comment: This mild form of hypothyroidism with ectopic thyroid glands is not always picked up by newborn TSH screening.

Manifestation: Clinical diagnosis is practically impossible before the third year of life.

Etiology: Unclear. As a rule, sporadic occurrence. Girls more frequently affected (ratio 70:30).

Frequency: Not so rare.

Course, prognosis: Favorable with early diagnosis and prompt initiation of replacement therapy.

Differential diagnosis: This disorder should no longer be confused with the epiphyseal and spondyloepiphyseal osteodysplasias.

Treatment: Immediate initiation of replacement therapy with L-thyroxine leads to rapid normalization of the pathological laboratory values, rapid advancement of ossification, catching-up of growth, and in some cases to distinct improvement of intellectual performance.

Illustrations:
1–3 and 5–7 an 11½-year-old girl; height 117.5 cm—below the third percentile.
4 A 4½-year-old girl. Short stature, 94 cm, below the third percentile.
8 X-ray of a 6-year-old patient.
9 X-ray of the same girl as in 8, 6 months after initiation of substitution therapy.

H.-R.W.

References:

Oldigs, H.-D., Schnakenburg, K. von, Wiedemann, H.-R. Zum Krankheitsbild der oligosymptomatischen Hypothyreose. *Med. Welt,* 32, 885 (1981).
Dessart, Y., Chaussain, J.L. et al. Le nanisme hypothyroidien isolé. Etude de 18 observations. *Arch. Fr. Pédiatr.,* 40, 375–378 (1983).
Rochiccioli, P., Dutau, G. et al. L'ectopie thyreoidienne, cause d'erreur du dépistage néonatal de l'hypothyroidie. *Arch. Fr. Pédiatr.,* 40, 405–406 (1983).
Grant, G.A., Carson, D.J. et al. Congenital hypothyroidism missed on screening. *Arch. Dis. Child.,* 61, 189–197 (1986).

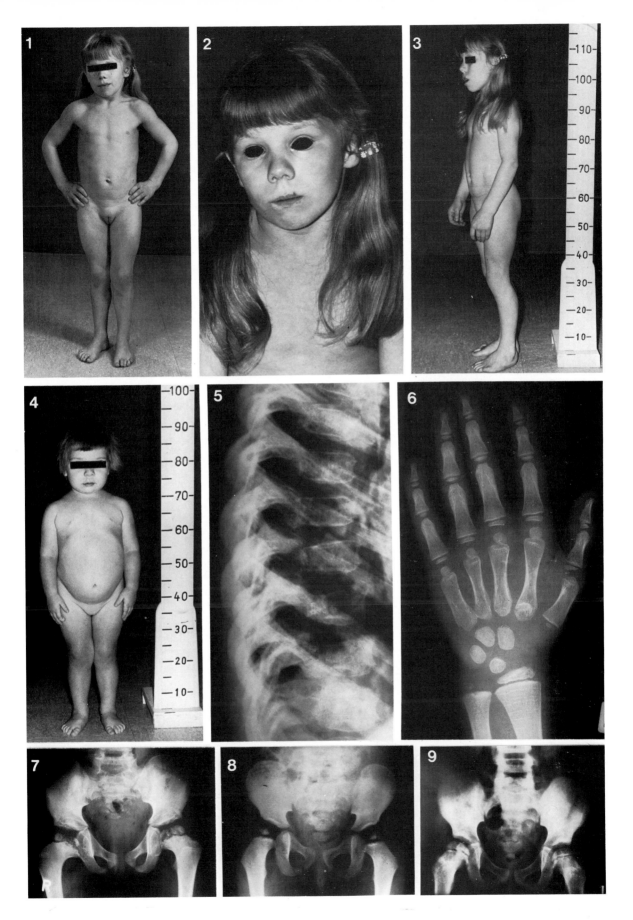

185

92. Short Stature Associated with Vitiligo and—in One Case—Chronic Hypoparathyroidism

Small stature associated with vitiligo in three siblings, one of whom in addition has chronic 'idiopathic' hypoparathyroidism.

Main signs:
1. Small stature: height of the 16-year-old girl (**2**) on the 15th percentile for her age; of her 12-year-old brother (**1**), below the 3rd percentile; and of her 10-year-old sister, on the 3rd percentile.
2. Vitiligo: typical depigmented patches below the knees in the 16-year-old (**5**), also symmetrically on the iliac crests (**2**), below the larynx, and on the lower back. The same affecting her brother on the eyelids, chin, inner surfaces of the upper arms, penis, distal lower legs, the backs of the feet, and other locations (**1, 4, 6, 7**). The same on the trunk of their younger sister.
3. Chronic idiopathic hypoparathyroidism (established biochemically and endocrinologically and controlled therapeutically with dihydrotachysterol) only in the mentally retarded, irritable boy; pseudohypoparathyroidism ruled out; to date, no evidence of autoimmune disease. Both girls of normal intelligence, normocalcemic, and euparathyroid.

Supplementary findings: Additional anomalies in the boy: asymmetric brachycephaly, dysplastic auricles, hypertelorism, epicanthic folds, and broad nasal root (**3**).

Manifestation: Small stature in the first decade of life. Vitiligo appearing in the 11th, 9th, and 10th years of life respectively. First seizure of the boy at 3 months; years later, the first clinical evidence of characteristic tetanic spasms.

Etiology: Uncertain.

Course, prognosis: Normal life expectancy with adequate treatment of hypoparathyroidism.

Comment: The small stature in these patients is familial (father, 1.67 m; mother 1.52 m; further persons of small stature in the mother's sibship). Generalized vitiligo as present in these siblings is considered an autosomal dominant defect with variable expression. Primary idiopathic hypoparathyroidism presenting in early childhood occurs in an X-linked recessive and in an autosomal dominant form, among others. Combinations of vitiligo with diverse endocrinopathies, including chronic idiopathic hypoparathyroidism, are known. The association of small stature and generalized vitiligo in the siblings shown here, one of whom has chronic hypoparathyroidism, will for now be considered as a chance combination.

Illustrations:
1, 3, 4, 6, and 7 A 12-year-old boy with early onset chronic idiopathic hypoparathyroidism, generalized vitiligo, and (familial) short stature.
2 and 5 One of his two euparathyroid sisters with short stature and generalized vitiligo, at age 16 years.

H.-R.W.

References:
Lerner, A.B. and Nordlund, J.J. Vitiligo. What is it? Is it important? *JAMA*, 239, 1183 (1978).
McBurney, E.I. Vitiligo. Clinical picture and pathogenesis. *Arch. Int. Med.*, 139, 1295 (1979).
Betterle, C., Mirakian, R. et al. Antibodies to melanocytes in vitiligo. *Lancet*, I, 159 (1984).
Halder, R.M. et al. Vitiligo in childhood . . . *J. Am. Acad. Dermatol.*, 16, 948–954 (1987).

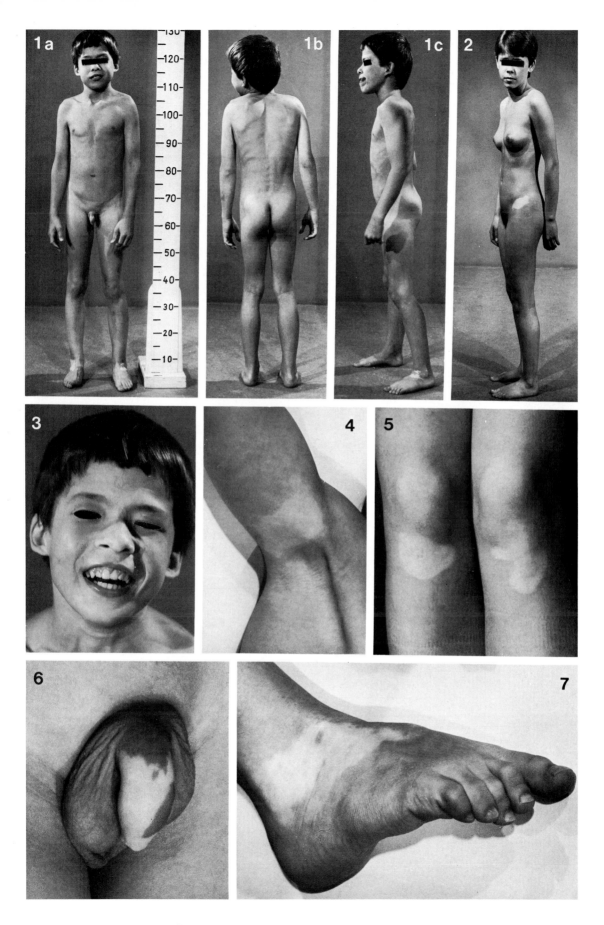

187

93. Pseudohypoparathyroidism

(Albright's Hereditary Osteodystrophy)

A hereditary syndrome of small stature; obesity; round face; brachydactyly due to abnormally short metacarpals, metatarsals, and phalanges; mental retardation; and in some cases seizures.

Main signs:
1. Short, stocky physique with short neck, short extremities, and round face (**1**). Adult height between about 1.38 and 1.52 m, although occasionally greater than this.
2. Obesity—usually moderately severe.
3. Short hands and/or feet due to abnormal shortness of one or more metatarsals and metacarpals—especially IV or V, III, and I—and/or distal phalanges (especially of the thumb) (**3–5**).
4. Mental retardation of variable severity, although not always present.

Supplementary findings: Manifestations of abnormal mineral metabolism including tetanic spasms or convulsions, delayed eruption of teeth, enamel defects, and ectopic calcification (e.g., in subcutaneous tissues, especially of the extremities and joints, see **2**; lenses of the eyes; the basal ganglia of the brain). Biochemically, typical findings of hypocalcemia/hyperphosphatemia, high serum level of immunoreactive parathormone, and parathormone resistance (diminished response of the kidneys to parathormone as determined by cAMP and phosphate excretion). Normocalcemic phases also possible.

Manifestation: Early childhood, but also frequently later in childhood. (Obesity, seizures, subcutaneous calcifications, 'osteomata cutis', accelerated bone age, osteoporosis, and coarse osseous trabeculations possibly as early as the first months of life.)

Etiology: Sex ratio of affected girls:boys = 2:1. The previous assumption of X-linked dominant transmission has had to be replaced by one of autosomal dominance with markedly decreased reproductive fitness in males.

Frequency: Low, although several hundred cases in the literature.

Course, prognosis: Normal life expectancy. No possibility of predicting whether mental retardation will occur.

Differential diagnosis: Shortening of the fourth and fifth metacarpals may also occur, for instance, in the Ullrich–Turner syndrome, which should not be difficult to exclude by the total clinical picture. Fibrodysplasia ossificans progressiva should also be considered.

Treatment: Symptomatic (vitamin D_3 medication, if indicated, as determined by experienced specialists). Genetic counseling after detailed clinical assessment.

Illustrations:
1 The 'round face' of a typically affected boy.
2 Subcutaneous calcium deposits above the right iliac wing.
3, 4, and 6 Typical shortening of, respectively, fingers, metacarpals, and toes.
5 An X-ray of the hands of an 11-year-old girl.

H.-R.W.

References:

Maroteaux, P. *Les maladies osseuses de l'enfant.* Flammarion, Paris, 1974.

Spranger, J.W., Langer, L.O., Jr., Wiedemann, H.-R. *Bone Dysplasias. An Atlas of Constitutional Disorders of Skeletal Development.* G. Fischer and W.B. Saunders, Stuttgart and Philadelphia, 1974.

Boscherini, B., Coen, G., Bianchi, G. et al. Albright's hereditary osteodystrophy. *Acta Pediatr. Scand.,* 69, 305 (1980).

Fitch, N. Albright's hereditary osteodystrophy: a review. *Am. J. Med. Genet.,* 11, 11–29 (1982).

Tsang, R.C., Venkataraman, P., Ho, M. et al. The development of pseudopseudohypoparathyroidism. *Am. J. Dis. Child.,* 138, 654–658 (1984).

Halal, F., Van Dop, C., Lord, J. Differential diagnosis in young women with oligomenorrhea and the pseudohypoparathyroidism variant of Albright's hereditary osteodystrophy. *Am. J. Med. Genet.,* 21, 551–568 (1985).

Kruse, K. Hypoparathyreoidismus und Pseudohypoparathyreoidismus. Neue Aspekte . . . *Monatschr. Kinderheilkd.,* 136, 652–666 (1988).

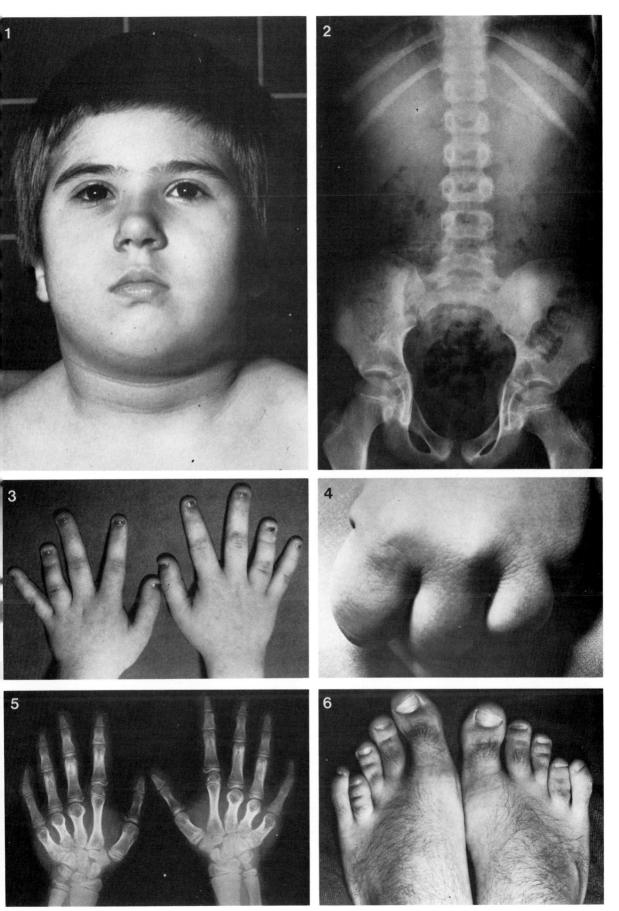

94. Acrodysostosis

(Acrodysostosis Type Maroteaux–Malamut; Maroteaux–Malamut Syndrome)

A syndrome of peripheral dysostosis, growth deficiency, hypoplasia of the nose, and mental retardation.

Main signs:
1. Considerably shortened hands and feet with short, stump-like fingers and toes; loose, wrinkled soft tissue on the dorsal surfaces; and short, broad nails (**1**).
2. Often small at birth; postnatal growth deficiency increasingly apparent. Relatively short forearms held in flexion with restricted extension at the elbows (**1**).
3. Characteristic facies: Hypoplasia of the nose with low nasal root; also, nose usually short and flat with a broad tip, which may have a median dimple; anteverted nares; long philtrum (**1**). In some cases, hypoplasia of the upper jaw, hypertelorism, epicanthic folds, prognathism, dysodontiasis, wide mandibular angle.
4. Mental retardation, of very variable severity, in about 75% of the cases.

Supplementary findings: Radiologically, hyperplasia of the first ray of the foot; severely shortened metacarpals and metatarsals with deformed epiphyses and shortened phalanges with cone-shaped epiphyses; frequent bowing and other malformations of the bones of the forearm (**2**).

Hearing defect in about two-thirds of the patients.

Manifestation: At birth or later, with increasingly apparent signs.

Etiology: The great majority of cases have occurred sporadically to date—predominantly in girls—but a genetic cause is most likely; autosomal dominant and autosomal recessive inheritance have both been described.

Frequency: Low (by 1988 at least 30 cases had been described).

Course, prognosis: Complicated by mental retardation, growth deficiency, increasing impairment of the hands, feet, and elbows, and by the facial disfigurement. Apparently normal life expectancy.

Comment: Pseudohypoparathyroidism (p.188) and acrodysostosis have been considered by some to represent different grades of severity of essentially the same clinical picture.

Treatment: Symptomatic. Plastic or cosmetic surgery may be indicated in cases with marked facial deformity.

Illustrations:
1 and 2 A 1.17 m-tall, 15-year-old girl with psychomotor retardation, the first child of nonconsanguineous parents. The patient shows the full clinical picture.

H.-R.W.

References:

Robinow, M., Pfeiffer, R.A., Gorlin, R.J. et al. Acrodysostosis. *Am. J. Dis. Child.*, 121, 195 (1971).

Ablow, R.C., Hsia, Y.E., Brandt, I.K. Acrodysostosis coinciding with pseudohypoparathyroidism and pseudopseudohypoparathyroidism. *Am. J. Roentgenol.*, 128, 95 (1977).

Niikawa, N., Matsuda, I. et al. Familial occurrence of a syndrome with mental retardation, nasal hypoplasia, peripheral dysostosis . . . *Hum. Genet.*, 42, 227–232 (1978).

Butler, M.G., Rames, L.J. et al. Acrodysostosis . . . with review of literature . . . *Am. J. Med. Genet.*, 30, 971–980 (1988).

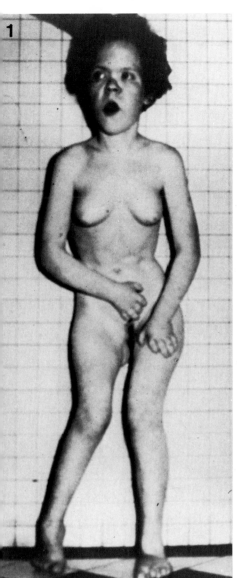

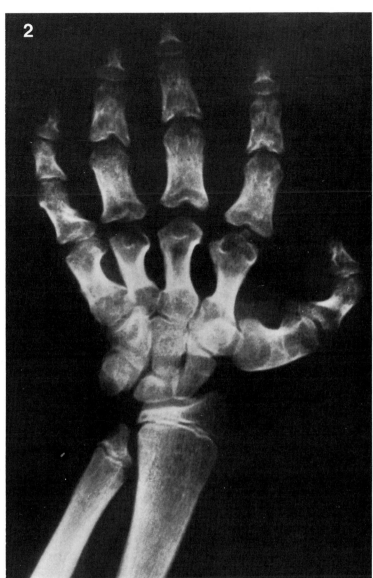

95. Ullrich–Turner Syndrome

(Turner Syndrome)

A malformation syndrome characterized especially by small stature, failure of puberty to occur, webbed neck, lymphedema of the hands and feet, and characteristic facies, all of which can be attributed to complete or partial absence of the X chromosome in phenotypic females.

Main signs:

1. Small stature, usually from birth, adult height usually around 145 cm. Failure of puberty to occur (along with insignificant pubertal growth spurt): absence of spontaneous breast development, poor development of further secondary sexual characteristics, primary amenorrhea; neck webbing, redundant skin folds, or edema of the neck; shield chest (**1, 7**).

2. Cubitus valgus; at birth, lymphedema of the dorsal surfaces of the hands and feet which usually regresses by late infancy (**9**); shortening of the fourth and fifth metacarpals; narrow, dysplastic, sometimes spoon-shaped or short nails (**9, 10**).

3. Somewhat expressionless ('sphinx') face. Ptosis of the eyelids, epicanthic folds (**1, 2, 4**); micrognathia (**1**), high and narrow hard palate with malpositioned teeth; low posterior hairline (**6**).

Supplementary findings: Gonadal dysgenesis with rudimentary 'streak' ovaries; renal anomalies (for the most part horseshoe kidney, unilateral renal agenesis); cardiac defect (usually coarctation of the aorta). Intellectual development within normal limits. Increased pigmented nevi and dermatofibromas (**4, 5**); prominent veins, especially on the arms; retarded bone age and osteoporosis; possible hearing defect (tendency to recurrent otitis). Low estrogen, high gonadotropin levels. Chromosomal findings are diagnostic.

Manifestation: At birth; however, the child may not come to medical attention until later on.

Etiology: Complete (in the majority of cases) or partial absence of an X chromosome—more precisely, complete or partial monosomy for the short arm of the X chromosome—in all or a proportion of the body cells.

Frequency: About 1:3,000 female births. No increased risk of recurrence for the affected family.

Prognosis: Dependent on the cardiac and renal anomalies. Increased tendency to thyroid disorders and diabetes.

Differential diagnosis: Noonan syndrome (p.196).

Treatment: Early treatment to promote growth (apparently best accomplished with a combination of HGH and oxandrolone) by an experienced pediatric endocrinologist. The latter can also determine an adequate schedule for therapy to develop the secondary characteristics and to initiate vaginal bleeding. Cardiac or renal surgery may be indicated. Plastic surgery and psychotherapy in some cases.

Illustrations:

1–4 Typical 'sphinx-like' facial expression in children of 3 months, 2½, 9, and 13 years.

4 and 5 A child with very marked neck webbing, pigmented nevi.

6 Same child as in 3: low posterior hairline.

7 and 8 7-year-old girl; shield chest, increased intermamillary distance, somewhat masculine habitus; height approximately corresponding to that of a 4½-year-old girl.

9 A 9-day-old newborn; marked lymphedema, short dysplastic nails.

10 A 1-day-old newborn; narrow, hyperconvex nails.

H.-R.W.

References:

Palmer, C.G. and Reichmann, A. Chromosomal and clinical findings in 100 females with Turner syndrome. *Hum. Genet.*, 35, 35 (1976).

Ranke, M.B., Pflüger, H. et al. Turner syndrome: spontaneous growth in 150 cases . . . *Eur. J. Pediatr.*, 141, 81–88 (1983).

Schwanitz, G., Tietze, H.U. et al. Gonadendysgenesie—Variationsbreite klinischer, hormoneller, zytogenetischer . . . Befunde. *Klin. Pädiatr.*, 195, 422–429 (1983).

Lyon, A.J., Preece, M.A. et al. Growth curve for girls with Turner syndrome. *Arch. Dis. Child.*, 60, 932–935 (1985).

Carr, R.E., Ochs, R.H. et al. Fetal cystic hygroma and Turner's syndrome. *Am. J. Dis. Child.*, 140, 580–583 (1986).

McCauley, E., Sybert, V.P. et al. Psychosocial adjustment of adult women with Turner syndrome. *Clin. Genet.*, 29, 284–290 (1986).

Nielsen, J. and Stradiot, M. Transcultural study of Turner's syndrome. *Clin. Genet.*, 32, 260–270 (1987).

Ranke, M.B., Blum, W.F. et al. Growth hormone, somatomedin levels and growth regulation in Turner's syndrome. *Acta Endocrinol.*, 116, 305–313 (1987).

Lin, T.-H., Kirkland, J.L. et al. Growth hormone assessment and short-term treatment with growth hormone in Turner syndrome. *J. Pediatr.*, 112, 919–922 (1988).

Rosenfeld, R.G., Hintz, R.L. et al. Three-year results of a randomized prospective trial of methionyl human growth hormone and oxandrolone in Turner's syndrome. *J. Pediatr.*, 113, 393–400 (1988).

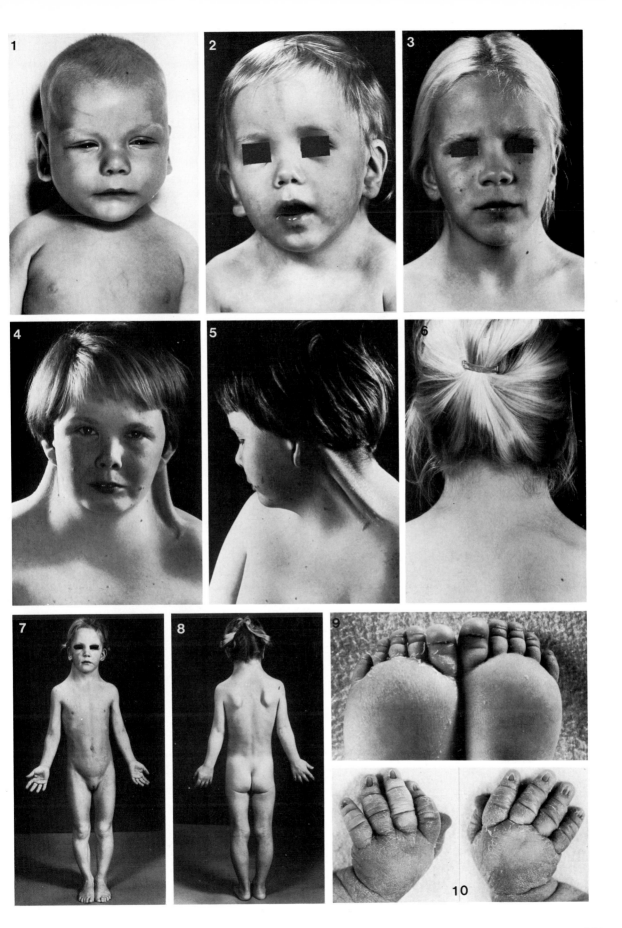

96. Aarskog Syndrome

A malformation syndrome occurring in males, with short stature, unusual facies, typical genital appearance, and other anomalies.

Main signs:
1. Small stature, frequently with a long trunk.
2. Round face characterized by a prominent forehead with large widow's peak, hypertelorism, sometimes slight antimongoloid slant of the palpebral fissures, and uni- or bilateral ptosis, hypoplasia of the midface, short and broad nose with anteverted nostrils and long broad philtrum, anomalies of the external ear, horizontal groove directly under the lower lip; prognathism (**1, 3**).
3. Shawl-like scrotal folds cranially enclosing the base of the penis, cryptorchidism (**2, 4**).
4. Short hands (with simian creases), and feet (metatarsus adductus; stubby toes). Short fingers due to hypoplasia of the distal phalanges, often with mild cutaneous syndactyly and an especially short fifth finger with often only one flexion crease. Unusual hyperextensibility of the proximal interphalangeal joints when the hands are extended at the metacarpophalangeal joints and the distal interphalangeal joints are flexed.

Supplementary findings: Pectus excavatum. Inguinal hernias.

Occasional anomalies of the cervical vertebral bodies, craniosynostoses.

Mild mental retardation in about 10% of cases.

Manifestation: At birth; retarded growth in height (usually normal birth measurements) during first year of life.

Etiology: X-linked recessive inheritance assumed to play the main role, since mothers and other female family members of affected boys often show partial manifestations of the syndrome (especially of the face and hands, and possibly also slight short stature). However, autosomal dominant—see captions to illustrations—and autosomal recessive inheritance have also been considered. Possible heterogeneity.

Frequency: Apparently not so low; about 100 cases were reported between the time of the first description, in 1970, and 1980.

Prognosis: Good. Although initial growth is around or below the third percentile, satisfactory height is usually attained after a normal puberty.

Differential diagnosis: Noonan syndrome (p.196), which does not include the penoscrotal anomaly, but includes pulmonary stenosis, pterygium, mental retardation. Robinow syndrome (p.210), q.v.

Treatment: Symptomatic. Genetic counseling.

Illustrations:
1 and 2 Case 1 at age 9 months (length 66 cm, corresponding to that of a 5-month-old boy). Broad, short hands, undescended testes. Bilateral simian creases. Premature closure of the sagittal suture (also present in his similarly affected sister). The father of both children shows mild signs of the syndrome.
3 and 4 Case 2 at 3¾ years. Height 95 cm, corresponding to that of a 3-year-old boy. Post-herniorrhaphy on the right; seizure disorder.

H.-R.W./J.K.

References:
Hoo, J.J. The Aarskog (facio-digito-genital) syndrome. *Clin. Genet.*, 16, 269 (1979).
Berry, C., Cree, J., Mann, T. Aarskog's syndrome. *Arch. Dis. Child.*, 55, 706 (1980).
Grier, R.-E., Farrington, F.H. et al. Autosomal dominant inheritance of the Aarskog syndrome. *Am. J. Med. Genet.*, 15, 39–46 (1983).
Meinecke, P. Das Aarskog-Syndrom. *Pädiatr. Prax.*, 28, 675–684 (1983).
Veoren, M.J. van de, Niermeijer, M.F. et al. The Aarskog syndrome . . . *Clin. Genet.*, 24, 439–445 (1983).
Bawle, E., Tyrkus, M. et al. Aarskog syndrome . . . *Am. J. Med. Genet.*, 17, 595–602 (1984).
Nielsen, K.B. Aarskog syndrome . . . *Clin. Genet.*, 33, 315–317 (1988).
Teebi, A.S., Naguib, K.K. et al. New autosomal recessive faciodigitogenital syndrome. *J. Med. Genet.*, 25, 400–406 (1988).

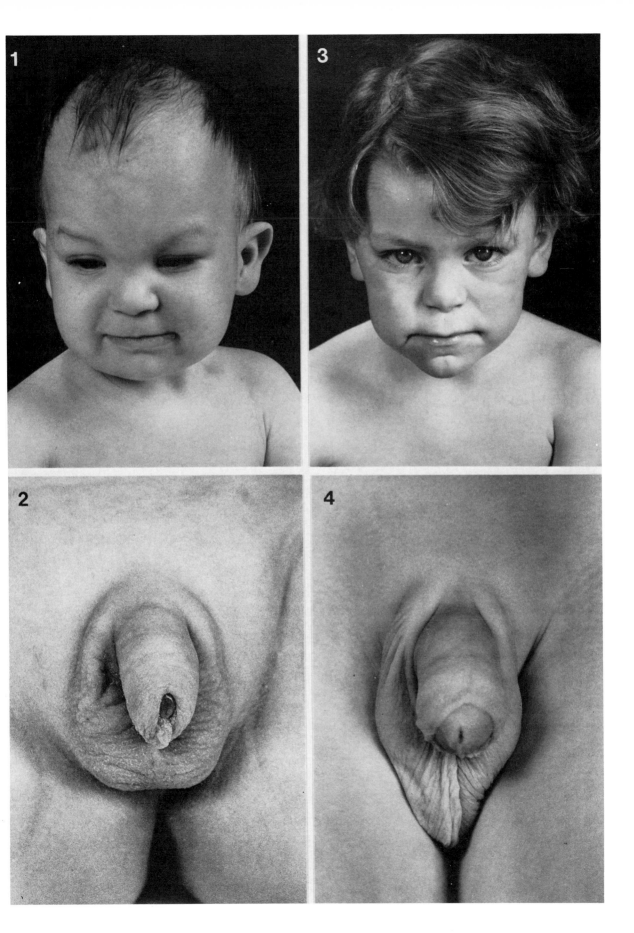

97. Noonan Syndrome

A probably heterogeneous malformation–retardation syndrome occurring in both sexes (without chromosomal aberration) with characteristic facies, short stature, cardiac defect, and multiple other, usually less severe, anomalies.

Main signs:

1. Usually mild, proportional short stature.
2. Not infrequently mild to moderate mental retardation; occasionally hearing defects.
3. Typical facies (**1, 2, 4, 6**), mainly characterized by hypertelorism, antimongoloid slant of the palpebral fissures, epicanthus, ptosis, down-turned corners of the mouth, and micrognathia.
4. Low posterior hairline, webbed neck or redundant skin of the lateral neck (**1, 7**); low-set ears with unusual rims; high palate.
5. Shield chest with pectus carinatum and/or excavatum.
6. Pulmonary stenosis (valvular, supravalvular, peripheral), rarely atrial septal defect, or other.
7. Frequently multiple pigment anomalies such as café-au-lait spots.

Supplementary findings: Cryptorchidism; undescended testes; possibly small testes (post pubertally). Delayed puberty in some cases; fertility possible in both sexes.

Cubitus valgus; short, radially curved fifth fingers; broad, short finger nails (**5**); lymphedema of the backs of the hands and feet in some cases.

Hypertrophic cardiomyopathy and, much less frequently, pulmonary lymphangiectasia may be present; chylothorax in isolated cases. A bleeding diathesis may be present.

Manifestation: At birth; however, the child may not come to medical attention until later in childhood.

Etiology: Genetically determined syndrome; probably heterogeneity. Extremely variable expression. Occurrence of autosomal dominant inheritance and probably other modes of inheritance. Many cases are sporadic.

Frequency: Quite common (many hundreds of patients); estimated 1 in 1,000 liveborn infants.

Course, prognosis: Essentially dependent on the possible cardiac defect and the mental development.

Treatment: Cardiac surgery, cryptorchidism surgery, or removal of webs may be indicated; hormone substitution. Genetic counseling.

Differential diagnosis:

1. Ullrich–Turner syndrome (p.192): marked growth retardation, usually normal intellect, failure of puberty to occur, frequent renal anomalies, and coarctation of the aorta as the usual cardiac defect. Chromosomal anomaly.
2. Multiple lentigines syndrome (LEOPARD syndrome, p.324): usually normal intelligence, skin covered by freckles, abnormal ventricular conduction on ECG, possible hearing defect, autosomal dominant transmission.
3. Aarskog syndrome (p.194).
4. Neurofibromatosis–Noonan syndrome (p.332).

Illustrations:

1 and 2 Patient 1 with quite typical facies, at age 16¾ years. Height 151 cm (average height of a 12½-year-old). Menarche at 14 years. Intelligence just within the normal range.

3–5 Patient 2 at age 6 years. Height 111 cm (third percentile). Birth measurements and heights at ages 11 months and 2¼ years within the norm. Testes not descended until after the second year of life. Infundibular and valvular pulmonary stenosis. Mild mental retardation.

6–7 Patient 3 at age 3 weeks. Definite psychomotor retardation at 6 months. Mild supravalvular pulmonary stenosis, marked septation of the left ventricle. Malrotation II.

H.-R.W.

References:

Wilroy, R.S., Jr., Summit, R.L., Tipton, R.E. et al. Phenotypic heterogeneity in the Noonan syndrome. *Birth Defects*, 15/5B, 305 (1979).
Duncan, W.J., Fowler, R.S., Farkas, L.G. et al. A comprehensive scoring system for evaluating Noonan syndrome. *Am. J. Med. Genet.*, 10, 37 (1981).
Allanson, J.E., Hall, J.G. et al. Noonan syndrome: the changing phenotype. *Am. J. Med. Genet.*, 21, 507–514 (1985).
Mendez, H.M.M. and Opitz, J. Noonan syndrome: a review. *Am. J. Med. Genet.*, 21, 493–506 (1985).
Witt, D.R., Keena, B.A. et al. Growth curves for height in Noonan syndrome. *Clin. Genet.*, 30, 150–153 (1986).
Allanson, J.E. Noonan syndrome. *J. Med. Genet.*, 24, 9–13 (1987).
Char, F.L. The halo iris of the Noonan syndrome. *Dysmorphol. Clin. Genet.*, 1, 71–72 (1987).
Witt, D.R., Hoyme, H.E. et al. Lymphedema in Noonan syndrome . . . *Am. J. Med. Genet.*, 27, 841–856 (1987).
Ranke, M.B., Heidemann, P. et al. Noonan syndrome: growth and clinical manifestations in 144 cases. *Eur. J. Pediatr.*, 148, 220–227 (1988).
Witt, D.R., McGillivray, B.C. et al. Bleeding diathesis in Noonan syndrome. *Am. J. Med. Genet.*, 31, 305–317 (1988).

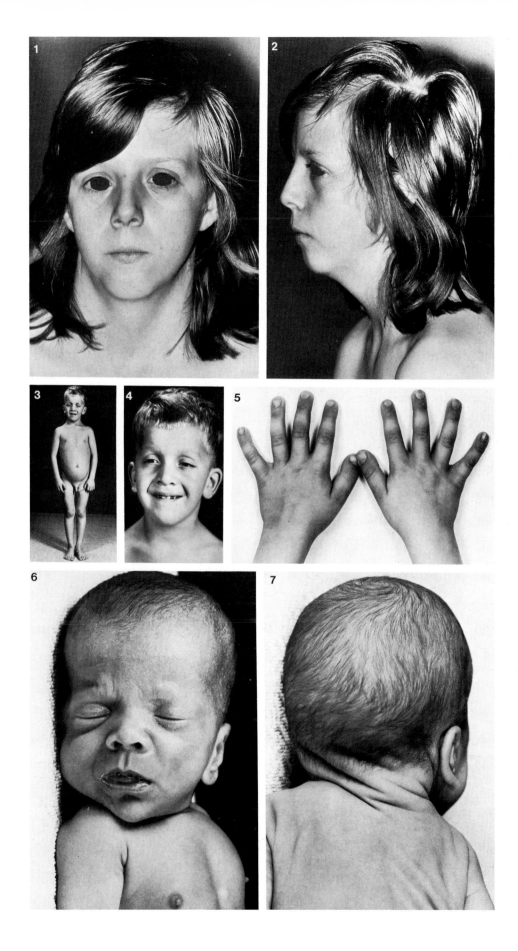

98. A Syndrome of Abnormal Facies, Short Stature, and Psychomotor Retardation

A syndrome of facial dysmorphism, short stature with thickset physique, and considerable mental retardation.

Main signs:
1. Facies: Flat and broad with wide, low-set nasal root, hypertelorism, short 'pug' nose, and high philtrum. Short, narrow palpebral fissures; epicanthic folds (left more pronounced than right). High narrow palate. Low-set dysplastic ears (1–6). Similarity of the boy's facial features with those of his father (7) and his father's father.
2. Short stature of prenatal onset, well below the third percentile. Short neck, thickset trunk, stubby hands and feet. Unusual stocky build during infancy and early childhood with extremities at first appearing too short, and later too long (3, 4).
3. Mental retardation.

Supplementary findings: Alternating convergent strabismus. Left lower extremity shorter (2½ cm) and thinner than the right. Mild clinodactyly of the little fingers (8).

Manifestation: At birth.

Etiology: Not known.

Course, prognosis: Overshadowed by the degree of mental retardation.

Comment: The clinical picture brought to mind several well-known syndromes, but could not be classified under any of them. Maternal alcoholism *non aderat*.

Treatment: Symptomatic.

Illustrations:
1, 3, and 5 The affected child at age 3½ years.
2, 4, 6–8 The same child at 6 years 10 months.
7 Together with his father. The third child of young, nonconsanguineous, healthy, but small (father 1.64 m; mother 1.52 m) parents. Two older siblings healthy and of normal height. Proband born 10 days before the expected date of delivery after a normal pregnancy, birth measurements 2600 g and 44 cm. At 6¾ years 104.5 cm. No evidence of large internal organs (blunted renal pelves on i.v. pyelography). Ocular fundi, EEG normal; pneumoencephalogram: Cysterna interventricularis et cavum septi pellucidi communicans. Blood chemistry and endocrinological investigations normal. Chromosome analysis (with banding) normal.

H.-R.W.

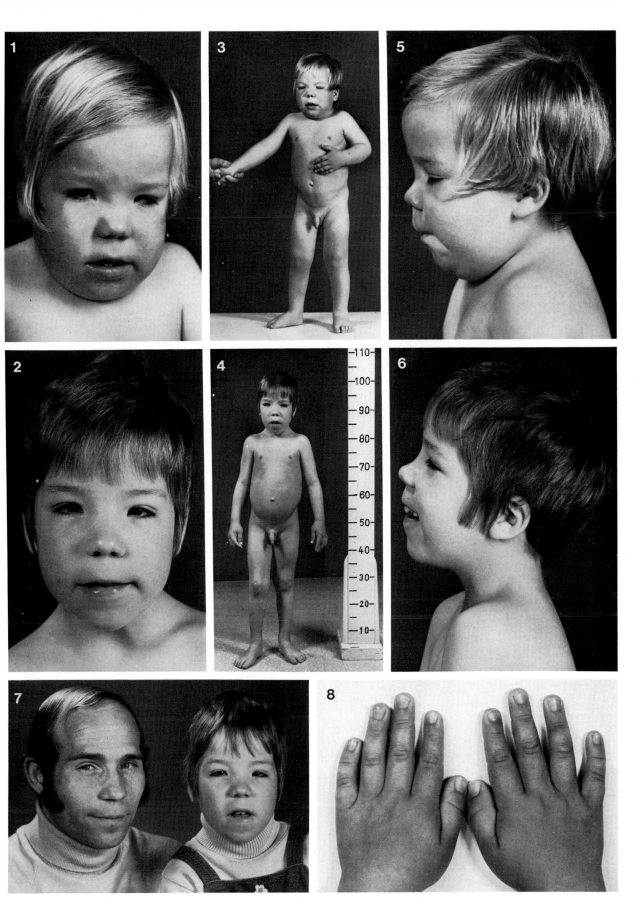

99. Pyknodysostosis

(Maroteaux, Lamy)

A characteristic hereditary disease of the skeleton with typical facial dysmorphism, short stature, and osteosclerosis.

Main signs:
1. Small stature from early childhood mainly due to shortness of the extremities. Adult height between 1.30 and 1.55 m.
2. Large, long, and narrow cranium with prominent forehead (**4, 5**), delayed closure of fontanelles and sutures (**7**), in part until adulthood; relatively small facial part of the cranium with prominent nose, hypoplasia of the lower jaw, micrognathia, and marked flattening or even extension of the submaxillary angle (**7**). Mild exophthalmos in some cases; bluish sclera.
3. Short, stubby hands (**8**) and feet, especially the fingers and toes, with abnormal, very brittle nails (**8**).
4. Frequently increased tendency to fractures (**6**).

Supplementary findings: Dysodontiasis (anomalies of eruption, malocclusion, and other). Radiologically generalized osteosclerosis. Hypoplasia of the clavicles. Dysplasia or acro-osteolysis of the distal phalanges of the fingers and toes (**9**), especially of the index fingers.

Manifestation: From infancy.

Etiology: Autosomal recessive disorder.

Frequency: Low. Up to now, at least 150 cases described in the literature.

Course, prognosis: Life expectancy normal or slightly reduced. Tendency to fractures varies from case to case. Fractures heal well.

Differential diagnosis: Cleidocranial dysplasia and, readily distinguishable, osteopetrosis.

Treatment: Early orthodontic supervision as needed.

Illustrations:
The same child at age 2½ (**1 and 4**), 5 (**2 and 5**), and 10 years (**3**); growth deficiency respectively of 4.5, 9.5, and 16 cm from the median for age.
7 Skull X-ray at 3½ years: Increased density of the base of the skull; increased density and bossing of the frontal and occipital bones; anterior fontanelle and lambdoid suture wide open; hypoplasia of the mandible with absence of the angle.
9 X-ray of the hand at 8 years: osteosclerosis; acro-osteolysis of the distal phalanges.
6 X-ray of the lower leg of an adult with pyknodysostosis showing several spontaneous fractures.

H.-R.W.

References:
Wiedemann, H.-R. Pyknodysostonse. *Fortschr. Röntgenstr.*, 103, 590 (1965).
Spranger, J.W., Langer, L.O., Jr., Wiedemann, H.-R. *Bone Dysplasias. An Atlas of Constitutional Disorders of Skeletal Development.* G. Fischer and W.B. Saunders, Stuttgart and Philadelphia, 1974.
Srivastava, K.K., Bhattacharya, A.K., Galatius-Jensen, F. et al. Pycnodysostosis (report of four cases). *Aust. Radiol.*, 22, 70 (1978).
M. de Almeida, L. A genetic study of pycnodysostosis. In: Papadatos, C.J. and Bartsocas, C.S. (eds.). *Skeletal Dysplasias.* Alan R. Liss, New York, pp.195–198 (1982).
Beighton, P. and Cremin, B.J. *Sclerosing Bone Dysplasias.* Springer, Berlin. 1980.
Mills, K.L.G. and Johnston, A.W. Pycnodysostosis. *J. Med. Genet.*, 25, 550–553 (1988).
Kumar, R., Misra, P.K. et al. An unusual case of pycnodysostosis. *Arch. Dis. Child.*, 63, 558–559 (1988).

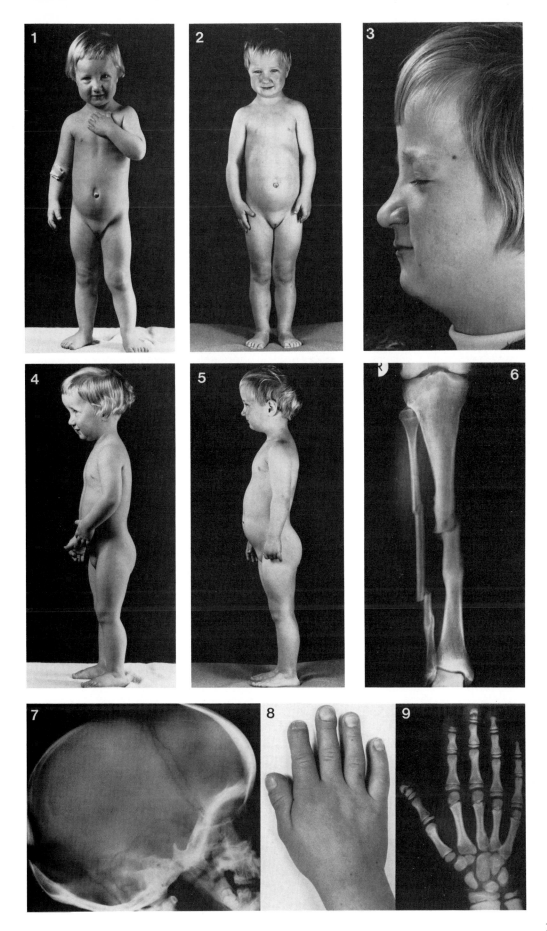

201

100. Dyschondrosteosis

(Léri–Weill Syndrome)

A syndrome of short forearms with Madelung's deformity and quite distinct shortening of the lower legs, resulting in disproportionate ('mesomelic') small stature.

Main signs:
1. Reducible dorsal subluxation of the distal ulna (Madelung's deformity, 1, 2) in both arms with limitation of movement.
2. Generally obvious short stature, disproportionate due to striking relative shortness of the slightly bowed forearms and in some cases also of the lower legs.

Supplementary findings: Occasionally short hands and feet; exostoses on the proximal tibia and fibula; hyperlordosis; bow-legs or knock-knees.
   Radiologically: shortening, bowing, broadening, and increased separation of the bones of the forearm, dorsal subluxation of the head of the ulna, pyramid-like compression of the carpal ossification centers at the wrist.

Manifestation: From infancy, but more frequently somewhat later in childhood, with small stature and wrist deformity; development of the full roentgenological picture of the Madelung's deformity by puberty.

Etiology: Autosomal dominant disorder, with more severe expression but only 50% penetrance(?) in female. Males:females = about 4:1.

Frequency: Relatively low.

Course, prognosis: Normal life expectancy. Adult height between about 135 and over 150 cm.

Treatment: Orthopedic measures in cases of increased fatigability and pain of the wrists (e.g., leather supports; exceptionally, surgery). Genetic counseling.

Illustrations:
1 and 2 A 15-year-old girl with dyschondrosteosis.
1 Reducible dorsal subluxation of the distal end of the ulna and bayonet-like volar displacement of the hand ('Madelung's deformity').
2 Shortening, bowing, and broadening of the radii; increased ulnar deviation of the distal radial epiphyses; ulna slender distally; angulation of the carpal bones.

H.-R.W.

References:

Spranger, J.W. and Wiedemann, H.-R. Dyschondrosteose. *Hdb. Kinderheilkd.*, Opitz, H. and Schmid, F. (eds.), vol VI, 204. Springer, Berlin Heidelberg New York (1967).
Spranger, J.W., Langer, L.O., Jr., Wiedemann, H.-R. *Bone Dysplasias. An Atlas of Constitutional Disorders of Skeletal Development.* G. Fischer and W.B. Saunders, Stuttgart and Philadelphia, 1974.
Lichtenstein, J.R., Sundaram, M., Burdge, R. Sex-influenced expression of Madelung's deformity in a family with dyschondrosteosis. *J. Med. Genet.*, 17, 41 (1980).
Koch, H.L. Die Dyschondrosteose Léri–Weill. *Fortschr. Röntgenstr.*, 138, 603–606 (1983).

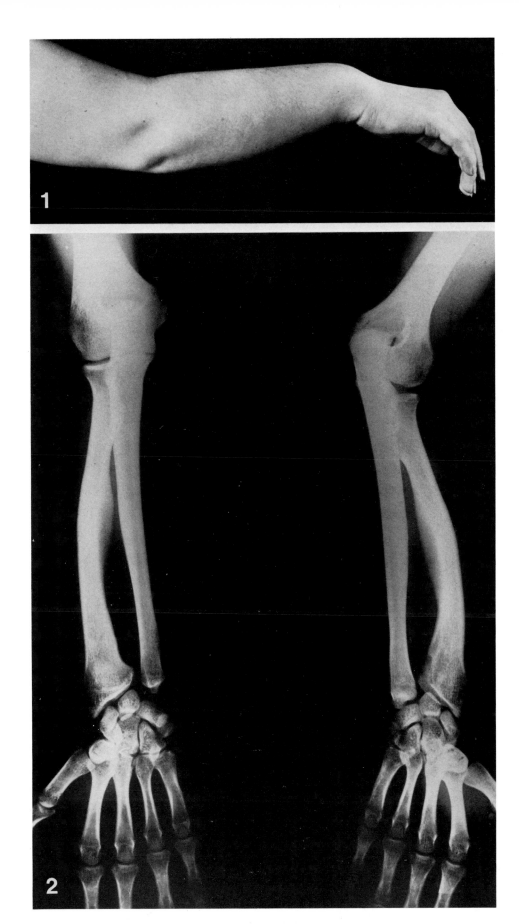

101. Mesomelic Dysplasia Type Langer

A hereditary disproportionate dwarfism due to severe shortening of the forearms and lower legs with characteristic radiological findings.

Main signs:
1. 'Mesomelic dwarfism' due to shortening (and bowing) of the forearms and lower legs with distinct ulnar deviation of the hands, possibly also malpositioning of the feet, and limited motion at the elbows, wrists, and possibly ankles (**1**).
2. Radiologically, profound symmetrical shortening, bowing, and broadening of the bones of the forearms and lower legs (**2, 3**) with unusual hypoplasia of the distal ulnae (**3**) and proximal fibulae (**2**).

Supplementary findings: Not infrequently, hypoplasia of the mandible. Increased lumbar lordosis.
Normal mental development.

Manifestation: At birth.

Etiology: Inherited disorder. In an increasing number of cases, both parents have been shown to be carriers of dyschondrosteosis (p.202); the proband could be regarded as homozygous for the dyschon-. drosteosis gene.

Frequency: Low.

Course, prognosis: Normal life expectancy. Adult height about 1.30 m.

Differential diagnosis: Other types of mesomelic dysplasia (p.206, p.210, p.264) and dyschondrosteosis (p.202); acrodysostosis (p.190).

Treatment: Physiotherapy; orthopedic treatment may be indicated in some patients. Genetic counseling.

Illustrations:
1–3 A toddler, the first living child of nonconsanguineous parents after three spontaneous abortions and two interrupted pregnancies (indications not clear). Both parents: dyschondrosteosis. Height of the proband at about the third percentile.

H.-R.W.

References:
Spranger, J.W., Langer, L.O., Jr., Wiedemann, H.-R. *Bone Dysplasias. An Atlas of Constitutional Disorders of Skeletal Development.* G. Fischer and W.B. Saunders, Stuttgart and Philadelphia, 1974.
Esperitu, C., Chen, H., Wooley, P.V. Mesomelic dwarfism as the homozygous expression of dyschondrosteosis. *Am. J. Dis. Child.,* 129, 375 (1975).
Kunze, J. and Klemm, T. Mesomelic dysplasia, type Langer—a homozygous state for dyschondrosteosis. *Eur. J. Pediatr.,* 134, 269 (1980).
Goldblatt, J., Wallis, C. et al. Heterozygous manifestations of Langer mesomelic dysplasia. *Clin. Genet.,* 31, 19–24 (1987).
Evans, M.I., Zador, I.E. et al. Ultrasonographic prenatal diagnosis . . . of Langer mesomelic dwarfism. *Am. J. Med. Genet.,* 31, 915–920 (1988).

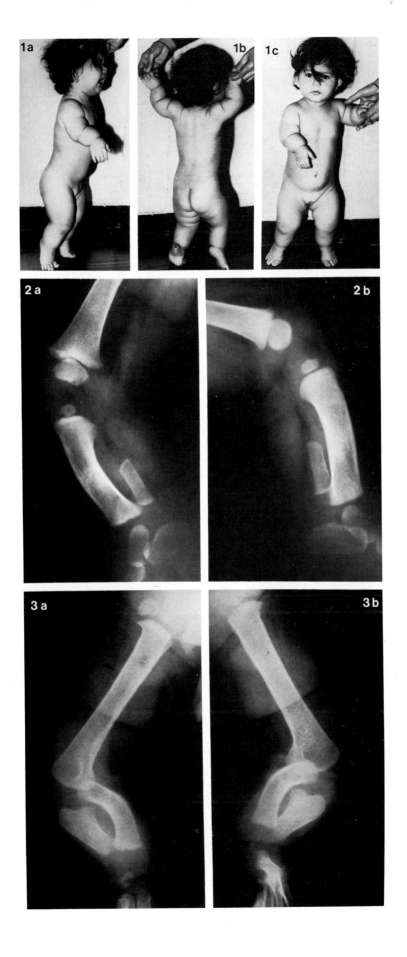

205

102. Nievergelt Syndrome

(Syndrome of Mesomelic Dysplasia, Nievergelt Type)

An autosomal dominant syndrome with severe shortening and deformity of the lower legs, occasionally also of the forearms, with characteristic X-ray findings in the lower extremities.

Main signs:
1. Short lower legs (**1, 2**) with occasional shortening of the forearms; sometimes atypical club feet. Motion may be limited at the elbows as a result of radioulnar synostosis; subluxation of the head of the radius.
2. Radiologically (**3, 4**) an almost triangular or rhomboid configuration of the short, broad tibiae (sometimes also of the radii), and to a lesser degree of the fibulae (possibly also of the ulnae). Development of synostoses of the tarsals. Radioulnar synostoses in some cases (see above).

Manifestation: At birth.

Etiology: Autosomal dominant disorder with very variable expression.

Frequency: Extremely low; only about 15 cases described since the original report (1944).

Course, prognosis: As a rule, general health is otherwise unimpaired.

Differential diagnosis: Other forms of congenital shortening of the lower legs/forearms can be differentiated radiologically.

Treatment: Surgical correction of club feet, in some cases. Further conservative operative orthopedic measures and general aids and care for the physically handicapped. Genetic counseling.

Illustrations:
1 and 2 A 7-year-old boy; height 1.05 m, with prosthesis for walking 1.23 m; length of lower leg about 11 cm (upper leg, 36 cm); genu valgus and curved legs, malpositioning of the feet, deformities of the toes. Arms normal.
3 and 4 X-rays of the same patient: massive shortening and somewhat rhomboidal broadening of the bones of the lower legs, oblique course of the terminal metaphyseal plates; synostoses of the tarsal bones.

H.-R.W.

References:

Solonen, K.A. and Sulamaa, M. Nievergelt syndrome and its treatment. *Ann. Chir. Gynaec. Fenn.*, 47, 142 (1958).
Spranger, J.W., Langer, L.O., Jr., Wiedemann, H.-R. *Bone Dysplasias. An Atlas of Constitutional Disorders of Skeletal Development.* G. Fischer and W.B. Saunders, Stuttgart and Philadelphia, 1974.
Young, L.W. and Wood, B.P. Nievergelt syndrome. *Birth Defects*, 11/5, 81 (1975).
Hess, O.M., Goebel, N.H., Streuli, R. Familiärer mesomeler Kleinwuchs (Nievergelt-Syndrom). *Schweiz. Med. Wochenschr.*, 108, 1202 (1978).

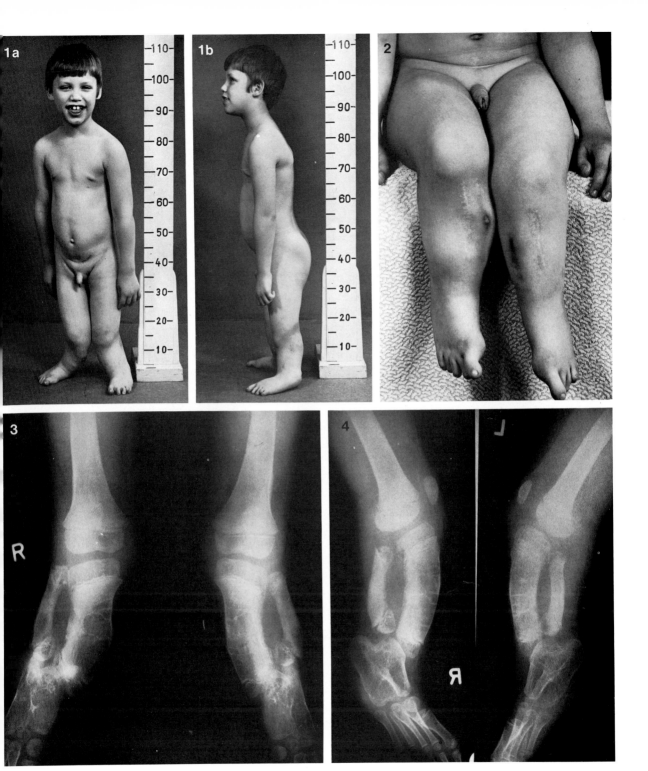

103. A 'New' Mesomelic Dysplasia Syndrome

A syndrome of mesomelic dysplasia with small stature, delayed ossification of the cranial vault, unusual facies, short neck, cardiac defect, and symmetrical flexion contractures of the fingers and toes.

Main signs:
1. Short, slightly bowed forearms. Lower extremities do not appear short, but are likewise bowed (1, 8, 10). Small stature, below the third percentile.
2. Bilateral, mostly symmetrical, flexion contractures of fingers II–V; bilateral fifth finger clinodactyly. Pes valgus and planus with mild malpositioning of the toes with flexion contractures (4, 5).
3. Large, round cranium with alopecia, except for a cockscomb-like abundant, bristly growth of hair over the region of the sagittal suture. (1–3). Frontal and sagittal sutures still completely open at age 9 months, wide open anterior fontanelle.
4. Unusual facies: broad, slightly prominent forehead; widely spaced eyes; slightly low-set ears; very broad, low nasal root; blue sclera; high narrow palate; microretrognathia (1–3). Short neck; loose nuchal skin, which can be drawn out as a pterygium.
5. Cardiologically: complete right bundle-branch block; large atrial septal defect, secundum type.
   Glandular hypospadias; bilateral cryptorchidism.

Supplementary findings: Normal mental and motor development.

Radiologically: subluxation of the elbows, bones of the forearms slightly bowed and short, with the right ulna showing a thornlike excrescence (9, 11). Tibiae a little short, slightly curved anteriorly. Fibulae relatively too long, thin, with marked anterior bowing and elevation of the distal ends (8, 10). Increased curvature and slight broadening of the clavicles.

Manifestation: At birth; small stature apparent in the toddler.

Etiology: A genetic basis certain; mode of inheritance not clear.

Frequency: Low.

Course, prognosis: Apparently favorable.

Differential diagnosis: The Robinow syndrome (p.210) shows similarities; however, it can be readily excluded.

Treatment: Symptomatic.

Illustrations:
1–11 The first child of healthy, young, nonconsanguineous parents, after two miscarriages. Birth measurements 3000 g and 51 cm.

H.-R.W.

Reference:
Löhr, H. and Wiedemann, H.-R. Mesomelic dysplasia—associated with other abnormalities. *Eur. J. Pediatr.*, 137, 313 (1981).

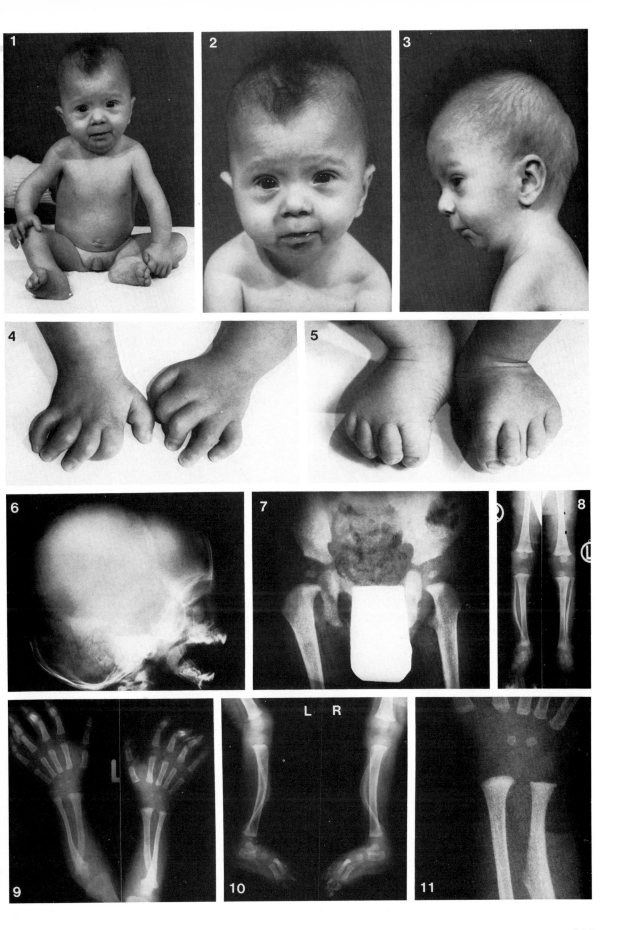

104. Robinow Syndrome

(Fetal Face Syndrome; Mesomelic Dysplasia, Robinow Type)

A syndrome of unusual facies, short forearms, genital hypoplasia and short stature.

Main signs:
1. 'Fetal face': a disproportionately large cranium with large anterior fontanelle and prominent forehead, the face being relatively small and flat with hypertelorism, wide palpebral fissures and correspondingly large-appearing eyes, antimongoloid slant of the palpebral fissures; mid-face hypoplasia, pug nose, long philtrum, relatively large triangular mouth with down-turned corners, micrognathia (1).
2. Mesomelic dysplasia of the upper extremities, the forearms being short. Brachydactyly with fifth finger clinodactyly. Lower legs comparatively less affected or normal (1).
3. Micropenis, with testes and scrotum usually unremarkable (1); hypoplasia of the clitoris and labia minora.
4. Small stature.

Supplementary findings: Mental development normal in over 80% of cases.

Radiologically, bowing of the radius with subluxation of the capitulum; obvious shortening of the ulna.

Clefts of the distal phalanges of the fingers in some cases; dysplasia of the nails.

Frequent anomalies of the vertebral column and/or ribs (hemi- or block vertebrae, fusion), in some cases resulting in scoliosis. Frequent dental anomalies and gingival hyperplasia.

Cryptorchidism not infrequent. Inguinal hernias.

Manifestation: At birth; birth lengths within normal limits, but falling to below the third percentile during the first years of life.

Etiology: Genetically determined, but variable syndrome. Autosomal dominant inheritance established. An autosomal recessive form, clinically indistinguishable, also occurs. Thus heterogeneity can be assumed.

Frequency: Low; between 1969 and 1987, barely 40 cases described.

Course, prognosis: With respect to general health, good in most cases. Less favorable for development of the penis. Adult height may be about normal. Data about reproduction, etc., still insufficient.

Differential diagnosis: Other forms of mesomelic dysplasia should not be difficult to rule out. A disturbingly striking overlap with the features of Aarskog syndrome (p.194), which however shows a peculiar type of scrotal dysplasia, as opposed to genital hypoplasia (in both sexes).

Treatment: Symptomatic. Orthopedic measures in some cases. Possible early trial of testosterone therapy to modify the micropenis, which may otherwise be treated by constructive plastic surgery. Psychological guidance. Genetic counseling.

Illustration:
1 A mentally normal 8-year-old boy, the third child of healthy, nonconsanguineous parents after two healthy children. Birth measurements 3200 g, 49 cm, head circumference 39 cm. Present height below the third percentile; cranial circumference in relation to his height, 98th percentile; frontal bossing. Micropenis of max. 3 cm length (after plastic surgery). Brachydactyly, clinodactyly; radiologically, slight clefts of the distal phalanges of the thumbs.

H.-R.W.

References:

Giedion, A., Battaglia, G.F., Bellini, F. et al. The radiological diagnosis of the fetal face (= Robinow) syndrome (mesomelic dwarfism and small genitalia). *Helv. Paediatr. Acta*, 30, 409 (1975).

Vogt, J., Reinwein, H., Fink, M. et al. Das Robinow-Syndrom. *Pädiat. Prax.*, 21, 103 (1979).

Lee, P.A., Migeon, C.J., Brown, T.R. et al. Robinow's syndrome. Partial primary hypogonadism in pubertal boys with persistence of micropenis. *Am. J. Dis. Child.*, 136, 327 (1982).

Shprintzen, R.J., Goldberg, R.B. et al. Male-to-male transmission of Robinow's syndrome. *Am. J. Dis. Child.*, 136, 594–597 (1982).

Bain, M.D., Winter, R.M. et al. Robinow syndrome without mesomelic 'brachymelia': a report of five cases. *J. Med. Genet.*, 23, 350–354 (1986).

Glaser, D., Herbst, J., Roggenkamp, K. et al. Robinow syndrome with parental consanguinity. *Eur. J. Pediatr.*, 148, 652–653 (1989).

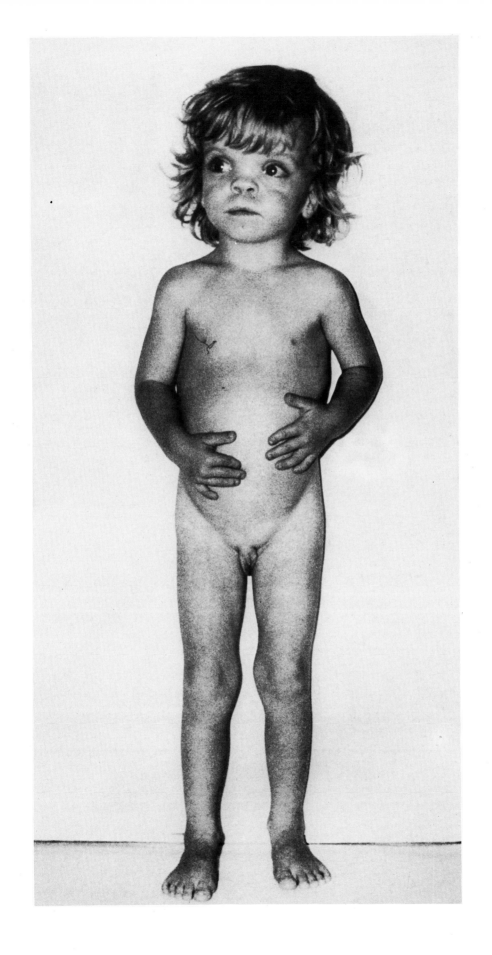

105. Achondrogenesis

An extremely severe congenital skeletal dysplasia with macrocephaly, extreme micromelia, and a variable degree of hydrops.

Main signs:
1. Macrocephaly, 'absent neck', short trunk with distended abdomen. Extremely short extremities, usually with varus positioning of the lower extremities.
2. Hydropic appearance (**1a**).

Supplementary findings: Normal number of fingers and toes. Radiologically, more or less absent ossification of vertebral bodies, sacrum, pubic bones, and ischia (**1b**). Comparatively well-developed cranial bones, especially the basilar bone.

Usually premature birth. Death in immediate postnatal period.

Manifestation: At birth.

Etiology: Hereditary disorder. Here, too, several forms that can be differentiated clinically–radiologically and histologically. Autosomal recessive mode of inheritance.

Frequency: Low; altogether at least 120 cases (of different types) have been described to date.

Course, prognosis: If not stillborn, death shortly after delivery.

Differential diagnosis: Thanatophoric dysplasia (p.214), and a few other skeletal dysplasias.

Treatment: At most, symptomatic. Genetic counseling. With subsequent pregnancies, prenatal diagnosis with ultrasonography.

Illustrations:

1a and b A child born 6 weeks prematurely (pregnancy complicated by hydramnios); length 28 cm.

H.-R.W.

References:

Wiedemann, H.-R., Remagen, W., Hienz, H.A., Gorlin, R.J., Maroteaux, P. Achondrogenesis within the scope of connately manifested generalized skeletal dysplasias. *Z. Kinderheilkd.*, 116, 223 (1974).
Spranger, J.W., Langer, L.O., Jr., Wiedemann, H.-R. *Bone Dysplasias. An Atlas of Constitutional Disorders of Skeletal Development.* G. Fischer and W.B. Saunders, Stuttgart and Philadelphia, 1974.
Kozlowski, K., Masel, J., Morris, L. et al. Neonatal death dwarfism. *Aust. Radiol.*, 21, 164 (1977).
Schulte, M.J., Lenz, W., Vogel, M. Letale Achondrogenesis: Eine Übersicht über 56 Fälle. *Klin. Pädiatr.*, 191, 327 (1978).
Andersen, P.E., Jr. Achondrogenesis type II in twins. *Brit. J. Radiol.*, 54, 61 (1981).
Chen, H., Lin, T., Yang, S.S. Achondrogenesis: a review . . . *Am. J. Med. Genet.*, 10, 379 (1981).
Smith, W.L., Breitweiser, T.D., Dinno, N. In utero diagnosis of achondrogenesis, type I. *Clin. Genet.*, 19, 51 (1981).
Whitley, C.B. and Gorlin, R.J. Achondrogenesis . . . genetic heterogeneity. *Radiology*, 148, 693–698 (1983).
Maroteaux, P., Stanescu, V. et al. Hypochondrogenesis. *Eur. J. Pediatr.*, 141, 14–22 (1983).
Borochowitz, Z., Ornoy, A. et al. Achondrogenesis II—hypochondrogenesis: variability versus heterogeneity. *Am. J. Med. Genet.*, 24, 273–288 (1986).
Kozlowski, K., Tsuruta, T. et al. A new type of achondrogenesis. *Pediatr. Radiol.*, 16, 430–432 (1986).
Horton, W.A., Machado, M.A. et al. Achondrogenesis type II . . . *Pediatr. Res.*, 22, 324–329 (1987).
Borochowitz, Z., Lachman, R. et al. Achondrogenesis type I: . . . identification of two distinct subgroups. *J. Pediatr.*, 112, 23–31 (1988).
Dilmen, U., Kaya, I.S. et al. Achondrogenesis type II. *Pediatr. Radiol.*, 19, 53 (1988).

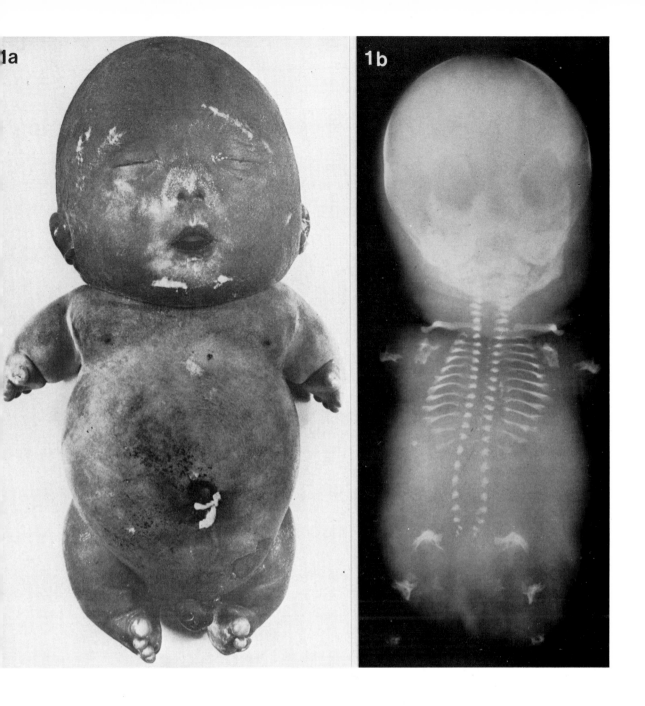

213

106. Thanatophoric Dysplasia

(Maroteaux, Lamy, Robert)

A severe congenital skeletal dysplasia with disproportionately large cranium, narrow thorax, and marked micromelia.

Main signs:
1. Macrocephaly (with wide fontanelles and sutures), with low nasal root and proptosis of the eyes.
2. Relatively normal trunk length with narrow thorax.
3. Micromelia (**1a**).

Supplementary findings: Radiologically: Short ribs with narrow thorax; marked platyspondyly with abnormal configuration of the vertebral bodies; narrow, short, and flat pelvis; long bones shortened, poorly shaped, and in part considerably bowed (the shape of the femur has been compared to that of a telephone receiver) (**1b**). Immediate development of the respiratory distress syndrome.

Manifestation: At birth (frequently hydramnios).

Etiology: Sporadic occurrence; autosomal dominant new mutation?

Frequency: Low (about 1:40,000–45,000 births; up to 1980 about 100 observations reported in the literature.

Course, prognosis: As a rule, death shortly after birth. Early ultrasonographic diagnosis should be carried out in subsequent pregnancies.

Differential diagnosis: The appearance of the children is very suggestive of achondroplasia in older individuals. However, the physical signs and radiological findings in newborns with the usual heterozygotic (and even with the rare homozygotic) achondroplasia are considerably milder.

Type II and several 'variants' of thanatophoric dysplasia, in addition to other severe congenital skeletal dysplasias, must be ruled out.

Illustrations:
1a and b A child (8-month gestation) who died on the second day of life, and an X-ray of the same.

H.-R.W.

References:

Spranger, J.W., Langer, L.O., Jr., Wiedemann, H.-R. *Bone Dysplasias. An Atlas of Constitutional Bone Disorders.* G. Fischer and W.B. Saunders, Stuttgart and Philadelphia, 1974.
Connor, J.M., Connor, R.A.C. et al. Lethal neonatal chondrodysplasias . . . *Am. J. Med. Genet.,* 22, 243–253 (1985).
Martinez-Frias, M.L., Ramos-Arroyo, M.A. et al. Thanatophoric dysplasia: an autosomal dominant condition? *Am. J. Med. Genet.,* 31, 815–820 (1988).
Young, I.D., Patel, I., Lamont, A.C. Thanatophoric dysplasia in identical twins. *J. Med. Genet.,* 26, 276 (1989).

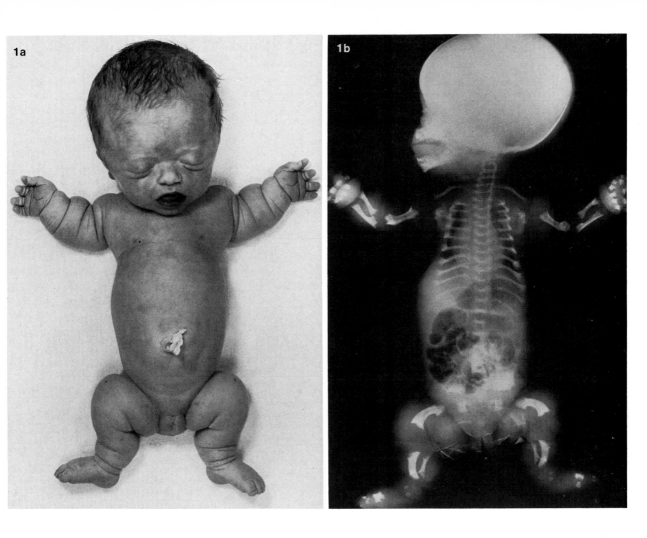

107. Thanatophoric Dysplasia Type II with Cloverleaf Skull

A form of thanatophoric dysplasia with cloverleaf skull, straight or minimally bowed femora, and less markedly flattened vertebral bodies.

Main signs:
1. Macrocephaly with cloverleaf-like deformity (large cranium with upward and outward protrusions; depressed nasal root; exophthalmos; and downward displacement of the ears, almost to the horizontal) (**1–5**).
2. Trunk of near-normal length, with narrow, often bell-shaped thorax and protruding abdomen (**2, 6**).
3. Micromelia with numerous skin folds; extremities held away from the trunk, femora abducted and externally rotated; very small fingers and toes (**2, 6**).

Supplementary findings:
1. Below average size in many cases.
2. Radiologically, short ribs with narrow thorax, unremarkable clavicles. Flattening of the vertebral bodies—but height of L2 (second lumbar) is 50% or more of the height of the adjacent L2–3 intervertebral disc.
   Characteristic pelvic shape of thanatophoric dysplasia. Shortening and partial bowing of the long bones—although the femora may be straight for the most part. The fibulae are shorter than the tibiae. Very short, broad phalanges of the fingers and toes (**6**).
3. Immediate development of the respiratory distress syndrome.

Manifestation: At birth (frequently hydramnios).

Etiology: With the exception of one set of siblings, all cases have been sporadic; parental consanguinity never demonstrated with certainty. Mode of inheritance still unclear. For the time being, the risk of recurrence may be considered very low.

Frequency: Low; about 25 cases have been reported in the literature.

Course, prognosis: As a rule, death shortly after birth from respiratory insufficiency. Early ultrasonographic diagnosis indicated in subsequent pregnancies.

Diagnosis, differential diagnosis: The example of type I thanatophoric dysplasia (p.215 with markedly bowed femora and severe platyspondyly) shows a very mild cloverleaf skull configuration. This is present only as an exception.

Illustrations: **1–6** A characteristically affected male newborn, born at term. Birth measurements: 47 cm, 3540 g, 39 cm (head circumference). Death at 5 days of age from respiratory insufficiency.

H.-R.W.

References:

Partington, M., Gonzalez-Crussi, F., Khakee, S.G. et al. Cloverleaf skull and thanatophoric dwarfism. Report of four cases, two in the same sibship. *Arch. Dis. Child.*, 46, 656–664 (1971).

Gemelli, M., Galatioto, S., Longo, M. et al. Nanismo tantoforo con cranio a trifoglio. *Min. Ped.*, 34, 977–982 (1982).

Horton, W.A., Harris, D.J., Collins, D.L. Discordance for the Kleeblattschädel anomaly in monozygotic twins with thanatophoric dysplasia. *Am. J. Med. Genet.*, 15, 97–101 (1983).

Isaacson, G., Blakemore, K.J., Chervenak, F.A. Thanatophoric dysplasia with cloverleaf skull. *Am. J. Dis. Child.*, 137, 896–898 (1983).

Elejalde, B.R. and Elejalde, M.M.de. Thanatophoric dysplasia: fetal manifestations and prenatal diagnosis. *Am. J. Med. Genet.*, 22, 669–683 (1985).

Langer, L.O., Jr., Yang, S.S., Hall, J.G. et al. Thanatophoric dysplasia and cloverleaf skull. *Am. J. Med. Genet.*, (Suppl.) 3, 167–179 (1987).

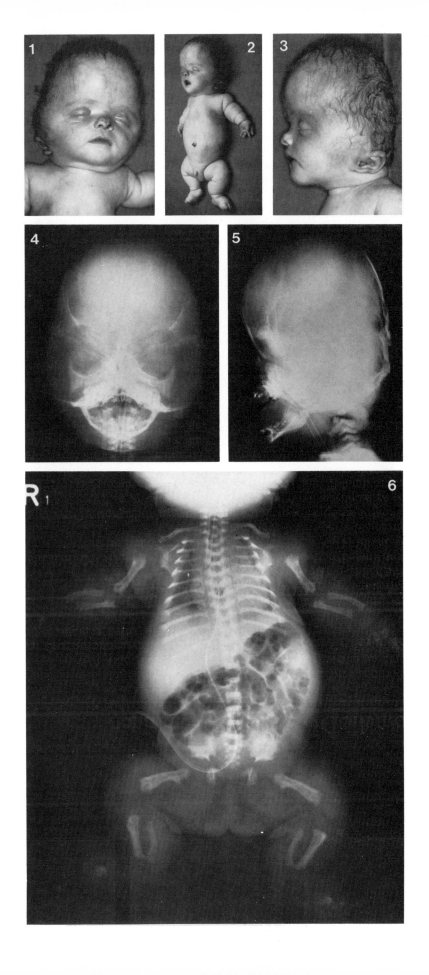

217

108. Saldino–Noonan Type of Short Rib–Polydactyly Syndrome

(Saldino–Noonan Syndrome)

A hereditary syndrome leading to perinatal death, with narrow thorax, very short ribs, brachymelia, polydactyly, anogenital anomalies, and characteristic radiological changes.

Main signs:
1. Severe narrowing of the thorax (with hypoplasia of the lungs) and distended abdomen (**1**). Respiratory insufficiency.
2. Brachymelia and usually postaxial polydactyly (**1**).
3. Anal atresia and/or genital hypoplasia or malformation.
4. Usually congenital hydrops.
5. Radiologically: short, horizontal ribs, anomalies of the scapulae and the pelvis, marked metaphyseal irregularities of the long bones, which are considerably shortened, and many other abnormalities (**1b**).

Supplementary findings: Round, flat face; absence of nails. At autopsy, anomalies of the heart, kidney, pancreas, and other organs are frequent.

Manifestation: At birth.

Etiology: Autosomal recessive disorder.

Frequency: Low; by 1987 over 60 observations had been reported.

Course, prognosis: Poor. If not stillborn, the infant dies shortly after birth from respiratory insufficiency.

Differential diagnosis: There are further rare short rib–polydactyly syndromes. In addition, the Ellis–van Creveld (p.244) and the D₁ trisomy (p.86) syndromes should be considered.

Treatment: Symptomatic. Genetic counseling; prenatal diagnosis with ultrasonography in subsequent pregnancies.

Illustrations:
1a and 1b A typically affected premature newborn (35.5 cm; 1300 g), the first child of young parents after one termination of pregnancy and a spontaneous abortion. Death immediately *post partum*. Postaxial polydactyly of the hands and feet. (Unusual additional finding: multiple frenulae between the upper lip and the alveolar process—as in Ellis–van Creveld syndrome, p.244).

H.-R.W.

References:

Spranger, J.W., Langer, L.O., Jr., Wiedemann, H.-R. *Bone Dysplasias. An Atlas of Constitutional Disorders of Skeletal Development.* G. Fischer and W.B. Saunders, Stuttgart and Philadelphia, 1974.

Krepler, R., Wießenbacher, G., Leodolter, S. et al. Nicht lebensfähiger mikromeler Zwergwuchs . . . *Monatschr. Kinderheilkd.,* 124, 167 (1976).

Richardson, M.M., Beaudet, A.L., Wagner, M.L. et al. Prenatal diagnosis of recurrence of Saldino–Noonan dwarfism. *J. Pediatr.,* 91, 467 (1977).

Rupprecht, E. and Gurski, A. Kurzrippen-Polydaktylie-Syndrom Typ Saldino–Noonan bei zwei Geschwistern. *Helv. Pediatr. Acta,* 37, 161 (1982).

Johnson, V.P., Petersen, L.P. et al. Midtrimester prenatal diagnosis of . . . Saldino–Noonan syndrome. *Birth Defects,* 18, 133–141 (1982).

Grote, W., Weisner, D. et al. Prenatal diagnosis of . . . Saldino–Noonan at 17 week's gestation. *Eur. J. Pediatr.,* 140, 63–66 (1983).

Toftager-Larsen, K. and Benzie, R.J. Fetoscopy in prenatal diagnosis of . . . Saldino–Noonan . . . *Clin. Genet.,* 26, 56–60 (1984).

Bernstein, R., Isdale, J. et al. Short rib-polydactyly syndrome: a single or heterogeneous entity? *J. Med. Genet.,* 22, 46–53 (1985).

Sillence, D., Kozlowski, K. et al. Perinatally lethal short rib-polydactyly syndromes . . . *Pediatr. Radiol.,* 17, 474–480 (1987).

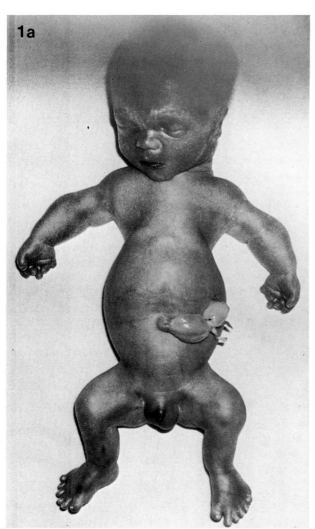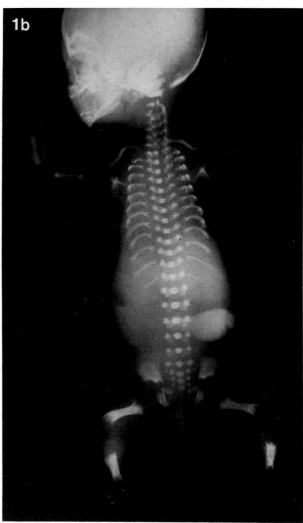

109. Chondrodysplasia Punctata, Autosomal Recessive Type

(Chondrodysplasia Punctata, Rhizomelic Type)

A hereditary disorder with primordial growth deficiency, unusual facies, severe psychomotor retardation, and not infrequently ichthyosiform skin changes.

Main signs:
1. Disproportionate short stature with predominantly symmetrical shortening of the arms and upper legs and multiple joint contractures (1).
2. Flat face; very full cheeks; broad, depressed nasal root. Altogether somewhat mongoloid appearance (1). Very short, broad neck.
3. Not infrequently, ichthyosiform skin changes, alopecia.
4. Marked psychomotor retardation, tetrasparosis, usually microcephaly.

Supplementary findings: Bilateral cataracts almost always present, occasional optic atrophy.

Radiologically, usually severe symmetrical shortening, metaphyseal flaring, and punctate calcification of the ends of the humerus and/or femur (2). Dysplasia of the pelvis. Little or no punctate calcification ('stippling') in the vertebral column; dorsal and ventral ossification centers of the vertebral bodies (on lateral view) not joined! (Disappearance of the calcium flecks usually during the first year of life; fusion of the vertebral ossification centers).

Manifestation: At birth.

Etiology: Autosomal recessive disorder, an X-linked recessive form has recently been reported; peroxisomal enzyme defect.

Frequency: Very low (about 60 observations in the literature).

Course, prognosis: Poor. The great majority of affected children die in infancy, usually of infections.

Differential diagnosis: Other types of chondrodysplasia punctata (pp.222 and 226) and other conditions that show or may show stippled epiphyses on X-ray in the newborn period, such as trisomy 18 and Down's syndromes (pp.88 and 90), CHILD, Smith–Lemli–Opitz, or Zellweger syndromes (pp.228, 494, and 514), fetal alcohol syndrome and coumarin (= 'Warfarin') embryopathy.

Treatment: Symptomatic. Genetic counseling. Ultrasonographic prenatal diagnosis.

Illustrations:
1 and 2 A newborn. Early death from pneumonia and hypoplastic lungs. Right clubfoot.

H.-R.W.

References:

Spranger, J.W., Langer, L.O., Jr., Wiedemann, H.-R. *Bone Dysplasias. An Atlas of Constitutional Disorders of Skeletal Development.* G. Fischer and W.B. Saunders, Stuttgart and Philadelphia, 1974.

Gilbert, E.F., Opitz, J.M., Spranger, J.W. et al. Chondrodysplasia punctata—rhizomelic form. *Eur. J. Pediatr.,* 123, 89 (1976).

Heymans, H.S.A., Oorthuys, J.W.E. et al. Rhizomelic chondrodysplasia punctata: another peroxismal disorder. *N. Engl. J. Med.,* 313, 187–188 (1985).

Heymans, H.S.A., Oorthuys, J.W.E. et al. Peroxismal abnormalities in rhizomelic chondrodysplasia punctata. *J. Inher. Metab. Dis.,* 9, 329–331 (1986).

Poulos, A., Sheffield, L. et al. Rhizomelic chondrodysplasia punctata . . . *J. Pediatr.,* 113, 685–690 (1988).

Bick, D., Curry, C.J.R. et al. Male infant with ichthyosis, Kallmann syndrome, chondrodysplasia punctata, and an Xp chromosome deletion. *Am. J. Med. Genet.,* 33, 100–107 (1989).

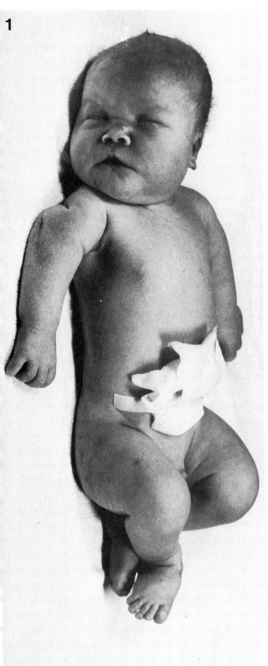

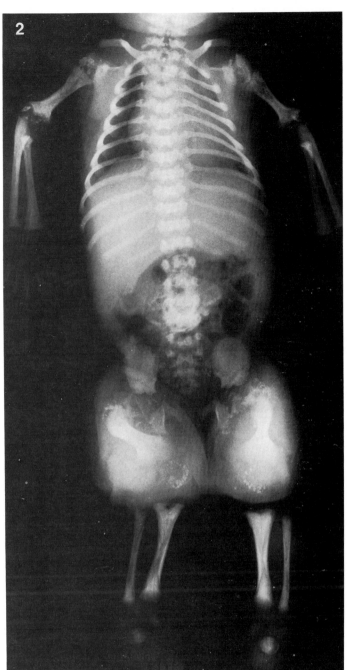

110. Chondrodysplasia Punctata, Autosomal Dominant Type

(Chondrodysplasia Punctata Type Conradi–Hünermann; Syndrome of Chondrodysplasia Calcificans; Conradi–Hünermann Syndrome)

A skeletal dysplasia syndrome with unusual facies, short extremities, and frequently curvature of the spine and small stature.

Main signs:
1. Facial dysmorphism with low broad nasal root, slight mongoloid slant of the palpebral fissures in some cases, hypoplasia of the midface, and frequently bilateral notches of the tip of the nose (1).
2. Small stature with symmetrical or slightly asymmetrical shortening of the extremities; frequent development of scoliosis, kyphosis.
   Dysplasia and contractures of the joints.

Supplementary findings: No cataracts; no obvious dermatoses.
   Radiologically, punctate or stippled calcifications of the ends of the long bones, the vertebral processes, the carpal and tarsal bones, and the ischial and pubic bones; eventual disappearance of these calcifications (2).

Manifestation: At birth. Scoliosis may develop later.

Etiology: Autosomal dominant inheritance; sporadic cases suggest of new mutation.

Frequency: Low.

Course, prognosis: Good, after survival of the hazardous first months of life.

Differential diagnosis: Personally, I consider that the existence of this form remains uncertain. At any rate, in every suspected case the other hereditary types of chondrodysplasia, coumarin embryopathy (p.224), alcohol damage to the fetus, etc., must be ruled out as completely as possible.

Treatment: Symptomatic orthopedic. Genetic counseling.

Illustrations:
1 and 2 A boy born at term, the first child of young parents. No evidence of possible teratogenic damage during pregnancy.
   Flat face with slight mongoloid slant of the palpebral fissures; low nasal bridge; hypoplastic, 'notched' nose with anteverted nostrils (1). Broad, short thorax. No recognizable shortening of the extremities. Clinodactyly of the fourth toe bilaterally. No dermatosis. No cataract. Normal karyotype. A Zellweger syndrome was excluded. Radiologically, 'stippling' of the epiphyses at the large joints and pronounced along the vertebral column (2). The father of the child shows degenerative skeletal changes; his mother, short stature.

H.-R.W.

References:
Spranger, J.W., Opitz, J.M., Bidder, U. Heterogeneity of chondrodysplasia punctata. *Hum. Genet.*, 11, 190–212 (1971).
Happle, R. Cataracts as a marker of genetic heterogeneity in chrondrodysplasia punctata. *Clin. Genet.*, 19, 64–66 (1981).

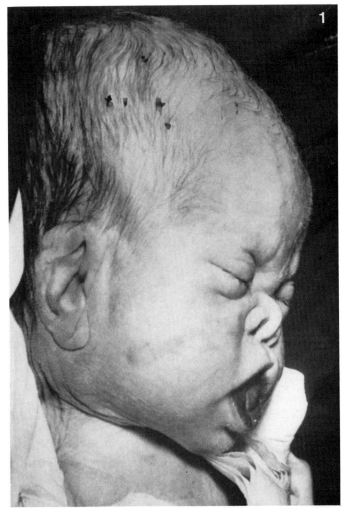

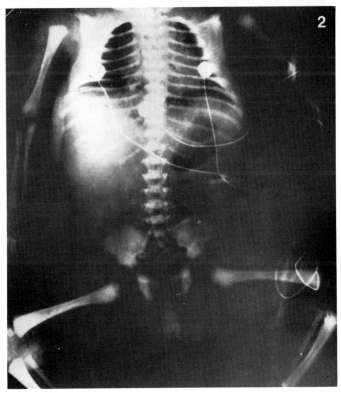

223

111. Coumarin Embryopathy

(Warfarin Embryopathy)

An embryopathy that can present a variably severe phenocopy of the autosomal dominant type of chondrodysplasia punctata.

Main signs:
1. Hypoplasia of the midface; low, broad root of the nose, initially with anteverted nares and with generally obvious notches between the tip of the nose and the alae nasi (**1–3**).
2. Prenatal growth retardation and postnatal small stature with symmetrical or slightly asymmetrical shortening of the extremities, especially the proximal portions (**4**).
3. In infancy, radiological punctate or stippled calcifications, especially of the carpal and tarsal bones, along the vertebral column, and in the proximal femur.

Eventual disappearance of these calcifications (see **7**—X-rays at different ages).

Supplementary findings: Frequently initial respiratory difficulties (due to choanal stenosis?). Frequently subsequent development of hyperlordosis or kyphosis, scoliosis (**4, 5**). Limited motion of the large joints. Brachydactyly, syndactyly (**6**). Hypoplasia of the nails. Mental impairment in some cases.

Manifestation: At birth.

Etiology: Coumarin exposure of the mother in the first trimester of pregnancy, especially between the sixth and the ninth weeks. (Later or prolonged exposure can cause marked CNS damage, especially to the eyes and vision.)

Frequency: Low; at least 50 cases are known.

Course, prognosis: Increased mortality in the perinatal period and in the first year of life, dependent on the severity. The nose improves in appearance with the passage of time (cf. **1–3**).

Differential diagnosis: Chondrodysplasia punctata, and occasionally some of the numerous other disorders that may show epiphyseal stippling on X-ray during the newborn period and infancy.

Treatment: Symptomatic, including orthopedic care.

Illustrations:
1–7 The same patient at age 2 months (**1** and **7**, left side), 13 months (**7**, right side), 8 years (**2** and **4**), and 31 years (**3, 5,** and **6**). At 2 months, length and weight below the third percentile, short arms and thighs, bent legs, and stippling of the vertebral column, most of the epiphyses of the bones of the arms and legs, and the tarsals and carpals. Height at 8½ years 105 cm (below the third percentile); right extremities somewhat shorter than the left; scoliosis, flattening of the vertebral bodies from T6 down; limited extension at both knees and elbows. At 31 years, disproportionate small stature of 154 cm; scoliosis, lordosis; brachydactyly, syndactyly. Normal intelligence. In 1954 the clinical picture was considered that of chondrodysplasia calcificans; subsequently that of an autosomal dominant type. When, in 1985, the patient's wife was expecting their first child and was quite concerned about the 50% risk, the medical records from 1953 of the patient's mother were checked. These showed that his mother had received coumarin therapy during the sixth to the ninth and eleventh to thirteenth weeks of gestation. Subsequent birth of a healthy child.

H.-R.W.

References:

Hall, J.G., Pauli, R.M., Wilson, K.M. Maternal et fetal sequelae of anticoagulation during pregnancy. *Am. J. Med.*, 68, 122–140 (1980).
Whitfield, W.F. Chondrodysplasia punctata after warfarin in early pregnancy. *Arch. Dis. Child.*, 55, 139–142 (1980).
Kleinebrecht, J. Zur Teratogenität von Cumarin-Derivaten. *Dtsch. Med. Wochenschr.*, 107, 1929–1931 (1982).
Tamburrini, O., Bartolomeo-De Iuri, A., Di Guglielmo, G.L. Chondrodysplasia punctata after warfarin. *Pediatr. Radiol.*, 17, 323–324 (1987).
Hosenfeld, D. and Wiedemann, H.-R. Chondrodysplasia punctata in an adult recognized as vitamin K antagonist embryopathy. *Clin. Genet.*, 35, 376–381 (1989).

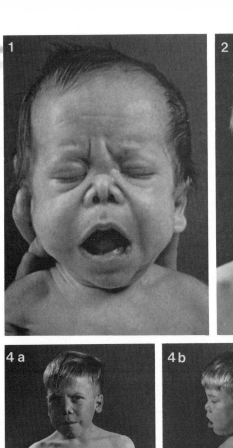
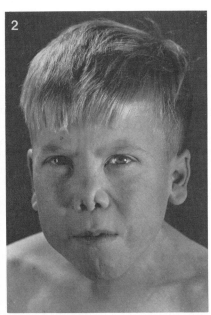
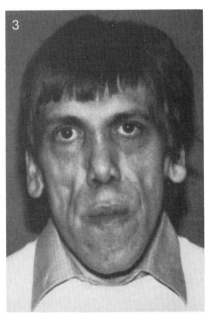
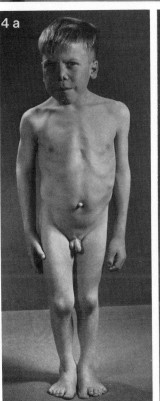
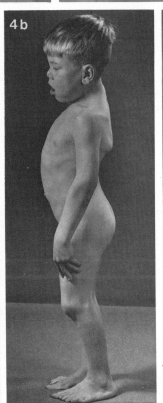
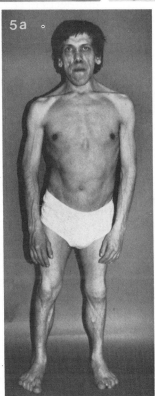
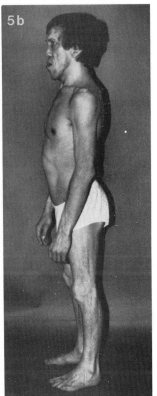
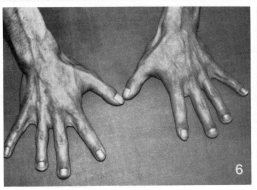
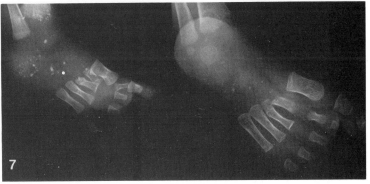

112. Chondrodysplasia Punctata, Sex-Linked Dominant Type

A dysplasia syndrome affecting only females with a mosaic pattern of skin changes and anomalies of the skeleton and eyes, generally with asymmetric distribution.

Main signs:
1. Asymmetric skeletal anomalies with congenital shortening of the long bones (most frequently the femur, then the humerus) (2); dysplasia and contracture of joints (hip, knee, ankle, and other) and in some cases dysplasia of the vertebral column, with secondary scoliosis. Unusual facies with low, broad nasal root, slight mongoloid slant of the palpebral fissures, possible marked asymmetry of the facial skeleton. Hexadactyly in some patients (3).
2. Congenital ichthyosiform erythroderma (4, 7) with patchy and striated areas of hyperkeratosis. Later, patchy and striated atrophy of the skin, especially affecting the hair follicles (particularly of the forearm); patchy areas of alopecia (6, 8) and areas of brittle, tortuous, coarse, lackluster hair (6); eyebrows and eyelashes sparse, growing in various directions (6). Older children frequently affected with ichthyosis (5).
3. Congenital or early cataracts in about two-thirds of cases, may be uni- or bilateral; if bilateral, usually one eye more severely affected than the other (1).

Supplementary findings: Systemic streaky pigmentation anomalies in some cases; nails may be flat, with tendency to split horizontally (3).

Frequent short stature, in part secondary to scoliosis. Normal intellect.

Radiologically, 'stippling' (punctate calcifications) in various areas of the skeleton, especially the epiphyses of the long bones. Early disappearance of the stippling; diagnosis also possible in its absence.

Manifestation: At birth.

Etiology: Presumably an X-linked dominant disorder with lethal effect of the gene on male embryos. The presence of mild cutaneous signs in the mothers of some probands (9) suggests there is also an incomplete manifestation of this hereditary form. Most cases are sporadic and should represent new mutations.

Frequency: Low. By 1980, 40 cases, exclusively in females, could be identified.

Course, prognosis: Good on the whole (patients handicapped by growth deficiency, scoliosis, and in some cases ocular defects). Spontaneous regression of the congenital ichthyosiform erythroderma during infancy with development of systemic atrophoderma.

Differential diagnosis: See p.220. A systemic anomaly of pigmentation may suggest the Bloch–Sulzburger syndrome (p.338) (transmitted by the same mode of inheritance), which should not be difficult to exclude by careful observation.

Treatment: Symptomatic (ophthalmological, orthopedic, etc.). Careful examination of the mother for mild signs of the disorder. Genetic counseling. Prenatal diagnosis.

Illustrations:
1–6 An affected girl as a newborn (4), at 6 months (1 and 3), at 6 years (2), and as an adolescent. Asymmetric thorax and asymmetrical shortening of the extremities; postaxial hexadactyly of the left hand. As a newborn, multiple foci of calcium in the epiphyses of the left leg and in the costal cartilages. Foci of alopecia and typical changes of the scalp hair.
7 and 8 An affected girl as a newborn (also 'stippling' on X-ray, skeletal asymmetry, and unilateral cataract) and as an adolescent.
9 Foci of alopecia of the scalp of the proband's mother.

H.-R.W.

References:
Manzke, H., Christophers, E., Wiedemann, H.-R. Dominant sex-linked inherited chondrodysplasia punctata: a distinct type of chondrodysplasia punctata. *Clin. Genet.*, 17, 107 (1980).
Happle, R. X-gekoppelt dominante Chondrodysplasia punctata. *Monatschr. Kinderheilkd.*, 128, 203 (1980).
Mueller, R.F., Crowle, P.M. et al. X-linked dominant chondrodysplasia punctata . . . *Am. J. Med. Genet.*, 20, 137–144 (1985).
Kozlowski, K., Bates, E.H. et al. Dominant X-linked chondrodysplasia punctata. *Am. J. Dis. Child.*, 142, 1233–1234 (1988).

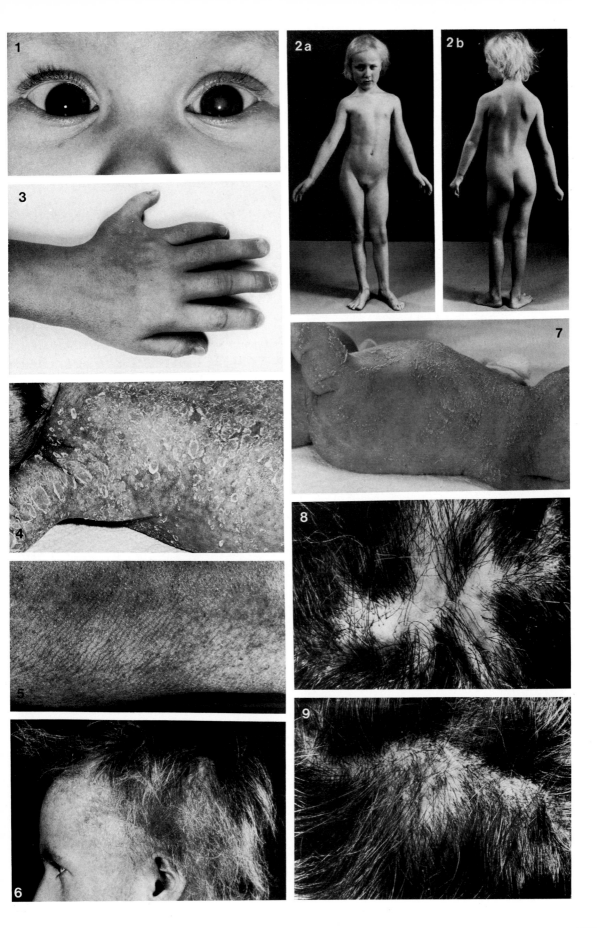

113. CHILD Syndrome

(Syndrome of Congenital Hemidysplasia with Ichthyosiform Erythroderma and Limb Defects)

A syndrome of unilateral ichthyosiform erythroderma and ipsilateral defects of variable severity of the limbs and skeleton.

Main signs:
1. Ichthyosiform erythroderma, which—more or less completely—affects one half of the body and is sharply outlined along the midline of the trunk (**1, 7**). Variable progression—the extent may parallel the severity of the skeletal and visceral defects. The face is usually spared. The nails may develop severe hyperkeratoses (**3, 4**).
2. Ipsilateral skeletal hypoplasia (**2, 2a**). Practically any part of the skeleton may be affected, in most cases usually the long bones are involved—varying from mere hypoplasia of phalanges to absence of a whole extremity. A hand and/or foot may be severely deformed.

Supplementary findings: The right side has been affected in the vast majority of cases observed to date (smaller anomalies may also occur contralaterally).

Secondary scoliosis in some cases (**2a**).

Ipsilateral anomalies of the internal organs (heart, lungs, kidneys, or other) or of the nervous system may occur.

Radiologically, in a few cases examined in the early postnatal period, epiphyseal calcium spots were demonstrated ipsilaterally in the limbs, the pelvis, or elsewhere.

Manifestation: At birth. The dermatosis may develop later, during the first months of life.

Etiology: Apparently a genetic syndrome. Almost exclusively girls affected. Possibly based on an X-linked dominant gene with lethal effect in males.

Frequency: Low (up to 1982, 25 observations were reported).

Course, prognosis: The dermatosis may remain constant in severity or may transiently vary in severity, it may affect new areas of skin, but may also show continuing spontaneous regression. Otherwise the prognosis depends on the presence and severity of internal and skeletal defects.

Differential diagnosis: With chondrodysplasia punctata of the X-linked dominant type (p.226), the dermatosis occurs on both sides of the body in a different pattern and (in older children) with signs of dermal atrophy. The Schimmelpenning–Feuerstein–Mims syndrome (p.314) shows a different type of dermatosis.

Treatment: No effective treatment for the dermatosis is known. Remedial measures, such as orthopedic, prosthetic, or plastic surgery. Treatment of internal organ anomalies in some cases. Handicap aids. Genetic counseling.

Illustrations:
1–6 An affected girl at ages 4 months (**1, 2,** and **2a**), 1 year (**3–5,** and 3 years (**6**). Hypoplasia of the extremities on the right (**2**) with flexion contracture of the elbow. Right-sided hypoplasia of the mandible, scapula, ribs, pelvis, and right vertebral bodies (note also vertebral clefts) with secondary scoliosis (**2 and 2a**). Dermatosis manifest at 2 months, sharply outlined along the midline of the trunk (**1**), the only areas spared being part of the face and head and the palmar and plantar surfaces. Right renal aplasia. Dermatosis for the most part resistant to therapy, but eventual spontaneous regression (**5 and 6**). Development of severe hyperkeratosis of and around the nails (**3 and 4**).
7 and 8 A 4-year-old girl with similar skeletal involvement and corresponding localized, medially outlined dermatosis in the right lumbar region (**7**) and an affected area on the left hand (**8**).

H.-R.W.

References:
Happle, R., Koch, H., Lenz, W. The CHILD syndrome. *Eur. J. Pediatr.*, 134, 27 (1980).
Happle, R. X-chromosomal vererbte Dermatosen. *Hautarzt*, 33, 73–81 (1982).
Christiansen, J.V., Petersen, H.O. et al. The CHILD-syndrome . . . *Acta Derm. Venereol.* (Stockh.), 64, 165–168 (1984).

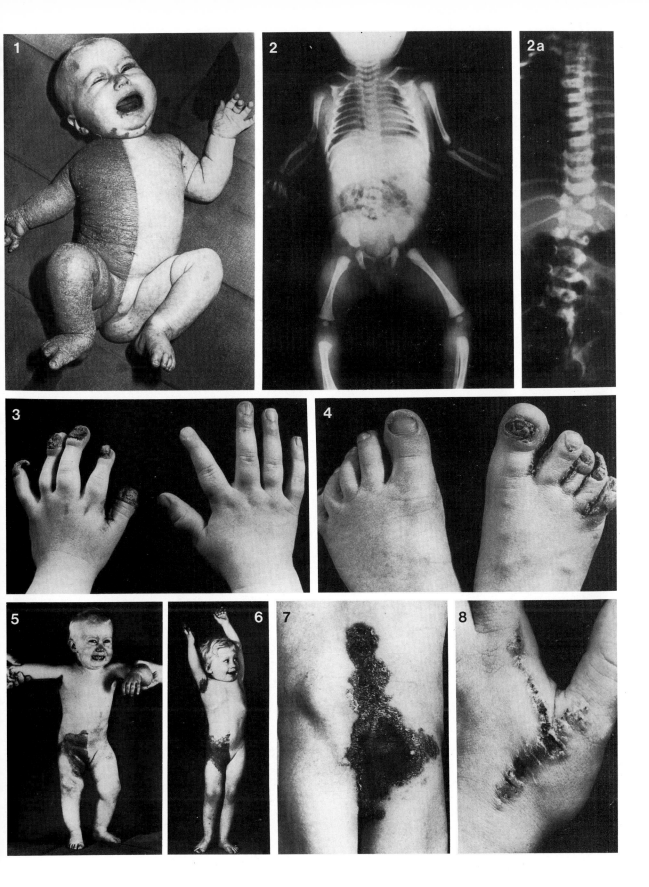

114. Keutel Syndrome

A characteristic syndrome of brachytelephalangism, abnormal cartilage calcification, impaired hearing, and unusual appearance.

Main signs:
1. Abnormally short distal phalanges of the fingers (**4**).
2. Abnormal calcification of cartilage in the tracheobronchial tree, in the epiphyses of the long bones (stippled epiphyses), and in the nose and ears (**3**).
3. Hearing defect of a mixed or conductive nature.
4. Facies characterized by hypoplasia of the midface with abnormally shaped nose (**1, 2**).

Supplementary findings: Increased susceptibility to infections of the respiratory tract, bronchiectasis or bronchial asthma (5 out of 6 affected children). Anomalies of the cardiovascular system (peripheral pulmonary stenosis, septal defect) in 3 out of 6 cases. Mental retardation (two-sixths); short stature (one-sixth).

Manifestation: At birth and later.

Etiology: Autosomal recessive disorder.

Frequency: Low; to date, 6 cases in the literature.

Course, prognosis: Mainly dependent on the involvement of the thoracic organs.

Diagnosis, differential diagnosis: To be considered in children with 'stippled epiphyses'.

Treatment: Cardiac surgery in some patients; otherwise symptomatic.

Illustrations:
1–4 Typical findings in a 13-year-old girl.

H.-R.W.

References:

Keutel, J., Jörgensen, G., Gabriel, P. A new autosomal recessive syndrome: peripheral pulmonary stenoses, brachytelephalangism, neural hearing loss, and abnormal cartilage calcification/ossification. In: Bergsma, D. (ed.) *The Clinical Delineation of Birth Defects: The Cardiovascular System.* Williams and Wilkins Co for the National Foundation—March of Dimes, Baltimore. *Birth Defects,* VIII(5), 60–68 (1972).

Fryns, J.P., Fleteren, A. van, Mattelaer, P. et al. Calcification of cartilages, brachytelephalangy and peripheral pulmonary stenosis. Confirmation of the Keutel syndrome. *Eur. J. Pediatr.,* 142, 201–203 (1984).

Cormode, E.J., Dawson, M., Lowry, R.B. Keutel syndrome: clinical report and literature review. *Am. J. Med. Genet.,* 24, 289–294 (1986).

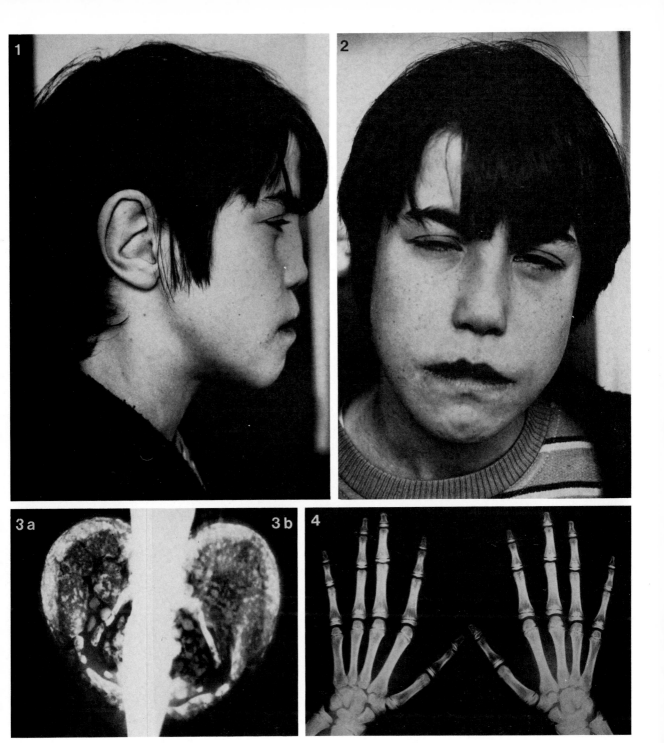

115. Camptomelic Dysplasia

(Camptomelic Syndrome)

An apparently uniform clinical picture of congenital symmetrical bowing and shortening of the lower extremities (with club feet), unusual facies, and usually early death of the child from respiratory insufficiency —to be differentiated from other disorders with congenital bowing of the long bones.

Main signs:
1. Disproportionate body at birth due to shortened extremities, especially the lower, which show symmetrical anterior bowing (**1**) with pretibial dimples and club feet. Arms may be shortened in some cases, and are only occasionally bowed.
2. Unusual facies: low nasal root, hypertelorism, narrow palpebral fissures, long philtrum, Robin sequence (micrognathia, glossoptosis, cleft palate, see p.68), usually relatively small mouth, anomalies of the external ears. Frequent macrodolichocephaly; wide open fontanelles (**1**).
3. Narrow thorax; respiratory problems are usual.
4. Radiologically short, broad, bowed tibiae; bowed femora of normal width. Absence of the distal femoral and proximal tibial epiphyses. Severe hypoplasia of the scapulae, of the fibulae, and other bones.

Supplementary findings: Birth usually at term with moderate low birth weight; hydramnios relatively frequent.

Muscular hypotonia. Possible dislocation of the hips, elbows, big toes, fingers (with mild brachydactyly of the hands).

Phenotypic females often show a male karyotype.

At autopsy, frequent hydronephrosis, cardiac anomalies, and anomalies of the olfactory nerve and trachea.

Manifestation: At birth.

Etiology: Usually sporadic occurrence; distinct preponderance of female cases; among these, frequently individuals with a male karyotype and absence of the HY-antigen. Currently, autosomal recessive inheritance is considered most likely.

Frequency: Low; over 100 cases had been reported by 1983.

Course, prognosis: Unfavorable; patients have respiratory and feeding problems and usually die within a few weeks of birth; as an exception, survival into adulthood.

Differential diagnosis: Other skeletal dysplasias with congenital bowing of the long bones.

Treatment: Symptomatic. Genetic counseling and ultrasonographic prenatal diagnosis in future pregnancies.

Illustrations:
1 and **2** A child with typical features of the syndrome.

H.-R.W.

References:

Hall, B.D. and Spranger, J. Campomelic dysplasia. *Am. J. Dis. Child.*, 134, 285 (1980).
Bricarelli, F.D., Fracaro, M., Lindsten, J. et al. Sex-reversed XY females with campomelic dysplasia are HY negative. *Hum. Genet.*, 57, 15 (1981).
Noyal, P., Vermeulin, G. et al. La dysplasie campomélique. *Arch. Fr. Pédiatr.*, 39, 621–624 (1982).
Balcar, I. and Bieber, F.R. Sonographic . . . findings in campomelic dysplasia. *AJR*, 141, 481–482 (1983).
Houston, C.S., Opitz, J.M. et al. The campomelic syndrome: review, report of 17 cases . . . *Am. J. Med. Genet.*, 15, 3–28 (1983).
Cooke, C.T., Mulcahy, M.T. et al. Campomelic dysplasia with sex reversal . . . *Pathology*, 17, 526–529 (1985).
Kapur, S. and Vloten, A.van. Isolated congenital bowed long bones. *Clin. Genet.*, 29, 165–167 (1986).
Nogami, H., Oohira, A. et al. Congenital bowing of long bones . . . *Teratology*, 33, 1–7 (1986).
Pazzaglia, U.E. and Beluffi, G. Radiology and histopathology of the bent limbs in campomelic dysplasia . . . *Pediatr. Radiol.*, 17, 50–55 (1987).

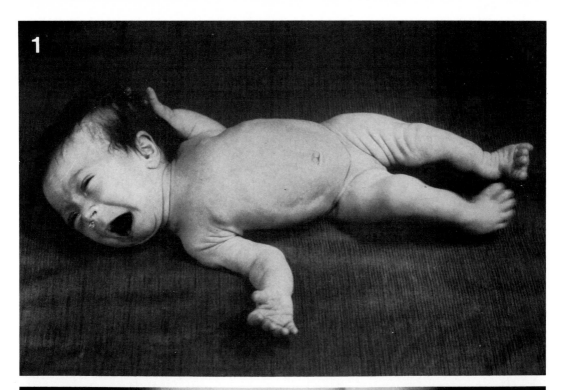

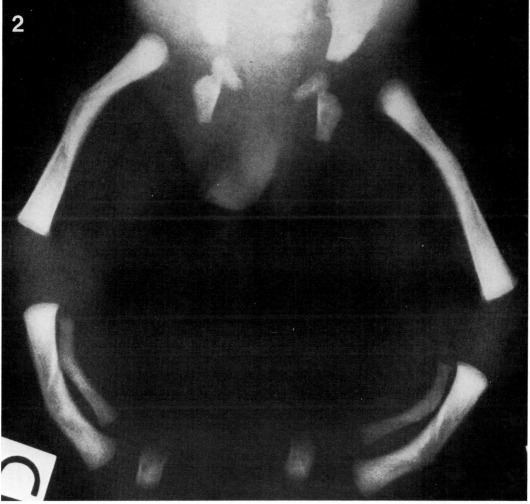

116. Achondroplasia

(Chondrodystrophia Fetalis, Parrot Syndrome)

A 'classic' generalized skeletal dysplasia with disproportionate short stature, large head, typical facial dysmorphism, and characteristic X-ray findings.

Main signs:

1. Primordial disproportionate small stature; the proximal parts of the extremities (upper arm, thigh) more severely shortened than the trunk (3–7). Average adult height for women 124 cm; for men 131 cm. Ulnar deviation of the hands, splayed fingers ('trident hand', 8). Limited extension at the elbows; genu varus, rarely valgus (3, 5, 6).

2. Head too large for the body and occasionally also for age, especially the cerebral cranium, which shows striking growth in the first years of life (men, around 60 cm and women, around 57 cm). Coarse facial features, depressed nasal root, prognathism, and hypoplasia of the midface (1, 3–7).

3. Flat thorax, frequently bell-shaped. Thoracolumbar kyphosis, lumbosacral lordosis (4, 5, 7).

4. Delayed motor, normal mental development. Occasional hearing impairment (conductive or sensori-neural).

Supplementary findings: Large cranium with frontoparietal bossing and relatively short base. Small foramen magnum, progressive narrowing of the lumbar spinal canal caudally (which, combined with progressive lumbosacral lordosis, may lead to corresponding signs of compression).

Broad flat pelvis, narrow pelvic inlet (generally dystocia), flat acetabula (9). Long bones shortened, with normal width (2), fibulae relatively too long.

Manifestation: At birth.

Etiology: Autosomal dominant disorder, with 80–90% of cases being new mutations (usually with above-average paternal age). Risk of recurrence after an affected child generally around 5%; with siblings affected (germinal mosaicism), risk of recurrence 20–35%; in the rare cases of familial occurrence, a labile premutation with reduced 'phenotrance' is still assumed. Affected homozygotes are rare; in these cases early death usual with extremely severe skeletal dysplasia.

Frequency: About 1:20,000–25,000.

Prognosis: Increased mortality in all age groups: under 4 years from brain stem compression; subsequently, up to about 25 years, from central nervous system causes or respiratory disorders (due to thoracic deformities, airway obstruction, or neurological defects [see above]); later from cardiac problems.

Differential diagnosis: Thanatophoric dysplasia (p.214), hypochondroplasia (p.260), pseudochondroplasia (p.268), and others.

Treatment: Symptomatic. Ultrasonography of the skull at regular intervals after birth and during infancy is recommended. Best measures possible to prevent obesity and kyphosis. Possible osteotomies and specific surgery for signs of neurological compression. Orthopedic care; aids for the physically handicapped. Genetic counseling. Ultrasonographic prenatal diagnosis.

Illustrations:

1 A 7-month-old infant.
2 X-ray of the left hand of a toddler.
3–5 An 8-year-old boy.
6–9 A 15-year-old boy.

H.-R.W./J.K.

References:

Silverman, E.N. Achondroplasia. *Prog. Pediatr. Radiol.*, vol 4. *Intrinsic Diseases of Bones*, p.94. Karger, Basel, 1973.

Spranger, J.W., Langer, L.O., Jr., Wiedemann, H.-R. *Bone Dysplasias. An Atlas of Constitutional Disorders of Skeletal Development.* G. Fischer and W.B. Saunders, Stuttgart and Philadelphia, 1974.

Lutter, L.D., Paul. S., Langer, L.O. Neurological symptoms in achondroplastic dwarfs—surgical treatment. *J. Bone. Jt. Surg.*, 59A, 87 (1977).

Horton, W.A., Rotter, J.I. et al. Standard growth curves for achondroplasia. *J. Pediatr.*, 93, 435–438 (1978).

Hall, J.G., Golbus, M.S., Graham, C.B. et al. Failure of early prenatal diagnosis in classic achondroplasia. *Am. J. Med. Genet.*, 3, 371 (1979).

Bland, J.D. and Emery, J.L. Unexpected death of children with achondroplasia . . . *Develop. Med. Child. Neurol.*, 24, 489–492 (1982).

Hall, J.G., Horton, W. et al. Head growth in achondroplasia . . . *Am. J. Med. Genet.*, 13, 105 (1982).

Aterman, K., Welch, J.P. et al. Presumed homozygous achondroplasia. *Path. Res. Pract.*, 178, 27–39 (1983).

Pauli, R.M., Conroy, M.M. et al. Homozygous achondroplasia . . . *Am. J. Med. Genet.*, 16, 459–473 (1983).

Stokes, D.C., Philips, J.A. et al. Respiratory complications of achondroplasia. *J. Pediatr.*, 102, 534–541 (1983).

Opitz, J.M. 'Unstable premutation' in achondroplasia: penetrance vs phenotrance. *Am. J. Med. Genet.*, 19, 251–254 (1984).

Reiser, C.A., Pauli, R.M. et al. Achondroplasia: unexpected familial recurrence. *Am. J. Med. Genet.*, 19, 245–250 (1984).

Thompson, J.N., Schaefer, G.B. et al. Achondroplasia and parental age. *N. Engl. J. Med.*, 314, 521–522 (1986).

Dodinval, P. and Marec, B.L. Genetic counselling in unexpected familial recurrence of achondroplasia. *Am. J. Med. Genet.*, 28, 949–954 (1987).

Hecht, J.T., Francomano, C.A. et al. Mortality in achondroplasia. *Am. J. Hum. Genet.*, 41, 454–464 (1987).

Editorial: Leg length in achondroplasia. *Lancet*, I, 1032 (1988).

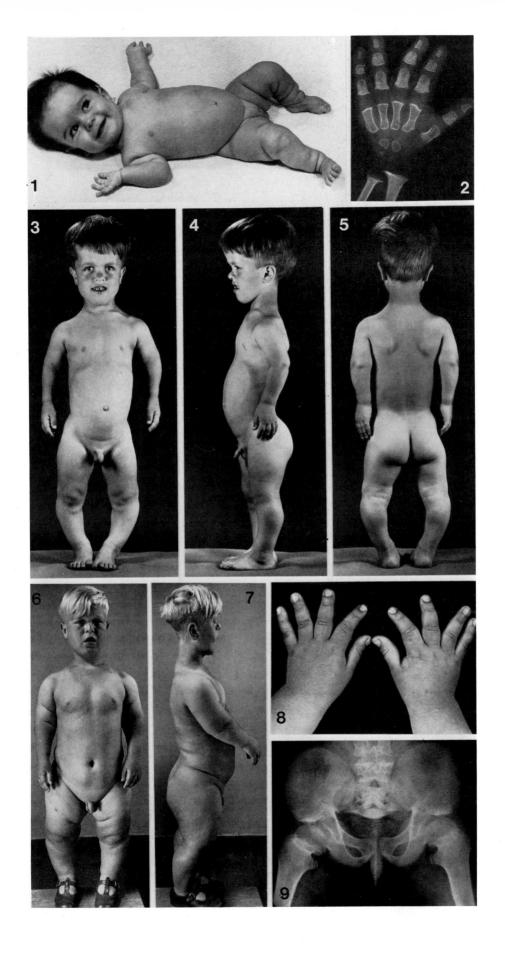

117. Diastrophic Dysplasia

A characteristic hereditary disorder of severe short stature, club feet, joint contractures, malpositioning of the thumbs and big toes, anomalies of the auricles, and cleft palate.

Main signs:
1. Micromelic short stature, birth measurements between 38 and 44 cm, with club feet, joint contractures (especially of the shoulders, elbows, hips, and interphalangeal joints) with abduction of the proximally displaced, hyperextensible thumbs ('hitchhiker thumb') and big toes (1–3, 6).
2. Anomalies of the external ear (development of cystic masses in early infancy; later, thickening and deformity) (5). Cleft palate in about 25% of cases.
3. In most cases progressive thoracolumbar kyphoscoliosis and cervical kyphosis (2b, 4).

Supplementary findings: Tendency to subluxation and dislocation of the joints, promoted by laxity of the muscles and ligaments. Stridor in about 25% of cases. Possible deafness as a result of fusion or absence of auditory ossicles. Absence of the flexion creases of the fingers due to intrauterine joint contractures (7).

Radiologically, severe epimetaphyseal changes of the—shortened—long bones and distension of the metaphyses; delayed ossification with deformity especially of the proximal femoral epiphyses; usually distinct fork-like deformity of the distal femoral and distal radial epiphyses and of the metatarsals; hook-shape changes of the lateral ends of the clavicles, ovoid deformity of first metacarpal in the young child, and other anomalies (8, 9).

Manifestation: At birth. Changes of the auricle usually develop in the first three months of life; kyphoscoliosis usually develops after infancy).

Etiology: Autosomal recessive disorder with very variable expression.

Frequency: Low (over 150 cases are known).

Course, prognosis: Increased early mortality due to respiratory disorders and in some cases cardiac defects. Later on, increased risk of the consequences of the severe kyphoscoliotic changes. Adult height may be under 1 meter, but occasionally may reach 1.40 m. Normal mental development.

Differential diagnosis: Pseudodiastrophic dysplasia, arthrogryposis.

Treatment: Symptomatic. Intensive orthopedic care mandatory. All appropriate aids for the physically handicapped. Genetic counseling. Prenatal diagnosis by ultrasound in subsequent pregnancies.

Illustrations:
1, 3, 5, and 6 A 4½-year-old boy.
2, 4, and 8 A 1½-year-old girl. Note micromelia, club feet, hypermobility or abduction (up to and including subluxation) of the thumbs and big toes, early thoracolumbar kyphosis (2b) and considerable cervical kyphosis (4), blunting and deformity of the hand bones (8).
7 and 9 Features of other typical cases.

H.-R.W.

References:
Walter, H. Der diastrophische Zwergwuchs. *Adv. Hum. Genet.*, 2, 31, Stuttgart, Thieme (1970).
Spranger, J.W., Langer, L.O., Jr., Wiedemann, H.-R. *Bone Dysplasias. An Atlas of Constitutional Disorders of Skeletal Development.* G. Fischer and W.B. Saunders, Stuttgart and Philadelphia 1974.
Horton, W.A., Rimoin, D.L., Lachman, R.S. et al. The phenotypic variability of diatrophic dysplasia. *J. Pediatr.*, 93, 609 (1978).
Bethem, D., Winter, R.B., Lutter, L. Disorders of the spine in diastrophic dwarfism. *J. Bone. Jt. Surg.*, 62A, 529 (1980).
Lachman, R., Sillence, D., Rimoin, D. et al. Diastrophic dysplasia . . . *Radiology*, 140, 79 (1981).
Horton, W.A., Hall, J.G., Scott, C.I. et al. Growth curves for height for diastrophic dysplasia . . . *Am. J. Dis. Child.*, 136, 316 (1982).
Gustavson, K.-H., Holmgren, G., Jagell, S. et al. Lethal and non-lethal diastrophic dysplasia. *Clin. Genet.*, 28, 321–334 (1985).
Butler, M.G., Gale, D.D., Meaney, F.J. Metacarpophalangeal pattern profile analysis in diastrophic dysplasia. *Am. J. Med. Genet.*, 28, 685–689 (1987).
Gollop, T.R. and Eigier, A. Prenatal ultrasound diagnosis of diastrophic dysplasia at 16 weeks. *Am. J. Med. Genet.*, 27, 321–324 (1987).
Krecak, J. and Starshak, R.J. Cervical kyphosis in diastrophic dwarfism: CT and MR findings. *Pediatr. Radiol.*, 17, 321–322 (1987).
Gembruch, U., Niesen, M. et al. Diastrophic dysplasia: a specific diagnosis by ultrasound. *Prenatal Diagnosis*, 8, 539–545 (1988).

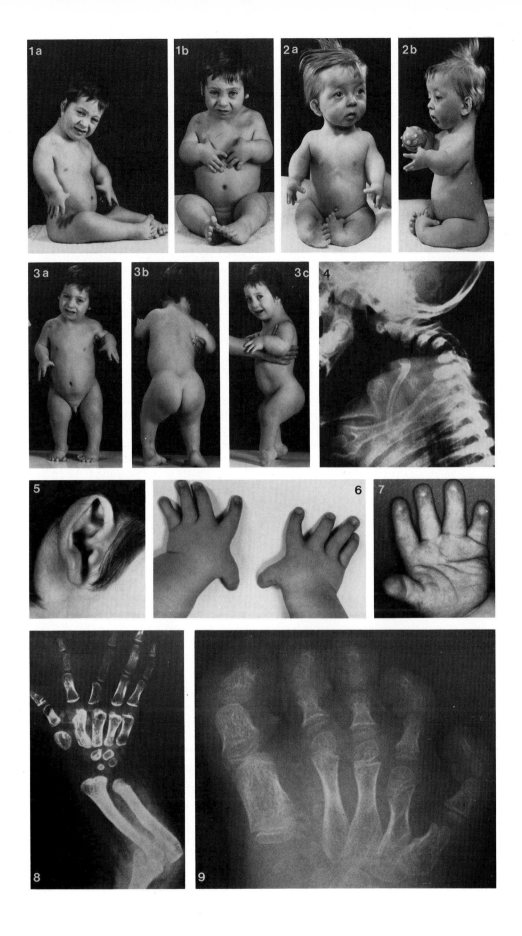

118. Pseudodiastrophic Dysplasia Burgio Type

A syndrome of short-limbed small stature with macrocranium and unusual facies, short neck, club feet, joint contractures and dislocation, large pinnae, and cleft palate.

Main signs:
1. Congenital short-limbed small stature. Large skull. Short neck. Bell-shaped (wider above) thorax. Almost angular dorsolumbar kyphosis or early scoliosis (1, 2, 4).
2. Peculiar facies with flat nose, hypertelorism, hypoplasia of the midface, and abnormally full cheeks. Cleft palate. Large deformed ears (1, 2).
3. Club feet. Limited motion at the metacarpal and metatarsal joints, the vertebral column, and to a lesser degree the knees and shoulders. Dislocation of both hips, both elbows, and characteristically, several finger joints (3).

Supplementary findings: Radiologically, all bones of the extremities shortened and bluntly shaped (3). Hypoplasia of the scapulae with dysplasia of the joint fossae; somewhat squarish, deformed ilia. Hypoplasia of the cervical vertebrae; platyspondyly of the lower vertebrae with narrowing of the interpedicular, widening of the intervertebral spaces.

Manifestation: At birth.

Etiology: Autosomal recessive disorder.

Frequency: Low (only about 10 cases known).

Course, prognosis: Increased early mortality. In cases surviving longer, problems arise as a consequence of severe kyphoscoliotic changes.

Differential diagnosis: Diastrophic dysplasia (p.236), arthrogryposis (p.402).

Comment: Although designated pseudodiastrophic dwarfism because of signs overlapping with those of diastrophic dysplasia, the similarities are limited to appearance; this syndrome is an independent entity, clinically, radiologically, and osteochondro-histologically and -histochemically.

Treatment: Symptomatic. Appropriate physiotherapeutic, orthopedic and, if indicated, neurosurgical care. Genetic counseling. Prenatal diagnosis by ultrasound in future pregnancies.

Illustrations:
1–4 The first child of healthy young nonconsanguineous parents. Birth measurements: 3120 g, 44 cm, and head circumference 38 cm. Progression of the kyphoscoliosis. The peculiar facies persisted unchanged. Chromosome analysis negative. Frequent episodes of fever of unknown origin (normal immunoglobulins). Sudden death at age 8 months. A female sibling born subsequently showing the same clinical picture died at age 4 days with idiopathic hyperthermia.

H.-R.W.

References:

Burgio, G.R., Belloni, C., Beluffi, G. Nanisme pseudodiastrophique. Etude de deux soeurs nouveaunées. *Arch. Franç. Péd.*, 31, 681 (1974).

Gorlin, R.J., Pindborg, J.J., Cohen, M.M., Jr. *Syndromes of the Head and Neck*, 2nd edn. McGraw–Hill Book Co., New York, 1976.

Kozlowski, K., Masel, J., Morris, L., Kunze, D. Neonatal death dwarfism (a further report). *Fortschr. Röntgenstr.*, 129, 626 (1978).

Stanescu, V., Stanescu, R., Maroteaux, P. Etude morphologique et biochemique du cartilage de criossance dans les osteochondrodysplasies. *Arch. Franç. Péd.*, (Suppl.), 1, 34 (1977).

Horton, W.A., Rimoin, D.L. et al. The phenotypic variability of diastrophic dysplasia. *J. Pediatr.*, 93, 609–613 (1978).

Canki, N., Sernec-Logar, B. et al. Le nanisme pseudodiastrophique . . . *J. Génét. Hum.*, 27, 247–252 (1979).

Gustavson, K.-L., Holmgren, G. et al. Lethal and non-lethal diastrophic dysplasia . . . *Clin. Genet.*, 28, 321–334 (1985).

Eteson, D.J., Beluffi, G., Burgio, G.R. et al. Pseudodiastrophic dysplasia: a distinct newborn skeletal dysplasia. *J. Pediatr.*, 109, 635–641 (1986).

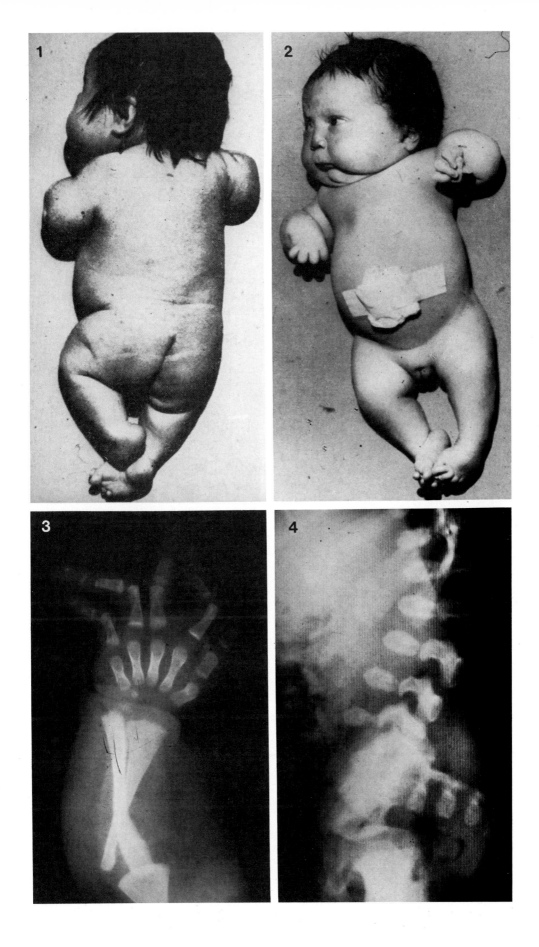

119. Metatropic Dysplasia

An inherited disorder leading to severe small stature with 'turnabout of proportions' during the course of childhood (initially, relatively short extremities; subsequently, more obvious shortening of the trunk) combined with limitation of motion of the large joints and frequently with a tail-like formation in the sacral area.

Main signs:

1. In the newborn and young child, a relatively long trunk with narrow thorax and short extremities (**1, 3**).
2. In the older child (and adults), 'truncal short stature' as a result of platyspondyly (**8**) and usually also severe progressive kyphoscoliosis, extremities now appearing abnormally long (**5, 7**).
3. Often a tail-like appendage medially over the sacral area (**3c, 5b, 7b**).
4. Restricted motion at the generally prominent large joints (**1, 5, 7**).

Supplementary findings: Secondary deformities of the thorax.

Hyperextensible finger joints.

Radiologically, aniso- and platyspondyly (**8**), striking anomalies in the size and form of the pelvic bones and proximal femora (**4**), severe epimetaphyseal disorders of the—shortened—tubular bones with broadening of the metaphyses and marked irregularities of the epiphyseal ossification centers (**2, 6**).

Manifestation: At birth and later by the change of proportions.

Etiology: Monogenic disorder; heterogeneity; occurrence of autosomal recessive and autosomal dominant transmission. Possibly three differentiable types:

1. non-lethal form with autosomal recessive transmission;
2. non-lethal form with autosomal dominant transmission;
3. lethal form with death shortly before or after delivery and autosomal recessive inheritance.

Frequency: Relatively low.

Course, prognosis: Increased early mortality as a consequence of the congenitally narrowed thorax. Later, patients at risk from the effects of severe kyphoscoliosis. In severe cases, adult height may lie between 1.10 and 1.20 m. Normal mental development.

Differential diagnosis: Particularly the Kniest syndrome (p.250) and Morquio's syndrome (p.124).

Treatment: Symptomatic. Intensive orthopedic supervision and in some cases therapy. All appropriate handicap aids. Genetic counseling.

Illustrations:

1 The same child at ages 1¼ years, 3 years, (**1c**), and 4 years (**1b**).
3 and 5 A girl at 10 months and again at 7 years ('turnabout of proportions').
6–8 A 7-year-old child, with X-rays of hand (**6**) and spine (**8**).
2 and 4 X-rays of a newborn.
Note the early onset of manifest kyphosis in **3a** and the severe progression in **5**. 'Tail formations' in **3c, 5b,** and **7b**.

H.-R.W.

References:

Maroteaux, P., Spranger, J., Wiedemann, H.-R. Der metatropische Zwergwuchs. *Arch. Kinderheilkd.*, 173, 211 (1966).
Spranger, J.W., Langer, L.O., Jr., Wiedemann, H.-R. *Bone Dysplasias. An Atlas of Constitutional Disorders of Skeletal Development.* G. Fischer and W.B. Saunders, Stuttgart and Philadelphia, 1974.
Miething, R., Stöver, B., Noeske, H. Metatroper Zwergwuchs. *Monatschr. Kinderheilkd.*, 128, 153 (1980).
Beck, M., Roubicek, M. et al. Heterogeneity of metatropic dysplasia. *Eur. J. Pediatr.*, 140, 231–237 (1983).
Boden, S.D., Kaplan, F.S. et al. Metatropic dwarfism. *J. Bone. Jt. Surg.*, 69A, 174–184 (1987).
Shohat, M., Lachman, R., Rimoin, D.L. Odontoid hypoplasia with vertebral cervical subluxation and ventriculomegaly in metatrophic dysplasia. *J. Pediatr.*, 114, 239–243 (1989).

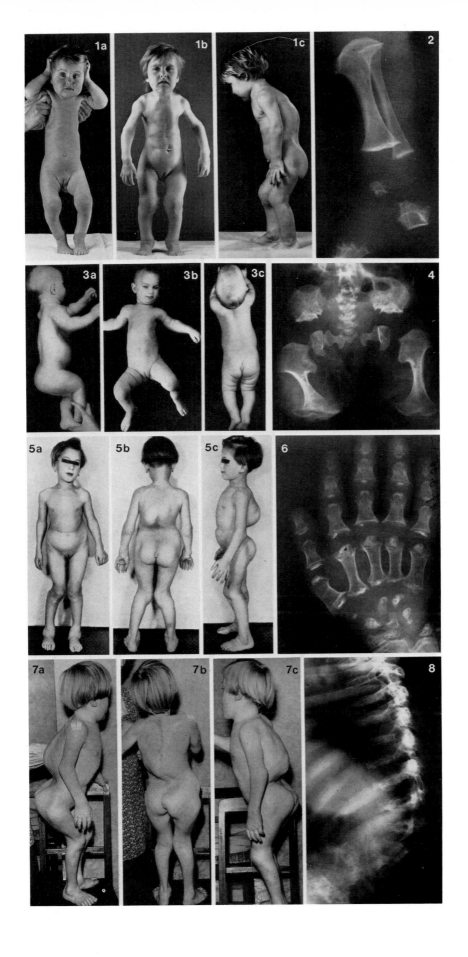

120. Fibrochondrogenesis

A rare familial, neonatally lethal, rhizomelic chondrodysplasia with broad dumb-bell-shaped long bones and pear-shaped vertebral bodies.

Main signs:
1. Mild brachycephaly, wide open fontanelles and sutures.
2. Facial dysmorphism: round face, hypertelorism, large prominent eyes, flat nasal root, anteverted nostrils, microstomia.
3. Short neck, flat thorax. Rhizomelic shortening of the arms and legs. Absence of the flexion and extension creases of the fingers.
4. Death from respiratory insufficiency in the neonatal period.
5. X-ray findings: wide fontanelles and cranial sutures. Long, thin clavicles. Short ribs with wide anterior ends. Cervical to lumbar vertebral bodies flat (platyspondyly). In the upper and mid vertebral column, ossification of only the anterior part of the vertebral body. In the lower thoracic spine and the lumbar region, the increased anterior ossification of the vertebral bodies lends them a pear-shaped appearance on lateral view. In the anteroposterior (AP) view, sagittal midline clefts of the vertebral bodies with broad defects of midline ossification. Hypoplastic pelvis with ovoid ilium, flat acetabulum with medially placed notch. The pubic and ischial bones are short and broad. The tubular bones are also short and broad with dumb bell-like distension of the metaphyses. Short fibulae.

Manifestation: Pre- and postnatally.

Etiology: Autosomal recessive inheritance probable. Take note of possible consanguinity.

Frequency: Five patients were known by 1988.

Prognosis: Unfavorable: death in the newborn period from respiratory insufficiency in spite of intensive medical measures.

Differential diagnosis: Metatropic dysplasia, Kniest dysplasia, atelosteogenesis, and SED congenita (spondyloepiphyseal dysplasia, congenital type).

Illustrations:
1–7 Typical features of an affected neonate.

J.K.

References:

Whitley, C.B., Langer, L.O., Jr., Ophoven, J. et al. Fibrochondrogenesis: Lethal autosomal recessive chondrodysplasia with distinctive cartilage histopathology. *Am. J. Med. Genet.*, 19, 265–275 (1984).
Eteson, D.J., Adomian, G.E., Ornoy, A. et al. Fibrochondrogenesis: radiologic and histologic studies. *Am. J. Med. Genet.*, 19, 277–290 (1984).

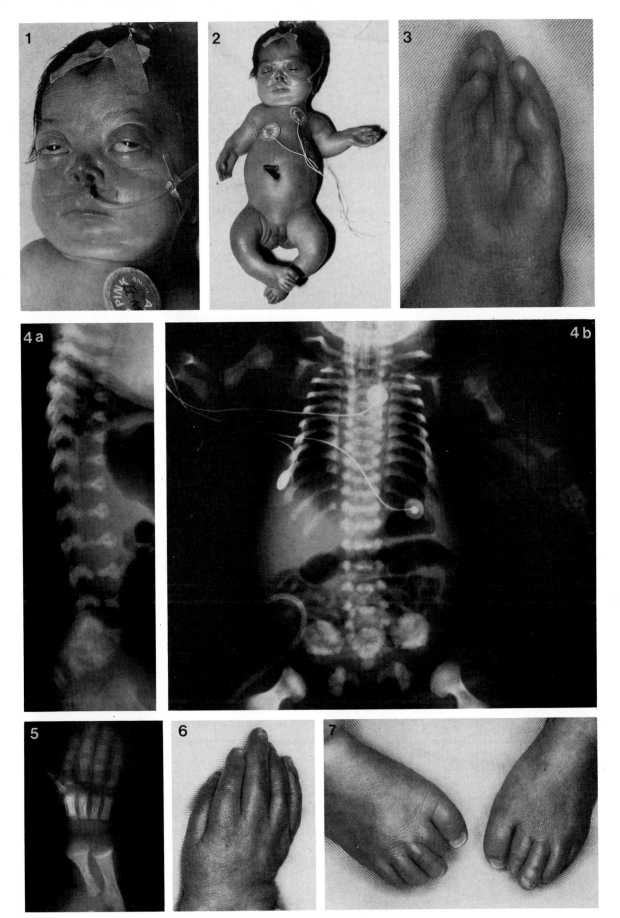

243

121. Chondroectodermal Dysplasia

(Ellis–van Creveld Syndrome)

A syndrome of congenital short-limbed small stature with postaxial polydactyly, hypoplasia of the nails, and abnormal frenula between the upper lip and the alveolar process.

Main signs:
1. Disproportionate, short-limbed small stature with more marked shortness of the extremities distally (**1, 2**).
2. Postaxial hexadactyly of the hands, occasionally also of the feet (**1, 2, 4, 5**).
3. Hypo- and dysplasia of the nails (**4, 5**).
4. Short upper lip, joined to the alveolar ridge by numerous, generally accessory frenula (**3**).
5. Dysodontiasis (possible congenital teeth; partial anodontia; small, early or late-erupting teeth; malpositioning of teeth).
6. In at least half of the cases, congenital cardiac anomaly (usually large atrial septal defects).

Supplementary findings: In some cases, narrow thorax (**1**); later, genu valgus.

Radiologically, increasing hypoplasia of the distal phalanges; possible bony fusion of metacarpals or phalanges, or of the capitate and hamate; and many other anomalies.

Manifestation: At birth.

Etiology: Autosomal recessive disorder with variable expression.

Frequency: Low (apart from the Lancaster County Amish in the USA for whom there are at least 5 cases per 1,000 births); altogether about 250 cases known to date.

Course, prognosis: In infancy, increased mortality as a consequence of pulmonary complications or cardiac defect. Adult height quite variable (between 1.05 and 1.60 m).

Differential diagnosis: The fully expressed syndrome should not cause diagnostic difficulties.

Treatment: Symptomatic. Orthopedic treatment of polydactyly and genu valgus. Early dental care. Surgical correction of cardiac defect may be indicated. Genetic counseling.

Illustrations:
1 A typically affected infant with hexadactyly; death at 24 days from respiratory insufficiency.
2–5 A 9-month-old boy, the first child of healthy, young, nonconsanguineous parents. The characteristically disproportionate development is more marked on the left side (**2, 4, 5**); ulnar deviation of the left hand; clinodactyly of the fifth and sixth fingers bilaterally. Considerable hypoplasia of the left wing of the ilium with dysplasia and subluxation of the hip. Bilateral talipes calcaneus and pes valgus. Delayed dentition. Small penis.

H.-R.W.

References:

McKusick, V.A., Egeland, J.A., Eldridge, R. et al. Dwarfism in the Amish. I. The Ellis–van Creveld syndrome. *Bull. Johns Hopkins Hosp.*, 115, 306–336 (1964).

Spranger, J.W., Langer, L.O., Jr., Wiedemann, H.-R. *Bone Dysplasias. An Atlas of Constitutional Disorders of Skeletal Development.* G. Fischer and W.B. Saunders, Stuttgart and Philadelphia, 1974.

Milgram, J.W. and Bailey, J.A. Orthopedic aspects of the Ellis–van Creveld syndrome. *Bull. Hosp. Joint. Dis.*, 36, 11 (1975).

Oliveira, E., Silva, D., Janovito, D. et al. Ellis–van Creveld syndrome. Report of 15 cases . . . *J. Med. Genet.*, 17, 349 (1980).

Rosemberg, S., Carneiro, P.C., Zerbini, M.C.N. et al. Chondroectodermal dysplasia (Ellis–van Creveld) with anomalies of CNS and urinary tract. *Am. J. Med. Genet.*, 15, 291–295 (1983).

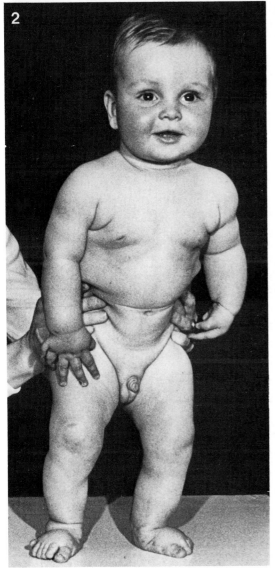

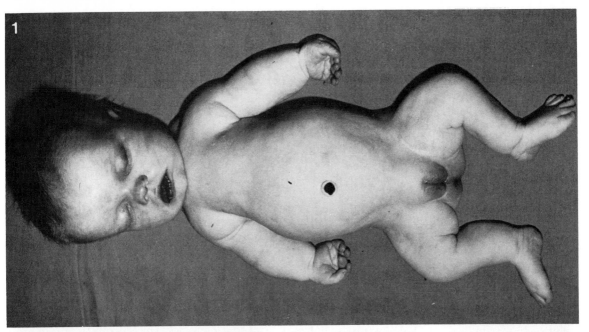

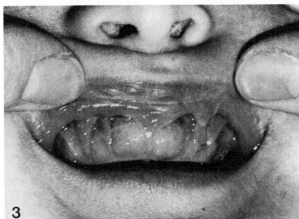

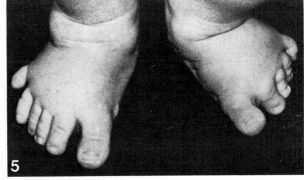

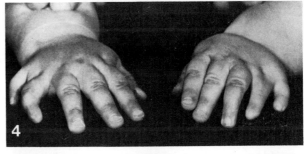

245

122. Spondyloepiphyseal Dysplasia Congenita

(SED Congenita = Spondyloepiphyseal Dysplasia Congenita)

A syndrome of disproportionate short stature with severe shortening of the vertebral column; barrel-shaped chest; deep lumbar lordosis; severe dysplasia of the epiphyses, especially those near the trunk; practically normal cranium, hands, and feet; frequent myopia or retinal detachment.

Main signs:

1. Disproportionate short stature with shortening especially of the vertebral column. Short neck, compressed-appearing trunk with barrel-shaped chest and pectus carinatum, lumbar hyperlordosis, possible kyphoscoliosis of the thoracic spine (**1a–1d**).

2. Relatively long extremities. Frequent waddling gait with severe hip dysplasia and marked coxa vara. Frequent genu valgus (less frequently varus). Normal-sized hands and feet (**1**).

3. Impaired vision due to myopia and/or retinal detachment in about half of the cases.

Supplementary findings: Flat face (occasional hypertelorism) (**1a, 1d**). Occasional cleft palate.

Fully mobile, sometimes hyperextensible joints (with the possible exception of hips, shoulders, and elbows). Lax ligaments. Muscular hypotonia in infancy. Occasionally club feet.

Delayed motor, normal mental development.

Sensorineural hearing impairment not unusual.

Radiologically, delayed ossification (see also 3), especially in the pelvic bones and hip joints (with severe coxa vara), flattening and diverse irregularities of the vertebral bodies with hypoplasia of the odontoid process, epimetaphyseal dysplasia of the long bones, relatively normal bones of the hands and feet.

Manifestation: At birth.

Etiology: For the great majority of cases autosomal dominant inheritance with considerably variable expression can be assumed. However, there may be heterogeneity; autosomal recessive transmission seems to occur too.

Frequency: Not particularly rare.

Course, prognosis: Since retinal detachment may occur relatively early, regular examination by an ophthalmologist is indicated. Danger of compression of the cervical medulla, from hypoplasia of the odontoid and laxity of the ligaments, which requires preventive orthopedic care. Adult height between 90 and 130 cm. Increasing arthritis of the large joints and corresponding handicaps in adulthood.

Differential diagnosis: The Morquio syndrome (later manifestation and other differences), see p.124; also, Stickler syndrome (p.532).

Treatment: Symptomatic. Early treatment of club feet when present; closure of cleft palate as required; careful neurological supervision and preventive orthopedic measures in view of the danger of spinal cord compression; coagulation treatment for retinal detachment may be indicated. All available aids and supports for the physical handicaps. Genetic counseling.

Illustrations:

1a–1d The same child at 6 months (height 14 cm below the average for age) and 7½ years (height deficit about 40 cm). Early kyphoscoliosis. Hypoplasia of the odontoid, with previously normal mobility at the atlantooccipital joint. Cleft palate.

2 X-ray of a hand of a patient, a 4-year-old girl (father similarly affected).

3 A hand X-ray of the child in 1 at age 5 years.

H.-R.W.

References:

Spranger, J.W., Langer, L.O., Jr., Wiedemann, H.-R. *Bone Dysplasias. An Atlas of Constitutional Disorders of Skeletal Development.* G. Fischer and W.B. Saunders, Stuttgart and Philadelphia, 1974.

Luthardt, T., Reinwein, H., Schönenberg, H., Spranger, J., Wiedemann, H.-R. Dysplasia spondyloepiphysaria congenita. *Klin. Pädiatr.,* 187, 538 (1975).

Kozlowski, K., Masel, J., Nolte, K. Dysplasia spondyloepiphysealis congenita Spranger–Wiedemann. *Aust. Radiol.,* 21, 260 (1977).

Horton, W.A., Hall, J.G., Scott, C.I. et al. Growth curves for height for diastrophic dysplasia, spondyloepiphyseal dysplasia congenita . . . *Am. J. Dis. Child.,* 136, 316 (1982).

Harrod, M.J.E., Friedman, J.M. et al. Genetic heterogeneity in spondyloepiphyseal dysplasia congenita. *Am. J. Med. Genet.,* 18, 311–320 (1984).

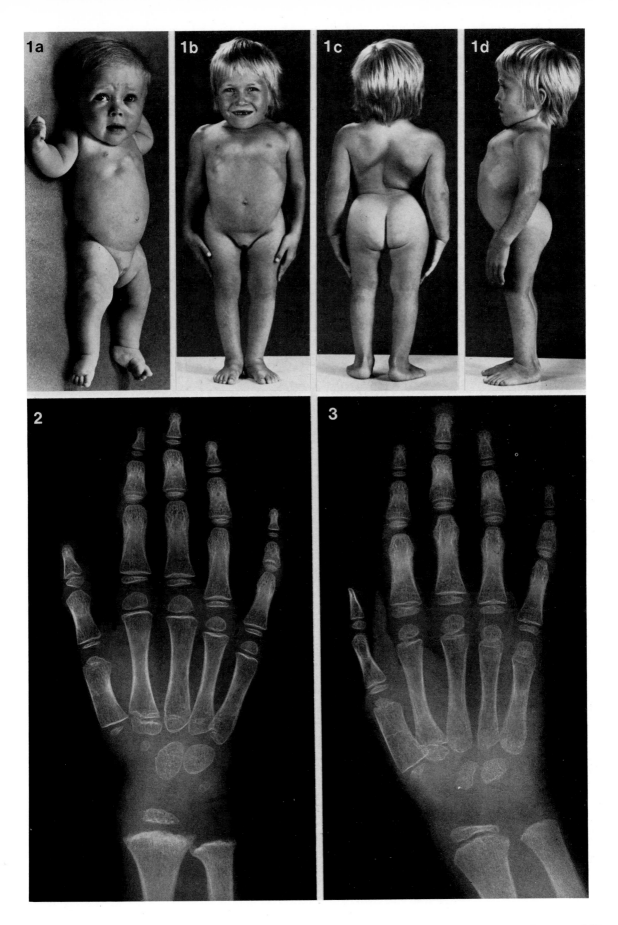

123. Spondyloepiphyseal Dysplasia Tarda

(SED Tarda)

A familial syndrome manifest between the 4th and 12th years of life with small stature, short vertebral column, prominent sternum, increased lumbar lordosis, and waddling gait with femoral epiphyseal dysplasia.

Main signs:
1. Short stature with shortened vertebral column, platyspondyly, increasing lumbar lordosis, sternal protrusion, broad thorax.
2. Extremities clinically unremarkable, hands and feet of normal size, narrow hips, complaints relating to the hip joints, waddling gait.

Supplementary findings: Calcification of the vertebral column may result in limitation of movements. Some patients show hyperextensible joints; a few have shown corneal dystrophy. Frequent early onset of arthritis.

Manifestation: Between the 4th and 12th years of life. Usually clinically recognized between the 6th and 8th years of life. Occasional early suspicion of 'hip disorder'.

Etiology: Heterogeneity: Usually X-linked recessive transmission, but autosomal dominant and autosomal recessive inheritance have also been described.

Frequency: Up to now, a rarely diagnosed disorder.

Course, prognosis: Adult height of the patients between 125 and 160 cm. Osteoarthritis of the hips and knees and calcification in the region of the vertebral column worsen the prognosis for freedom of movement in later years.

Differential diagnosis: Several authors have classified SED tarda into four groups, A–D:
1. brachyrachia (A);
2. brachyolmia (B);
3. classic X-linked recessive SED tarda (C); and
4. autosomal dominant and autosomal recessive SED tarda (D).
It is important to consider Morquio syndrome in the differential diagnosis.

Treatment: Orthopedic care, physiotherapy.

Illustrations:
1 A 7¾-year-old patient with short stature and hyperlordosis.
2 Slightly reduced height of the vertebral bodies, flattening of the anterior marginal crests; suggestion of tongue-like anterior extensions of L I–IV.
3 Flattening of the epiphyses of metacarpals II–IV; clinodactyly of the little fingers.
4 Pelvis and hip joints of the boy at age 4 years.

J.K.

References:

Spranger, J.W., Langer, L.O., Jr., Wiedemann, H.-R. *Bone Dysplasias*. Gustav Fischer Verlag, Stuttgart, 1974.

Byers, P.H., Holbrook, K.A., Hall, J.G. et al. A new variety of spondyloepiphyseal dysplasia characterized by punctate corneal dystrophy and abnormal dermal collagen fibrils. *Hum. Genet.*, 40, 157–169 (1978).

Pina Neto, J.M.de, Bonfim, M.D., Ferrari, I. Classic X-linked spondyloepiphyseal dysplasia tarda in a woman with normal karyotype. In: *Skeletal Dysplasias*. Papadatos, C.J. and Bartsocas, C.S. (eds.). Alan Liss, New York, pp. 127–132 (1982).

Al-Awadi, S.A., Farag, T.I., Naguib, K. et al. Spondyloepiphyseal dysplasia tarda with progressive arthropathy. *J. Med. Genet.*, 21, 193–196 (1984).

Harrod, M.E.J., Friedman, J.M., Currarino, G. et al. Genetic heterogeneity in spondyloepiphyseal dysplasia congenita. *Am. J. Med. Genet.*, 18, 311–320 (1984).

Iceton, J.A. and Horne, G. Spondylo-epiphyseal dysplasia tarda. The X-linked variety in three brothers. *J. Bone Jt. Surg.*, 68-B, 616–619 (1986).

Kohn, G., Elrayyes, E.R., Makadmah, I. et al. Spondyloepiphyseal dysplasia tarda: a new autosomal recessive variant with mental retardation. *J. Med. Genet.*, 24, 366–377 (1987).

Szpiro-Tapia, S., Sefiani, A. et al. Spondyloepiphyseal dysplasia tarda: linkage . . . from the distal short arm of the X chromosome. *Hum. Genet.*, 81, 61–63 (1988).

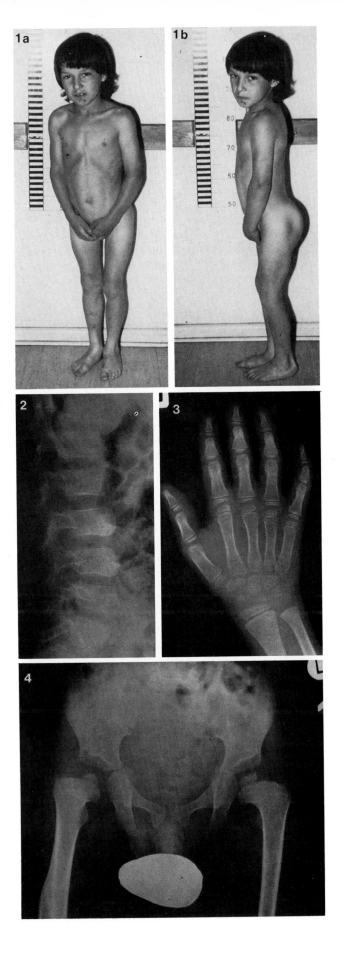

124. Osteodysplasia Kniest Type

(Kniest Syndrome, Kniest Disease)

An inherited disorder of disproportionate short stature with kyphoscoliosis, flat facies, often with hearing and visual impairment, and characteristic X-ray findings.

Main signs:

1. Disproportionate short stature with short trunk, wide thorax, marked lumbar lordosis and thoracic kyphoscoliosis, and short extremities, which appear swollen at the joints and too long relative to the trunk (1). Final height between about 100 and 145 cm.
2. Flat facies, possibly with widely spaced eyes and proptosis due to flat orbits, flat nasal root, and (in about half the cases) cleft palate.
3. Frequently limited motion at the joints (especially marked at the hips); long fingers.
4. Frequent hearing impairment (conductive and/or sensorineural defect), frequent high-grade myopia with retinal degeneration and danger of glaucoma, cataract, and retinal detachment with loss of sight.

Supplementary findings: Often umbilical and inguinal hernias.

Radiologically, striking anomalies in shape and size of the pelvic and femoral bones. Platyspondyly, short clavicles, marked changes of the long bones—broadening of the metaphyses and irregularities of the epiphyses and metaphyses in the form of honeycombed, porous translucencies and delayed ossification (especially of the femoral heads).

Manifestation: At birth (short, deformed extremities, disorders of joint mobility) and later. Delayed motor development.

Etiology: Autosomal dominant disorder. Heterogeneity cannot be excluded with certainty.

Frequency: Low.

Course, prognosis: Probably life expectancy is about average, but with moderate to severe physical handicaps—articular, respiratory, and in some cases ocular and auditory.

Differential diagnosis: Mainly metatropic dysplasia (p.240) and spondyloepiphyseal dysplasia congenita (p.246). Morquio syndrome (p.532) and diastrophic and pseudodiastrophic dysplasias (pp. 236 and 238) should be fairly easy to rule out.

Treatment: Starting at an early age, regular follow-up with ophthalmological and audiometric examinations. Closure of cleft palate and speech therapy if required. Orthopedic care of joint contractures and kyphoscoliosis. All appropriate aids for the physically handicapped. Genetic counseling.

Illustration:

1 A 7-year-old with Kniest syndrome and his healthy twin brother.

H.-R.W.

References:

Spranger, J.W., Langer, L.O., Jr., Wiedemann, H.-R. *Bone Dysplasias. An Atlas of Constitutional Disorders of Skeletal Development.* G. Fischer and W.B. Saunders, Stuttgart and Philadelphia, 1974.
Lachman, R.S., Rimoin, D.L., Hollister, D.W. et al. The Kniest syndrome. *Am. J. Roentgenol.,* 123, 805 (1975).
Kniest, W. and Leiber, B. Kniest-Syndrom. *Monatschr. Kinderheilkd.,* 125, 970 (1977).
Silengo, M.C., Davi, G.F. et al. Kniest disease . . . *Pediatr. Radiol.,* 13, 106–109 (1983).
Wynne-Davis, R., Hall, C.M. et al. *Atlas of Skeletal Dysplasias.* Churchill–Livingstone, Edinburgh, 1985.

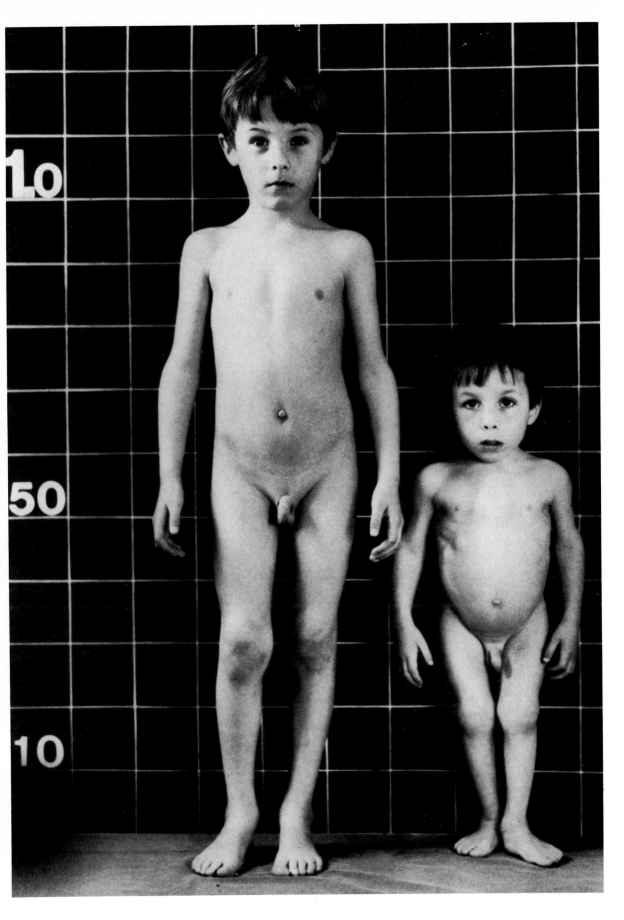

251

125. Hypophosphatasia

A familial disorder with deficient calcification of the bones, absent calcification of the calvaria (craniotabes), late closure of the anterior fontanelle, craniosynostosis, premature loss of deciduous teeth, bowed long bones, fractures, hypercalcemia, and nephrocalcinosis.

Main signs: Very variable expression (congenital lethal (or fetal), infantile, late infantile–juvenile, and adult forms).
1. Absent calcification of the calvaria (craniotabes), late fontanelle closure, craniosynostosis, oxycephaly.
2. Fractures and bowing of the long bones, genu valgum.
3. Rickets-like radiological changes: absent calcification of the skeletal system of varied severity, rachitic rosary, broad metaphyses, 'notching' or 'fraying' of the ends of the long bones. Biochemically: decreased or absent alkaline phosphatase; frequent hypercalcemia; hypercalcuria; increased phosphoethanolamine excretion in the urine.

Supplementary findings: Muscular hypotonia, failure to thrive, respiratory disorders, seizures, anemia, nephrocalcinosis, exophthalmos, increased intracranial pressure, vomiting, bone pains, increased tendency to infections, growth retardation.

Manifestation: Fetal form: intrauterine. Prenatal diagnosis from absent calcification of the cranium (differentiate from anencephaly), decreased alkaline phosphatase in amniotic fluid and cells.
Infantile form: at birth and thereafter.
Late infantile–juvenile form: after the third year of life.
Adult form: After puberty. 'Rickets' history.

Etiology: As a rule, autosomal recessive inheritance. Diagnosis of heterozygotes difficult (decreased alkaline phosphatase, increased phosphoethanolamine excretion in the urine). Autosomal dominant inheritance has been observed in a few families. Gene localized to chromosome 1.

Frequency: By 1972 more than 120 cases had been published. Adult cases are frequently not recognized.

Course, prognosis: Fetal form: intrauterine death, stillbirth.
Infantile form: lethal in 50% of cases.
Juvenile form: good chance of survival, orthopedic and dental problems.
Adult form: spontaneous fractures.
No clear boundaries between the individual forms.

Treatment: To date, no effective means of treatment. Vitamin D resistance. Cortisone not consistently effective. High doses of phosphate administered orally have been tried. Prenatal diagnosis in future pregnancies.

Differential diagnosis: Achondrogenesis and thanatophoric dysplasia with the neonatal forms. Osteogenesis imperfecta.

Illustrations:

1a and 1b Fetal form, intrauterine death. Absent calcification of the skull; barely mineralized, thin ribs. Vertebrae and pelvic bones barely distinguishable. Partial calcification of the long bones, flaring of the metaphyses.
2a 5-month-old infant, early craniostenosis, thoracic in-drawing.
2b Defective calcification of the skeleton, osteomalacia.

J.K./H.-R.W.

References:

Mulivor, R.A., Mennutti, M., Zackai, E.H. et al. Prenatal diagnosis of hypophosphatasia: genetic, biochemical, and clinical studies. *Am. J. Med. Genet.*, 30, 271–282 (1978).

Rasmussen, H. Hypophosphatasia. In: Stanbury, J.B., Wyngaarden, J.B., Fredrickson, D.S., Goldstein, J.L., Brown, M.S. (eds.): *The Metabolic Basis of Inherited Disease*, 5th edn. McGraw–Hill, pp. 1497–1507 (1983).

Terheggen, H.G. and Wischermann, A. Die kongenitale Hypophosphatasie *Monatschr. Kinderheilkd.*, 132, 512–522 (1984).

Fallon M.D. et al. Hypophosphatasia: clinicopathologic comparison of the infantile, childhood, and adult forms. *Medicine*, 63, 12–24 (1984).

Ornoy, A., Adomian, G.E., Rimoin, D.L. Histologic and ultrastructural studies on the mineralization process in hypophosphatasia. *Am. J. Med. Genet.*, 22, 743–758 (1985).

Warren, R.C. et al. First trimester diagnosis of hypophosphatasia with monoclonal antibody to the liver/bone/kidney isoenzyme of alkaline phosphatase. *Lancet*, II, 856–858 (1985).

Whyte, M.P., Magill, H.L., Fallon, M.D. et al. Infantile hypophosphatasia: normalization of circulating bone alkaline phosphatase activity followed by skeletal remineralization. *J. Pediatr.*, 108, 82–88 (1986).

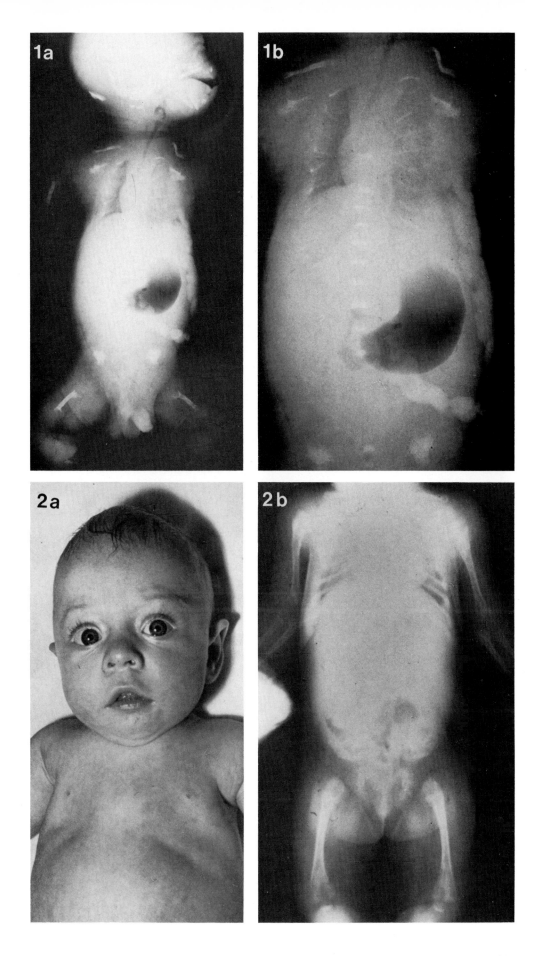

126. Familial Hypophosphatemic Rickets

(So-called Vitamin D-Resistant Rickets, Phosphate Diabetes)

A hereditary metabolic disorder with short stature and rachitic bone changes.

Main signs:
1. Moderately short stature with abnormalities of the lower extremities; pronounced bowlegs, less frequently knock-knees (1, 2, 4). Waddling gait, coxa vara. In childhood, also other rachitic bone changes (rachitic rosary, enlargement of the wrists and ankles, etc.).
2. Dental changes such as defects of enamel and dentin, delayed eruption, dental abscesses, early loss.
3. Abnormal curvature of the spine in adulthood.
4. Occasionally, craniosynostosis.

Supplementary findings: Osteomalacia in adulthood; also, bony protruberances at the sites of tendon attachments.

Radiologically, changes as in vitamin D-deficiency rickets (3); however, the pelvic and spinal regions are spared.

Hypophosphatemia hyperphosphaturia—these, together with slightly short stature, are the only signs of the mild form of the disorder—increased serum alkaline phosphatase, normal serum calcium and parathormone.

Manifestation: Biochemically, during the course of the first six months of life. Clinically, usually between 6 and 18 months, or later.

Etiologically: X-linked dominant disorder; correspondingly milder manifestations of the disease in affected girls. Combined disorder of phosphate reabsorption and of regulation of $1,25\text{-}(OH)_2D$ secretion in the proximal renal tubules.

Frequency: About 1:25,000.

Course, prognosis: Improvement of the signs of florid rickets with the physiological slowing and cessation of growth. Adult height between about 1.30 and 1.60 meters. Frequent back and joint pain and complaints of stiffness in adulthood.

Differential diagnosis: Vitamin-deficiency rickets (here, elevated parathormone and low 25-hydroxy-vitamin D in serum; no positive family history), and other forms of rickets. The metaphyseal chondrodysplasia syndrome, Schmid type and cartilage–hair hypoplasia should also be considered.

Treatment: Clinically and biochemically, good results from daily administration of vitamin D analogs ($1\alpha\text{-}OHD_3$, $1,25\text{-}(OH)_2D_3$) with careful monitoring of blood chemistries. Many authors have seen a positive effect on growth. Correction of the leg deformities by orthopedic surgery preferably after cessation of growth.

Illustrations:
1 and 2 Two children (different parents) at ages 5 and 3 years. Both have a height deficit of 9 cm.
3 The radiological bone changes of a 1-year-old patient.
4 A father and daughter with phosphate diabetes; the small stature of the child led to diagnostic clarification; the father has a history of corrective surgical procedures.

H.-R.W.

References:

Stanbury, J.B., Wyngaarden, J.B., Fredrickson, D.S. et al. *The Metabolic Basis of Inherited Disease.* McGraw–Hill Book Co., 1983, p.1743.

Carlsen, N.L.T., Krasilnikoff, P.A., Eiken, M. Premature cranial synostosis in X-linked hypophosphatemic rickets . . . *Acta Pediatr. Scand.*, 73, 149–154 (1984).

Mimouni, F., Mughal, Z. et al. Picture of the month: X-linked dominant hypophosphatemic rickets. *Am. J. Dis. Child.*, 142, 191–192 (1988).

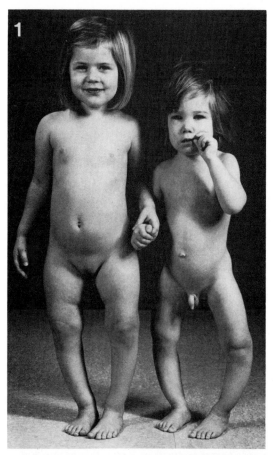

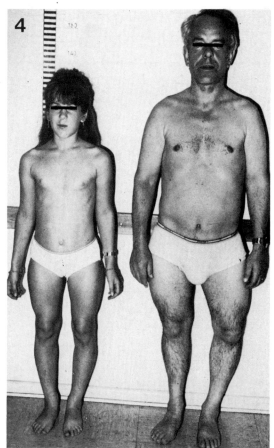

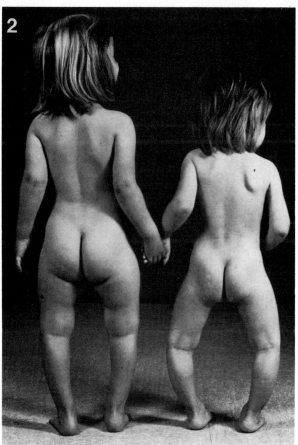

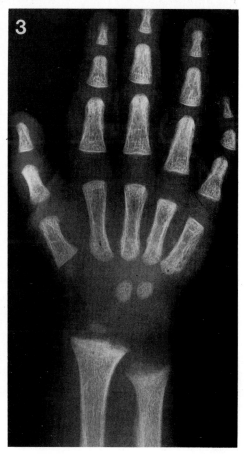

255

127. An Unknown Syndrome of Short Stature with Striking Distal Inhibition of Ossification

A syndrome of short stature, severe infantile scoliosis and other skeletal anomalies, with severely delayed ossification of the bones of the hands and feet.

Main signs:
1. Marked short stature.
2. Marked infantile scoliosis with corresponding abnormal proportions and other secondary changes (11–13).
3. On X-ray, markedly delayed ossification in bones of the hands and feet ('empty wrist') (6, 7).

Supplementary findings: Normal mental development for age.

Radiologically, numerous wormian bones of the skull (3, 4). Possible evidence of malformations of the vertebral column or other regions.

Manifestation: At birth or in early childhood.

Etiology: Not established (receptor defect in the bone matrix?). Genetic basis probable.

Course, prognosis: Unclear, certainly very dependent on the skeletal problems and whether the scoliosis is amenable to therapy.

Treatment: Adequate orthopedic care.

Illustrations:
1–13 A 4½-year-old boy, the sixth child of healthy, consanguineous Turkish parents. A similarly affected sister: mental development normal for age; short stature; severe right convex scoliosis of the thoracic spine, allegedly since 3 years of age, with wedge-shaped vertebrae and synostoses; torsion defect of the lower leg. Other living siblings healthy.

In the proband, the deformities of the spine and thorax (bulging rib cage on the right) were said to be present at birth. Normal mental, delayed motor development. Currently, short stature, well below the third percentile, with short neck, abnormal orientation of the ribs, extremities relatively too long, and severe right convex scoliosis of the thoracic spine (sloping of shoulders and pelvis). Round cranium and numerous wormian bones in the sagittal and especially the lambdoid sutures. Mild coxa vara; torsion defect of the upper and lower leg; lateral dislocation of the patellae; pes adductus with various positional anomalies of the toes. Radiologically, practically 'empty' wrists and delayed ossification of the metacarpals and phalanges but approximately normal epiphyses for age at the pelvis and knees. Also, marked delay in development of the bones of the feet. Exhaustive laboratory examinations, including endocrinological, were normal.

H.-R.W.

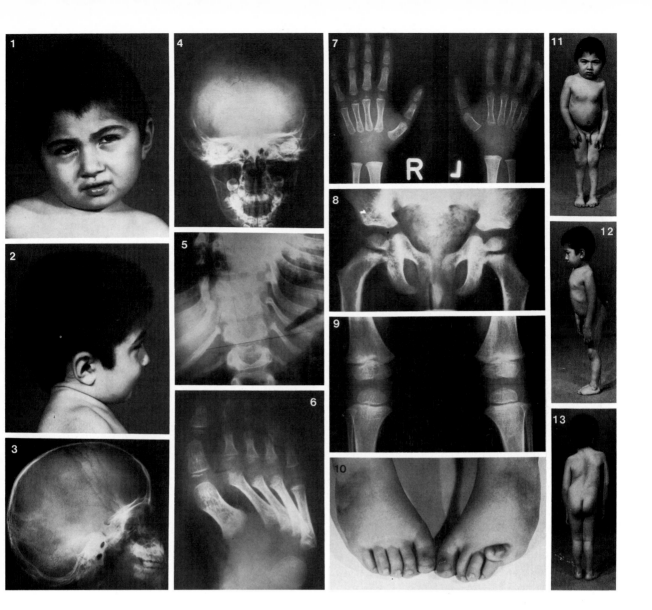

128. Joint Dysplasia–Short Stature–Erythema Telangiectasia

An unusual syndrome with multiple congenital joint dysplasias, short stature, and telangiectatic erythema of the face.

Main signs:
1. Congenital, not completely symmetrical anomalies of the joints and skeleton: dysplasia of the hips, limited extension of the knees, and small club feet, bilateral malformation of the distal humeri with dislocation of the humeroulnar and radioulnar joints, relatively short forearms, limited mobility of the wrists, campto- and sometimes clinodactyly of fingers II–V (**4, 6–8**). No skin dimples.
2. Primary ($001 secondary) short stature, below the third percentile (at 12 years and 2 months around 1.30 m; twin brother: about 1.60 m).
3. Starting at age 2 years and for about the next 6 years, butterfly-like distribution of a paranasally localized telangiectatic erythema of the face, minimally also on the forearms, that may have been aggravated by sunlight (**1** and **2**; in **3** and **5** at age 12 years, only mild residual spots on the left cheek).

Supplementary findings: Dolichocephaly, long narrow face with prominent nose and slightly receding chin (**3, 5**).
   Kyphoscoliosis, lumbar hyperlordosis (**4**).
   At 12 years, still no signs of onset of puberty.
   X-rays of the hands and feet: hypoplasia of the distal ends of the ulnae with absence of the styloid processes; considerable bilateral brachymesophalangy of fingers II–V, severe brachymesophalangy of toes II–V.

Manifestation: At birth and later.

Etiology: Undetermined.

Comment: Bloom syndrome (p.360) is apparently not present. Larsen syndrome (p.404) could be ruled out. Classification as arthrogryposis multiplex congenita (p.402) did not seem to be justified here.

Treatment: Intensive orthopedic-surgical and physiotherapeutic efforts required. Promotion of intellectual development, adequate vocational training and psychological guidance. Genetic counseling.

Illustrations:
1–8 A mentally normal girl, a twin child (brother quite unremarkable) of healthy, nonconsanguineous parents after two older siblings. Father was 47 years old and mother 40 at the proband's birth. Unremarkable family history. Birth measurements 3000 g, 49 cm; no problems of any kind in first year of life.
1 The patient as a young pre-school child.
2 As a young school girl.
3–8 At age 12¼ years. Flexion and adduction contractures of the hips with deviation of the thighs to the left; contracted talipes equinovarus. Chromosome analysis normal.

H.-R.W.

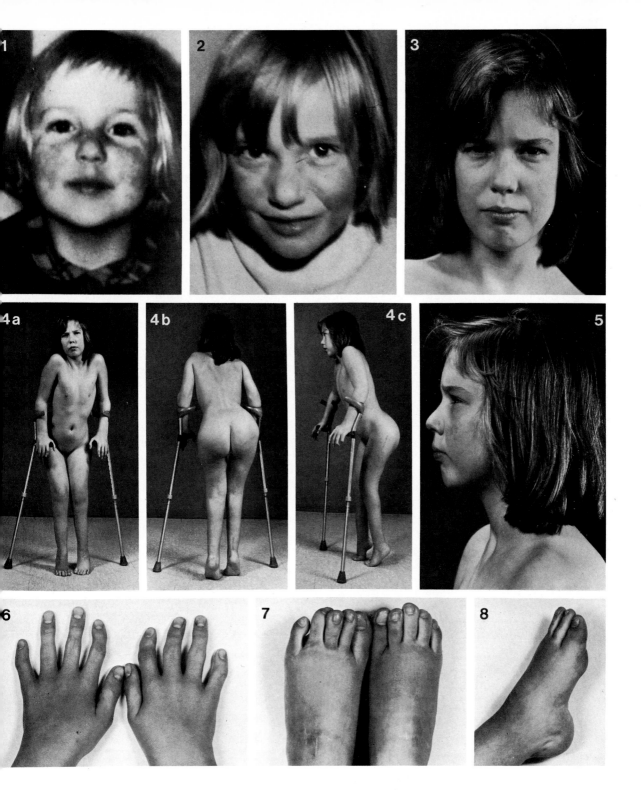

129. Hypochondroplasia

An achondroplasia-like hereditary condition with short-limbed small stature of milder expression.

Main signs:
1. Short stature with disproportionately short extremities—which are usually clinically obvious—and broad, short hands (without 'trident' appearance) and feet (**1–6**). Adult height between about 1.15 and 1.50 m.
2. Cranium normal or oversized, often with prominent forehead. Root of the nose is not low and the facial formation is otherwise essentially normal (**1–5**).
3. Limitation of motion of the elbows (with regard to full extension and supination). Frequently increased lumbar lordosis (**4b**) and genu varus with bow-legs (**2, 3, 4a**).

Supplementary findings: Radiologically (**6, 7**), signs of a somewhat 'attenuated achondroplasia'. Square pelvis with narrow inlet (often leading to dystocia), short and broad femoral necks, disproportionately long fibulae, brachydactyly, etc.

Occasional, usually mild, mental retardation (in about 10% of cases).

Manifestation: At birth (length usually about 48 cm) and thereafter. Sporadic cases are first noted by family members during the early pre-school years.

Etiology: Hereditary disorder, autosomal dominant, of very variable expression, may even appear very similar to achondroplasia. Many sporadic cases representing new mutations, frequently associated with increased paternal age.

Frequency: Not particularly rare.

Course, prognosis: Normal life expectancy. Final height of males between about 1.35 and 1.55 m, in females between about 1.25 and 1.50 m.

Differential diagnosis: Achondroplasia (p.234; here typical facial dysmorphism, markedly shortened upper arms, trident hands, etc.), metaphyseal chondrodysplasia Schmid type (p.262; here, quite different X-ray findings) and other forms of short stature.

Treatment: Symptomatic. Genetic counseling. Prenatal diagnosis may be possible.

Illustrations:
1–5 Children and adults with hypochondroplasia: a 1-year-old; an 11-year-old boy; a mother and daughter; a 12-year-old; and a 16-year-old girl.
6 X-rays of the left hand of a further child at 6 and at 13 years.
7 X-ray of the lower extremities of the girl in 3.

H.-R.W.

References:
Spranger, J.W., Langer, L.O., Jr., Wiedemann, H.-R. *Bone Dysplasias. An Atlas of Constitutional Disorders of Skeletal Development.* G. Fischer and W.B. Saunders, Stuttgart and Philadelphia, 1974.
Oberklaid, F., Danks, M., Jensen, F. et al. Achondroplasia and hypochondroplasia. *J. Med. Genet.*, 16, 140 (1979).
Hall, B.D. and Spranger, J. Hyperchondroplasia: clinical and radiological aspects in 39 cases. *Radiology*, 133, 95 (1979).
Stoll, C., Manini, P. et al. Prenatal diagnosis of hypochondroplasia. *Prenatal Diagnosis.*, 5, 423–426 (1985).
Maroteaux, P. and Falzon, P. Hypochondroplasie. Revue de 80 cas. *Arch. Franc. Pédiatr.*, 45, 105–109 (1988).

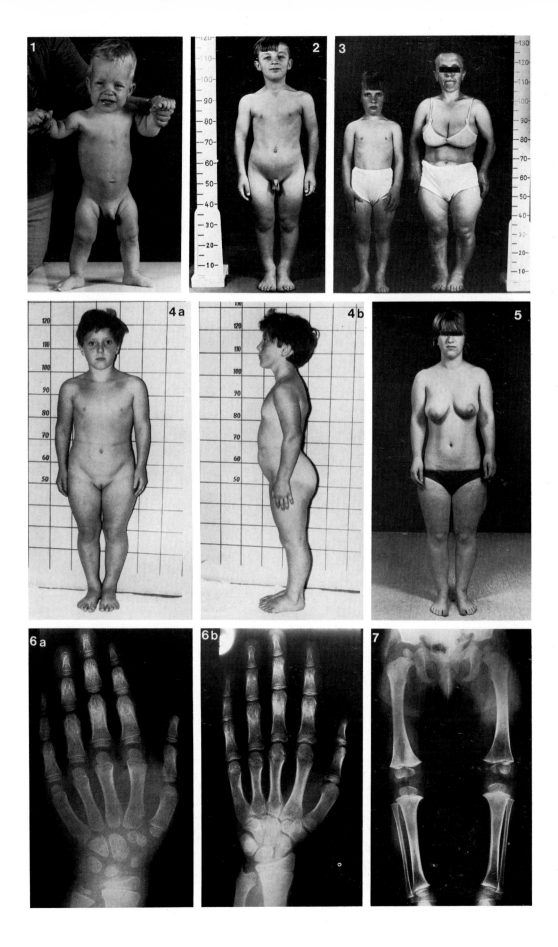

130. Metaphyseal Chondrodysplasia Schmid Type

(Dysostosis Metaphysaria Schmid Type)

An autosomal dominant disorder of short stature, relatively short legs with bowed appearance, waddling gait, and a pseudorachitic X-ray appearance of the metaphyses of the long bones.

Main signs:

1. Shortness of stature with short legs and unremarkable cranium, face, and trunk. Fairly marked bowlegs (**1a, 1b**). Waddling gait. Large joints usually freely mobile. No muscular hypotonia.

2. Radiologically, shortening of the long bones with variable rachitic-like changes of the metaphyses (but without mineral depletion) especially in the lower extremities, and mostly in the femora (distally > proximally). Coxa vara; enlarged epiphyses of the femoral heads in early childhood; short femoral necks (**1c**).

Vertebral column is not involved.

Supplementary findings: Normal blood and urine analyses.

Manifestation: Second year of life.

Etiology: Autosomal dominant disorder.

Frequency: Low (about 55 comparable cases in the literature up to 1988).

Course, prognosis: Favorable. Even though the varus deformity of the lower extremities usually persists, joint function is generally normal. Adult height between about 1.30 and 1.60 m.

Differential diagnosis: Syndrome of hereditary vitamin D-resistant rickets and other forms of rickets, which show appropriate biochemical abnormalities. Cartilage–hair hypoplasia (p.264) and other metaphyseal chondrodysplasias.

Treatment: After closure of the epiphyses, osteotomy to correct the bowlegs. Vitamin D therapy not indicated. Genetic counseling.

Illustrations:

1a–1c An affected child at ages 1 year (**a, c**) and 10 years. Micromelic short stature; bowed legs; swelling of some of the joints. X-ray shows broad, dense metaphyses with irregular borders; separate epiphyseal ossification centers of normal configuration.

H.-R.W.

References:

Spranger, J.W., Langer, L.O., Jr., Wiedemann, H.-R. *Bone Dysplasias. An Atlas of Constitutional Disorders of Skeletal Development.* G. Fischer and W.B. Saunders, Stuttgart and Philadelphia, 1974.

Lachman, R.S., Rimoin, D.L., Spranger, J. Metaphyseal chondrodysplasia, Schmid type . . . with a review of the literature. *Pediatr. Radiol.,* 18, 93–102 (1988).

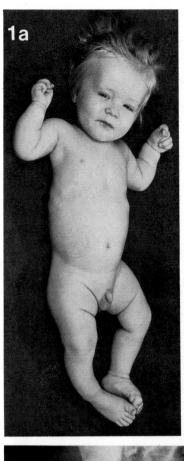

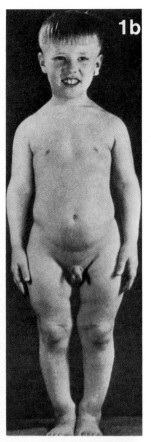

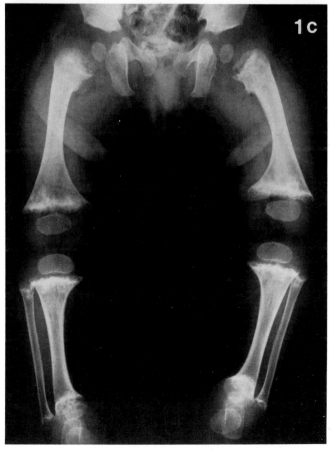

131. Cartilage–Hair Hypoplasia

(Cartilage–Hair Hypoplasia = CHH; Metaphyseal Chondrodysplasia McKusick Type)

A hereditary disorder, quite characteristic when fully expressed, comprising short stature, especially due to short extremities, combined with fine, sparse hair and short, pudgy hands and feet.

Main signs:
1. Short stature of the micromelic type with unremarkable cranial and facial configuration (**1a, 1b**).
2. Short, stubby hands and feet (**1a**) with hyperextensible wrist, ankle, and finger joints.
3. Sparse, fine, light, relatively brittle scalp hair; eyebrows, eyelashes, beard, and body hair may show similar characteristics.

Supplementary findings: In some cases, moderately severe deformity of the thorax. Narrow pelvis. Slightly curved legs (crura vara). Limited extension at the elbows. Short, sometimes brittle, finger- and toenails.

Radiologically, shortened tubular bones with metaphyseal dysplasia (**1c**), the metaphyseal irregularities are generally more distinct in the knee region than in the proximal femora. Disproportionately long fibulae, especially distally.

Possible signs of malabsorption in early childhood (tending to improve spontaneously); also Hirschsprung's disease. Severe combined immune defect, T-cell defects have been described.

Decreased intelligence in some cases.

Manifestation: Usually at birth.

Etiology: Autosomal recessive disorder; very variable expression.

Frequency: Low (apart from special isolates with inbreeding).

Course, prognosis: Limited vitality and a decreased average lifespan have been recorded. Adult height between about 1.10 and 1.45 m. With pregnancy, cesarian section needed because of narrow pelvis.

Differential diagnosis: Metaphyseal chondrodysplasia Schmid type (p.262) does not show correspondingly short, pudgy hands and feet (nor nail changes), but shows more pronounced crura vara, radiological abnormalities, and a different mode of inheritance.

All forms of rickets can be clinically differentiated from the fully expressed syndrome; in addition, they are easily ruled out biochemically.

Treatment: Avoidance of smallpox vaccination and, as far as possible, of exposure to varicella. Genetic counseling.

Illustrations:
1a–1d A now 23-year-old patient with the full picture of cartilage–hair hypoplasia. Small stature since birth; height now 130 cm. Short, broad hands with short nails. Scalp hair short, brittle, thin, sparse and blond. Secondary hair growth sparse. Hyperextensible wrists; limited extension of the elbows.
1c Knee joint with moderate metaphyseal irregularities, at 8 years of age.
1d The same joint at 23 years. Both show hypoplasia of the lateral portion of the femoral epiphysis.

H.-R.W.

References:
Wiedemann, H.-R., Spranger, J., Kosenow, W. Knorpel-Haar-Hypoplasie. *Arch. Kinderheilkd.*, 176, 74 (1967).
Spranger, J.W., Langer, L.O., Jr., Wiedemann, H.-R. *Bone Dysplasias. An Atlas of Constitutional Disorders of Skeletal Development.* G. Fischer and W.B. Saunders, Stuttgart and Philadelphia, 1974.
Steele, R.W., Britton, H.A. et al. Severe combined immunodeficiency with CHH . . . *Pediatr. Res.*, 10, 1003–1005 (1976).
Virolainen, M., Savilahti, E. et al: Cellular and humoral immunity in cartilage hair hypoplasia. *Pediatr. Res.*, 12, 961–966 (1978).
Seige, M. Metaphysäre Chondrodysplasie vom Typ McKusick. *Monatschr. Kinderheilkd.*, 128, 157–159 (1980).
Harris, R.E., Baehner, R.L. et al. Cartilage–hair hypoplasia . . . *Am. J. Med. Genet.*, 8, 291–297 (1981).
Trojak, J.E., Polmar, S.H. et al. Immunologic studies of cartilage hair hypoplasia . . . *John Hopkins Med. J.*, 148, 157–164 (1981).
Ashby, G.H. and Evans, D.I.K. Cartilage hair hypoplasia . . . *J. Roy. Soc. Med.*, 79, 113–114 (1986).
Lischka, A., Frisch, H. et al. Radiologische Veränderungen bei metaphysärer Chondrodystrophie Typ McKusick . . . *Monatschr. Kinderheilkd.*, 132, 550–553 (1986).

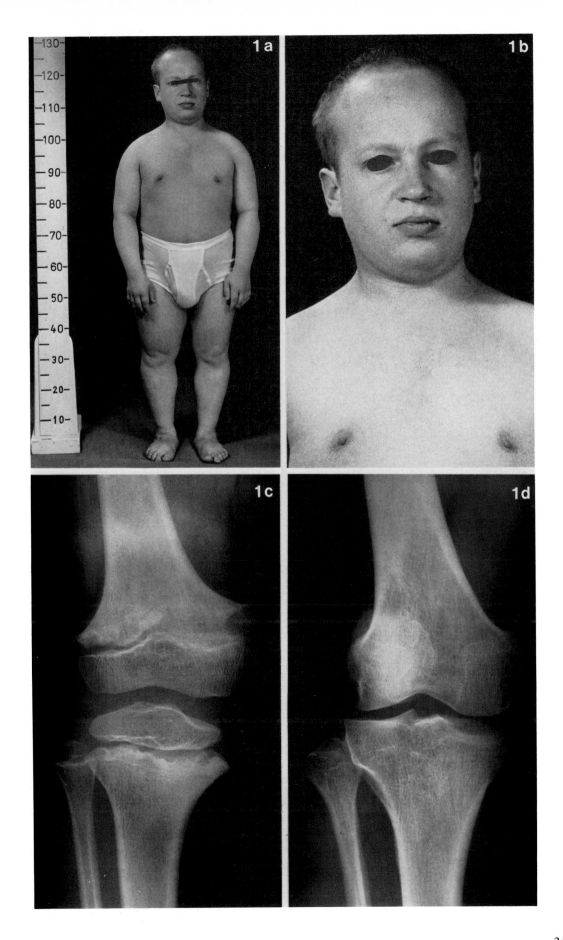

132. Metaphyseal Dysplasia Wiedemann–Spranger Type

A congenital skeletal dysplasia with short-limbed, small stature presenting during the first decade of life, the metaphyses of the long bones on X-ray appear similar to pseudorickets, a somewhat unusual physical appearance, and a good prognosis.

Main signs:
1. Congenital disproportionate small stature due to shortening, especially of the proximal extremities, and to crura vara (**1**). Short neck (**1**). Limited movement at the hips; initial swelling of the knees, wrists, and ankles.
2. Antimongoloid slant of the palpebral fissures (**1, 2**).
3. Radiologically, marked pseudorachitic structural anomalies of the metaphyses of the long bones (**3, 7**) and on lateral view, deformities of the vertebral bodies in part suggesting a reclining hourglass (**5**).
4. Gradual improvement of proportions, resulting in an unremarkable neck, straightening of the legs, extensive compensation of the initial radiological changes, (**2, 4, 6, 8**) and catch-up of growth.

Supplementary findings: Hypermobility of the shoulder and wrist joints. Unremarkable slender hands and feet.

Increased lumbar lordosis.

Somewhat delayed motor development, initially with pronounced waddling gait.

No characteristic metabolic abnormalities.

Manifestation: At birth.

Etiology: Little doubt of a genetic basis; mode of inheritance not clear.

Frequency: Probably low.

Course, prognosis: Favorable. Adult height about normal. Normal life expectancy.

Differential diagnosis: Other metaphyseal chondrodysplasias (e.g., Schmid type, p.262), which, however, are easily differentiated because they are usually manifest later in life.

Treatment: Symptomatic.

Illustrations:
1–8 The first child of healthy, tall, and well-proportioned, possibly consanguineous parents, born about 6 weeks prematurely with length 41 cm, birth weight 2000 g (**3** and **7** at 5 months, **1** at 10 months, **5** at 13 months, **4** and **8** at 13 years, **2** and **6** at 18 years). Gradual compensation of his growth deficiency during his early school years; adult height 1.66 m.

H.-R.W.

References:

Wiedemann, H.-R. and Spranger, J. Chondrodysplasia metaphysaria (Dysostosis metaphysaria)—ein neuer Typ? *Z. Kinderheilkd.*, 108, 171 (1970).
Several similar observations have been made known to the first author in the meantime (Maroteaux and others).

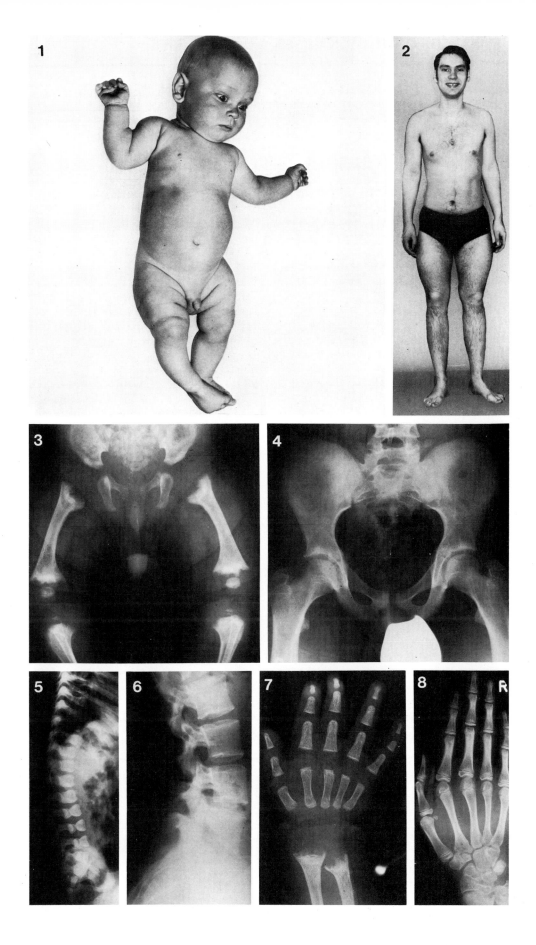

267

133. Pseudoachondroplasia

In appearance, achondroplasia-like short stature, but manifest postnatally, with normal craniofacial skeleton and a marked disorder of epiphyseal ossification on X-ray.

Main signs: Considerable short-limbed small stature with disproportionately long trunk. Craniofacial skeleton unremarkable. Lumbar hyperlordosis. Genu valgus or bowing of the legs. Hypermobility of most joints except the elbows (possibly also the hips and the knees) (1–3).

Supplementary findings: Weakness of joint capsules and ligaments. Not infrequently development of scoliosis.

Normal mental development.

Radiological changes of the vertebral bodies; severe developmental defects of the head of the femur and other epimetaphyseal areas (4, 5).

Manifestation: During the second year of life or later with the onset of a waddling gait and growth retardation (with corresponding radiological changes).

Etiology: Monogenic disorder with severe and mild forms; heterogeneity. Apparently, there are autosomal dominant and autosomal recessive types, each with a mild and a severe form. These at present cannot be differentiated—neither clinically, radiologically, nor biochemically—except by the growth deficiency being more marked in the autosomal recessive form.

Frequency: Not particularly low.

Course, prognosis: Normal life expectancy. Adult height between about 0.90 and 1.40 m. Early development of arthritis, especially of the hip and knee joints.

Differential diagnosis: Achondroplasia (p.234; manifested congenitally, abnormal cranial configuration, etc.); congenital spondyloepiphyseal dysplasia (p.246; manifestation at birth); hypochondroplasia (p.260).

Treatment: Symptomatic–orthopedic. Corrective surgery of bow legs towards the end of the growth period. Arthroplasties may be needed eventually. Psychological guidance with the best possible vocational training. Genetic counseling.

Illustrations:
1 A 14-year-old boy.
2 and 3 Two girls of about the same age. Height of each well below the third percentile (height difference from the average for age: about 40 cm for the girl in **3**; and about 70 cm for the child in **1**).

The boy in **1** was normally proportioned as an infant and could walk without support at 9 months. Manifestation at about 2 years.
4 and 5 X-rays of the child in **3**.

H.-R.W.

References:

Kopits, S.E., Lindstrom, J.A., McKusick, V.A. Pseudoachondroplastic dysplasia: pathodynamics and management. *Birth Defects*, 10/12, 341 (1974).

Spranger, J.W., Langer, L.O., Jr., Wiedemann, H.-R. *Bone Dysplasias. An Atlas of Constitutional Disorders of Skeletal Development.* G. Fischer and W.B. Saunders, Stuttgart and Philadelphia, 1974.

Hall, J. Pseudoachondroplasia. *Birth Defects*, 11/6, 187 (1975).

Heselson, N.G., Cremin, B.J., Beighton, P. Pseudoachondroplasia, a report of 13 cases. *Brit. J. Radiol.*, 50, 473 (1977).

Maroteaux, P., Stanescu, R., Stanescu, V. et al. The mild form of pseudoachondroplasia. *Eur. J. Pediatr.*, 133, 227 (1980).

Horton, W.A., Hall, J.G., Scott, C.I. et al. Growth curves for height for diastrophic dysplasia, spondyloepiphyseal dysplasia congenita, and pseudoachondroplasia. *Am. J. Dis. Child.*, 136, 316 (1982).

Stanescu, V., Maroteaux, P. et al. The biochemical defect of pseudoachondroplasia. *Eur. J. Pediatr.*, 138, 221–225 (1982).

Young, I.D. and Moore, J.R. Severe pseudoachondroplasia with parental consanguinity. *J. Med. Genet.*, 22, 150–153 (1985).

Wynne-Davies, R., Hall, C.M. et al. Pseudoachondroplasia . . . comparison of autosomal dominant and recessive types . . . review of 32 patients . . . *J. Med. Genet.*, 23, 425–434 (1986).

Hall, J.G., Dorset, J.P. et al. Gonadal mosaicism in pseudoachondroplasia. *Am. J. Med. Genet.*, 28, 143–151 (1987).

Nores, J.M., Maroteaux, P. Evolution sur 40 ans d'un cas de pseudo-achondroplasie. *Presse Méd.*, 17, 43: 2283–2286 (1988).

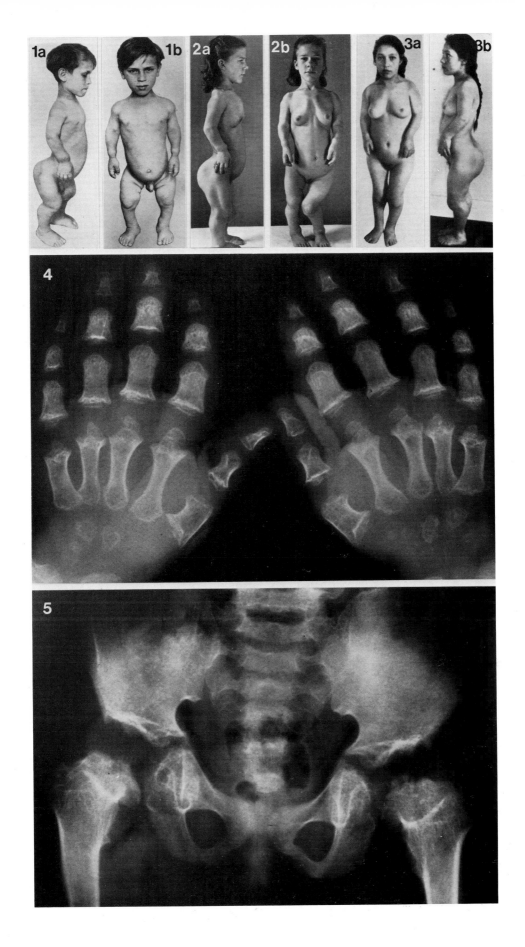

134. Progeria

(Gilford Syndrome, Hutchinson–Gilford Syndrome)

A highly characteristic syndrome comprising post-natal growth deficiency and premature ageing.

Main signs:
1. Growth deficiency manifesting after the first year of life.
2. Concomitant, increasing 'senescence': loss of hair (3–5), of subcutaneous fat—including that of the earlobes (7, 8), and of the normal thickness and elasticity of the skin; flexion contractures of the large joints (1, 6) and the finger joints; dystrophy of the nails (9); prominent scalp veins (4, 5, 7, 8). Development of a sharp, beak-like nose jutting out from the small face with receding chin, slightly protruding eyes, and relatively large cranium, defining a 'bird face', protruding abdomen.

Supplementary findings: Skin changes of diffuse scleroderma, in some cases.

Radiologically, hypoplastic skeleton with persistence of the anterior fontanelle, atrophy of the lateral portions of the clavicles and of the terminal phalanges (acromicria, 10); coxa valga.

Delayed and irregular dentition.

Absence or delay of sexual development (1, 6). High squeaky voice.

Intelligence in the normal range.

Insulin resistance, increased metabolic rate, serum lipid and collagen anomalies. No growth hormone deficiency.

Etiology: Appears certain that an autosomal recessive mode of inheritance exists.

Frequency: Very low; about 1 case in 250,000 live births estimated. Over 100 cases have been described to date (three of them in Germany).

Course, prognosis: Attained height barely over 1.15 m, attained weight barely 15 kg. Usually premature development of atherosclerosis. Death usually in the second decade of life as a result of atherosclerotic complications (coronary occlusion).

Diagnosis, differential diagnosis: Fully expressed clinical picture unmistakable. Exclusion of the Cockayne (p.166), the Hallermann–Streiff–François (p.530), the congenital cutis laxa (p.274), the de Barsy (p.276), and the Wiedemann–Rautenstrauch (p.272) syndromes should not cause any particular difficulties.

Treatment: Only symptomatic treatment is possible (psychological guidance, possibly a wig, etc.).

Illustrations:
1 Progeria in a 17-year-old from H. Gilford (1897/1904).
2–10 A German patient at 10 months (2), 18 months (3) (demonstrating growth deficiency, loss of hair), 3½ years (4) and 7½ years (5), and 14½ years (6–10). 6 Height of a 7-year-old, no signs of puberty; thin, tense, yellow-brownish, irregularly hyperpigmented skin; sclerosed radial artery; calcification of one of the heart valves; cardiac death at 15¾ years.

H.-R.W.

References:

Wiedemann, H.-R. Syndrome mit besonderem 'Altersaspekt': Progerie (Hutchinson–Gilford–Syndrom). *Handbuch der Kinderheilkunde*, vol. 1, part 1, p.828 ff. Springer, Heidelberg, 1971.
De Busk, F.L. The Hutchinson–Gilford progeria syndrome. *J. Pediatr.*, 80, 697 (1972).
Brown, W.T., Darlington, G.J., Arnold, A. et al. Detection of HLA antigens on progeria syndrome fibroblasts. *Clin. Genet.*, 17, 213 (1980).
Wiedemann, H.-R. Progeria. In: *Neurocutaneous Diseases*. Gomez, M.R. (ed.). Butterworths, Boston, 1987, pp. 247–253.
Trevas Maciel, A. Evidence for autosomal recessive inheritance of progeria . . . *Am. J. Med. Genet.*, 31, 483–487 (1988).
Khalifa, M.M. Hutchinson–Gilford progeria syndrome . . . autosomal recessive inheritance. *Clin. Genet.*, 35, 125–132 (1989).

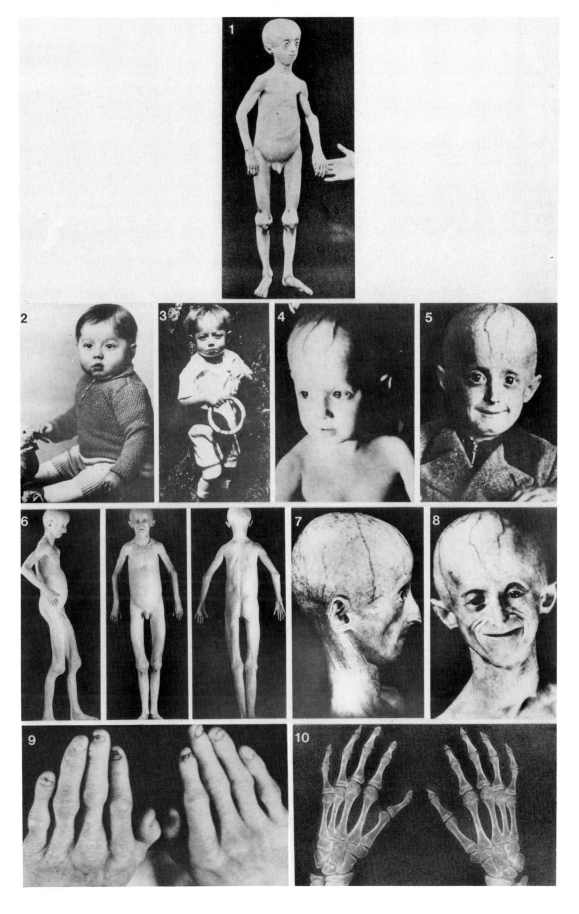

135. Congenital Pseudohydrocephalic Progeroid Syndrome

(Neonatal Progeroid Syndrome, Wiedemann–Rautenstrauch Syndrome)

A congenitally manifest syndrome of pre- and postnatal growth deficiency, pseudohydrocephalus, small senile-appearing face, 'congenital teeth', and extensive deficiency of adipose tissue.

Main signs:

1. Small, somewhat triangular, senile-appearing face and hydrocephaloid cranium with wide-open sutures, persistent anterior fontanelle, prominent venous markings, and sparse scalp hair (1–9). Relatively low-set ears, deep-set eyes, scanty eyebrows and eyelashes (possible entropion). Small upper jaw, protruding chin; 'congenital' incisors.

2. Relatively large hands and feet or fingers and toes.

3. Striking generalized deficiency of subcutaneous adipose tissue, apart from the possible development of paradoxical caudal accumulations of fatty tissue on the buttocks and flanks or in the anogenital area (10–13).

Supplementary findings: Congenital small size with at birth term. Failure to thrive. Deficient growth and development. Loss of the congenital and of newly erupted dysplastic teeth.

Progressive development of a beak-like nose in infancy (4–6).

Delayed motor development; possible appearance of neurological signs such as ataxia, dysmetria, nystagmus. Mental development generally severely impaired, but possibly within normal limits.

Radiologically, possible congenital ossification disorders with tendency to normalize.

Manifestation: At birth.

Etiology: Hereditary defect presumably with autosomal recessive transmission (one pair of affected siblings; one child of a consanguineous marriage).

Frequency: Extremely low; to date, seven published cases; a number of further cases, thought to have this syndrome, have been made known to us.

Course, prognosis: Mainly dependent on the presence and severity of a mental and/or neurological impairment. Long-term observations are not yet available.

Differential diagnosis: Primarily the Hallermann–Streiff–François syndrome (p.530) and congenital generalized lipodystrophy (p.280) must be ruled out, which is not difficult clinically. Hutchinson–Gilford syndrome, the true progeria, is not as a rule manifest congenitally, but develops during the early postnatal period (p.270).

Treatment: Symptomatic.

Illustrations:

1–3 Three different children, all a few weeks of age.
4–6 The development of a somewhat beak-like nose (4 and 5: the same child at ages 6 weeks and 8 months respectively).
7–9 Three children at age 8 months.
10–13 Absent subcutaneous adipose tissue, except for paradoxical accumulations of fat caudally, the latter especially apparent in 13.
(1, 7, 8, 11 from Rautenstrauch et al.—see below.)

H.-R.W.

References:

Rautenstrauch, T., Snigula, F., Krieg, T. et al. Progeria: A cell culture study and clinical report of familial incidence. *Eur. J. Pediatr.*, 124, 101 (1977).

Wiedemann, H.-R. An unidentified neonatal progeroid syndrome: Follow-up report. *Eur. J. Pediatr.*, 130, 65 (1979).

Devos, E.A., Leroy, J.G., Fryns, J.P. et al. The Wiedemann–Rautenstrauch or neonatal progeroid syndrome. *Eur. J. Pediatr.*, 136, 245 (1981).

Snigula, F. and Rautenstrauch, T. A new neonatal progeroid syndrome. *Eur. J. Pediatr.*, 136, 325 (1981).

Leung, A.K.C. Natal teeth. *Am. J. Dis. Child.*, 140, 249–251 (1986).

Ohashi, H., Eguchi, T. et al. Neonatal progeroid syndrome . . . *Jpn. J. Hum. Genet.*, 32, 253–256 (1987).

Rudin, C., Thommen, L. et al. The neonatal pseudohydrocephalic progeroid syndrome (Wiedemann–Rautenstrauch). *Eur. J. Pediatr.*, 147, 433–438 (1988).

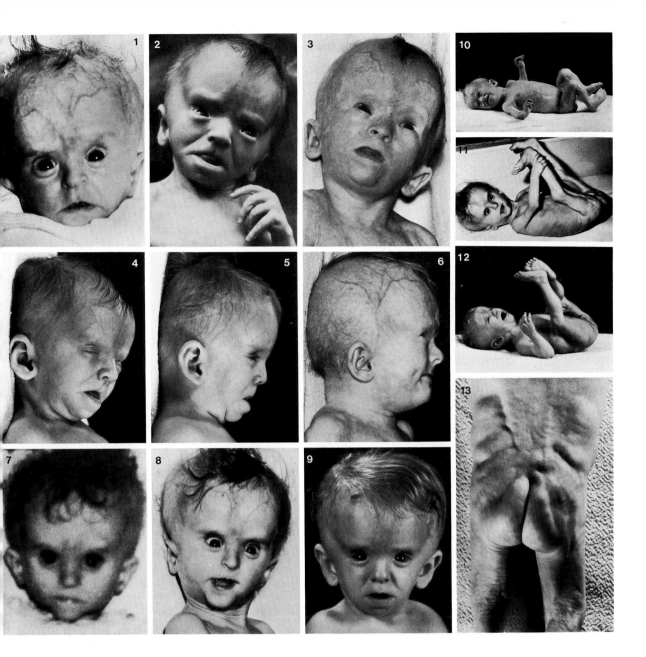

136. Congenital Cutis Laxa Syndrome

(Dermatochalasis Connata)

A hereditary disorder comprising cutis laxa with corresponding 'aged' appearance which may be associated with numerous other defects.

Main signs: Generalized cutis laxa: too much skin—soft, slack, pendulous, and wrinkled (1–3)—giving, especially in the face, the impression of premature aging, even senility, and possibly grotesque appearance.

Supplementary findings: Depending on the biological type (see below), the following may be present: congenital small size; postnatal growth retardation and general developmental delay; deficiency of subcutaneous adipose tissue and muscle weakness; hypertelorism (3a); micrognathia (1c) and other skeletal dysmorphism or deformities; delayed closure of the fontanelles; dislocation of the hips; generalized hyperextensibility of the joints and tendency to dislocation. Internal changes may include laxity of the vocal cords, emphysema of the lungs, vascular wall aneurysms and vascular stenoses, multiple gastrointestinal diverticula, hernias and prolapses. Thus, laxity of the skin may be only one, external, sign of a systemic mesenchymal disorder.

Manifestation: At birth.

Etiology: The syndrome (a still poorly delineated 'umbrella' term) comprises a number of monogenic hereditary disorders; thus, heterogeneity. Probably several autosomal recessive types of different expression and severity; a milder autosomal dominant type; and probably also X-linked types.

Formal pathogenesis: Histologically, deficiencies of elastic fibers have been demonstrated repeatedly, partly as a fairly generalized elastolysis (with degeneration and decomposition of elastic fibers). In many cases defects of various enzymes or enzyme inhibitors have been demonstrated, or abnormalities of copper metabolism, with the basic defect still unknown.

Frequency: Low. But well over 100 reports in the literature.

Course, prognosis: Dependent on the type. Potentially early lethal course especially with the recessive types (e.g., as a result of cor pulmonale).

Differential diagnosis: De Barsy syndrome (p.276). Certain cases from the broad field of the Ehlers–Danlos syndrome.

Treatment: The use of cosmetic plastic surgery in patients with mild forms of the disorder should be carefully considered. Genetic counseling.

Illustrations:
1–3 A congenitally undersized 6-year-old boy (his first-born brother died post partum with the identical clinical picture). Growth deficiency of about 15%; markedly delayed closure of the fontanelles; bilateral dislocated hips; generalized weakness of the ligaments, capsules, and muscles with further dislocations. Hypoplasia of the iris, tortuous fundal vessels. Sudden death at age 7 years.

H.-R.W.

References:

Wiedemann, H.-R. Über einige progeroide Krankheitsbilder und deren diagnostische Einordnung. *Z. Kinderheilkd.*, 107, 91 (1969).
Beighton, P. Cutis laxa. A heterogeneous disorder. *Birth Defects*, 10, 126 (1974).
Wilsch, L., Schmid, G., Haneke, E. Spätmanifeste Dermatochalasis. *Dtsch. Med. Wochenschr.*, 102, 1451 (1977).
Agha, A., Sakati, N.O. et al. Two forms of cutis laxa presenting in the newborn period. *Acta. Ped. Scand.*, 67, 775 (1978).
Sakati, N.O. and Nyhan, W.L. Congenital cutis laxa and osteoporosis. *Am. J. Dis. Child.*, 137, 452–454 (1983).
Sakati, N.O., Nyhan, W.L. et al. Syndrome of cutis laxa, ligamentous laxity, and delayed development. *Pediatrics*, 72, 850–856 (1983).
Karrar, Z.A. Cutis laxa . . . *Pediatrics*, 72, 903–904 (1984).
Fitzsimmons, J.S., Fitzsimmons, E.M. et al. Variable clinical presentation of cutis laxa. *Clin. Genet.*, 28, 284–295 (1985).
Allanson, J., Austin, W. et al. Congenital cutis laxa with retardation of growth and motor development . . . *Clin. Genet.*, 29, 133–136 (1986).
Gardner, L.I., Sanders-Fay, K. et al. Congenital cutis laxa syndrome . . . *Arch. Dermatol.*, 122, 1241–1243 (1986).
Rogers, J. and Danks, D. Congenital cutis laxa. *Clin. Genet.*, 30, 345 (1986).
Patton, M.A., Tolmie, J. et al. Congenital cutis laxa . . . *J. Med. Genet.*, 24, 556–561 (1987).
Taieb, A., Aumailley, M. et al. Collagen studies in congenital cutis laxa. *Arch. Dermatol. Res.*, 279, 308–314 (1987).
van Maldergem, L., Vamos, E. et al. Severe congenital cutis laxa with pulmonary emphysema . . . *Am. J. Med. Genet.*, 31, 455–464 (1988).
Goldblatt, J. Wallis, C. et al. Cutis laxa . . . *Dysmorphol. Clin. Genet.*, 1, 142–144 (1988).
Chabrolle, J.P., Caillez, D. et al. Cutis laxa . . . *Arch. Fr. Pediatr.*, 46, 129–132 (1989).

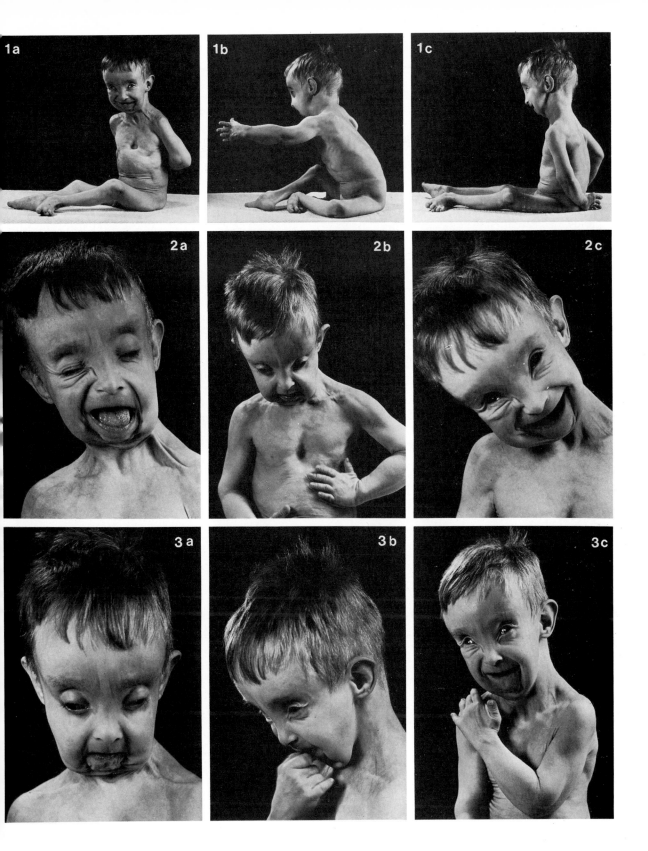

137. De Barsy Syndrome

An autosomal recessive progeroid syndrome with progressive mental impairment, cutis laxa, atrophy of the skin, decrease of subcutaneous fatty tissue, hyperextensibility of the small joints, eye changes, and small stature.

Main signs:
1. Postnatal onset of growth deficiency.
2. Progeroid facies with pronounced nasolabial folds, decrease of subcutaneous adipose tissue.
3. Large, dysplastic, prominent ears.
4. Corneal clouding, cataract.
5. Cutis laxa, skin atrophy with pigment anomalies.
6. Mental impairment.

Supplementary findings: Thin lips, hyperextensibility of the small joints, muscular hypotonia with increased tendon reflexes, accentuation of the mid-forehead, microcephaly, small stature, hypertrichosis, synophrys.

Manifestation: Corneal clouding present at birth; cutis laxa apparent by 6 months of age, at the latest.

Etiology: Autosomal recessive disorder.

Frequency: Low. To date only six isolated cases and two families with (three and four) affected siblings reported.

Course, prognosis: Progressive mental impairment leading to helplessness and confinement to bed.

Differential diagnosis: Can be readily differentiated from Berardinelli–Seip progressive lipodystrophy, Hutchinson–Gilford progeria, Wiedemann–Rautenstrauch neonatal progeroid syndrome, Cockayne syndrome, Hallermann–Streiff syndrome, and cutis laxa syndrome.

Treatment: Symptomatic.

Illustrations:
1–4 Siblings.
1, 1a, and 1b A 6-month-old male infant; bilateral corneal clouding, hyperelastic, wrinkled atrophic skin.
2 and 2a His 7½-year-old sister who has had corneal surgery; hypertrichosis; hyperextensibility of the small joints; thin, hyperpigmented atrophic skin.
3 and 3a Their 10-year-old sister, the same appearance; mental impairment.
4, 4a, and 4b Their 20-year-old brother; very marked signs of skin aging; distinct mental impairment.

J.K.

References:

Kunze, J., Majewski, F., Montgomery, P. et al. De Barsy syndrome—an autosomal recessive progeroid syndrome. *Eur. J. Pediatr.*, 144, 348–354 (1985).

Pontz, B.F. et al. Biochemical, morphological, and immunological findings in a patient with cutis laxa-associated inborn disorder (De Barsy syndrome). *Eur. J. Pediatr.*, 145, 428–434 (1986).

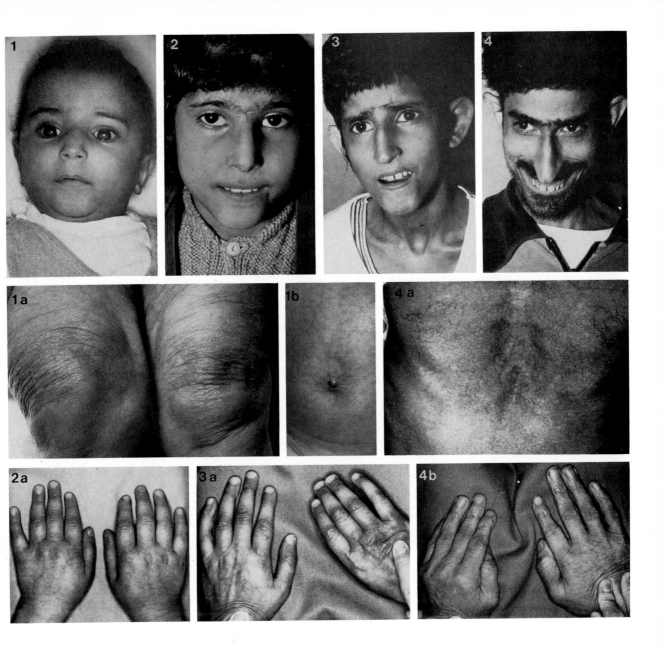

138. A Rare Progeroid Syndrome with Cardiac Anomaly

A syndrome of elderly appearance, extremely lean build, sparse hair growth, joint abnormalities, cardiovascular anomalies, and delayed maturation.

Main signs:
1. Narrow face, appearing generally 'too old', with hypotelorism, short palpebral fissures; somewhat deep-set eyes; prominent, narrow, slightly aquiline nose; prominent ears; high palate; and microretrognathia particularly in infancy (1–3, 5, 6). Dimpled chin (2, 5).
2. Premature closure of the fontanelles with the cranium remaining generally small (52.5 cm at 14 years). Mental development normal for age.
3. Extremely scanty development of scalp hair, eyebrows, and eyelashes during infancy (1–3). Subsequently also, relatively thin and delicate hair growth; at 14 years still almost no body hair and a deficiency of other signs of maturity (4–6).
4. Markedly poor development of musculature and subcutaneous adipose tissue (weight of this 14-year-old boy of normal height (1.60 m) is only 35 kg).
5. Knee and elbow joints not fully extensible since birth; other large joints hyperextensible. Unusually long fingers and toes, especially in infancy (7, 8), with 'acrogeria' (7–9); at 14 years, slight flexion contractures of the distally tapered distal phalanges of the fingers. Asymmetrically elevated shoulders with prominent scapulae; increased thoracic kyphosis. Dimples over most of the large joints.
6. Cardiac anomaly (ventricular septal defect, subvalvular pulmonary stenosis—both surgically corrected at 14 years—pulmonary vascular anomalies); no decrease of exercise tolerance.

Supplementary findings: Ophthalmological examination normal.

Radiologically, no skeletal malformations; slightly delayed ossification.

Blood chemistries unremarkable.

Karyotype 46 XY.

Unilateral cryptorchidism.

Manifestation: At birth.

Etiology: Unknown.

Course, prognosis: Apparently favorable.

Differential diagnosis: Many similarities with the observation of Ruvalcaba et al. (see below); however the progeroid manifestations occurred considerably later in their cases.

Treatment: Symptomatic.

Illustrations:
1–9 The second child of young, healthy, apparently nonconsanguineous parents (first child unremarkable). Pregnancy normal; birth at term with normal measurements.
1–3, 7 and 8 The proband at age 6 months;
4–6 and 9 At age 14 years.
2 The remainder of an ossified cephalohematoma on the left.

H.-R.W

References:
Ruvalcaba, R.H.A., Churesigaew, S., Myhre, S.A. et al. Children who age rapidly—progeroid syndromes. *Clin. Pediatr.*, 16, 248 (1977).

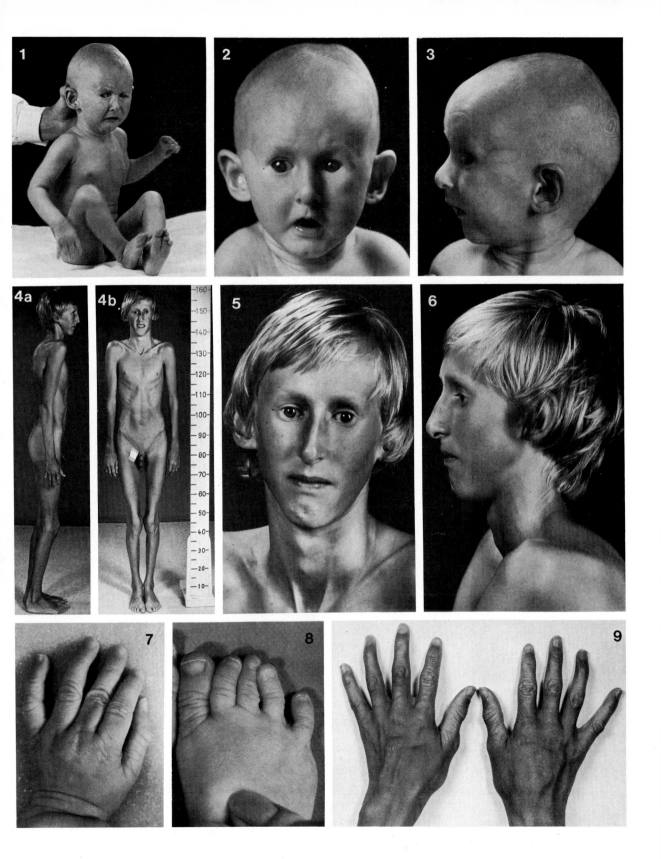

139. Congenital Generalized Lipodystrophy

(Berardinelli–Seip Syndrome)

A hereditary disorder with generalized deficiency of adipose tissue beginning at an early age, muscular hypertrophy, tall stature, acromegaly, encephalopathy, and other anomalies.

Main signs:
1. Generalized lipoatrophy (**1, 2**).
2. Muscular hypertrophy, possibly giving the child an athletic appearance.
3. Hyperpigmentation, acanthosis nigricans; overabundant, curly scalp hair (**2**) or generalized hypertrichosis; dilated cutaneous veins (**1b, 2b**).
4. Increased length or macrosomia at birth, or several years of postnatal tall stature. Acromegaloid facial dysmorphism, relatively large ear lobes, abnormally large hands and feet (**1b, 2b**); possible hypertrophy of the penis or clitoris, and polycystic ovaries.
5. 'Encephalopathy' of a nonprogressive nature with about half of the cases showing mental retardation (mild to severe) associated with, usually, demonstrable partial dilatation of the cerebral ventricles or cisterns.

Supplementary findings: Hepatomegaly (fatty liver) in most cases; cardiomegaly, nephromegaly also frequent.

Postnatal tall stature is accompanied by corresponding acceleration of ossification and dentition.

Increased metabolic rate. Disorder of fat and carbohydrate metabolism; extreme insulin resistance, hyperlipemia.

Development of nonketotic diabetes mellitus with lipoatrophy (starting at about the beginning of the second decade of life).

Manifestation: At birth and thereafter.

Etiology: Autosomal recessive disorder. Insulin receptor defect?

Frequency: Low (fewer than 100 observations in the literature).

Course, prognosis: Premature closure of the epiphyses; normal adult height. Onset of puberty at about the expected age. Prognosis complicated by hypertrophic cardiomyopathy and possibility of diabetic vascular complications.

Differential diagnosis: Acquired generalized lipodystrophy; partial lipodystrophies.

Treatment: Symptomatic, including psychological guidance and, when indicated, cosmetic measures. Genetic counseling.

Illustrations:
1 and 2 Typically affected siblings (18 months and 6 years old). Tall stature; bone age of the 6-year-old equivalent to a 12-year-old; hepatomegaly in both children; enlargement of the third ventricle and the basal cistern respectively on pneumoencephalogram.

H.-R.W.

References:

Seip, M. Generalized lipodystrophy. *Ergeb. Inn. Med. Kinderheilkd. N. F.*, 31, 59 (1971).

Wiedemann, H.-R. Dienzephale Syndrome des Kindesalters. *Pädiatr. Prax.*, 11, 95 (1972).

Oseid, S., Beck-Nielsen, H. et al. Decreased binding of insulin to its receptor in . . . congenital generalized lipodystrophy. *N. Engl. J. Med.*, 296, 245–248 (1977).

Huseman, C.A., Johanson, A.J. et al. Congenital lipodystrophy . . . with polycystic ovarian disease. *J. Pediatr.*, 95, 72–74 (1979).

Bjørnstad, P.G., Semb, B.K.H. et al. Echocardiographic assessment of cardiac function and morphology in patients with generalized lipodystrophy. *Eur. J. Pediatr.*, 144, 355–359 (1985).

Lestradet, C., Massol, J. et al. Lipodystrophie généralisée congénitale. *Arch. Fr. Pédiatr.*, 42, 705–707 (1985).

Mørk, N.J., Rajka, G. et al. Treatment of acanthosis nigricans with etretinate . . . in generalized lipodystrophy. *Acta Derm. Venereol.* (Stockh.), 66, 173–174 (1986).

Rheuban, K.S., Blizzard, R.M. et al. Hypertrophic cardiomyopathy in total lipodystrophy. *J. Pediatr.*, 109, 301–302 (1986).

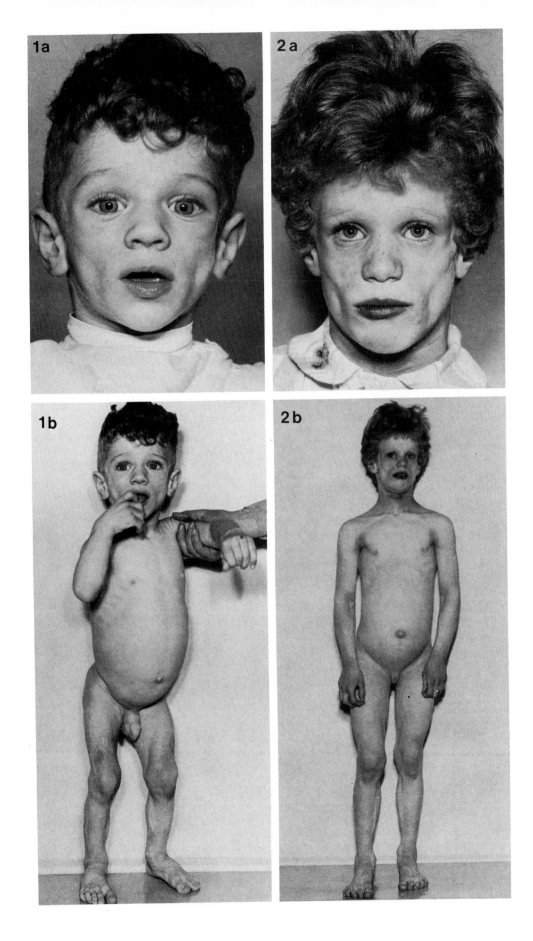

140. A Syndrome of Partial Lipoatrophy Associated with Juvenile Diabetes Mellitus in Monozygotic Twin Brothers

A lipodystrophy beginning in the lower extremities and subsequently affecting the upper extremities and the face, associated with juvenile diabetes mellitus.

Main signs:
1. Lipoatrophy of insidious onset in the second or third year of life (proband I = child in **1**) and in the fourth year of life (proband II = child in **4**), affecting the right foot and lower leg, beginning distally in proband I; and both feet, lower legs, and lower thighs, beginning distally, in proband II. In the meantime, proband II shows advanced lipoatrophy of the thighs and new areas on both hands, the distal half of both forearms, and in the buccal areas bilaterally (right side more than the left; severe disfigurement). Possible corresponding onset in the buccal area in proband I.
2. Easily controlled insulin-dependent diabetes mellitus in both children (manifest in proband I at 3½ years, in proband II at 13 months with pre-coma).

Supplementary findings: In areas of lipoatrophy, thin skin with very prominent veins (**1–6**).

Normal musculature.

In part, the lipoatrophy has been directly preceded by 'transient itchy flushing of the skin' as well as painless nodular indurations of the tissues.

Differentiating laboratory findings in the children. In proband II, in conformity with the greater acuteness of the process, considerably increased gamma globulins and IgG; C_3 complement elevated.

Manifestation: Early childhood.

Etiology: Not clear. Genetic basis assumed, the patients being monozygotic twins. The precise nature of the process still not known.

Comment: Highly unusual course for a lipodystrophy; the association with juvenile diabetes mellitus is also unusual.

Course, prognosis: Further progression of the lipoatrophy can be expected.

Differential diagnosis: Other forms of lipodystrophy.

Treatment: Only symptomatic treatment possible (including immunosuppression).

Illustrations:
1–6 Four-year-old monozygotic twin brothers of normal mental development, in whom subjective well-being is unaffected; no further internal or neurological findings. No acceleration of growth in height, ossification, or dentition. They are the second and third children of young, healthy, nonconsanguineous parents; a 16-year-old brother of the father has had insulin-dependent diabetes mellitus since 12 years of age.

H.-R.-W.

References:

Peters, M.S. and Winkelmann, R.K. Localized lipoatrophy (atrophic connective tissue disease panniculitis). *Arch. Dermatol.*, 116, 1363 (1980).
Billings, J.K., Milgraum, S.S. et al. Lipoatrophic panniculitis: a possible autoimmune inflammatory disease of fat. *Arch. Dermatol.*, 123, 1662–1666 (1987).

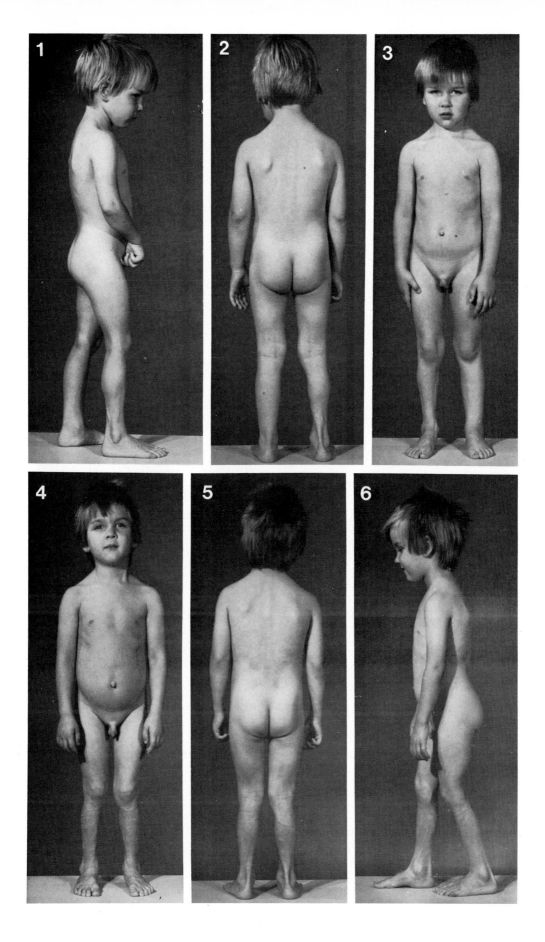

283

141. Diencephalic Tumor–Emaciation Syndrome of Infancy

(Russell)

A syndrome of severe wasting of fatty tissue; pseudo-anemic pallor and vomiting with good food intake; feeling of well-being to euphoria; behavior ranges from lively to hyperactive.

Main signs:
1. Progressive emaciation (**1**) in spite of good food intake (even hyperphagia).
2. Undiminished alertness, sprightliness to euphoria.
3. Increased liveliness to hyperactivity.
4. Vomiting (occasional or frequent). Striking pallor without anemia.
5. Nystagmus (in 50%).

Supplementary findings: Excitability, tremor, sweating. Diabetes insipidus in some cases.

Possible accelerated growth with acromegalic features (hands, feet, genitalia) (**1a**).

Characteristically, definite neurological signs tend to be absent for a long time.

Manifestation: From early infancy to about the end of the second year of life (rarely later).

Etiology: A slowly growing glioma in the anterior hypothalamus (usually an astrocytoma).

Frequency: Low. About 100 cases described in the literature.

Course, prognosis: To a great extent depends on how soon recognized and on the treatment (see below). Average survival of untreated cases after first manifestation, about 12 months.

Diagnosis: When suspected, ultrasonography, CT scan, or further neuroradiological examinations in addition to CSF protein determination and cell count.

Treatment: Where indicated, surgery and/or radiotherapy (which may prolong life considerably).

Illustrations:
1a–1c A 2-year-old boy with 'diencephalic lipodystrophy' of several months duration (underweight by 3.4 kg in relation to height; wasting, 'tobacco-pouch buttocks'). Cranium normal for age (but appearing relatively too large). Large ears, thick protruding lips, large penis, and large feet. Pseudoanemic pallor. Lively, friendly behavior (**1a**). Neurological examination superficially unremarkable. Suspected tumor on brain scintiscan and angiography. Operatively confirmed hypothalamic spongioblastoma.

H.-R.W.

References:

Wiedemann, H.-R. Dienzephale Syndrome des Kindesalters. *Päediatr. Prax.*, 11, 95 (1972).

Burr, I.M., Slonim, A.E., Danish, R.K., Gadoth, N., Butler, I.J. Diencephalic syndrome revisited. *J. Pediatr.*, 88, 439 (1976).

Andler, W., Stolecke, H., Sirang, H. Endocrine dysfunction in the diencephalic syndrome of emaciation in infancy. *Helv. Pediatr. Acta*, 33, 393 (1978).

Drop, S.L.S., Guyda, H.J., Colle, E. Inappropriate growth hormone release in the diencephalic syndrome of childhood: case report and a 4-year endocrinological follow-up. *Clin. Endocrinol.*, 13, 181 (1980).

Blanc, J.F., Chatelan, P. et al. Diagnostic echographique d'une tumeur diencéphalique cachectisante. *Arch. Fr. Pediatr.*, 40, 575–577 (1983).

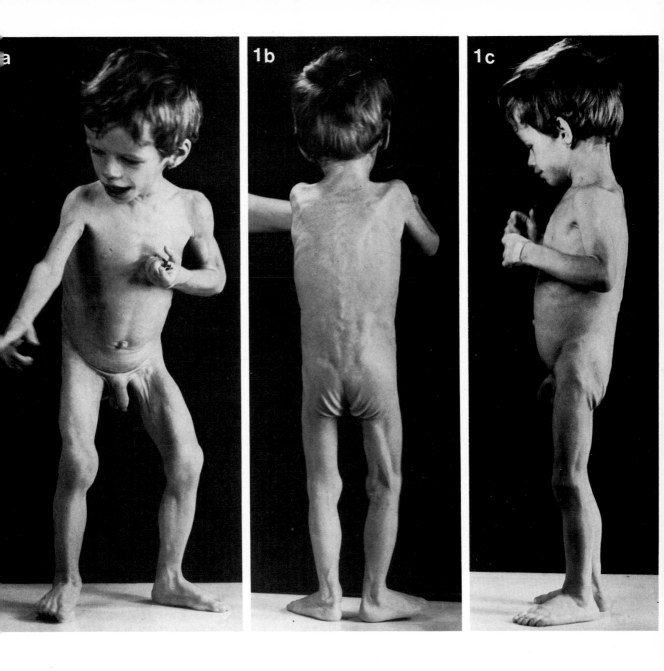

285

142. Prader–Willi Syndrome

(Prader–Labhart–Willi Syndrome; Prader–Willi–Labhart Syndrome)

A syndrome of mental retardation, small stature, obesity, and hypogonadism—after initial marked muscular hypotonia in infancy.

Main signs: Small stature (3–6), increasing obesity with hyperphagia, psychomotor retardation (usually quite severe); hypogenitalism: scrotal hypoplasia and frequent cryptorchidism (3, 5, 6, 7), or absence of the labia minora and underdevelopment of the labia majora; hypogonadism in both sexes.

Supplementary findings: A relatively narrow forehead with prominent forehead, frequent strabismus, almond-shaped eyes in some patients, and a triangular, open mouth may yield a quite typical facies in young children. Hypoplasia of enamel in some patients; early severe caries (8, 9).

Small hands and feet (acromicria) (10, 11). Frequent hypopigmentation. Frequent development of kyphoscoliosis.

Development of prediabetic metabolism; later nonketotic diabetes (usually after the second decade).

Manifestation: Congenital muscular hypotonia (possibly after weak fetal movements in utero and breech presentation, frequently low birth weight) often with extreme hypokinesia (1, 2) and respiratory and feeding problems. Gradual improvement of muscle tone around the second half of the first year of life. Obesity, hyperphagia, and growth retardation manifest after infancy.

Etiology: Genetic syndrome, usually sporadic; risk of recurrence minimal. In 50% of cases, deletion of band q11–13 (or rearrangement) of chromosome 15. Paternal origin of this abnormal chromosome leads to Prader–Willi syndrome; maternal origin leads to Angelman Syndrome?

Frequency: Not low, at least 1:10,000 births.

Course, prognosis: Often obesity is very difficult to control, and may increase to a grotesque extent. Decreased life expectancy. Often, delayed or incomplete puberty; no voice change in males. Frequent psychosocial problems in adolesence and adulthood. Infertility.

Diagnosis, differential diagnosis: Initially, other forms of early manifest muscular hypotonia ('floppy infant') must be ruled out. Later, diagnosis facilitated by the two-phase course, i.e., the history of congenital muscular atony and initial failure to thrive. Thus, Bardet–Biedl syndrome (which also has polydactyly, retinitis pigmentosa), Fröhlich adipsogenital dystrophy (with no mental retardation, but progressive CNS signs), and Cohen syndrome, can be readily eliminated.

Treatment: Limitation of the hyperphagia as far as possible, especially in view of the disposition to diabetes. Special nursery schools, special schooling, etc., may be indicated.

Illustrations:

1 and 2 A 4-month-old infant with severe muscular hypotonia, hypokinesia, and hyporeflexia; weak crying, sucking, and swallowing; expressionless face with triangular, open ('fish') mouth; micrognathia; psychomotor retardation.

3 and 7 The same child at age 5 years.

3–6 Children aged 5, 5, 6, and 7 years, all mentally retarded, with short stature, respectively 6.5, 9, 11, and 24 cm less than the average for age. Cryptorchidism in all three boys. Hyperglycemia of the boy in **6** after age 4 years and manifest diabetes after age 6.

8 Same child as in **6**.

10 and 11 A hand and a foot of a Prader–Willi patient (right) compared with those of a healthy child of the same age (left).

H.-R.W.

References:

Prader, A., Labhart, A., Willi, H. Ein Syndrom von Adipositas, Kleinwuchs, Kryptorchismus und Oligophrenie nach myatonieartigem Zustand im Neugeborenenalter. *Schweiz. Med. Wochenschr.*, 86, 1260 (1956).

Schinzel, A. Approaches to the prenatal diagnosis of the Prader–Willi syndrome. *Hum. Genet.*, 74, 327 (1986).

Cassidy, S.B. Recurrence risk in Prader–Willi syndrome. *Am. J. Med. Genet.*, 28, 59–60 (1987).

Greenswag, L.R. Adults with Prader–Willi syndrome: a survey of 232 cases. *Develop. Med. Child Neurol.*, 29, 145–152 (1987).

Ledbetter, D.H., Greenberg, Fr., Holm, V. et al. Second annual Prader–Willi syndrome scientific conference. *Am. J. Med. Genet.*, 28, 779–790 (1987).

Lee, P.D.K., Wilson, D.M., Rountree, L. et al. Linear growth response to exogenous growth hormone in Prader–Willi syndrome. *Am. J. Med. Genet.*, 28, 865–871 (1987).

Wenger, S.L., Hanchett, J.M., Steele, M.W. et al. Clinical comparison of 59 Prader–Willi patients with and without the 15(q12) deletion. *Am. J. Med. Genet.*, 28, 881–887 (1987).

Caldwell, M.L. and Taylor, R.L. *Prader–Willi syndrome*. Springer, Heidelberg, 1988 (120 pp).

Greenswag, L.R. and Alexander, R.C. *Management of Prader–Willi syndrome*. Springer, Heidelberg, 1988 (250 pp.).

Whitman, B.Y. and Accardo, P. Emotional symptoms in Prader–Willi syndrome adolescents. *Am. J. Med. Genet.*, 28, 897–905 (1987).

Zellweger, H. Can women with the Prader–Labhart–Willi syndrome (PLWS) reproduce? Does the deletion (15)(q11–13) occur in individuals not affected with PLWS? *Am. J. Med. Genet.*, 29, 669–672 (1988).

Knoll, J.H.M., Nicholls, R.D. et al. Angelman and Prader–Willi syndromes share a common chromosome 15 deletion but differ in parental origin of the deletion. *Am. J. Med. Genet.*, 32, 285–290 (1989).

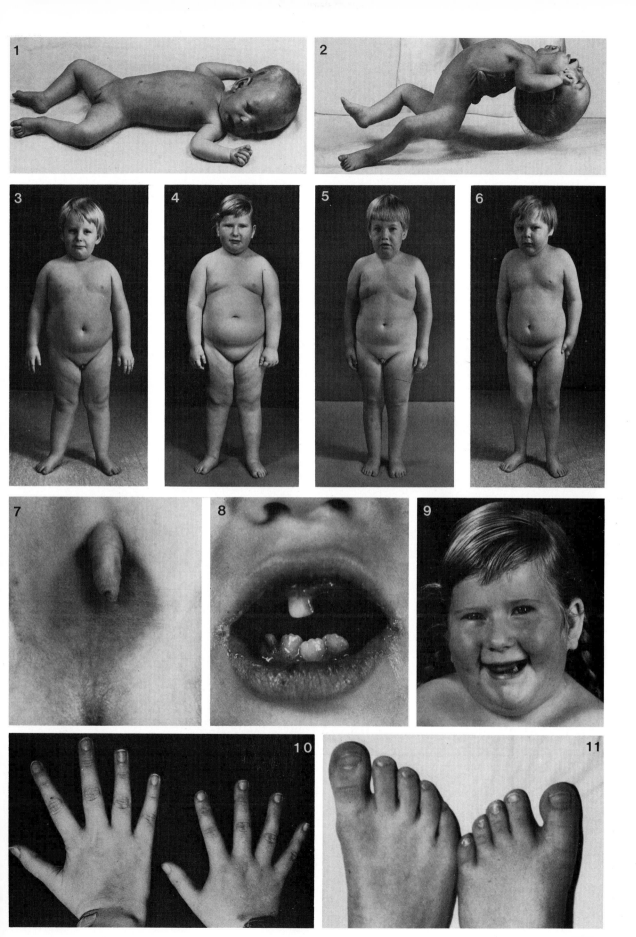

143. Bardet–Biedl Syndrome

A hereditary disorder with polydactyly, hypogenitalism, obesity, impaired vision, and mental retardation.

Main signs:
1. Obesity, mainly of the trunk, usually of early onset, frequently increasing (**1, 6**).
2. Hypogenitalism (with normal and decreased gonadotrophin levels), small genitalia (**4**), undescended testes, bifid scrotum, hypospadias. Little or no development of the secondary sex characteristics. Amenorrhea.
3. Distinct mental impairment. Occasionally defective hearing.
4. Ulnar or fibular polydactyly, varying from rudimentary appendages to functioning sixth fingers or toes (**2, 3**), usually of the feet. Possible middle syn- and/or brachydactyly.

Supplementary findings: Usually moderate small stature.

Retinitis pigmentosa (but also sine pigmento) as a very constant characteristic; nystagmus; other ophthalmological findings possible.

Frequently, small, poorly functioning kidneys with progressive decrease of function (to uremia); also malformations of the urinary tract, fibrosis of the liver.

Manifestation: Hexadactyly and possibly increased body weight at birth, retinopathy and distinct truncal obesity in early childhood, hypogenitalism from birth onwards.

Etiology: Autosomal recessive disorder of variable expression.

Frequency: Less than 1:160,000.

Course, prognosis: Determined by the degree of mental retardation and by the progression of the retino- and neuropathy.

Diagnosis, differential diagnosis: Symptomatic overlap with a number of other syndromes. The Prader–Willi syndrome, which is much more frequent, does not show polydactyly and retinopathy.

Treatment: Symptomatic; regular ophthalmological follow-up, urinary cultures, measurement of blood pressure. Genetic counseling.

Illustrations:
1–6 The same patient at ages 7 and 33 years. Overweight since infancy. Mild mental retardation. Rudimentary sixth rays of the hands and feet. Retinitis pigmentosa. Hypogenitalism.

H.-R.W.

References:
Pagon, R.A., Haas, J.E. et al. Hepatic involvement in the Bardet–Biedl syndrome. *Am. J. Med. Genet.*, 13, 373–381 (1982).
Schachat, A.P. and Maumenee, I.H. Bardet–Biedl syndrome and related disorders. *Arch. Ophthalmol.*, 100, 285–288 (1982).
Linné, T., Wikstad, I., Zetterström, R. Renal involvement in the Laurence–Moon–Biedl syndrome. *Acta Pediatr. Scand.*, 75, 240–244 (1986).
Harnett, J.D., Green, J.S. et al. The spectrum of renal disease in Laurence–Moon–Biedl syndrome. *N. Engl. J. Med.*, 319, 615–618 (1988).
Ritchie, G., Jequier, S., Lussier-Lazaroff. Prenatal renal ultrasound of Laurence–Moon–Biedl syndrome. *Pediatr. Radiol.*, 19, 65–66 (1988).
Editorial. Laurence–Moon and Bardet–Biedl syndromes. *Lancet*, II, 1178 (1988).

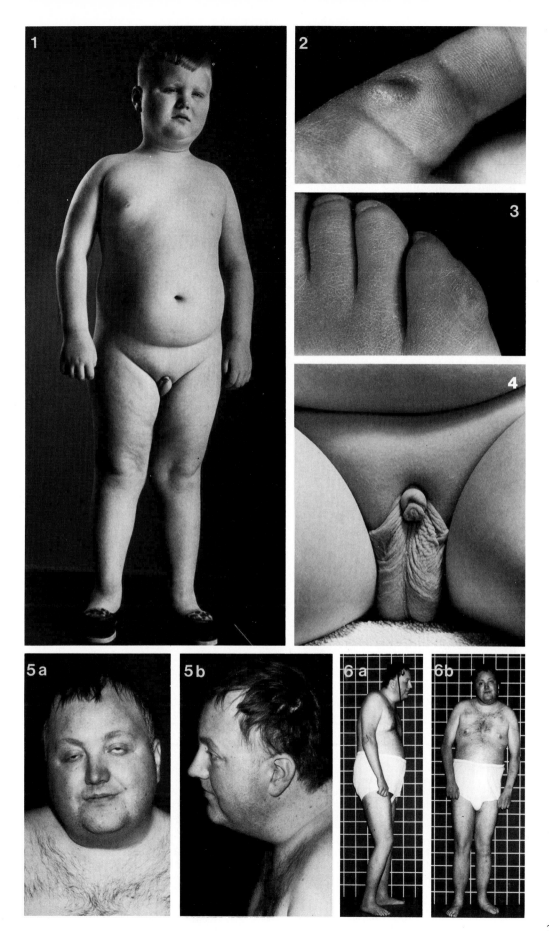

144. Cohen Syndrome

A syndrome of characteristic facies, mental retardation with microcephaly, muscular hypotonia, small stature, obesity, and anomalies of the hands and feet.

Main signs:
1. Facies: Possible slight antimongoloid slant of the palpebral fissures with broad, prominent nasal root; fairly prominent ears; prominence of the premaxilla, middle incisors, and upper lip with high narrow palate, short philtrum, and open mouth; micrognathia (1–3).
2. Mild microcephaly in about 50% of cases. Mental retardation (IQ between about 30 and 70) practically without exception.
3. Hypotonic and flaccid musculature and joints.
4. Small stature in about 70%.
5. Mild to moderate truncal obesity in about 70% of cases(1).

Supplementary findings: Hands and feet strikingly narrow with long, thin fingers and toes; possible syndactyly, simian crease. Cubitus valgus, genu valgum.

Possible strabismus, refractive error, and other ocular anomalies; abnormal electroretinogram.

Possible development of scoliosis, mitral valve prolapse, hiatal hernia.

Manifestation: At birth and later. Onset of obesity usually in mid-childhood.

Etiology: Hereditary disorder with variable expression; autosomal recessive connective tissue disease?

Frequency: Low; about 50 cases known up to 1988.

Differential diagnosis: Primarily Prader–Willi syndrome (p.286) and Bardet–Biedl syndrome (p.288).

Treatment: Symptomatic.

Illustrations:
1–3 The first and second children of healthy, young, nonconsanguineous parents. The 11-year-old girl and her 10-year-old brother are slightly microcephalic, mentally retarded, of small stature, and obese and show the characteristic facies. The boy is hypotonic; the girl has had a focal seizure disorder since early childhood.

H.-R.-W.

References:
Cohen, M.M., Jr., Hall, B.D., Smith, D.W. et al. A new syndrome with hypotonia, obesity, mental deficiency, and facial, oral, ocular, and limb anomalies. *J. Pediatr.*, 83, 280 (1973).
Ferré, P., Fournet, J.P., Courpotin, C. Le syndrome de Cohen . . . *Arch. Fr. Pédiatr.*, 39, 159 (1982).
Goecke, T., Majewski, F., Kauther, K.D., et al. Mental retardation . . . (Cohen syndrome). *Eur. J. Pediatr.*, 138, 338–340 (1982).
Friedman, E. and Sack. J. The Cohen syndrome. Report of five cases and a review of the literature. *J. Craniofac. Genet. Biol.*, 2, 193–200 (1982).
Norio, R., Raitta, Chr. et al. Further delineation of the Cohen syndrome . . . *Clin. Genet.*, 25, 1–14 (1984).
North, C., Patton, M.A. et al. The clinical features of the Cohen syndrome . . . *J. Med. Genet.*, 22, 131–134 (1985).
Young, I.D. and Moore, J.R. Infrafamiliar variation in Cohen syndrome. *J. Med. Genet.*, 24, 488–492 (1987).
Méhes, K., Kosztolányi, G. et al. Cohen syndrome: a connective tissue disorder? *Am. J. Med. Genet.*, 31, 131–133 (1988).

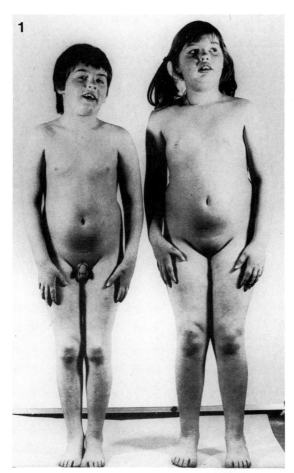

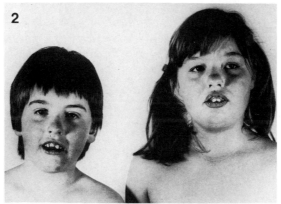

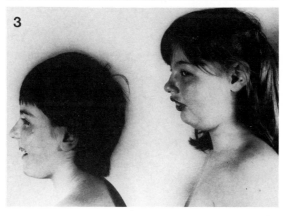

145. Aicardi Syndrome

A characteristic complex of malformations with ocular defects, costovertebral malformations, infantile nodding spasms, agenesis of the corpus callosum, and progressive psychomotor retardation, occurring only in females.

Main signs:
1. Practically limited to females (to date only two boys reported with Aicardi syndrome; of these, one Australian case with 47XXY karyotype).
2. Microphthalmia. Numerous pathognomonic lacunar chorioretinopathic foci; usually peripapillary and bilateral, less often peripheral. The foci are pigment-free; the lacunae, pale to ivory-colored.
3. Costovertebral malformations, fusion of vertebral bodies, hemivertebrae, clefts, absent ribs, fused ribs.
4. Infantile nodding spasms within the first 2 to 4 months of life; less frequently, may be as early as the first days of life. Clinically, variable pattern of seizures, possibly with focal signs.
5. Partial or total agenesis of the corpus callosum.
6. Progressive psychomotor retardation, asymmetric hypotonic tetraplegia or diplegia. Microcephaly in 75% of cases.

Supplementary findings: Cortical heterotopia, poly- and microgyria, deformity of the ventricles, as in the Dandy–Walker syndrome, in some cases.

Normal electroretinogram. Absent pupillary reaction; strabismus, nystagmus, cataract, synechiae of the iris, ptosis.

Characteristic EEG pattern: so-called burst-suppression pattern (groups of high theta and delta waves with enclosed hypersynchronic potentials, interrupted by stretches of flat activity of only a few seconds).

Manifestation: At birth. Seizures beginning in the second to fourth months of life.

Etiology: Probably an X-linked dominant disorder with lethality in males. The Australian case with XXY bears out this assumption. All patients have been single observations in their families. New mutations.

Frequency: Over 100 patients have been described to date.

Course, prognosis: Progressive psychomotor retardation, decreased vision. The oldest known patient is 14 years old.

Differential diagnosis: The oculo-vertebral syndrome of Weyers–Thier, which has dysplasia of the roof of the orbit; no lacunar chorioretinopathy; no sex limitation; no seizure disorder; no anomalies of the corpus callosum.

Treatment: Symptomatic treatment of the salaam spasms. Measures to promote development: physiotherapy; occupational therapy; visual training.

Illustrations:
1 A typically affected female newborn; short neck, microphthalmia on the right.
2 Her chest X-ray, showing hemivertebrae, tilted and oblique vertebrae, fused vertebrae, unequal number of ribs on the two sides, scoliosis.

Malformations also of the cervical vertebrae.

J.K.

References:
Bertoni, J.M., v. Loh, S., Allen, R.J. The Aicardi syndrome: report of 4 cases and review of the literature. *Ann. Neurol.*, 5, 475–482 (1979).
Köhler, B., Mayer, H., Osswald, H. Das Aicardi–Syndrom. *Pädiatr. Prax.*, 29, 45–58 (1983/84).
Yamamoto, N. et al. Aicardi syndrome: report of 6 cases and a review of Japanese literature. *Brain Dev.*, 7, 443–449 (1985).
Besenski, N., Bosnjak, V. et al. Cortical heterotopia in Aicardi's syndrome ... *Pediatr. Radiol.*, 18, 391–393 (1988).
Donnenfeld, A.E., Packer, R.J. et al. Clinical, cytogenetic, and pedigree findings in 18 cases of Aicardi syndrome. *Am. J. Med. Genet.*, 32, 461–467 (1989).

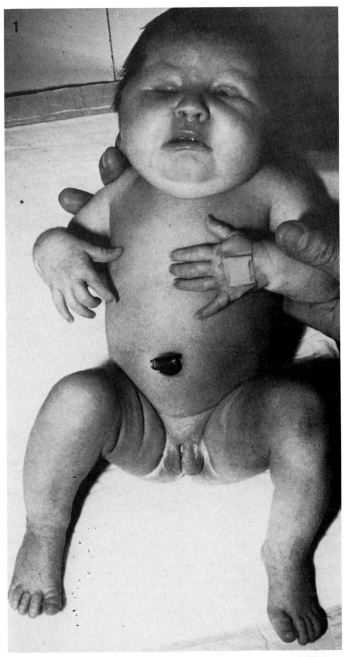

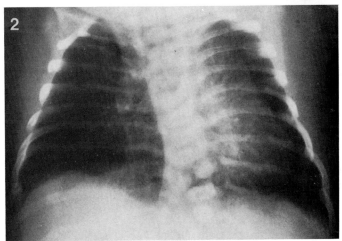

146. Spondylocostal Dysostosis

(Spondylocostal Dysplasia, Spondylothoracic Dysplasia/Dysostosis, Costovertebral Dysplasia, Jarcho–Levin Syndrome, Polydysspondyly, Occipito–Facio–Cervico–Thoraco–Abdomino–Digital Syndrome)

An etiologically heterogeneous clinical picture with vertebral and rib anomalies due to a disorder of segmentation in the axial skeleton.

Main signs:
1. Shortened trunk; opisthotonus position of the head; short neck; broad, asymmetrical, barrel-shaped thorax; protruberant abdomen; diastasis recti; slender, elongated extremities; hypotonic musculature.
2. Multiple hemi-, wedge-shaped, and block vertebrae; spina bifida.
3. Rib anomalies: particularly of number and shape, as well as synostoses.

Supplementary findings: Additional malformations occur occasionally: renal anomalies (aplasia, hydronephrosis, megaureter, double ureter, horseshoe kidney), cardiac defect (tetralogy of Fallot, pulmonary stenosis). Scoliosis, lordosis, camptodactyly, polydactyly, syndactyly, club feet.

Manifestation: At birth.

Etiology: Heterogeneous. Very often autosomal recessive, but also autosomal dominant inheritance described; part of a genetic malformation syndrome (costovertebral segmentation defect with mesomelia = COVESDEM); sporadic cases. Possible receptor defect in sclerotome development.

Frequency: Over 70 published cases.

Course, prognosis: Normal mental development; stable vertebral column. But also perinatal/early-infantile death from cardiopulmonary complications.

Differential diagnosis: Differentiation from the Klippel–Feil syndrome with its anomalies and synostoses in the cervical spine region. The VATER association shows additional malformations.

Treatment: Orthopedic care. Prenatal diagnosis possible.

Illustrations:
1a A characteristically affected male newborn.
1b Severe skeletal changes in the thoracic region of this child.
2 X-ray of the trunk region of another newborn with this syndrome.

J.K.

References:

Gassner, M. and Grabs, S.G. Kostovertebrale Dysplasie. Ein Rezeptordefekt der Sklerotomentwicklung? *Schweiz. Med. Wochenschr.,* 112, 791–797 (1982).
Pfeiffer, R.A., Hansen, H.G., Böwing, B. et al. Die Spondylocostale Dysostose. Bericht über 5 Beobachtungen einschließlich Geschwister und einen atypischen Fall. *Monatschr. Kinderheilkd.,* 131, 28–34 (1983).
Aymé, S. and Preus, M. Spondylocostal/spondylothoracic dysostosis: the clinical basis for prognosticating and genetic counseling. *Am. J. Med. Genet.,* 24, 599–606 (1986).
Ohashi, H., Sugio, Y. et al. Spondylocostal dysostosis: report of three patients. *Jpn. J. Hum. Genet.,* 32, 299–307 (1987).
Tolmie, J.L., Whittle, M.J., McNay, M.B. et al. Second trimester prenatal diagnosis of the Jarcho–Levin syndrome. *Prenatal Diagnosis,* 7, 129–134 (1987).

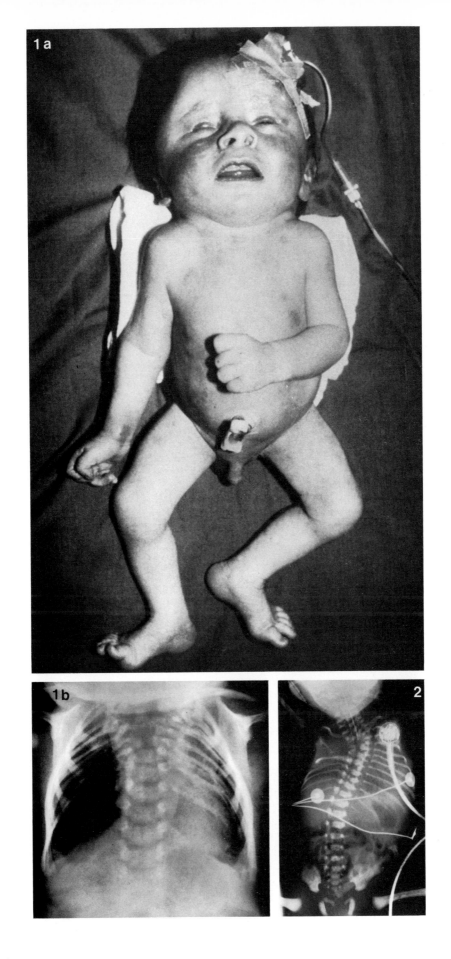

295

147. Klippel–Feil 'Syndrome'

A malformation complex particularly of the cervical spine with short neck and possible impairments of mobility, posture, and neurological function.

Main signs:
1. Short neck (**1a, 1b**) to 'necklessness', with low nuchal hairline. Usually, limited (painless) motion of the head, especially sidewards (**1a**). Thorax may be barrel-shaped, with high rounded hump. Possible elevation of the shoulders.
2. Radiologically: block vertebrae for a variable extent of the cervical spine (possible wedge-shaped or hemivertebrae or anomalies of the neural arches), sometimes with malformations of the lower spine or ribs (**2, 3**) and scoliosis. A classification into different types according to the nature, severity, and localization of the malformations has been undertaken.

Supplementary findings: Possibly, more extensive disorders of posture and mobility, and signs of nerve damage or loss of function.

Anomalies of and around the ears, cleft palate, micrognathia.

Diverse malformations of the extremities, congenital anomalies of the urogenital tract (ultrasonography of the kidneys is advisable), and cardiac defects possible.

In up to a third of cases, hearing impairment or even deafness.

Manifestation: At birth and later, depending on the severity of the malformations.

Etiology: Not uniform. Mostly isolated cases (may represent a disruption sequence due to embryonic vascular disturbance of the subclavian artery). Autosomal dominant and recessive transmission also observed.

Frequency: Low (estimated about 1:50,000).

Prognosis: Dependent on the severity of the anatomical disorder.

Treatment: For the most part symptomatic orthopedic treatment. Early auditory evaluation and adequate therapy if indicated.

Illustrations:
1a and **1b** A 6-month-old male infant with short neck, limited sideways motion of the head, somewhat barrel-shaped chest, normal psychomotor development.
2 AP cervical spine X-ray of the same boy, showing hemivertebrae and partial block vertebrae at the junction of the cervical and thoracic spines; bilateral hypoplasia of the upper ribs.
3 Lateral X-ray of the cervical spine of a 12-year-old girl with Klippel–Feil syndrome. Extensive block vertebrae with partial inclusion of the neural arches and spinal processes.

H.-R.W./J.K.

References:

Gunderson, C.H., Greenspan, R.H., Glaser, G.H., Lubs, H.A. The Klippel–Feil syndrome: genetic and clinical reevaluation of cervical fusion. *Medicine*, 46, 491 (1967).
Palant, D.I. and Carter, B.L. Klippel–Feil syndrome and deafness. *Am. J. Dis. Child.*, 123, 218 (1972).
Helmi, C. and Pruzansky, S. Craniofacial and extracranial malformations in the Klippel–Feil syndrome. *Cleft Palate J.*, 17, 65 (1980).
Fragoso, R., Cid-Garcia, A. et al. Frontonasal dysplasia in the Klippel–Feil syndrome . . . *Clin. Genet.*, 22, 270–273 (1982).
de Silva, E.O. Autosomal recessive Klippel–Feil syndrome. *J. Med. Genet.*, 19, 130–134 (1982).
Nagib, M.G., Maxwell, R.E. et al. Klippel–Feil syndrome in children: clinical features and management. *Child's Nerv. Syst.*, 1, 255–263 (1985).
Brill, C.B. Peyster, R.G. et al. Isolation of the right subclavian artery with subclavian steal in a child with Klippel–Feil anomaly . . . *Am. J. Med. Genet.*, 26, 933–940 (1987).

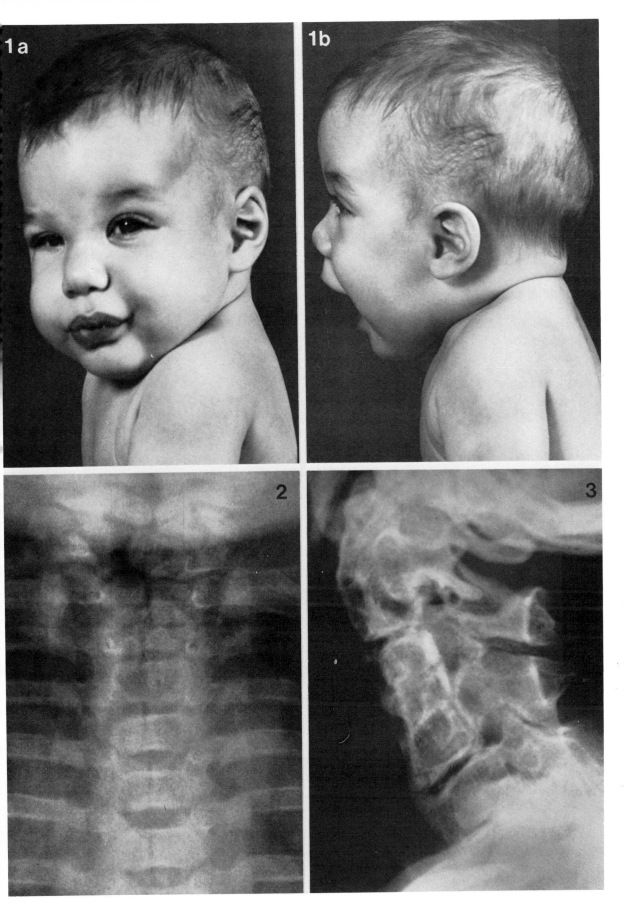

297

148. Wildervanck Syndrome

(Cervico-oculo-acoustic Syndrome)

A complex of anomalies including short neck, similar to that in Klippel–Feil 'syndrome' (p.296), facial anomalies, and hearing impairment, occurring almost exclusively in females.

Main signs:
1. Those of the Klippel–Feil 'syndrome' (p.296).
2. Usually, facial asymmetry, possibly with torticollis, uni- or less frequently bilateral paralysis of the abducens nerve and bulbar retraction (Duane syndrome), hypoplasia of the upper jaw, micrognathia, narrow or possibly cleft palate.
3. Uni- or bilateral, moderate to severe, conductive hearing impairment. Occurrence of outer and inner ear malformations.

Supplementary findings: Mental development normal as a rule. Unilateral epibulbar dermoids may occur (and heterochromia iridis, cleft palate, pterygium colli, renal aplasia have been noted in individual cases).

Manifestation: At birth; hearing impairment possibly later.

Etiology: Genetic situation not clear. Since the vast majority of those affected are female, sex-linked dominant inheritance has been considered, although multifactorial inheritance is also a possibility.

Frequency: Not particularly rare (about 1:3,000 deaf children); several hundred cases in the literature.

Course, prognosis: Favorable for life expectancy, after a potentially difficult neonatal course.

Diagnosis, differential diagnosis: Differential from the Goldenhar 'syndrome' (p.52) can be very difficult, if not impossible, as in the case presented here. Similar difficulties encountered in ruling out the Klippel–Feil 'syndrome' (p.296). Exclusion of mandibulofacial dysostosis (p.48) not difficult.

Treatment: Initial care as with the Pierre Robin sequence (q.v.) may be indicated. Early evaluation of hearing and, when indicated, prompt application of special hearing and speech aids. Orthopedic surgery, cosmetic surgery, or orthodontic corrective measures may be required.

Illustrations:
1–6 A 6-year-old girl with a faciovertebral anomaly complex. Bony malformation at the atlanto-occipital junction, block formation of second to fourth cervical vertebrae and synostoses of the spinous processes to C6. Low nuchal hairline. Marked limitation of movement of the neck. Mild facial asymmetry, relatively narrow and somewhat oblique left palpebral fissure (no epibulbar dermoid). Hypoplasia of the upper jaw (which has a double row of teeth), narrow palate, immobile soft palate, well-corrected horizontal clefts of the cheeks. Unremarkable external ears. Conductive hearing impairment.

H.-R.W./J.K.

References:
Sherk, H.H. and Nicholson, J.T. Cervico-oculo-acusticus syndrome. *J. Bone Jt. Surg.*, 54A, 1776 (1972).
Konigsmark, B.W. and Gorlin, R.J. *Genetic and Metabolic Deafness.* W.B. Saunders, Philadelphia, 1976.
Wildervanck, L.S. The cervico-oculo-acusticus syndrome. In: Vinken, P.J., Bruyn, G.W., Myrianthopulos, N.C. (eds.) *Handbook of Clinical Neurology*, vol 32. North Holland, Amsterdam, 1978, pp.123–130.
Strisciuglio, P., Raia, V. et al. Wildervanck's syndrome with bilateral subluxation of lens and facial paralysis. *J. Med. Genet.*, 20, 72–73 (1983).

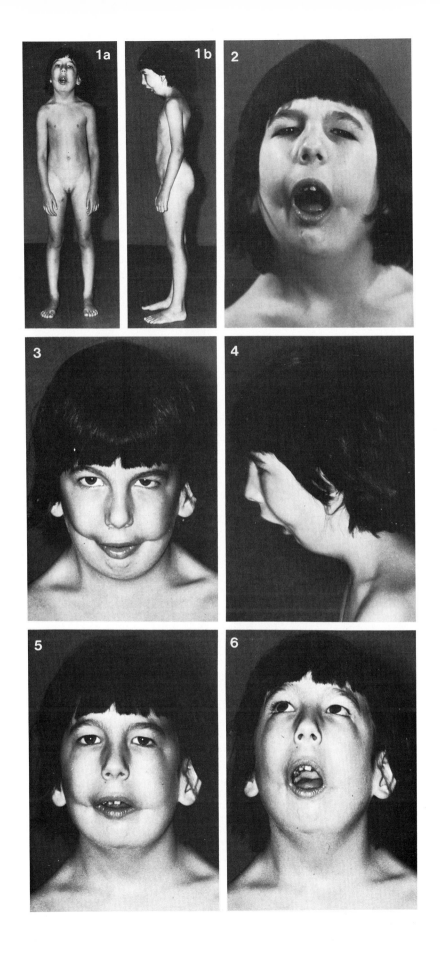

299

149. Aplastic Abdominal Musculature 'Syndrome'

(Prune Belly 'Syndrome')

A condition seen in males at birth with a slack, wrinkled abdominal wall; undescended testes; and urinary tract anomalies. (Analogous dysplasia of the abdominal muscles occurs in females only rarely.)

Main signs:
1. A thin, slack, and, especially in early life, wrinkled and shrivelled ('prune-like') abdominal wall with persistent furrow-like umbilicus (**1, 3**), protruding over 'wobbly' abdominal organs. (Basis: hypo- and aplasia of the abdominal wall musculature, not necessarily symmetrical.)
2. Bilateral cryptorchidism.
3. Fairly extensive, marked anomalies of the urinary tract: megacystis, megaureter, cystic dysplasia of the kidneys, hydronephrosis (**4**).

Supplementary findings: Quite frequently, malrotation or other additional abnormalities (e.g., of hips, feet, or heart).

Manifestation: Intrauterine or at birth.

Etiology: Not clear. Probably heterogeneous pathological complex (polytropic field defect). One theory is that it results from intrauterine urethral obstruction, to which male fetuses are far more susceptible. A few familial observations. The risk of recurrence in further offspring is a few per cent at the most.

Frequency: About 1:40,000 live births. Well over 800 cases described in the literature.

Course, prognosis: Dependent on the severity of the anomalies. A large proportion of those affected die within the first years of life.

Treatment: Exact assessment of the urodynamics. Prompt primary decompression may be required, e.g., by cystostomy. Measures to prevent urinary tract infection. Follow-up care by a pediatric urologist. Genetic counseling (see above). Prenatal diagnosis with chromosomal analysis ('prune belly' also occurs with trisomies) and with ultrasonography in subsequent pregnancies (looking for megacystis and fetal ascites). The question of possible antenatal decompression requires very careful consideration.

Illustrations:
1 A very severely affected male newborn; lethal form.
2–4 A further male infant, the second child of healthy parents (the first pregnancy resulted in a stillbirth at seven months, cause not known). Birth of the proband after an unremarkable pregnancy; extensive aplasia of the abdominal wall musculature, megacystis, megaureter, and undescended testes. Resection of a urethral polyp at 4 months. Apart from initial urinary tract infections, normal development of the child, who has since reached school age, his renal collecting system and total renal tubular function are now normal and his testes following surgery, are in a normal position.
4 Urogram in the newborn period showing extreme megaureter.

H.-R.W.

References:

Pagon, R.A., Smith, D.W., Shepard, T.H. Urethral obstruction malformation complex: a cause of abdominal muscle deficiency and the 'prune belly'. *J. Pediatr.*, 94, 900 (1979) + ibid. 96, 776, 777 (Letters to the Editor).

Aaronson, I.A. and Cremin, B.J. Prune belly syndrome in young females. *Urol. Radiol.*, 1, 151 (1979/80).

Kösters, S., Horwitz, H., Ritter, R. Typische röntgenologische Veränderungen an Nieren und Harntrakt beim Bauchmuskelaplasie-Syndrom. *Pädiatr. Prax.*, 22, 125 (1979/1980).

Straub, E. and Spranger, J. Etiology and pathogenesis of the prune belly syndrome. *Kidney Int.*, 20, 695–699 (1981).

Lubinsky, M. and Rapoport, P. Transient fetal hydrops and 'prune belly' in one identical female twin. *N. Engl. J. Med.*, I, 256–257 (1983).

Oliveira, G., Boechat, M.I., Ferreira, M.A. Megacystis-microcolon-intestinal hypoperistalsis syndrome in a newborn girl whose brother had prune belly syndrome: common pathogenesis? *Pediatr. Radiol.*, 13, 294–296 (1983).

Belohradsky, B.H. and Henkel, C. Das Prune-Belly-Syndrom. *Ergeb. Inn. Med. Kinderheilkd.*, 52, 157–205 (1984).

Burton, B.K. and Dillard, R.G. Prune belly syndrome: observations supporting the hypothesis of abdominal overdistension. *Am. J. Med. Genet.*, 17, 669–672 (1984).

Moerman, P., Fryns, J.-P., Goddeeris, P. et al. Pathogenesis of the prune belly syndrome: a functional urethral obstruction caused by prostatic hypoplasia. *Pediatrics*, 73, 470–475 (1984).

Nakayama, D.K., Harrison, M.R., Chinn, D.H. et al. The pathogenesis of prune belly. *Am. J. Dis. Child.*, 138, 834–836 (1984).

Kawamoto, K., Ikeda, T. Matsuo, T. et al. Prune belly syndrome: report of twelve cases and possible pathogenesis. *Cong. Anom.*, 25, 1–15 (1985).

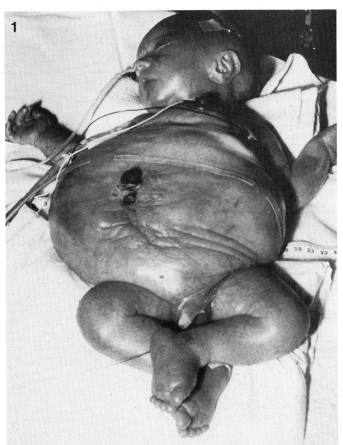

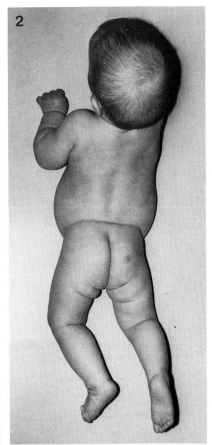

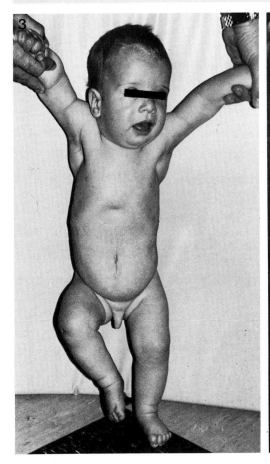

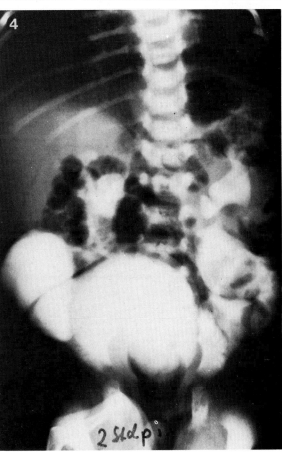

150. Autosomal Recessive Polycystic ('Infantile') Kidney Disease

A clinical picture of early abdominal distension, palpable 'giant tumors', often rapidly progressive course in the neonatal period, and fibrosis of the liver of variable severity with portal hypertension and arterial hypertension.

Main signs:
1. Protuberant and bulging abdomen with markedly enlarged kidneys (1, 2).
2. Liver fibrosis of varying degrees of severity, with hepatomegaly and signs of portal hypertension to the extent of bleeding from esophageal varices.
3. In the very severe form, 'Potter syndrome' as the result of oligo- or ahydramnios, or respiratory insufficiency from upward displacement of the diaphragm and hypoplasia of the lungs.
4. Fairly rapid development and progression of renal insufficiency, arterial hypertension.

Supplementary findings: Sonographic evidence of kidney enlargement with high echogenicity; intravenous pyelogram shows radially arranged, narrow collecting tubules filled with contrast medium (2).

Larger single cysts not typical, at least not in the neonatal period; eventual loss of a uniform picture. Presence or development of corresponding urinary, serum, and circulatory abnormalities.

Manifestation: Prenatal manifestation as 'Potter syndrome' possible; otherwise in neonatal period. Rarely presents in childhood or adolescence; only exceptionally present in adulthood.

Etiology: Autosomal recessive disorder. Various clinical forms probably due to multiple alleles.

Frequency: Not clear; about 1:20,000–1:40,000.

Course, prognosis: Life expectancy distinctly reduced depending on the age at presentation. Poor prognosis with early presentation.

Comment, differential diagnosis: Differentiation from early presentation of the autosomal dominant ('adult') form is occasionally possible solely by a positive family history (ultrasonographic examination of both parents) or by demonstration of hepatic fibrosis.

Treatment: Symptomatic. In later stages, dialysis or transplantation may be required. Genetic counseling. Ultrasonographic prenatal diagnosis may be attempted in future pregnancies, although this is often unsuccessful in the first half of pregnancy.

Illustrations:
1 and 2 The first child of young, healthy, nonconsanguineous parents. Birth at about term after an unremarkable pregnancy, 3170 g; breech presentation, markedly protuberant abdomen and symmetrical, firm kidney 'tumors' extending from the costal arch into the true pelvis. Intravenous pyelogram on the seventh/eighth day of life: after 2 hours, widely separated, markedly dilated renal pelvic systems vaguely recognizable; and 19 hours after injection, clearly visible renal parenchymal shadows of 10 cm and 6 cm diameter, with axes converging caudally (2). Cystography: unremarkable efferent urinary tract. During a 10-week hospital stay, initial edema, elevation of urinary nitrogen, hematuria, erythrocyturia, leukocyturia, and mild proteinuria. With symptomatic treatment, clearing of these signs and subsequent good progress.
1 The proband at 3 years 4 months. At 5 years 7 months, 112.5 cm and 20.5 kg (average for age); palpably enlarged kidneys, liver 3 cm below the costal margin; urine negative; blood pressure with medication normal, occasionally to 135/80 mmHg. Meanwhile, the boy is about to start school and has three healthy brothers.

K. Zerres/H.-R.W.

References:

Blyth, H. and Ockenden, B.G. Polycystic disease of kidneys and liver presenting in childhood. *J. Med. Genet.*, 8, 257 (1971).
Zerres, K. Genetics of cystic kidney disease. Criteria for classification and genetic counselling. *Pediatr. Nephrol.*, 1, 397–404 (1987).
Kääriäinen, H., Koskimies, O. et al. Dominant and recessive polycystic kidney disease in children: evaluation of clinical features and laboratory data. *Pediatr. Nephrol.*, 2, 312 (1988).
Neumann, H.P.H., Zerres, K. et al. Late manifestation of autosomal recessive polycystic kidney disease in two sisters. *Am. J. Nephrol.*, 8, 194–197 (1988).
Zerres, K. Genetics of cystic kidney diseases . . . *Pediatr. Nephrol.*, 1, 397–404 (1988).
Zerres, K., Hansmann, M. et al: Autosomal recessive polycystic kidney disease. Problems of prenatal diagnosis. *Prenatal Diagnosis*, 8, 215–229 (1988).

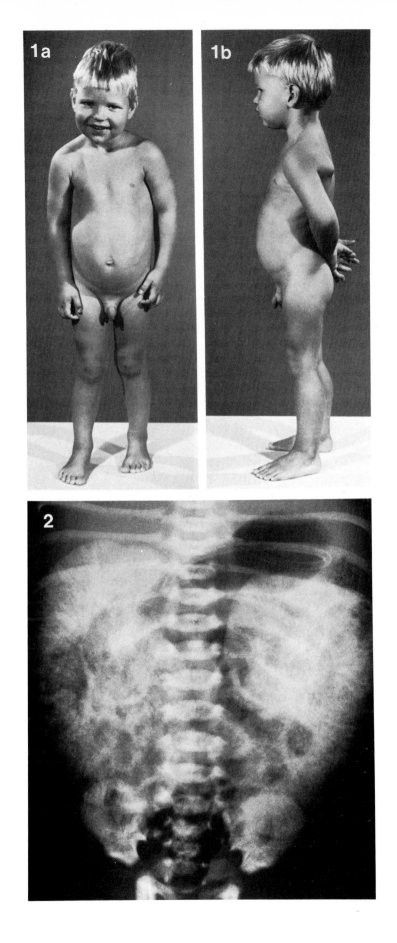

303

151. Gaucher's Disease Type I

('Classic', chronic visceral form of Gaucher's disease)

A chronic lysosomal 'storage' disease, which spares the nervous system, with hepatosplenomegaly, dyshematopoiesis, and characteristic orthopedic complications.

Main signs:
1. Hepatosplenomegaly, which may be considerable (**1b**).
2. Dyshematopoiesis ('splenogenic marrow depression', thrombocytopenia, leukopenia, anemia); pallor, possibly hemorrhages.
3. Periodic bone and joint pain, especially in the long tubular bones; pseudo-osteomyelitic or pseudo-arthritic pathologic fractures, sometimes with aseptic necrosis; epiphysiolysis. Usually found in: femur (on X-ray showing an 'Erlenmeyer flask deformity' distally); necrosis of the femoral head is particularly characteristic (**1c, 2**); also destruction of vertebral bodies and other areas.
4. In children, frequent short stature, delayed puberty (**1a**).

Supplementary findings: Mental development and nervous system normal.

Yellowish-brownish coloration of the skin in some patients, especially of the face, back of the neck, hands, and extensor surfaces of the lower legs and—in adults—yellowish spots ('pingueculae') of the sclera.

Elevation of the (tartrate-resistant) serum acid phosphatase; demonstration of Gaucher cells in bone marrow aspirates or other tissue preparations; or demonstration of a cerebroside-beta-glucosidase defect in leukocytes, which is simpler and diagnostic.

Manifestation: Possible at any age (from early childhood).

Etiology: Autosomal recessive disorder especially affecting Jewish individuals (Ashkenazim): homozygote affected 1:2,500, heterozygotes 4%. Heterogeneity.

Course, prognosis: Patients may live to an old age. The sequelae to fractures of the neck of the femur with necrosis of the femoral head are, when damage is irreversible, often considered as the greatest problem in adults.

Treatment: Careful orthopedic supervision. Exemption from school sports. Promotion of intellectual development and adequate vocational guidance. For acute attacks of pain, immobilization suffices. For previous severe hip damage, possible operative reduction and more extensive revision at a later date. Splenectomy for marked signs of abdominal displacement and marked dyshematopoiesis. Psychological guidance. Genetic counseling. Heterozygote test and prenatal diagnosis via enzyme assay. Gene therapy as a result of progress in molecular genetics may be possible in the future.

Illustrations:
1 and 2 A 14-year-old girl (one parent Ashkenazi). 'Coxitis' on the left at age 5 years, further attacks of hip pain at 11 and, bilaterally, at 13 years, Protuberant abdomen due to both hyperlordosis (**1b**) and upper abdominal organomegaly. Post-splenectomy (typical Gaucher histology); hepatomegaly to the level of the umbilicus. Growth deficiency (here below the third percentile) with overlong extremities; delayed puberty (no menarche to date); bone age retarded about 3 years. 'Limping' for months: dislocated left hip with necrosis of the left femoral head and severe destruction of the neck of the femur (for which a reduction was carried out); storage deposits also in the right femur below the lesser trochanter (**2**); no further skeletal foci found (nor evidence of lung involvement). Enzyme defect demonstrated by leukocyte test.

H.-R.W.

References:
Any comprehensive pediatric or internal medicine text book. In addition:
Tjhen, K.Y. and Zillhardt, H.W.M. Gaucher Typ 1. *Pädiatr. Prax.*, 18, 247 (1977).
Goldblatt, J., Sacks, S., Beighton, P. The orthopedic aspects of Gaucher disease. *Clin. Orthopaed.*, 137, 208 (1978).
Choy, F.Y.M. Gaucher disease . . . *Am. J. Med. Genet.*, 21, 519–528 (1985).
Grabowski, G.A., Goldblatt, J. et al. Genetic heterogeneity in Gaucher's disease . . . *Am. J. Med. Genet.*, 21, 529–549 (1985).
Beaudet, A.L. Gaucher's disease. *N. Engl. J. Med.*, 316, 619–620 (1987).
Hobbs, J.R., Jones, K.H. et al. Beneficial effect of pretransplant splenectomy on displacement bone marrow transplantation for Gaucher's syndrome. *Lancet*, I, 1111–1115 (1987).
Matoth, Y., Chazan, S. et al. Frequency of carriers of chronic (type 1) Gaucher disease . . . *Am. J. Med. Genet.*, 27, 561–565 (1987).
Choy, F.Y.M. Intrafamilial clinical variability of type 1 Gaucher disease . . . *J. Med. Genet.*, 25, 322–325 (1988).
Goldblatt, J. Type 1 Gaucher disease. *J. Med. Genet.*, 25, 415–418 (1988).
Zlotogora, J., Sagi, M. et al. Gaucher disease type 1 and pregnancy. *Am. J. Med. Genet.*, 32, 475–477 (1989).

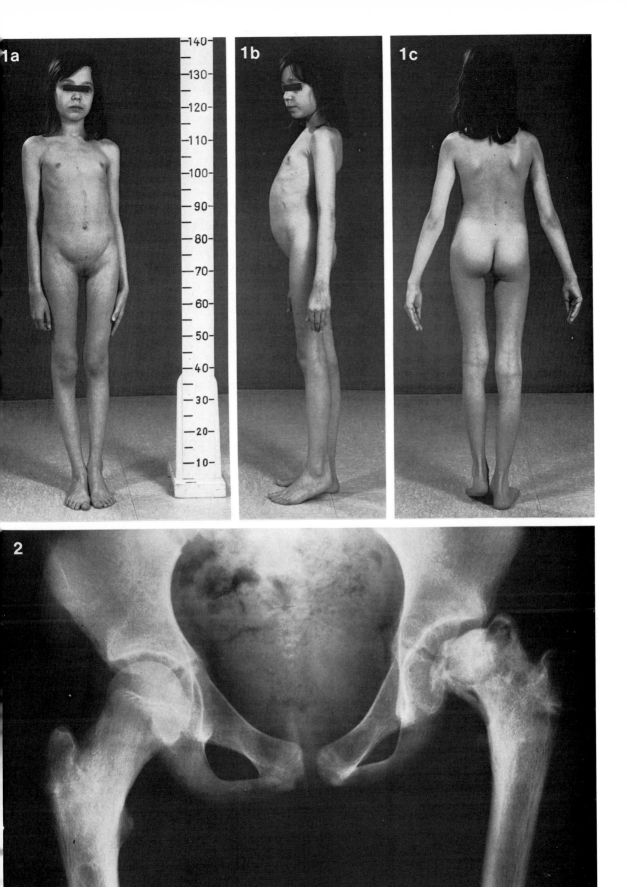

305

152. Caudal Dysplasia 'Syndrome'

(Sacrococcygeal agenesis 'syndrome'; Caudal regression 'syndrome')

A sequence of hypo- or aplasia of the caudal spine of variable severity—with developmental defect of the corresponding spinal segments—and hypo- or dysplasia of the pelvis and lower extremities.

Main signs:

1. Shortening, narrowing, or atypical configuration of the lower part of the trunk, especially apparent dorsally, the buttocks often appearing flat with dimples and a shortened gluteal fold (**1b**). Distinctly disproportionate short stature possible, due to short trunk and long extremities, especially the arms (**1a, 1b**).

2. Weakness and atrophy, with possible malformation or hypoplasia, of the legs. Hips frequently dislocated (**2, 3**). Flexion contractures of the hips and knees. Club feet. Frequent paralysis of the pelvic floor muscles and sphincters with urinary and fecal incontinence; frequent areflexia of the legs (motor and sensory defects need not correspond). Thus, total neurological impairment may vary between a slight disorder of bladder control and total paralysis below the defect.

Supplementary findings: Radiologically, lumbosacrococcygeal vertebral defects of variable severity. Possible malformation and narrowing of the pelvis with narrowly spaced hypoplastic ilia, which are directly apposed dorsally (**2, 3**). Dislocated hips, femoral hypoplasia possible.

Possible malformation of the gastrointestinal tract, the abdominal organs, the heart, or other organs.

Maternal diabetes mellitus in some cases.

Manifestation: At birth.

Etiology: Not uniform. Mostly isolated cases. At least 15% of cases have mothers with poorly controlled diabetes; in these, the syndrome falls within the spectrum of a 'diabetic embryopathy'.

Frequency: Not particularly low. The majority of cases are not associated with maternal diabetes; about 1% of children of diabetic mothers are affected.

Course, prognosis: Dependent on the severity of the dysplasia and on the quality and consistency of care and multidisciplinary rehabilitation.

Illustrations:

1–3 A 14-year-old girl whose mother had been diabetic for 13 years at the time of the patient's birth. Growth deficiency of about 20 cm from the average height for age due to caudal shortening of the trunk. Narrowly spaced ilial wings; abnormal configuration of the lower back and gluteal region (**1b**) with shortened gluteal folds and dimples. Waddling gait with complete bilateral dislocated hips; contracted knee joints; muscle wasting and abundant fat in the lower extremities, the former especially of the calves; absent patellar reflex; sensation in the legs intact. Urinary incontinence (previously also fecal incontinence). Relatively good physical rehabilitation after surgery for club feet and other orthopedic measures, after surgery for congenital valvular and subvalvular pulmonary stenosis and an atrial septal defect, and under pediatric urological care. Very good psychosocial adjustment. X-rays (**2** and **3** at 5½ and 8 years respectively): absence of the fourth and fifth lumbar vertebrae, all of the sacrum, and the coccyx. Ilial wings small and directly apposed dorsally; small heart-shaped pelvis and extremely narrow pelvic outlet. Severe bilateral dysplasia of the hip joints; lateralized capital femoral epiphyses, coxa vara.

H.-R.W.

References:

Price, D.L., Dooling, E.C., Richardson, E.P., Jr. Caudal dysplasia (caudal regression syndrome). *Arch. Neurol.*, 23, 212 (1970).

Amendt, P., Goedel, E., Amendt, U., Becker, G. Mißbildungen bei mütterlichem Diabetes mellitus unter besonderer Berücksichtigung des kaudalen Fehlbildungssyndroms. *Zbl. Gynäk.*, 96/30, 950 (1974).

Andrish, J., Kalamchi, A., MacEwen, G.D. Sacral agenesis: a clinical evaluation of its management, heredity, and associated anomalies. *Clin. Orthopaed.*, 139, 52 (1979).

Stewart, J.M. and Stoll, S. Familial caudal regression anomalad and maternal diabetes. *J. Med. Genet.*, 16, 17 (1979); and ibid. 17, 57 (1980).

Mitnick, J., Kramer, E. et al. Radiological case of the month: syndrome of caudal regression ... *Am. J. Dis. Child.*, 136, 637–638 (1982).

Fuhrmann, K., Reiher, H. et al. Prevention of congenital malformations in infants of insulin-dependent diabetic mothers. *Diabetes Care*, 6, 219–223 (1983).

Lausecker, M. and Stögmann, W. Stellen Sie die Diagnose. *Pädiatr. Pädol.*, 22, 73–77 (1987).

Mills, J.L., Knopp, R.H. et al. Lack of relation of increased malformation rates in infants of diabetic mothers to glycemic control during organogenesis. *N. Engl. J. Med.*, 318, 671–676 (1988).

Bergman, M., Newman, S.A. et al. Letters: Diabetic control and fetal malformations. *N. Engl. J. Med.*, 319, 647–649 (1988).

Editorial. Congenital abnormalities in infants of diabetic mothers. *Lancet*, I, 1313–1315 (1988).

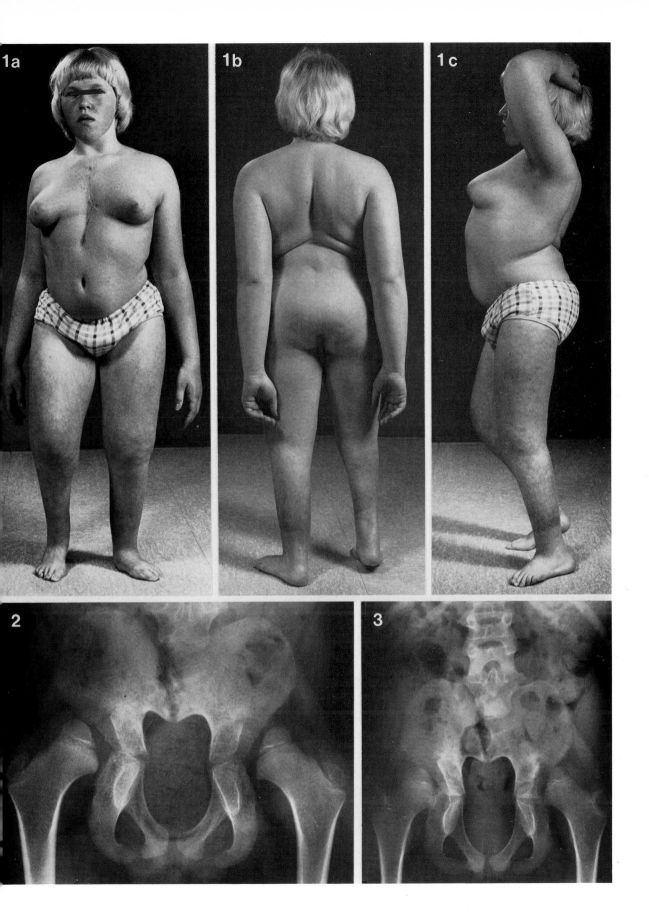

153. Syndrome of Multiple Benign Ring-Shaped Skin Creases

(Michelin Tire Baby Syndrome)

A familial syndrome, manifesting in childhood with multiple benign ringlike constrictions of the skin that do not lead to amputation and that are mostly lost in adulthood.

Main signs: Deep ringlike constrictions of the skin, especially over the extremities, fingers, and toes without signs of strangulation or amputation. Less prominent rings on the trunk. No lymphedema. Nails unremarkable.

Supplementary findings: Minor anomalies such as medial epicanthus, mongoloid slant of the palpebral fissures, auricular peculiarities, hypertelorism, or micrognathia may be present.

The three patients pictured here showed in addition:
1 Neuroblastoma, cleft palate.
2 Ureteroceles, cleft palate.
3 Complicated febrile seizures.

Manifestation: At birth.

Etiology: Autosomal dominant inheritance.

Frequency: Higher than previously reported, especially in its milder form.

Course, prognosis: The ring-shaped constrictions become less distinct during childhood and are barely demonstrable in the adult.

Differential diagnosis: No relation to amniotic bands.

Treatment: None.

Comment: The designation 'Michelin tire baby syndrome' is a misnomer and should be avoided.

Illustrations:
1a–1c A female neonate (6 days old).
2a and 2b A 4-month-old female infant.
3a A 9-month-old boy.
3b The child's father at age 10 months.

J.K./H.-R.W.

References:

Kunze, J. and Riehm, H. A new genetic disorder: autosomal-dominant multiple ring-shaped skin creases. *Eur. J. Pediatr.*, 138, 301–303 (1982).
Niikawa, N., Ishikiriyama, S., Shikimani, T. Letter to the editor: The 'Michelin tire baby' syndrome—an autosomal dominant trait. *Am. J. Med. Genet.*, 22, 637–638 (1985).
Kunze, J. Letter to the editor: The 'Michelin tire baby syndrome': An autosomal-dominant trait. *Am. J. Med. Genet.*, 25, 169 (1986).
Niikawa, N. and Ishikiriyama, S. Letter to the editor: response to Dr. Kunze. *Am. J. Med. Genet.*, 25, 171 (1986).
Wiedemann, H.-R. Letter to the editor: multiple benign circumferential skin creases on limbs—a congenital anomaly existing from beginning of mankind. *Am. J. Med. Genet.*, 28, 225–226 (1987).

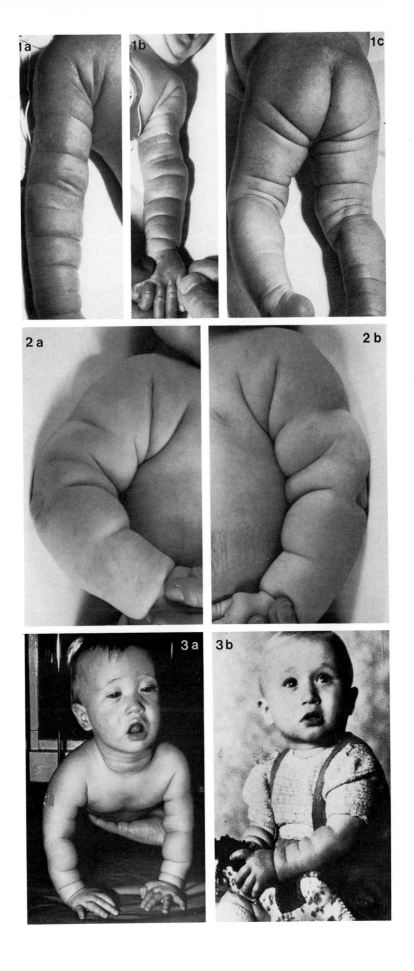

309

154. Gingival Fibromatosis–Hypertrichosis Syndrome

(Gingival Fibromatosis with Hypertrichosis)

A hereditary disorder with early manifestation of generalized hypertrichosis and gingival fibromatosis.

Main signs:
1. Generalized hypertrichosis, usually with dark hair (even in families with otherwise fair complexions) (**1, 3**).
2. Gingival fibromatosis, which more or less covers the teeth, delays eruption, overgrows the crowns, and may bring about loss of teeth (**4–6**). In some cases, protrusion of the lips and jaws and other secondary mechanical effects.

Supplementary findings: Epilepsy and/or mental retardation are often present, especially in the infrequent sporadic cases (see below; recessive inheritance?).

Manifestation: Development of generalized hypertrichosis in the first two years of life; the gingival changes also present in infancy or early childhood.

Etiology: Hereditary disorder, usually autosomal dominant. Possibly also an autosomal recessive form; heterogeneity is therefore likely.

Frequency: Low.

Prognosis: Favorable with respect to the gingival hyperplasia, assuming adequate treatment. The prognosis depends on the patient's mental development.

Comment: In a rare type, in which mode of inheritance is uncertain and which cannot be definitely identified before sexual maturity, female carriers, develop mammary fibroadenomatosis with a tendency to malignant degeneration.

Treatment: Very meticulous oral hygiene; gingivectomy; in some cases, extraction of teeth and prosthetic measures. Depilation. Genetic counseling.

Illustrations:
1–4 A boy with typical development of the syndrome; very heavily developed eyebrows, hyperplasia of the eyelashes (three rows), apparent small size of the teeth.
5 and 6 Further demonstration of gingival hyperplasia in two other cases.

H.-R.W.

References:
Synder, C.H. Syndrome of gingival hyperplasia, hirsutism, and convulsions . . . *J. Pediatr.*, 67, 499–502 (1965).
Witkop, C.J., Jr. Heterogeneity in gingival fibromatosis. *Birth Defects*, 7, 210 (1971).
Horning, G.M., Fisher, J.G. et al. Gingival fibromatosis with hypertrichosis . . . *J. Periodontol.*, 56, 344–347 (1985).

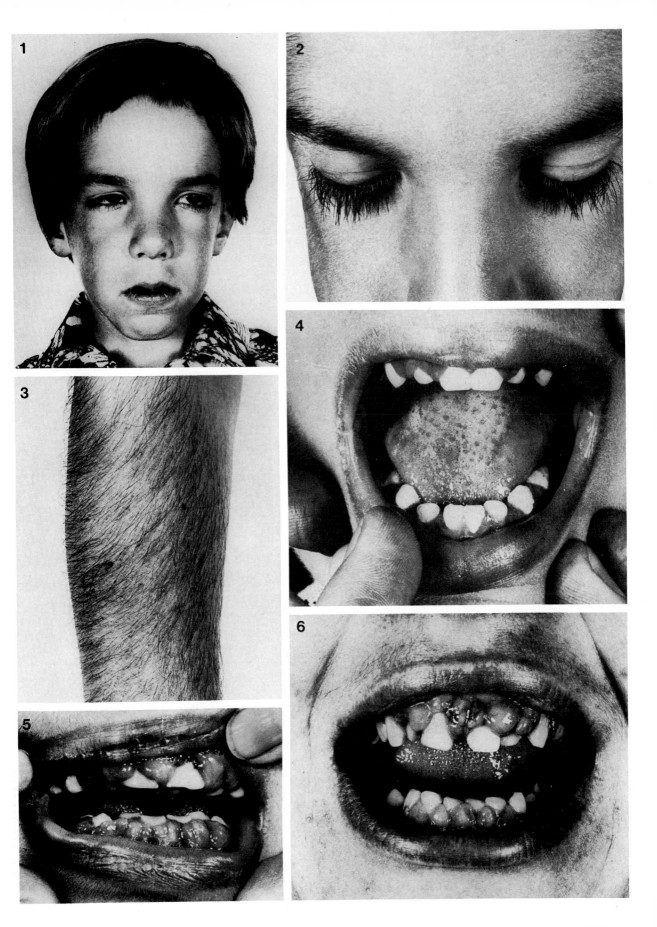

155. 'Syndrome' of Giant Hairy Nevus with Satellite Nevi

(Melanophacomatosis)

Extensive congenital melanocytic nevus which may be associated with leptomeningeal melanocytosis (then: 'neurocutaneous melanoblastosis').

Main signs: Skin changes: usually intensive black-brown macular or partially raised and nodular/wartlike; usually with coarse hairs; with bilaterally symmetrical or asymmetrical distribution ('bathing suit', 'bathing trunk', 'cap', 'neck poultice', 'stocking' nevus, etc.) with multiple corresponding smaller nevi (1, 2).

Supplementary findings: Development of hydrocephalus, CNS seizures, or other neurological or psychological features indicate progressive meningocerebral involvement.

Manifestation: Hairy nevi present at birth. Although cerebral signs may appear as early as infancy, they generally begin at a pre-school age, and occasionally not until much later.

Etiology: Unclear. Usually sporadic occurrence, familial as an exception (affected family members usually have multiple small nevi only); possibly, multifactorial inheritance. Basic defect unknown.

Frequency: Up to 1987, only about 100 reported cases of neurocutaneous melanosis; of these, at least 35 with malignant meningeal meningioma (see below).

Course, prognosis, treatment: CNS involvement or its progression may lead to death in infancy or early childhood. (Extensive hairy nevi of the head or neck region are frequently associated with meningeal melanocytosis, with unfavorable prognosis.) In the region of the skin nevus and the correspondingly affected intracranial area, there is an increased risk of developing a malignant melanoma, which usually presents within the first five years of life. The *treatment* of choice is complete resection of the entire giant skin nevus (as well as the satellites) with grafting; when not feasible, as is often the case, the most extensive possible excision. Such a procedure may be carried out more successfully after infancy. Definite cosmetic improvement is accomplished by planing, although such dermabrasion can hardly decrease the risk of melanoma developing in deeper portions. Considering the associated risk, a hairy nevus requires frequent regular careful follow-up (preferably with photographic documentation of the course); the patient and in some cases family members require appropriate psychological help and guidance.

Illustrations:

1a–1d A newborn with 'bathing trunk' giant hairy nevus and numerous satellite nevi. Relatively large cranium. No pathological growth of the skull or other neurological signs.

2a–2c A 6½-year-old boy. Hairy nevus with satellites. Recent onset of focal seizures.

H.-R.W.

References:

Voigtländer, V. and Jung, E.G. Giant pigmented hairy nevus in two siblings. *Humangenetik*, 24, 79 (1974).
Lamas, E., Diez Lobato, R. et al. Neurocutaneous melanosis. *Acta. Neurolchirurgica*, 36, 93 (1977).
Solomon, L.M. The management of congenital melanocytic nevi. *Arch. Derm.*, 116, 1017 (1980).
Hecht, F., LaCanne, K.M., Carroll, D.B. Inheritance of giant pigmented hairy nevus . . . *Am. J. Med. Genet.*, 9, 177 (1981).
Fleissner, J., Kleine, M., Bonsmann, G. et al. Dermabrasion eines großflächigen kongenitalen Pigmentnävus . . . *Pädiatr. Prax.*, 26, 505 (1982).
Konz, B. Problem der angeborenen pigmentierten Nävi. *Pädiatr. Prax.*, 26, 106 (1982).
Müller-Holzner, E., Weiser, G. et al. Neurokutane Melanose. *Medwelt*, 1984, 1184–1187.
Cazzani, M., Lampertico, P. et al. La melanosi neurocutanea. *Min. Ped.*, 39, 43–51 (1987).
Drepper, H. and Hundeiker, M. Beurteilung und Behandlung angeborener Pigmentzellnaevi. *Monatschr. Kinderheilkd.*, 135, 406–410 (1987).
Schnyder, U.W., Schneider, B.V. et al. Kongenitale Naevuszellnaevi als Melanomprekursoren der Haut. *Monatschr. Kinderheilkd.*, 135, 259–264 (1987).
Schrudde, J. and Steffens, K. Tierfellnävi . . . *Pädiatr. Prax.*, 35, 279–286 (1987).
Pascual-Castroviejo, I. Neurocutaneous melanosis. In: Gomez, M.R. (ed.) *Neurocutaneous Diseases*. Butterworths, Boston, 1987, pp. 329–334 (chapter 36).

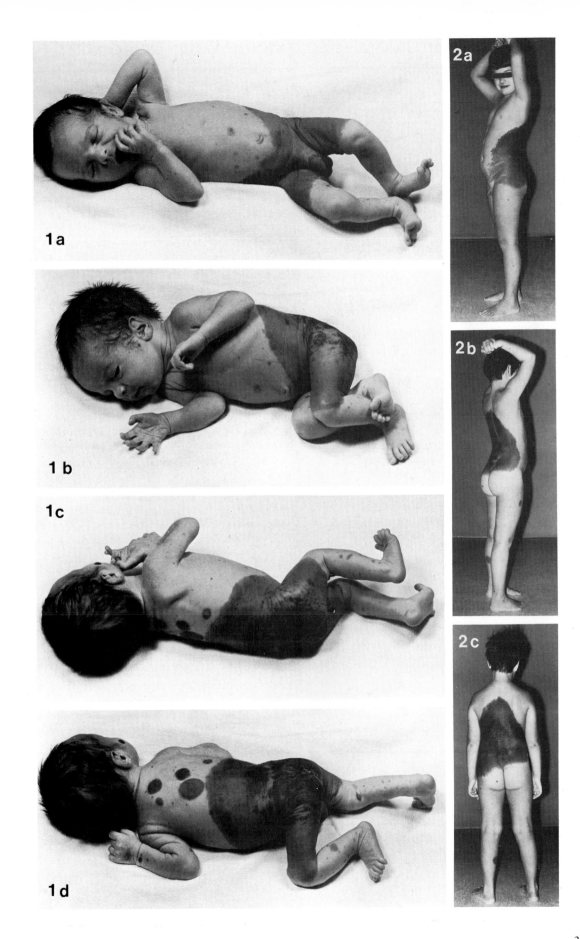

313

156. Schimmelpenning–Feuerstein–Mims 'Syndrome'

(Linear Sebaceous Nevus 'Syndrome')

A syndrome of streak-like Jadassohn sebaceous nevus usually involving the middle of the face, cerebral seizures, and mental retardation.

Main signs:

1. Sebaceous nevus of Jadassohn; uni- or bilateral; localized mainly on the head (with focal alopecia), around the ears, on the forehead and temples, often extending to the tip of the nose or to the rest of the face, also possibly elsewhere on the body; changes varying from narrow and pale to broad, conspicuous stripes. Yellow-brown appearance; greasy warty consistency (1–3). Often additional, quite widely distributed, pigmented nevi (1, 2).

2. Cerebral seizures, usually in the form of focal epilepsy, of variable severity.

3. Very variable mental or psychomotor retardation present in some cases. Frequently behavioral disorder also present.

Supplementary findings: Congenital involvement of one or both eyes in about 50% of cases: coloboma of the iris (sometimes involving chorioretina or lid); lipodermoids of the conjunctiva and possibly cornea.

Often markedly asymmetrical development of the two sides of the head and face. Hemimacrocephaly, eye anomalies, dilated ventricles and focal EEG findings with probably hamartomatous cerebral involvement and atrophy which is, as a rule ipsilateral to the main nevus involvement.

Frequent excrescences of the oral mucosa and dysodontiasis of variable severity (5).

Possible osteodystrophy with pathologic fractures (Milkman phenomenon). Small stature in some cases.

Manifestation: Nevus usually congenital (additional pigmentary anomalies and verrucous changes of the nevus occur later). Cerebral seizures, usually focal, may occur early in infancy—or sometimes much later. Mental retardation.

Etiology: Not clear. Sporadic occurrence. Somatic mutation?

Frequency: Low; by 1980, about 80 cases reported.

Course, prognosis: Seizures and developmental defects are especially likely when linear sebaceous nevus affects the middle of the face. The course is very variable, depending on the severity of mental retardation and epilepsy. The former need not be severe; the latter may improve spontaneously or be controlled medically. The Jadassohn nevus is subject to verrucous hyperplasia in childhood and adolescence and may pose a serious cosmetic problem (1). Difficult dental problems may arise early on (5).

In adulthood, development in the nevus of malignant tumors, e.g., basal cell epithelioma, must be anticipated (approximately 15% of cases). In addition, this syndrome may be associated with tumor development (renal hamartoma, nephroblastoma, cystic adenoma of the liver, fibroangioma, osteoclastic tumors of the jaw) in isolated cases.

Differential diagnosis: Encephalocraniocutaneous lipomatosis (p.318), Proteus syndrome (p.352), and other phacomatoses.

Treatment: Symptomatic. Early resection of the nevus as far as possible. Appropriate anticonvulsive medication when indicated. Dental care. Cosmetic attention as needed.

Illustrations:

1–5 A 12-year-old boy, the second child of young, nonconsanguineous parents after a healthy sibling. Congenital Jadassohn nevus in broad stripes bilaterally and asymmetrically on the face, scalp (there, alopecia), and neck (1: post-planing; 3); narrow streaks on the abdomen; right leg and foot; spotty hyperpigmentation of the trunk and arms (2). Onset of left focal seizures in the second year; dilated left cerebral ventricle; mental retardation (Hawick IQ 78). Also, neurogenic hemiatrophy (left-sided for the head and tongue, 1b, 4, 5; below that, right-sided, 2a) with dysphagia, abnormal motor function, and dysreflexia of the atrophic side. Excrescences of the oral mucosa, numerous pathologic fractures or Looser zones, and small stature, below the third percentile. Eyes normal. Father of the patient has a neuromotor disability, one arm covered in pigmental moles, and a family history of focal seizure disorders.

H.-R.W.

References:

Schimmelpenning, G.W. Klinischer Beitrag zur Symptomatologie der Phakomatosen. *Rö Fo*, 87, 716 (1957).
Feuerstein, R.C. and Mims, L.C. Linear nevus sebaceous with convulsions and mental retardation. *Am. J. Dis. Child.*, 104, 675 (1962).
Leiber, B. Schimmelpenning–Feuerstein–Mims-Syndrom. *Monatschr. Kinderheilkd.*, 127, 585 (1979).
Schimmelpenning, G.W. Langjährige Verlaufsuntersuchung . . . *RöFo*, 139, 63 (1983).
Prensky, A.L. Linear sebaceous nevus. In: Gomez, M.R. (ed.) *Neurocutaneous Diseases.* Butterworths, Boston, 1987 (chapter 37).

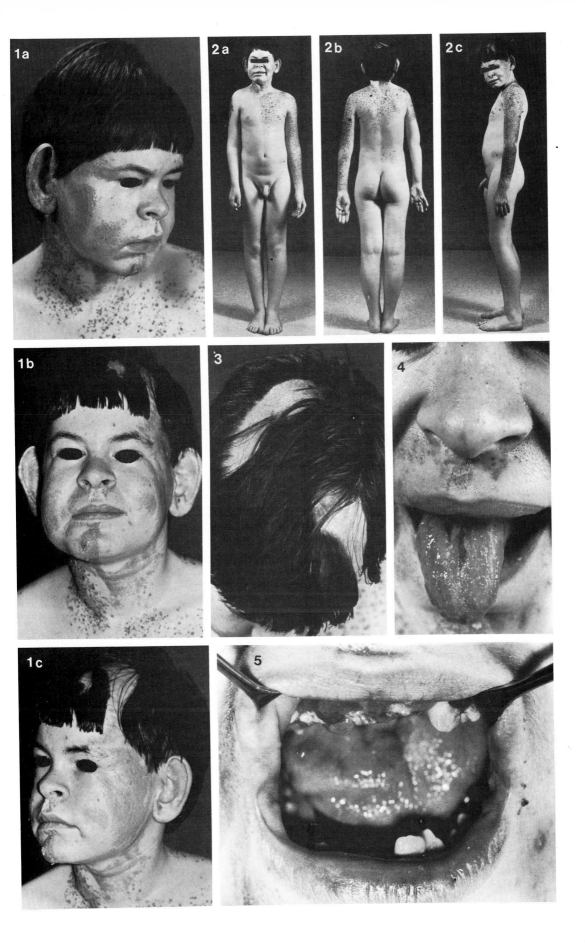

157. Syndrome of Partial Macrosomia, Linear Nevus, Macrocranium with Signs of Cardiac Overload from Intracranial A-V Shunt, Parietal Soft-Tissue Swelling with Alopecia, Psychomotor Retardation, and Small Stature

A syndrome of congenital macrosomia of one lower extremity, linear verrucous nevus on the trunk, macrodolichocephaly with signs of cardiac overload (without evidence of cardiac malformation) from intracranial arteriovenous (A-V) fistula, biparietal soft-tissue swelling with alopecia, psychomotor retardation, and short stature.

Main signs:

1. Congenital macrosomia of the left leg (**1**), from which a cavernous hemangioma of the thigh was removed at 2 years. Excess length over right leg: 2 cm at 3 years; 4 cm at 4 years. Livid discoloration of the left leg with padding-like swelling, especially of the back of the foot. Secondary contractures of the hip and knee. Systolic murmur over the femoral artery, but absence of a significant A-V fistula on angiogram.

2. Linear hyperpigmented verrucous nevus of the thorax, extending to the midline, then continuing downwards (**1, 3**: note biopsy scar on upper abdomen: epitheliomatous nevus).

3. Macrodolichocephaly (at 2¾ years 53 cm, at 4¾ years 55 cm) with signs of cardiac overload and cardiomegaly with barrel-shaped chest, without evidence of cardiac malformation. Continuous systolic–diastolic murmur over the cranium. Evidence of an intracranial A-V fistula of the great vein of Galen and dilatation of the neighboring venous sinuses (**4**).

4. Biparietal soft-tissue swelling with alopecia present since the first weeks of life (**2**). (Biopsy: 'anetoderma'.)

5. Physical and psychomotor retardation with muscular dystonia. (No cerebral seizure disorder.)

6. Short stature (below the third percentile).

Supplementary findings: High forehead with bossing. Antimongoloid slant of the palpebral fissures, especially the right.

High narrow palate; bifid uvula.

Bony protuberance of the lateral rim of the left orbit; on skull X-ray, irregular translucent areas and densities of the parietal cortex. Oval cystic translucency on the left femur distally.

Slight pareses of the left facial and abducens nerves with strabismus. Ocular fundi hyperpigmented, otherwise normal.

Manifestation: At birth and later.

Etiology: Uncertain; presumably a genetic basis.

Course: Death of the child at age 5 years from intracranial bleeding.

Comment: The clinical picture of this child suggests the Schimmelpenning–Feuerstein–Mims 'syndrome' (p. 314), encephalocraniocutaneous lipomatosis (p. 318), or an observation by Goldschmidt et al. (see below); however, it does not completely correspond to any of these; cf. also p. 34 and p. 400.

Illustrations:

1–4 A 3-year-old boy, the first child of young, healthy, nonconsanguineous parents. Features as described above.

H.-R.W.

Reference:

Goldschmidt, H., Thiede, G., Pfeiffer, R.A. et al. Hemihypertrophie, Naevus sebaceus, multiple Knochenzysten und zerebroretinale Angiomatose: eine komplexe Phakomatose. *Helv. Paediatr. Acta*, 31, 487 (1976).

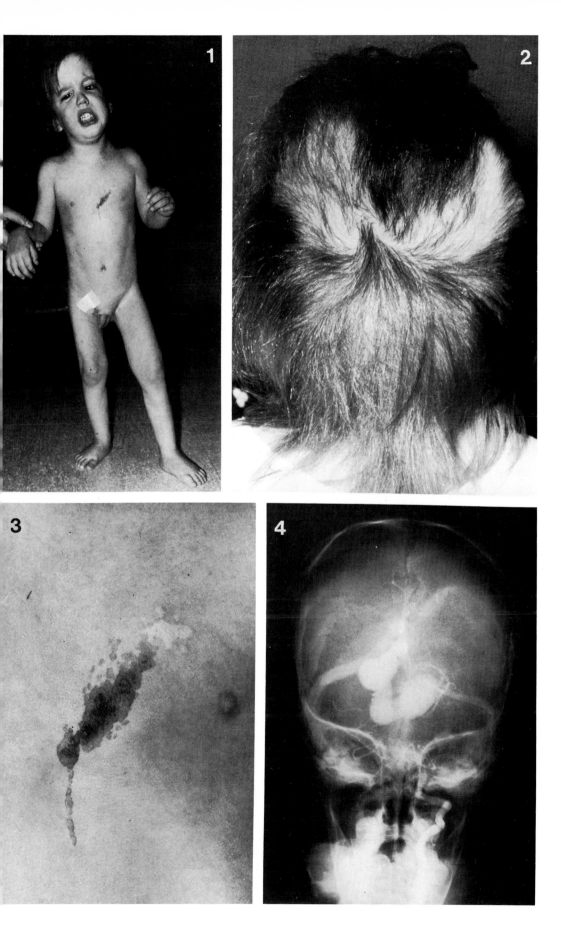

158. Encephalocraniocutaneous Lipomatosis

A clinical picture including macrocephaly, soft-tissue tumors of the head and eyes, unilateral porencephalic cyst with focal CNS seizures, psychomotor retardation, and cerebral hemiatrophy with lipomatosis.

Main signs:
1. Congenital or postnatally manifest macrocrania, which may be clearly asymmetrical, and possibly with distinct progression and signs of hydrocephaly (1–5).
2. Soft-tissue swellings, small or large, single or multiple, uni- or bilateral, of the parieto-occipital, fronto-temporal, or other parts of the cranial or facial part of the skull; alopecia of the affected area; lipomatous on biopsy (1–5). Bony growths possible (exostoses).
3. Possible soft-tissue tumors involving conjunctiva, sclera, cornea and/or eyelids; lipodermoid on biopsy.
4. Focal CNS seizures, manifest early.
5. Psychomotor retardation of various grades of severity, in some cases with hemispasticity, etc.
6. A unilateral porencephalic cyst of variable size communicating with the ventricular system, with ipsilateral atrophy of the brain, can be demonstrated. Autopsy may show fairly extensive intracranial (and possibly intraspinal) lipomatosis, possibly involving the cranial bones.

Supplementary findings: Additional small 'connective tissue nevi', angiofibromas, or fibrolipomas possible in the craniofacial area.

Xanthochromia and increased protein in the cerebrospinal fluid in some cases.

Manifestation: At birth and postnatally.

Etiology: Not certain; presumably a genetic basis.

Frequency: Low, only a few cases described in the literature.

Course, prognosis: Unfavorable.

Differential diagnosis: Proteus syndrome and Schimmelpenning–Feuerstein–Mims 'syndrome' (pp.352 and 314). We consider encephalocraniocutaneous lipomatosis as a form of Proteus syndrome with more localized, encephalocraniofacial, manifestations. Although there is definite overlap with Schimmelpenning–Feuerstein–Mims syndrome, the particular histopathological findings would seem to justify separate classification.

Treatment: Symptomatic.

Illustrations:
1–5 The first child of young, healthy, nonconsanguineous parents (1 and 2 at 4 weeks, 3–5 at 2½ years). Congenital macrodoliochocephaly (41.5 cm) with signs of increasing intracranial pressure, xanthochromia and increased protein in the cerebrospinal fluid. Severe congenital soft-tissue swelling of the left cheek; (hamartoma of the right upper eyelid). Very early focal CNS seizures. Psychomotor retardation with signs of cerebral palsy. Ophthalmologically: localized accumulations of chorioretinal pigmentation in the left eye; otherwise normal. CT scan showed severe porencephalic dilatation of the left ventricular system. Ventriculo-cardiac shunt. Head circumference at 2½ years 62.5 cm; very high forehead. Removal of a lipoma from the left cheek. Death of the child at 3¼ years.

H.-R.W.

References:

Haberland, C. and Perou, M. Encephalocraniocutaneous lipomatosis. *Arch. Neurol.*, 22, 144 (1970).

Fishman, M.A., Chang, C.S.C., Miller, J.E. Encephalocraniocutaneous lipomatosis. *Pediatrics*, 61, 580 (1978).

Sanchez, N.P., Rhodes, A.R., Mandell, F. et al. Encephalocraniocutaneous lipomatosis: a new neurocutaneous syndrome. *Br. J. Dermatol.*, 104, 89 (1981).

Schlack, H.G. and Skopnik, H. Encephalocraniocutane Lipomatose und lineärer Naevus sebaceus. *Monatschr. Kinderheilkd.*, 133, 235–237 (1985).

Wiedemann, H.-R. and Burgio, G.R. Encephalocraniocutaneous lipomatosis and Proteus syndrome. *Am. J. Med. Genet.*, 25, 403–404 (1986).

Fishman, M.A. Encephalo-cranio-cutaneous lipomatosis. In: Gomez, M.R. (ed.) *Neurocutaneous Diseases*. Butterworths, Boston, 1987, pp.349–355 (chapter 39).

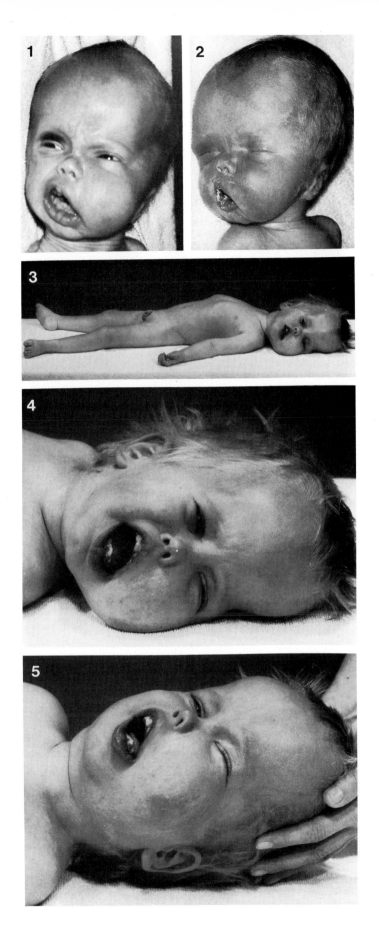

319

159. McCune–Albright Syndrome

(Albright Syndrome; Weil–Albright Syndrome)

A characteristic syndrome of fibrous dysplasia of the bone, irregular brown hyperpigmentation of the skin, and precocious puberty (almost exclusively in girls).

Main signs:
1. Café au lait or darker-colored hyperpigmented areas with irregular, sharp map-like borders (1), often unilateral along the midline, preferentially on the buttocks, thighs, back, and neck. (In rare cases these features may be absent.)
2. Precocious menarche, followed by premature development of secondary sexual characteristics (in boys precocious puberty only exceptionally).
3. Spontaneous fractures and variable degree of skeletal deformity, usually in the lower extremities, especially the proximal femur, with polyostotic fibrous dysplasia lesions and corresponding X-ray findings (2).

Supplementary findings: In some cases, accelerated growth in height and skeletal maturity; premature closure of the epiphyses may eventually result in short stature.

Serum calcium and phosphate levels normal; alkaline phosphatase normal or elevated.

Manifestation: Pigmented areas present at birth or shortly thereafter, and subsequently grow proportionally. Menarche may even occur in infancy (regular menses usually do not occur until a few years later); further sexual characteristics may develop subsequently. Bony defects manifest mainly during the first decade of life.

Etiology: Sporadic occurrence. Hypothesis: this clinical picture results from an autosomal dominant lethal gene that can only be expressed phenotypically in mosaic combination with healthy cells. No increased risk for siblings, no transmission to the next generation. Precocious puberty in girls apparently brought about by gonadotropin-independent estrogen secretion of the ovaries, which show cystic changes.

Frequency: Relatively low (up to 1980, about 160 case reports in the literature).

Course, prognosis: The number and extent of bone changes usually progress slowly while the child is growing, becoming stationary after the second to third decade of life as a rule. Life expectancy is normal on the whole (a few cases developing sarcomas during adolescence). Fractures tend to heal well.

Treatment: Cyproterone acetate, alone or in combination with luteinizing hormone releasing hormone (LHRH) analogs; operative ovarian cystectomy? Avoidance of stress damage, care of pathological fractures, and orthopedic care of skeletal deformities. Attempts at therapeutic application of ionizing radiation *contraindicated*. Gestagen administration in some cases.

Illustrations:
1 A 13¼-year-old girl: pigmentation anomalies since birth, vaginal bleeding since infancy, secondary characteristics since early childhood. On X-ray: polyostotic fibrous dysplasia with foci in the pelvis and upper leg, left tibia, left scapula, the proximal humeral metaphyses, and both temporal bones.
2 X-ray of the patient. Pelvis oblique and tilted; coxa vara; pathologic fracture of the left medial femoral neck; cystic and honeycomb-like changes in the iliosacral region bilaterally, in the region of the left anterior iliac spine, and in both proximal femora, the epiphyses being largely spared; cortical thinning of the broadened left diaphysis due to marked cystic expansion.

H.-R.W./J.K.

References:

Boenheim, F. and McGavack, T.H. Polyostotische fibröse Dysplasie. *Erg. Inn. Med. Kinderheilkd.*, 3, 157 (1952).
Hauke, H. Osteofibrose. *Handbuch der Kinderheilkunde*, Bd 6, Springer, Heidelberg, 1967, p.389ff.
Spranger, J.W., Langer, L.O., Jr., Wiedemann, H.-R. *Bone Dysplasias. An Atlas of Constitutional Disorders of Skeletal Development.* G. Fischer and W.B. Saunders, Stuttgart and Philadelphia, 1974.
Giovannelli, G., Bernasconi, S., Banchini, G. McCune–Albright syndrome in a male child: a clinical and endocrinologic enigma. *J. Pediatr.*, 92, 220 (1978).
Grant, D.B. and Martinez, L. The McCune–Albright syndrome without typical skin pigmentation. *Acta Pediatr. Scand.*, 72, 477–478 (1983).
Foster, C.M., Feuillan, P. et al. Ovarian function in girls with McCune–Albright syndrome. *Pediatr. Res.*, 20, 859–863 (1986).
Mauras, N. and Blizzard, R.M. The McCune–Albright syndrome. *Acta Endocrinol. Suppl.*, 279, 207–217 (1986).
Danon, M. and Crawford, J.D. The McCune–Albright syndrome. *Erg. Inn. Med. Kinderheilkd.*, 55, 82–115 (1987).
Happle, R. The McCune–Albright syndrome: a lethal gene surviving by mosaicism. *Clin. Genet.*, 29, 321–324 (1986).
Stier, B. and Ranke, M.B. Pubertas praecox bei McCune–Albright-Syndrom . . . *Klin. Pädiatr.*, 199, 376–381 (1987).

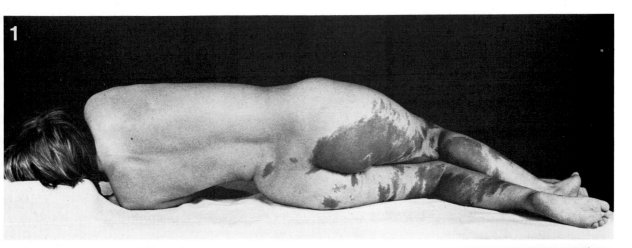

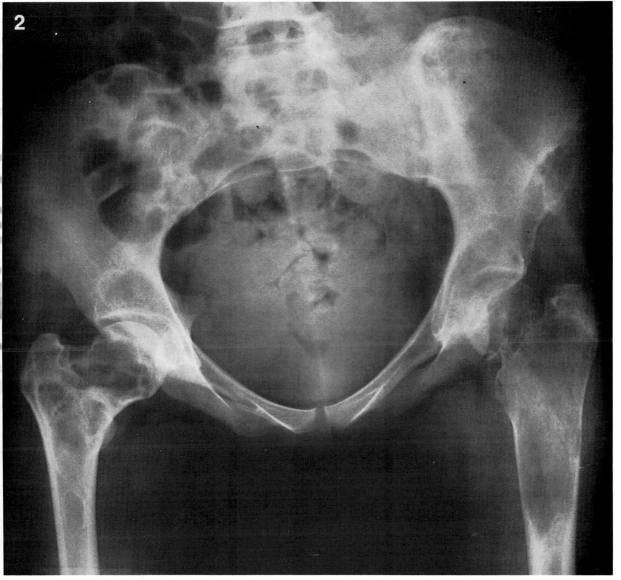

160. Miescher Syndrome

(Bloch–Miescher Syndrome; Mendenhall Syndrome; Rabson–Mendenhall Syndrome)

A syndrome—closely resembling congenital generalized lipodystrophy—of congenital acanthosis nigricans, hypertrichosis, failure to thrive and short stature, dysmorphism especially of the jaws and oral cavity, insulin-resistant diabetes mellitus, and a characteristic general appearance.

Main signs:

1. Acanthosis nigricans especially of the neck, axillary, inguinal, and genital regions (2–4, 6–8).
2. Lanugo-type hypertrichosis of the trunk (5), possibly also of the extremities; overabundant scalp hair in some cases (3, 7).
3. Poor physical and possibly also mental, growth with deficiency of adipose tissue (2), aged appearance (4, 7, 8), and short stature.
4. Relatively coarse facial features with prognathism (3, 4, 7, 8), poorly formed, malpositioned teeth (9, 11), and large, relatively low-set ears (7, 8).

Supplementary findings: High palate, fissured tongue (10); oral mucous membranes coarse, velvety, and of milky opacity.

Simply formed fingers and toes.

Goiter (3, 4), frequently nodular. (Hyperplasia of the pineal body.)

Insulin-resistant diabetes with little tendency to ketosis.

Manifestation: At birth and in subsequent years; diabetes manifest during childhood or adolescence.

Etiology: Autosomal recessive disorder. Insulin receptor defect.

Frequency: Very low.

Course, prognosis: Decrease in intensity and extent of the acanthosis nigricans possible after many years. Diabetes relatively benign.

Illustrations:

1–11 Siblings with the Miescher syndrome. Latent diabetes mellitus in the father. Both children of short stature. The distinctly more severely affected 13½-year-old boy has manifest diabetes and nodular goiter; his 11½-year-old sister, latent diabetes. (6, 10, 11: the boy; 9: the girl.)

H.-R.W.

References:

Miescher, G. Zwei Fälle von congenitaler familiärer Akanthosis nigricans, kombiniert mit Diabetes mellitus. *Derm. Z.*, 32, 276 (1921).

Mason, H.H. and Sly, G.E. Diabetes mellitus: report of a case resistant to insulin . . . *JAMA,* 108, 2016 (1937).

Mendenhall, E.N. Tumor of pineal body with high insulin resistance. *J. Indiana M.A.*, 43, 32 (1950).

Rabson, S.M. and Mendenhall, E.N. Familial hypertrophy of pineal body . . . *Am. J. Clin. Pathol.*, 26, 283 (1956).

Wiedemann, H.-R., Spranger, J., Mogharei, M. et al. Über das Syndrom . . . und Miescher-Syndrom im Sinne dienzephaler Syndrome. *Z. Kinderheilkd.*, 102, 1 (1968).

Seip, M. Generalized lipodystrophy. *Ergeb. Inn. Med. Kinderheilkd.*, 31, 59 (1971).

Dumas, R., Rolin, B., de Paulet, P.C. et al. Trois observations de diabète lipoatrophique familial. *Ann. Pédiatr.*, 21, 625 (1974).

Barnes, N.D., Palumbo, P.J., Hyles, A.B. et al. Insulin resistance, skin changes, and virilization . . . *Diabetologia*, 10, 285 (1974).

West, R.J., Lloyd, J.K., Turner, W.M.L. Familial insulin-resistant diabetes, multiple somatic anomalies . . . *Arch. Dis. Child.*, 50, 703 (1975).

Holmes, J. and Tanner, M.S. Premature eruption and macrodontia associated with insulin-resistant diabetes . . . *Br. Dent. J.*, 141, 280 (1976).

West, R.J. and Leonard, J.V. Familial insulin resistance . . . *Arch. Dis. Child.*, 55, 619 (1980).

Colle, M., Doyard, P., Chaussain, J.-L. et al. Acanthosis nigricans, hirsutisme et diabète insulino-resistant. *Arch. Franç. Pédiatr.*, 36, 518 (1979).

Rüdiger, H.W., Dreyer, M. et al. Familial insulin-resistant diabetes secondary to an affinity defect of the insulin receptor. *Hum. Genet.*, 64, 407–411 (1983).

Dreyer, M. and Rüdiger, H.W. Erbliche Rezeptordefekte als Krankheitsursache. *Dtsch. Med. Wochenschr.*, 111, 465–471 (1986).

Rittey, C.D.C., Evans, T.J. et al. Melatonin state in Mendenhall's syndrome. *Arch. Dis. Child.*, 65, 852–854 (1988).

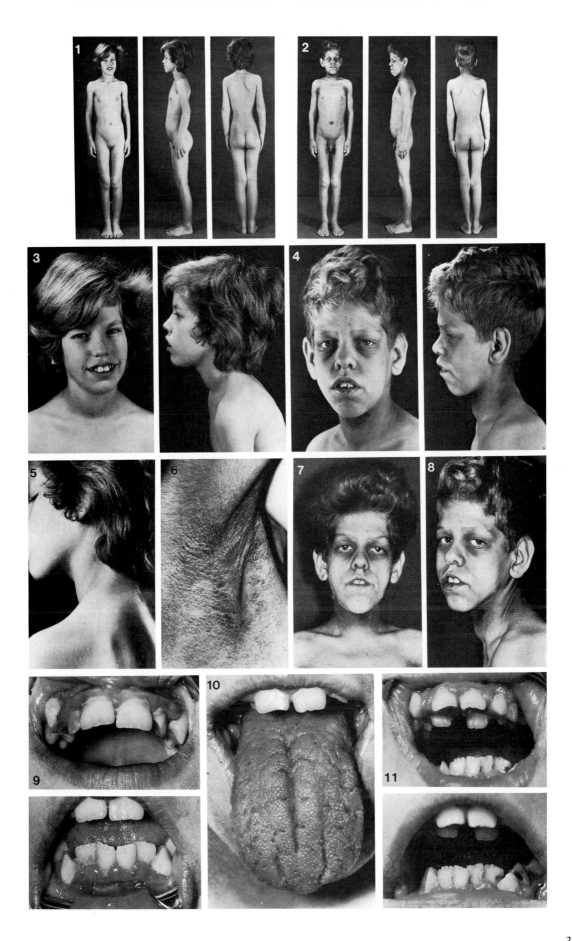

161. Multiple Lentigines

(LEOPARD Syndrome; Lentiginosis; Lentiginosis–Deafness–Cardiomyopathy Syndrome)

A complex hereditary syndrome involving skin, cardiac, and other manifestations and with relatively typical facial dysmorphism.

Main signs:
1. Multiple lentigines of the skin (dark brown, up to 5 mm diameter), most common on the back of the neck and upper trunk (3–6). Face, scalp, palms, soles, and genitalia may also be affected. Mucous membranes not involved.
2. Cardiac anomalies (7)—usually mild pulmonary stenosis and/or subaortic stenosis, or hypertrophic obstructive cardiomyopathy—with various ECG changes (e.g., conduction disorders).
3. Hypertelorism and 'coarse' facies (2); large ears, pouting lips, prominent lower jaw.

Supplementary findings: Growth and skeletal abnormalities: short stature; possible anomalies of thoracic shape (pectus excavatum or carinatum), winging of the scapula, kyphosis, and generalized connective tissue laxity.

Genital dysplasia (cryptorchidism, hypospadias) or delayed puberty. Sensorineural hearing impairment in some cases. Mild mental retardation found in a few cases.

Manifestation: Lentigines present at birth, or appear in the first years of life, increasing continuously in number (3, 4). Hearing impairment may be congenital or of early onset, when present. Cardiac disorder according to severity.

Etiology: Autosomal dominant disorder. Variable expression. Several sporadic cases.

Frequency: Low (about 100 cases reported by 1978).

Course, prognosis: Increasing number of lentigines. Degree of impairment otherwise dependent essentially on the type, development, and possible operative correction of the cardiac defect as well as on a possible hearing or mental impairment; also on the extent of possible growth deficiency and delay in sexual maturation.

Differential diagnosis: von Recklinghausen neurofibromatosis (p.332). Occasionally, additional single (and rather dark) café au lait spots have been found with the LEOPARD syndrome. Noonan syndrome (p.196).

Comment: The designation LEOPARD syndrome is taken from the initials of the most important signs: Lentigines; Electrocardiographic conduction defects; Ocular hypertelorism; Pulmonary stenosis; Abnormalities of genitalia; Retardation of growth; Deafness.

Illustrations:
1–7 An affected child at ages 7½ (1, 3), 10 (4), 11 (2, 5, 6), and 12 years (7). Note coarsening of the facies (1, 2) and increase in the number of lentigines (3, 4). Cardiac defect recognized since birth; later demonstrated as marked stenosis of the pulmonary valve along with a left heart anomaly (probably severe subaortic stenosis); X-ray: markedly enlarged and deformed heart shadow (7); ECG: pathological right heart pattern with deep Q_3 and extremely high ventricular peaks on the limb leads; extreme right and left ventricular hypertrophy with conduction defect and severe impairment of repolarization. Lentigines increasing continuously since birth. No hearing impairment. Increasing growth deficit (at 7½ years about 17 cm, at 12 years about 20 cm, below the average for age). Slight mental retardation (attended special school). High, narrow cranium (2), epicanthic folds, gothic palate, short neck (5, 6), winging of the scapula, coxa valga. Death due to heart failure in the middle of the second decade of life.

H.-R.W.

References:
Voron, D., Hatfield, H., Kalkhoff, R. Multiple lentigines syndrome. *Am. J. Med.*, 60, 447 (1976).
Sutton, S.J., Tajik, A.J. et al. Hypertrophic obstructive cardiomyopathy and lentiginosis . . . *Am. J. Cardiol.*, 47, 214–217 (1981).
Senn, M., Hess, O.M. et al. Hypertrophe Kardiomyopathie und Lentiginose. Schweiz. Med. Wochenschr., 114, 838–841 (1984).
Hagler, D.J. Lentiginosis–deafness-cardiopathy syndrome. In: Gomez, M.R. (ed.) *Neurocutaneous Diseases*. Butterworths, Boston, 1987, pp.80–84.

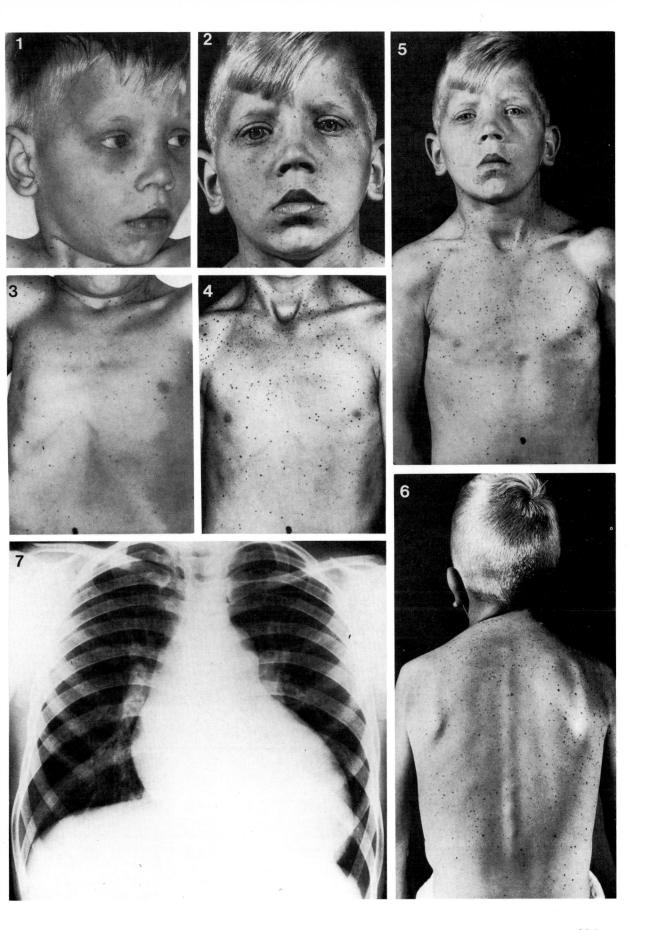

325

162. Peutz–Jeghers Syndrome

(Mucocutaneous Pigmentation and Intestinal Polyposis Syndrome; Pigment Spots–Polyposis)

An autosomal dominant disorder of conspicuous pigmentation predominantly of the face and oral mucosa associated with intestinal polyposis.

Main signs: Dark, brown- or bluegrey-black pigmented spots on the skin of the face—especially around the orifices, on the oral mucosa, extremities (including nail beds), and occasionally other areas (1–5).

Supplementary findings: With appropriate studies, usually extensive polyposis of the gastrointestinal tract—especially the jejunum—and occasionally of the mucosa of the respiratory and/or urogenital tracts.

Manifestation: The melanin spots may be present at birth, otherwise they appear in early childhood. Manifestations of intestinal polyposis—colicky pain, intestinal bleeding with possible development of anemia, in some cases recurrent signs of intussusception—occur frequently in early childhood.

Etiology: Autosomal dominant disorder with almost 100% penetrance and decreased expression of the pathological gene.

Frequency: Not particularly low; over 500 cases reported.

Course, prognosis: The extent of the pigmentation of the oral mucosa does not help predict the extent of visceral polyposis. The pigmented spots of the skin tend to fade after early adulthood. Possible danger of malignant transformation of the polyps, usually after childhood, with different familial risks. Occasional development of extraintestinal tumors (e.g., lung, breast, kidney, ovary, or testes).

Differential diagnosis: Freckles: different distribution and no involvement of the mucous membranes. The latter is also true for the LEOPARD syndrome (p.324). Addison disease: pigmentation of the skin more diffuse or more pronounced in the skin folds (oral mucosa may show similar spots, however).

Treatment: Intussusception, etc., may require surgery, resection of polypous segments of the intestine may be necessary. Regular follow-up. Genetic counseling.

Illustrations:
1–5 A 9-year-old boy. Pigmented macules noted in the second year of life. Since school age, recurrent signs of early ileus. Also, polyposis demonstrated in the stomach and large intestine. Father of the boy died of ileus secondary to intestinal polyposis; he allegedly had shown no pigmentation anomalies of the skin.

H.-R.W.

References:

Jeghers, H., McKusick, V.A., Katz, K.H. Generalized intestinal polyposis and melanin spots of the oral mucosa, lips, and digits. A syndrome of diagnostic significance. *N. Engl. J. Med.*, 241, 993 (1949).

Klostermann, G. *Pigmentfleckenpolypose.* Thieme, Stuttgart, 1960.

Long, J.A., Jr. and Dreyfuss, J.R. The Peutz–Jeghers syndrome: a 39-year clinical and radiographic follow-up report. *N. Eng. J. Med.*, 297, 1070 (1977).

Burdick, D. and Prior, J.T. Peutz–Jeghers syndrome . . . *Cancer*, 50, 2139–2146 (1982).

Rasenack, U. and Caspary, W. Das Peutz–Jeghers-Syndrom. *Dtsch. Med. Wochenschr.*, 108, 389–391 (1983).

Solh, H.M., Azoury, R.S. et al. Peutz–Jeghers Syndrom . . . *J. Pediatr.*, 103, 593–595 (1983).

Tovar, J.A., Eizaguirre, I. et al. Peutz–Jeghers syndrome in children . . . review of the literature. *J. Pediatr. Surg.*, 18, 1–6 (1983).

Walecki, J.K., Hales, E.D. et al. Ultrasound contribution to diagnosis of Peutz–Jeghers syndrome . . . *Pediatr. Radiol.*, 14, 62–64 (1984).

Shields, H.M. Peutz–Jeghers syndrome . . . *Gastroenterology*, 93, 1135–1141 (1987).

Giardiello, F.M., Welsh, S.B. et al. Increased risk of cancer in the Peutz–Jeghers syndrome, *N. Engl. J. Med.*, 316, 1511–1514 (1987).

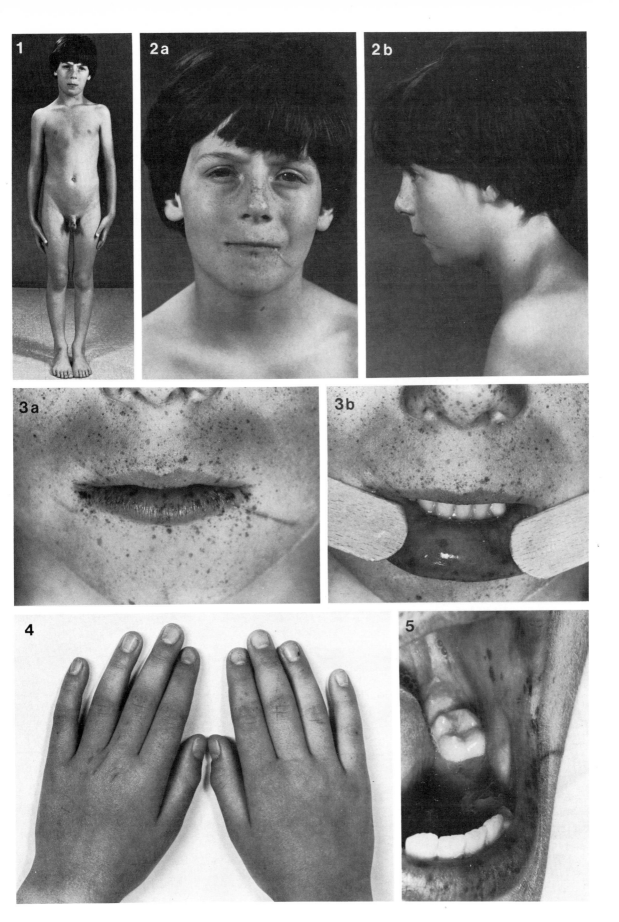

163. Rothmund–Thomson Syndrome

(Congenital Poikiloderma)

A hereditary disorder of early onset of 'mottling' of the skin frequently combined with development of cataracts, growth deficiency, and other anomalies.

Main signs:
1. 'Poikiloderma' (mottled skin) as a result of erythema with subsequent patchy atrophy, hyper- and depigmentation, and reticular telangiectasia involving the face, ears, back of the hands, underarms, extensor surfaces of the legs, and other areas exposed to light. Photosensitivity. Possibly absence of most of the eyebrows (as a sign of atrophy), involvement of the prolabium, eventual development of spotty hyperkeratoses of the backs of the hands and fingers (1–2).
2. Bilateral cataract in some cases.
3. Frequently proportional short stature (very variable; 'triangular' face with prominent forehead and low nasal root; small hands and feet with brachydactyly.

Supplementary findings:
Frequent generalized or partial hypotrichosis; anomalies of nails and teeth.

Cryptorchidism and other signs of hypogonadism.

Skeletal anomalies, especially of the extremities (e.g., hypo- or aplasia of the first ray of the upper extremities) in about half of the cases.

Manifestation: Development of skin changes in early childhood (early infancy), of cataracts usually between the second and eighth years of life.

Etiology: Inherited disorder, autosomal recessive transmission (uniformity of the syndrome? genetic heterogeneity of cases with and without cataract?). Substantially more frequent in females—up to 75% of observed cases.

Frequency: Low (around 100 cases described).

Course, prognosis: Life expectancy normal—unless skin cancer is induced as a result if marked photosensitivity combined with the atrophic skin and hyperkeratoses, which is unusual.

Differential diagnosis: Bloom syndrome (p.360).

Treatment: Symptomatic. Protection from the sun. Oncological surveillance when indicated. Genetic counseling.

Illustrations:
1 and 1a A 5-year-old girl with typical poikiloderma congenitum.
2 A 4½-year-old girl similarly affected.

H.-R.W.

References:
Rodermund, O.-E. and Hausmann, D. Das Rothmund-Syndrom. Z. Hautkr., 52, 129 (1977).
Hall, J.G., Pagon, R.A. et al. Rothmund–Thomson syndrome with severe dwarfism. Am. J. Dis. Child., 134, 165–169 (1980).
Dechenne, C., Chantraine, J.M. et al. A Rothmund–Thomson case with hypertension. Clin. Genet., 24, 266–272 (1983).
Nathanson, M., Dandine, M. et al. Syndrome de Rothmund–Thomson avec glaucome. Ann. Pédiatr., 30, 520–525 (1983).
Starr, D.G., McClure, J.P. et al. Non-dermatological complications and genetic aspects of the Rothmund–Thomson syndrome. Clin. Genet., 27, 102–104 (1985).
Pagon, R.A. Rothmund–Thomson syndrome. In: Gomez, M.R. (ed.) Neurocutaneous Diseases. Butterworths, Boston, 1987 (chapter 12).
Vanscheidt, E., Wolff, G. et al. Rothmund–Syndrom oder Thomsen-Syndrom . . . Monatsch. Kinderheilkd., 136, 264–269 (1988).

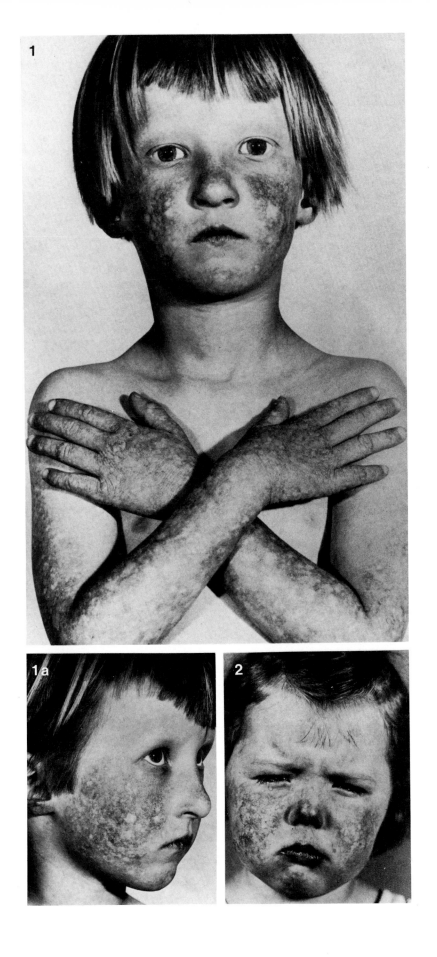

164. Xeroderma Pigmentosum

A hereditary disorder of hypersensitivity to sunlight and photophobia starting early in life, development of pigment anomalies, and early development of skin cancer or precancerous lesions.

Main signs:

1. Hypersensitivity to sunlight and photophobia (to ultraviolet light) from birth.
2. Development of hyper- and depigmentation (**1, 2**).
3. Development of precancerous lesions and of skin cancer in the light-damaged areas.
4. Especially endangered areas are the lips and the eyes (with possible development of keratitis and corneal scars, and of malignant growths on the conjunctiva and eyelids).

Manifestation: Photophobia from birth; skin changes from early to late infancy.

Etiology: Hereditary disorder. Usually autosomal recessive inheritance (eight different types, usually endonuclease defects—excision repair defects—with the same clinical course). A much rarer autosomal dominant type with less severe course, longer life expectancy, ability to reproduce.

Frequency: Relatively low in Europeans.

Course, prognosis: Unfavorable. Progressive disorder. Some patients develop neurological disorders, mental deterioration, cerebral atrophy, choreoathetosis, ataxia, spasticity (the minor DNA repair disorders are found in this group of cases). Death usually before age 20 years. Patients in the other groups (with the most marked DNA disorders) do not show neurological signs and live longer.

Treatment: As far as possible, avoidance of exposure to sunlight; regular application of a sunscreen lotion (Contralum®*) early excision of precancerous lesions. Oral administration of high doses of isotretinoin seems to be effective in preventing skin cancer. Genetic counseling of the parents.

Illustrations:

1 and 2 A 5-year-old boy. Development of hypersensitivity to sunlight early in life; appearance of pigmented moles and telangiectases on the face and hands starting in the second year of life. Now all sunlight-exposed areas of the skin are covered with small hyper- and depigmented spots and telangiectases. Up to this age, ten precancerous lesions. Additional development of numerous hemangiomas and multiple keratoacanthomas.

H.-R.W./J.K.

---

* A special ointment for treating xeroderma pigmentosum, manufactured in Germany but available in other countries.

References:

Any dermatology text book.

Maher, V.M., Rowan, L.A. et al. Frequency of UV-induced neoplastic transformation of diploid human fibroblasts is higher in xeroderma pigmentosum cells . . . *Proc. Natl. Acad. Sci.*, 79, 2613–2617 (1982).

Welshimer, K. and Swift, M. Congenital malformations and developmental disabilities in . . . xeroderma pigmentosum families. *Am. J. Hum. Genet.*, 34, 781–793 (1982).

Imray, P., Hockey, A. et al. Sensitivity to ultraviolet radiation in a dominantly inherited form of xeroderma pigmentosum. *J. Med. Genet.*, 23, 72–78 (1986).

Robbins, J.H. Xeroderma pigmentosum. In: Gomez, M.R. (ed.) *Neurocutaneous Diseases*. Butterworths, Boston, 1987 (chapter 10).

Kraemer, K.H., DiGiovanna, J.J. et al. Prevention of skin cancer in xeroderma pigmentosum with the use of oral isotretinoin. *N. Engl. J. Med.*, 318, 1633–1637 (1988).

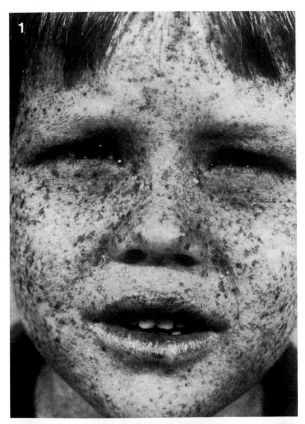

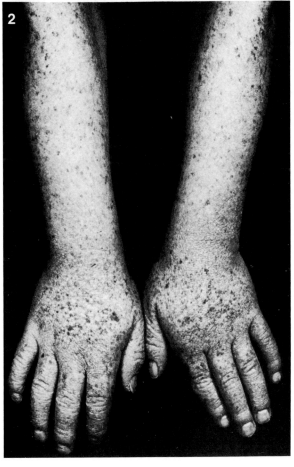

165. Von Recklinghausen Neurofibromatosis

A characteristic hereditary disorder of multiple café au lait spots, skin tumors, and skeletal, neurological, and other signs.

Main signs:

1. Variable numbers of café au lait spots, especially on the trunk; also various other pigmentation anomalies (1–9, 12).

2. Multiple fibromas or neurofibromas and other dysplastic intra- and subcutaneous growths along the peripheral nerves and other locations (e.g., optic glioma) (11, 12).

3. Frequent neurological or ocular disorders (e.g., due to nerve compression) (1, 2).

4. Frequent skeletal anomalies: congenital pseudarthrosis of the tibia, club foot, dislocation of the hip; development of kyphoscoliosis; cystic-sclerotic lesions (seen on X-ray) (9, 3, 4). Partial macrosomia in some cases (1, 10).

5. Mental retardation in about 10%, seizure disorder in about 15% of cases.

Supplementary findings: Macrocrania and ocular changes are frequent (neurofibroma of the eyelid, corneal clouding; Lisch nodules of the iris in over 90% of school-age or older patients). Possible precocious puberty or development of pheochromocytoma.

Manifestation: From birth onwards. Initially often only café au lait spots or freckle-like pigmentation, with gradual increase in size and number.

Etiology: Autosomal dominant disorder with 100% penetrance, but very variable expression. About half of the cases represent new mutations. Gene probably located on chromosome 17.

Frequency: relatively high. Estimation: 1 case in every 2,500–3,300 births.

Course, prognosis: In principle, progression can be expected. Blindness, paresis or paralysis, signs of paraplegia, etc., may occur. Possibility of developing dysplastic tumours also on the deep-lying peripheral nerves; on sympathetic nerves, on the spinal roots, cranial nerves, or retina; in the brain or intraspinally; on the adrenals, kidneys, and other locations. Also danger of later development of malignancy in these sites in over 5% of cases.

Diagnosis: At least six café au lait spots of more than 1.5 cm diameter can be considered diagnostic of neurofibromatosis. Lisch nodules of the iris (slit lamp) and pigmented moles of the axilla (axillary freckling) are diagnostically valuable.

Differential diagnosis: Multiple lentigenes syndrome (p.324); perhaps also McCune–Albright syndrome (p.320). Patients showing signs of classic neurofibromatosis as well as of Noonan syndrome (p.196) are said to have 'neurofibromatosis–Noonan syndrome'. It is still unclear whether this represents a variant of neurofibromatosis I or is an independent autosomal dominant disorder.

Note: The above applied to the 'classic' (so-called von Recklinghausen, peripheral, or type I) form of neurofibromatosis. Additional forms, especially the so-called acoustic or central type, or type II, with the main sign being bilateral acoustic neuromas occurring in the second to third decade of life, show only minimal skin changes, and no Lisch nodules. Type II is at least 100 times less common than type I.

Treatment: Symptomatic. Genetic counseling.

Illustrations:

1 A pre-school child from a neurofibromatosis kindred. Clusters of café au lait spots; small tumors of the head and left leg; tumorous macrosomia of the right leg (histologically: neurofibromatosis); intraspinal space-occupying lesion; hypertrophy of the clitoris; congenital dislocation of hips.

2 and 12 A 5-year-old patient, fibroma on the left thigh, multiple smaller tumors and xanthoma tuberosum. Macrocephaly, ataxia; mild mental retardation. Coxa vara. Neurofibromatosis kindred.

3 A 10-year-old patient: multiple café au lait spots, kyphoscoliosis, mental retardation.

4 A 13-year-old patient: hyperpigmented areas, up to palm size; fibromas; bulbous deformity of the nose; thoracic gibbus; mild mental retardation.

5–8 A 12-year-old patient; short stature, kyphosis, bilateral Lisch nodules; pigmentary anomalies of the fundus.

9 A 5-year-old patient; neurofibromatosis kindred; sacrococcygeal deformity; café au lait spots, short stature, congenital heart defect, hypertelorism, strabismus, prominent optic disc on the left, mental retardation.

10 Left-sided macrodactyly in a 12-year-old patient studded with café au lait spots; hypertelorism, facial asymmetry, fibroma.

11 The back of a woman from a neurofibromatosis kindred.

H.-R.W.

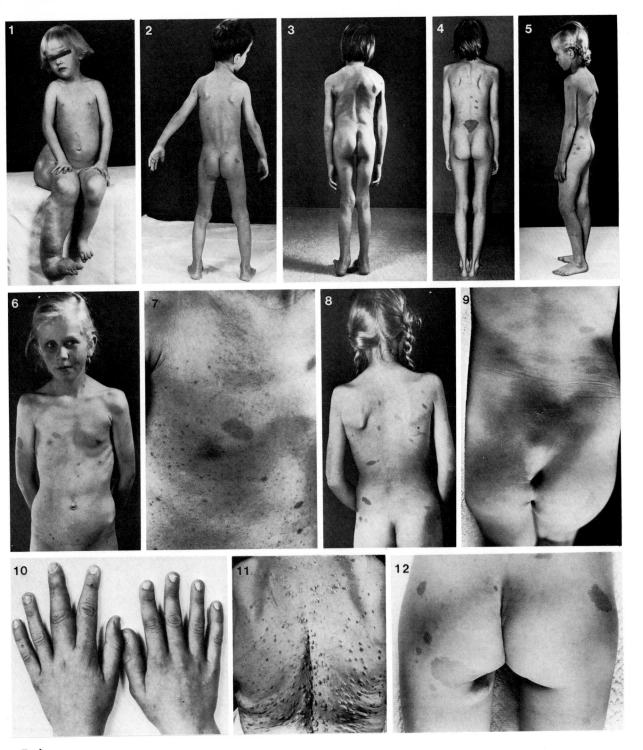

References:

Flüeler, U. and Boltshauser, E. Iris hamartomata as diagnostic criterion in neurofibromatosis. *Neuropediatrics*, 17, 183–185 (1986).

Boltshauser, E. Letter to the editor. *Klin. Pädiatr.*, 199, 385 (1987).

Meinecke, P. Evidence that the 'Neurofibromatosis–Noonan syndrome' is a variant of von Recklinghausen neurofibromatosis. *Am. J. Med. Genet.*, 26, 741–745 (1987).

Quattrin, T., McPherson, E. et al. Vertical transmission of the neurofibromatosis/Noonan syndrome. *Am. J. Med. Genet.*, 26, 645–649 (1987).

Riccardi, V.M. Neurofibromatosis. In: Gomez, M.R. (ed.) *Neurocutaneous Diseases*. Butterworths, Boston, 1987, pp.11–29.

Abuelo, D. and Meryash, D. Neurofibromatosis with fully expressed Noonan syndrome. *Am. J. Med. Genet.*, 29, 937–941 (1988).

DiSimone, R.E., Berman, A.T. et al. The orthopedic manifestations of neurofibromatosis. *Clin. Orthopaed.*, 230, 277–283 (1988).

Stambolian, D. and Zackai, E.H. Gene location in neurofibromatosis. *Am. J. Med. Genet.*, 29, 963–965 (1988).

Leading article: Genetic markers for neurofibromatosis. *Lancet*, II, 719–720 (1988).

166. Goltz–Gorlin Syndrome

(Focal Dermal Hypoplasia)

A complex mesoectodermal hereditary defect characterized by focal dermal atrophy with hernias of adipose tissue, associated with a multitude of skeletal, dental, eye, and other anomalies.

Main signs:
1. Approximately lentil-sized areas of dermal atrophy in an irregular—netlike, wormlike, or striped—or a systematic distribution, together with corresponding larger foci with hernias of adipose tissue (1). Also, pigmentation changes, telangiectases, scars (from congenital skin defects) and possible papillomas of the lips, gums, and genital and/or anal regions.
2. Skeletal anomalies: syndactyly (2, 3); hypo- and/or aplasia of rays of the fingers and/or toes (5) in addition to more extensive dysmelia. Hypo- and aplasia also of the truncal skeleton, in some cases leading to kyphoscoliosis, etc.
3. Malpositioning and hypo- and aplasia of the teeth. Hypo- and dysplasia of the nails (2b, 5). Disorders of hair growth (hypotrichosis or local alopecia).
4. Possible eye anomalies such as coloboma, aniridia, microphthalmos, and other.

Supplementary findings: Microcephaly, mental retardation, short stature, asymmetry or hemihypoplasia, ear anomalies, and many other developmental defects may occur.

Radiologically, characteristic longitudinal striation of the metaphyses of the long bones.

Manifestation: Skin changes usually present at birth or developing shortly thereafter from erythematous areas. Papillomas usually develop later.

Etiology: Genetically determined syndrome with very variable expression; predominantly sporadic cases, with females almost exclusively affected. The assumption is of X-linked dominance of the mutated gene with intrauterine lethal effect, almost without exception, in males.

Frequency: Low; about 100 cases reported up to 1985 (of these, 9 were boys).

Course, prognosis: Dependent on the type and severity of non-cutaneous involvement.

Differential diagnosis: Mainly the Bloch–Sulzberger syndrome (p.338).

Treatment: Symptomatic (multidisciplinary care may be needed). Genetic counseling.

Illustrations:
1–5 The second child of healthy young nonconsanguineous parents. Typical skin changes and additional anomalies much more pronounced on the right side (2, 4: diaphragmatic hernia, 5). Partial 2/3 syndactyly and fifth finger clinodactyly of the right hand (2b). Aplasia of the twelfth rib on the right. Aplasia of two rays of the right foot (5). Radiologically: typical 'osteopathia striata'.

H.-R.W.

References:

Braun-Falco, O. and Hoffmann, C. Das Goltz–Gorlin-Syndrom. *Hautarzt*, 26, 393 (1975).
Happle, R. and Lenz, W. Striation of bones in focal dermal hypoplasia . . . *Br. J. Dermatol.*, 96, 113 (1977).
Fryns, J.P., Dhondt, F., Lindemans, L. et al. Focal dermal hypoplasia (Goltz's syndrome) in a male. *Acta Paed. Belg.*, 31, 37 (1978).
Kunze, J., Heyne, K., Wiedemann, H.-R. Diaphragmatic hernia in a female newborn with focal dermal hypoplasia and marked asymmetric malformations (Goltz–Gorlin syndrome). *Eur. J. Pediatr.*, 131, 213–218 (1979).
Römke, C., Gödde–Salz, E., Grote, W. Investigations of chromosomal stability in the Gorlin–Goltz syndrome. *Arch. Dermatol. Res.*, 277, 370–372 (1985).
Wechsler, M.A., Papa, C.M. et al. Variable expression in focal dermal hypoplasia. *Am. J. Dis. Child.*, 142, 297–300 (1988).

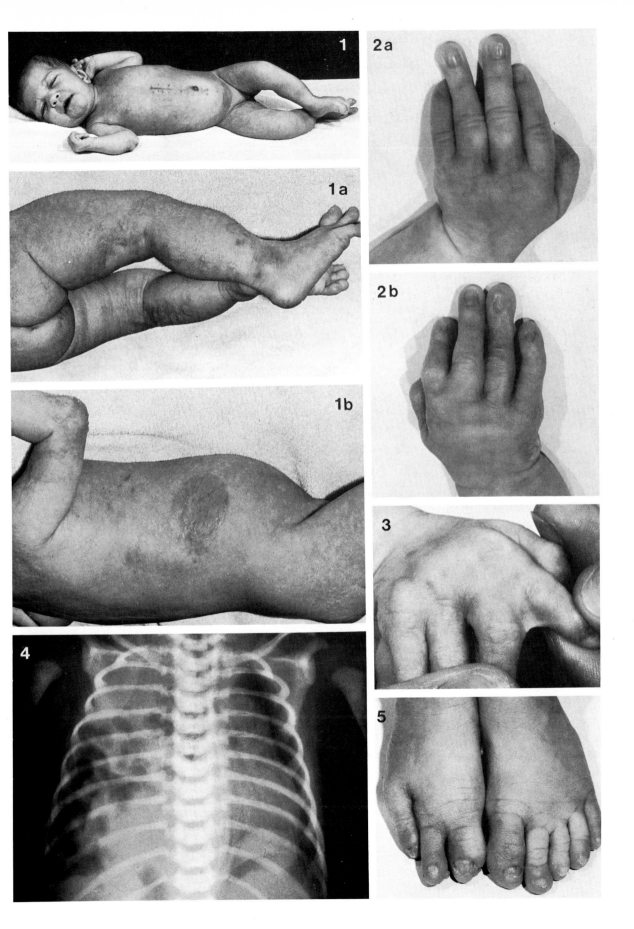

335

167. Syndrome of Hemihypoplasia and Symmetrical Localized Dermal Atrophy of the Hands and Feet

A clinical picture of congenital general hemihypoplasia, symmetrical foci of atrophied skin and subcutaneous fat on the hands and feet, and other anomalies.

Main signs:
1. Right-sided hemitrophy affecting the entire half of the body clinically and radiologically, with marked shortening of the tibia (humerus, radius, and ulna about 4–5 mm, femur about 6 mm, fibula about 7 mm, and tibia about 11 mm shorter than the opposite side) (**1–4**).
2. Atrophy of subcutaneous fatty tissue and overlying skin, which is thin and wrinkled and never showed vesicular or other changes, symmetrically over the extensor surfaces of the wrists and ankles, more pronounced on the right than the left (**3**, **4**). No fat herniation, no telangiectasis. Skin of the right abdominal region somewhat less pigmented than that of the left; fine, diffuse hemangioma-like changes on the back, more pronounced on the right; one café au lait spot each on the left shoulder, the left elbow, and the right arm.

Supplementary findings: Flat face with widely spaced eyes, epicanthus. Left supernumerary nipple. Short thumbs bilaterally, deep insertion of the big toes; toe malpositioned and occasionally incurved, more so on the right than the left.

Radiologically, distinct aortic configuration of the heart. Kidneys normal on pyelogram. Skeletal survey negative for calcium flecks ('stippling') and longitudinal striation of the metaphyses.

Manifestation: At birth.

Etiology: Not established with certainty.

Course: At age 8 years, height below the second percentile; the right arm now 2 cm shorter, and the right leg about 5 cm shorter than the left. Small cranium, eyes normal, small triangular mouth, severe malpositioning of the teeth. Widely spaced nipples. Atrophic lesions of the skin and subcutaneous fat unchanged. Faint depigmentations on all extremities. Expressionless face, mental retardation; no seizures or physical handicap. Bone age delayed about three years in the right hand and two years in the left.

Comment: Goltz–Gorlin syndrome (p.334) had to be considered in the case presented here; however, in addition to other signs, the characteristic fat hernias and striations of the metaphyses on X-ray were not present. Most likely to be the result of early varicella infection of the embryo (the so-called congenital varicella syndrome), although no evidence at all from the maternal history of a corresponding viral infection.

Illustrations:
1–4 A 7-month-old girl, the second child of healthy parents. Birth after an otherwise unremarkable full-term twin pregnancy, length 48 cm, weight 2800 g, and head circumference 34 cm. Slightly retarded statomotor development, mental development initially considered normal. Measurements (including head circumference) in the low–normal range. Ocular fundi normal; neurological examination normal. Chromosome analysis normal. Laboratory chemistries and serological examinations normal.

H.-R.W.

References:
Schlotfeldt-Schäfer, I., Schaefer, P. et al. Congenitales Varicellensyndrom. *Monatsch. Kinderheilkd.*, 131, 106–108 (1983).
König, R., Gutjahr, P. et al. Konnatale Varizellen-Embryo-Fetopathie. *Helv. Pediatr. Acta*, 40, 391–398 (1985).
Unger-Köppel, J., Kilcher, P. et al. Varizellenfetopathie. *Helv. Paediatr. Acta*, 40, 399–404 (1985).
Alkalay, A.L., Pomerance, J.J. et al. Fetal varicella syndrome. *J. Pediatr.*, 111, 320–323 (1987).

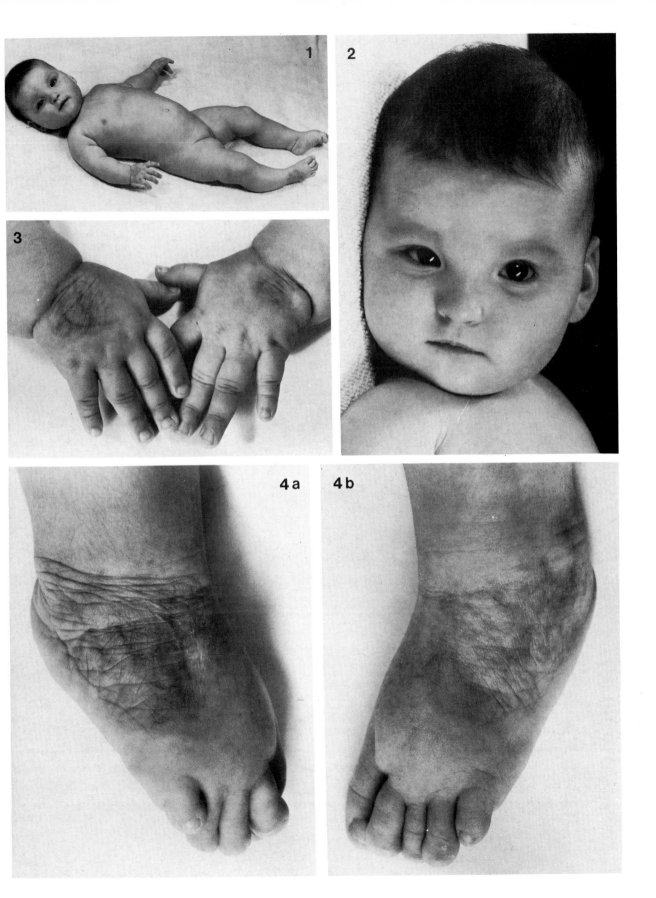

337

168. Incontinentia Pigmenti

(Bloch–Sulzberger Syndrome)

A hereditary dermatosis—herpetiform dermatitis, patchy or verrucous hyperkeratosis and/or streaky hyperpigmentation—with anomalies of the dentition, central nervous system, and eyes.

Main signs:

1. Skin manifestations can be divided into three stages:

I Papules, vesicles, and pustules on an erythematous base, frequently linear distribution, usually sparing the face, present at birth or appearing during the first months of life, persisting or taking an intermittent course for several months (1), occasionally for years.

II Somewhat macular or verrucous pigmented hyperkeratoses following the lesions in stage I, also usually lasting several months (2, 3), occasionally years.

III Dirty-brown, streaky, garland-like distribution of hyperpigmentation, frequently symmetrical, preferentially affecting the lateral trunk, axillae, groin, and thighs (3–6).

The stages occur consecutively with overlap. Stage III may occur on previously normal skin, usually healing completely by the third decade of life, occasionally with residual depigmentation.

2. Dental anomalies almost always present (delayed eruption, malformed teeth, hypodontia). Focal alopecia common; nail deformities less common.

Supplementary findings: In about 30%, eye anomalies (strabismus, cataract, pseudoglioma, and others) and CNS disorders (spastic tetraplegia, seizure disorder, mental retardation, and others), microcephaly.

In stage I, up to 50% blood eosinophils; eosinophilic granulocytes in the vesicles.

Manifestation: Stage I, at birth and in early infancy. Stage II, principally in the 2nd–6th week and stage III in the 12th–26th week of life.

Etiology: The prevailing view is of an X-linked dominant disorder. The mutated gene is usually lethal *in utero* for males, so that girls are affected almost exclusively (about 97%).

Frequency: About 1:40,000 girls. Over 650 cases, 16 of them male, became known in the past 50 years.

Course, prognosis: In the absence of severe neurological impairment, life expectancy normal,

Differential diagnosis: Goltz–Gorlin syndrome (p.334), Ito syndrome (p.340), among others.

Treatment: None known, even for the skin disorder. Genetic counseling; prenatal diagnosis by means of DNA analysis.

Illustrations:

1 Patient 1 at age 2 weeks; male infant, but with Klinefelter syndrome (XXY sex chromosomes). Tooth buds present. Neurologically unremarkable.
2 and 3 Patient 2 at ages 2 months and 16 months. Hypodontia. Seizure disorder since the seventh week of life. Normal intelligence.
4 Patient 3 at age 19 months, up to then normal psychological development. Delayed dentition, hypodontia.
5 and 6 Patient 4 at 12 years. Malformed teeth, microdontia. Seizure disorder since the fourth week of life, right-sided spastic hemiparesis.

H.-R.W.

References:

Carney, R.G., Jr. Incontinentia pigmenti. *Arch. Dermatol.*, 112, 535 (1976).
Kunze, J., Frenzel, U.H. et al. Klinefelter's syndrome and incontinentia pigmenti . . . *Hum. Genet.*, 35, 237–240 (1977).
Hohenauer, L. and Wilk, F. Incontinentia pigmenti. *Paediatr. Prax.*, 19, 417 (1977/78).
Korting, G.W. and Bechtold, M. Alternierende Manifestationsäquivalente der Incontinentia pigmenti in 2 Generationen. *Med. Welt.*, 31, 759 (1980).
Kurczynski, T.W., Berns, J.S. et al. Studies of a family with incontinentia pigmenti variably expressed in both sexes. *J. Med. Genet.*, 19, 447–451 (1982).
Lenz, W., Ullrich, E., Witkowski, R. et al. Halbseitige Incontinentia pigmenti . . . *Pädiatr. Pädol.*, 17, 187 (1982).
Hecht, F. and Hecht, B.K. The half chromatid mutation model and bidirectional mutation in incontinentia pigmenti. *Clin. Genet.*, 24, 177–179 (1983).
Sommer, A. and Liu, P.H. Incontinentia pigmenti in a father and his daughter. *Am. J. Med. Genet.*, 17, 655–659 (1984).
Avrahami, E., Harel, S. et al. Computed tomographic demonstration of brain changes in incontinentia pigmenti. *Am. J. Dis. Child.*, 139, 372–374 (1985).
O'Brien, J.E. and Feingold, M. Incontinentia pigmenti: a longitudinal study. *Am. J. Dis. Child.*, 139, 711–712 (1985).
Hodgson, S.V., Neville, B. et al. Two cases of X/autosome translocation in females with incontinentia pigmenti. *Hum. Genet.*, 71, 231–234 (1985).
Larsen, R., Ashwal, S. et al. Incontinentia pigmenti: association with anterior horn cell degeneration. *Neurology*, 37, 446–450 (1987).
Rosman, P. Incontinentia pigmenti. In: Gomez, M.R. (ed.) *Neurocutaneous Diseases*. Butterworths, Boston, 1987 (chapter 32).
Sefiani, A., Sinnett, D. et al. Linkage studies do not confirm the cytogenic location of continentia pigmenti on Xp11. *Hum. Genet.*, 80, 282–286 (1988).

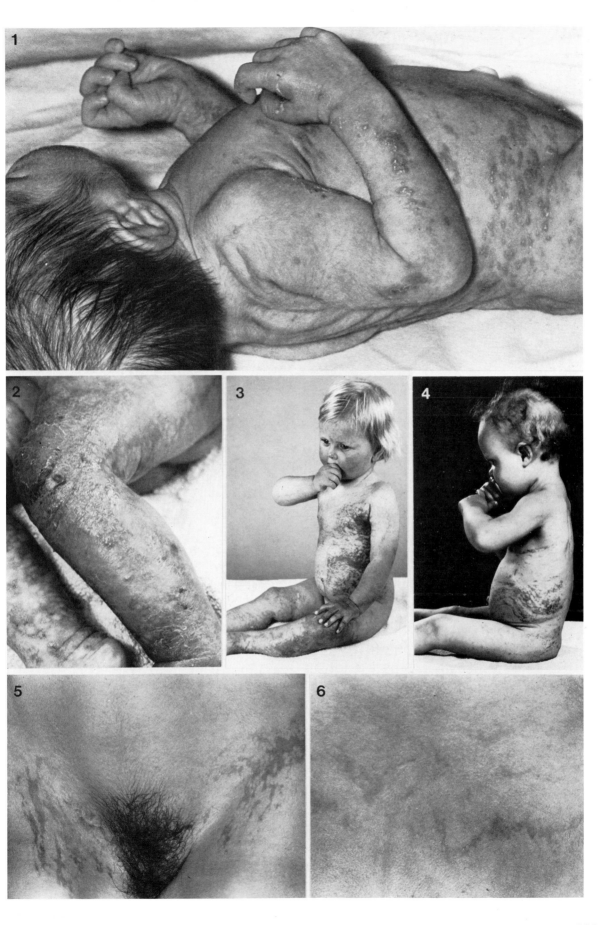

169. Hypomelanosis Ito

(Ito Syndrome; Incontinentia Pigmenti Achromians)

A hereditary neurocutaneous syndrome of streaky, patchy, or spray-like depigmentation of the skin, frequently associated with other diverse anomalies.

Main signs:
1. Systemic leukoderma, with bizarre, usually symmetrical (but occasionally unilateral) depigmented streaks, patches, whorls, or sprays. The changes follow Blaschko's lines (1–3), occurring most commonly on the trunk (not crossing the midline), less frequently on the face; mainly an axial course and on the flexor surfaces in the extremities. Apart from the hypopigmentation and occasional hyperkeratosis follicularis, the skin is unremarkable. No preceding or accompanying vesico-bullous or verrucous changes.
2. Associated noncutaneous anomalies in about half of the cases. Especially: CNS seizures or seizure disorders; psychomotor retardation; ophthalmological findings (strabismus, myopia, changes of the fundus, and others); dyscrania (e.g., macrocrania).

Supplementary findings: Hypertelorism, anomalies of the external ears, 'coarse' facies, sometimes with hypertrichosis; high or cleft palate possible. Hamartomatous growths on the upper and lower incisors.

Legs possibly of unequal lengths, or other asymmetries, scoliosis, hip dysplasia, and other skeletal anomalies.

Manifestation: Birth or early or late infancy. Obviously, the changes appear lighter and more marked in people with a dark complexion than in those with fair skin (in doubtful cases, examine under a Wood's lamp). During early childhood the depigmented areas may at least give the impression of spreading.

Etiology: Almost exclusively sporadic occurrence. Various chomosomal defects have been described. Sex ratio males : females about 1 : 2.5. For affected males, somatic mosaicism for an autosomal dominant gene defect that is lethal for ectoderm and its derivitives, has been suggested; this would imply no risk for the offspring of affected males. For affected females, X-linked dominant inheritance has been assumed.

Frequency: Considered low; about 100 cases reported.

Course, prognosis: Dependent on the presence and severity of associated anomalies. The depigmented skin areas may darken with time.

Differential diagnosis: Bloch–Sulzberger syndrome (p.338), which has been described as the 'negative' of Ito syndrome. However, 'incontinentia pigmenti' hyperpigmentation is the residual of an inflammatory process (with a different histological picture and mode of inheritance).

Treatment: Symptomatic. Genetic counseling.

Illustrations:
1–3 A 5-year-old boy with typical Ito syndrome. Depigmentation noted in the first year of life, which subsequently increased in size and area. In early infancy, abnormal growth of skull (hydrocephalus); insertion of a shunt. A focal seizure disorder starting in infancy, eventually well controlled. Tapetoretinal degeneration with poor visual acuity; strabismus, nystagmus. Hearing normal. Delayed statomotor, good intellectual development. Sturdy, stocky body build; dark complexion. No hyperpigmented lesions. Follicular hyperkeratoses of the arms and back. Foci of alopecia on the top of the head; mild hypertrichosis of the face and back. Macrocranium; CT scan now normal. Impaired motor coordination, right more than left; EEG still with focal changes. IQ (for language) 112. Slight mongoloid slant of the palpebral fissures, epicanthi, high palate, malpositioning of the teeth, and long, narrow, peglike front teeth. Short, broad neck with low nuchal hairline. Increased dorsal kyphosis and compensatory lumbar lordosis. Elevation of the right gluteal fold, hypoplasia of the right gluteal region. Loose excessive tissue in the left flank. Scrotum palmatum (surgically corrected); small penis with true phimosis. Small hands with abnormally abductable thumbs; small feet with zygodactyly.

H.-R.W.

References:
Pfeiffer, R.-A., Happle, R., Stupperich, G. Das Syndrom von Ito . . . *Klin. Pädiatr.*, 188, 181 (1976).
Schwartz, M.F., Jr., Esterly, N.B., Fretzin, D.F. et al. Hypomelanosis of Ito . . . *J. Pediatr.*, 90, 236 (1977).
Ortonne, J.-P., Coiffet, J., Floret, D. Hypomélanose de Ito, *Ann. Dermatol. Venereol.*, 106, 47 (1979).
Happle, R. and Vakilzadeh, F. Hamartomatous dental cups in hypomelanosis of Ito. *Clin. Genet.*, 21, 65 (1982).
Rosemberg, S., Arita, F.N. et al. Hypomelanosis of Ito . . . *Neuropediatrics,* 15, 52–55 (1984).
Meinecke, P., Müller, E.P. et al. Das Ito-Syndrom. *Pädiatr. Prax.*, 32, 129–137 (1985/86).
Happle, R. Tentative assignment of hypomelanosis of Ito to 9q33 → qter. *Hum. Genet.*, 75, 98–99 (1987).
Moss, C. and Burn, J. Genetic counselling in hypomelanosis of Ito . . . review. *Clin. Genet.*, 34, 109–115 (1988).

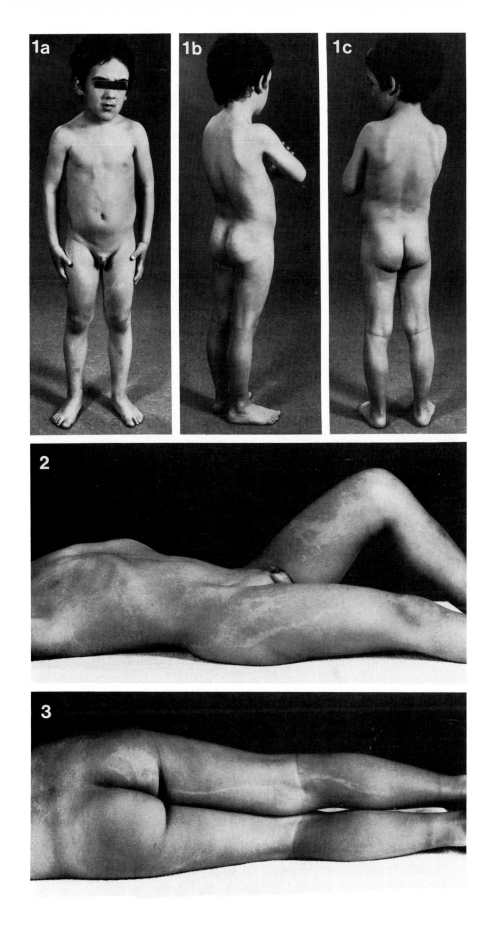

170. Tuberous Sclerosis

(Bourneville Syndrome)

A characteristic hereditary disorder comprising skin changes, mental retardation, and epileptic manifestations.

Main signs:
1. Skin changes:
a. Varying numbers of 'white spots': irregular but sharply outlined leaf- or lancet-shaped areas of depigmentation 0.5–3.0 cm in diameter on the trunk and/or extremities (1).
b. Butterfly-like yellow-red nodular paranasal rash also on the cheeks and chin (so-called adenoma sebaceum, Pringle type; 2–6).
c. Possible fibroepitheliomas, shagreen patch (lumbosacral, also facial), sub- or periungual angiofibromas (8a, 8b).
2. Mental retardation—frequent and often severe.
3. Seizure disorder (initially very often as jacknife of salaam spasms, then possibly grand mal or any of the other forms). Possible spastic pareses.

Supplementary findings: Occasionally, tumors of the lids or nodules of the conjunctiva. Frequent mushroom- or mulberry-like nodules in the optic disc or elsewhere in the fundus.

Not infrequently, pit-like enamel defects of the teeth, depigmented tufts of hair.

Often renal tumors and cysts (usually bilaterally (9); often angiomyolipomas) and/or rhabdomyomas of the heart.

Tumor-like nodules of the cerebral cortex, ventricular or subependymal hamartomas (7)—possibly leading to obstructive hydrocephalus, malignant degeneration, etc.—with strong tendency to calcify.

Manifestation: White spots usually the first cutaneous abnormality, often from birth (in up to 90% of cases, seen in the first years of life). Usually early onset of seizures (first two years of life). 'Adenoma sebaceum' rarely in infancy, usually not until later (2–6).

Etiology: Autosomal dominant disorder, variable expression, incomplete penetrance. New mutation in two-thirds of cases. Gene localized to the long arm of chromosome 9.

Frequency: Not low; estimated 1:20,000–40,000.

Course, prognosis: Essentially progressive. The mental status—in some cases normal—may deteriorate at any time (whereas seizures are more readily controlled or decrease with increasing age). Death (in status epilepticus, from cardiac rhabdomyoma, or as a result of renal tumors) not infrequently before adulthood.

Diagnosis: Jacknife of salaam spasms and white spots in an infant should suggest tuberous sclerosis. In light-skinned individuals, a Wood's lamp may be needed to identify white spots. Intracranial foci can now be detected more easily and earlier by CT and NMR scan. Also in potential gene carriers. (In rare cases, CT scan of the parents negative, but further offspring affected suggesting reduced penetrance.)

Treatment: Symptomatic (possibly including cosmetic skin surgery). Genetic counseling.

Illustrations:
1, 5, 6, and 8a A child at age 10 and 12 years. Multiple white spots on the trunk, increasing adenoma sebaceum, periungual fibroma of the big toe. Fine macular skin depigmentation and fibromatous plaques. Increased intracranial pressure, unilateral exophthalmos, diplopia, and facial paresis; intracranial calcification; space-occupying lesion in one kidney.
2 and 8b A 4-year-old boy with primary Pringle nevus, subungual fibroma, white spots, macrocephaly, choreoathetosis.
3 A 3-year-old patient with distinct Pringle nevus, white spots, hamartoma in the nasal meatus; macrocephaly, markedly decreased visual acuity, tumors of the fundus.
4 and 9 A 7½-year-old patient, microcephaly, secondarily increased intracranial pressure; palpable kidney tumors, possible cardiac involvement.
7 Pneumoencephalogram (PEG) of a 7-year-old patient with white spots, Pringle nevus, shagreen patch, and fundal involvement; lateral indentation of the right lateral ventricle.

Mental retardation and a history of epilepsy in all five children (in **3**, onset with infantile spasms).

H.-R.W.

References:
Flinter, F.A. and Neville, B.G.R. Examining the parents of children with tuberous sclerosis. *Lancet*, II, 1167 (1986).
Connor, J.M., Stephenson, J.B.P. et al. Non-penetrance in tuberous sclerosis. *Lancet*, II, 1275 (1986).
McLaurin, R.L. and Towbin, R.B. Tuberous sclerosis diagnostic and surgical considerations. *Pediatr. Neurosci.*, 12, 43–48 (1986).
Fryer, A.E., Connor, J.M. et al. Evidence that the gene for tuberous sclerosis is on chromosome 9. *Lancet*, I, 659–660 (1987).
Gomez, M.R. Tuberous sclerosis. In: *Neurocutaneous Diseases*. Butterworths, Boston, 1987, pp.30–52.
Terwey, B. and Doose, H. Tuberous sclerosis: magnetic imaging of the brain. *Neuropediatrics*, 18, 67–69 (1987).
Narla, L.D., Slovis, T.L. et al. The renal lesions of tuberosclerosis . . . screening with sonography and computerized tomography. *Pediatr. Radiol.*, 18, 205–209 (1988).

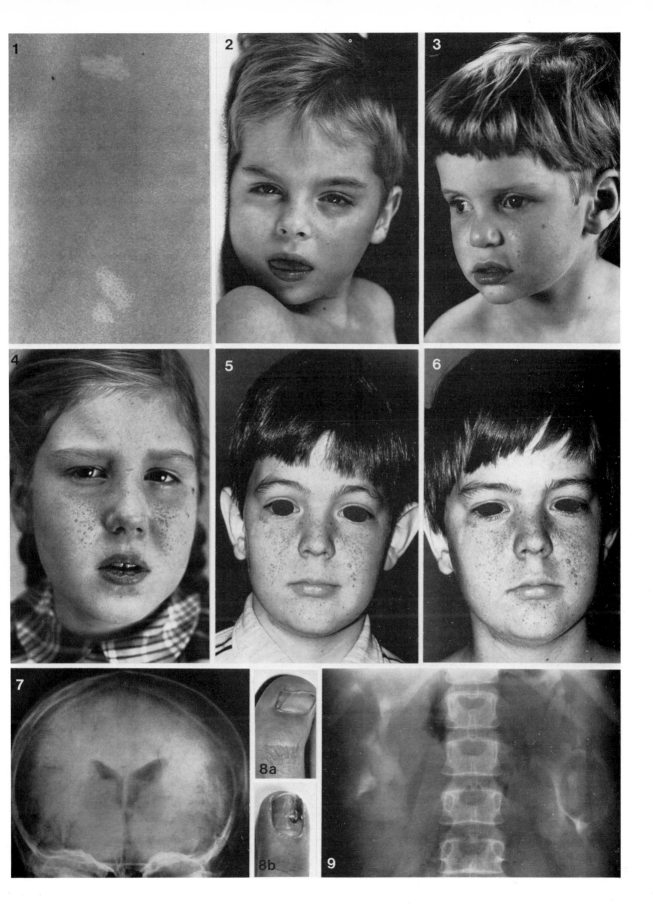

171. Waardenburg Syndrome Types I and II

Syndrome with facial anomalies, partial albinism, and possible deafness.

Main signs: Lateral displacement of the inner corners of the eyes ('dystopia canthorum' resulting in short palpebral fissures) and of the lacrimal ducts, both in type I only; broad, high nasal root and bridge (**1–3**); eyebrows quite pronounced medially, possible synophrys; strands of white hair above the midforehead (**1, 4**) and/or other signs of partial albinism; in some cases, congenital sensorineural hearing impairment (apparently much more frequent with type II, without dystophia canthorum; frequently bilateral and severe; altogether in about 40% or more of cases).

The facial appearance may be quite distinctive (see below).

Supplementary findings: Apart from a white forelock, partial albinism may be manifest as: pale blue coloring—or heterochromia—of the iris; depigmented areas of skin; pigment-free strands of hair elsewhere on the head; or pigmentation anomalies of the retina.

A relatively small cranium, thick heavy scalp hair with low anterior hairline, relative hypoplasia of the alae nasi, protrusion of the lower jaw and full lower lip may be present. Furthermore, hyperopia, Marcus Gunn ptosis; cleft lip and palate, occasionally combined with Hirschsprung disease (in types I and II); relatively short stature, diverse skeletal anomalies of the upper extremities (this sign apparently in a further variant or type). Occasional mental retardation.

Manifestation: At birth (for the malformations including hearing impairment). The white forelock may be present at birth and darken later on. Also, possible premature greying or whitening of the scalp hair, either generalized or localized.

Etiology: Genetic basis. Heterogeneity. Mode of transmission for both types autosomal dominant with considerably variable penetrance and expression. High paternal age favors new mutations.

Frequency: Estimation for Holland of 1:42,000 individuals, and of 4% of total cases with congenital deafness (1951); the latter figure for Thuringia approximately the same (1965); more than 1,300 reported cases by 1977.

Prognosis: Normal life expectancy. Crucial to the prognosis is whether a hearing impairment is present, whether uni- or bilateral, how severe, and whether progressive.

Diagnosis: From appearance (especially type I) and details of clinical findings, including an audiogram. Early diagnosis is important so that hearing can be evaluated and treatment started if impairment present (to avoid possible deaf-mutism and incorrect diagnosis of mental retardation).

Treatment: Symptomatic and as above. Genetic counseling.

Illustrations:
1 A 9-year-old girl and her mother, both with Waardenburg syndrome (probably type II). Note the striking facies in the child, with broad, coarsely formed nose, high nasal root, and white forelock (the forelock being more pronounced in the mother and her similarly affected twin sister). Further findings in the child: low anterior hairline and very thick hair; bluish sclerae; macular depigmentation of the trunk; increased lanugo hair on the back; small cranium; somewhat short stature; kyphoscoliosis; asymmetry of the thorax and slight coxa valga; high palate and caries; hyperopia; mild mental retardation; audiogram normal so far; normal female karyotype.
2–4 Two siblings, 3 years 4 months and 2 years 3 months old, with type I Waardenburg syndrome. Typical facies in both (distinct telecanthus—distance between the inner canthi 42 and 37 mm, characteristically formed nose with prominent root and broad, flat tip, synophrys; **2, 3**), but white forelock, which both girls showed at birth, no longer present (**4**: the younger sister). Right-sided severe and moderately severe sensorineural hearing impairment in both children; the younger also showing heterochromia of the iris (right blue, left green). The father of the girls and his mother both show the syndrome (white forelock, heterochromia of the iris), as does her mother, and the father's younger sister, and both of her children (typical facies, telecanthus, median white forelock).

H.-R.W.

References:

Ahrendts, H. Das Waardenburg-Syndrom, dargestellt in fünf Familien. *Z. Kinderheilkd.*, 93, 295 (1965).

De Haas, E.B.H. and Tan, K.E.W.P. Waardenburg's syndrome. *Docum. Ophthalmol.*, 21, 239 (1966).

Hageman, M.J. and Delleman, J.W. Heterogeneity in Waardenburg syndrome. *Am. J. Hum. Genet.*, 29, 468 (1977).

Meinecke, P. Das Waardenburg Syndrom Typ I. *Klin. Pädiatr.*, 194, 112 (1982).

Yoshino, M., Nakao, M. et al. Incidences of dystopia canthorum and some other signs in a family with Waardenburg syndrome type I. *Jpn. J. Hum. Genet.*, 31, 373–378 (1986).

Meire, F., Standaert, L., De Laey, J.J. et al. Waardenburg syndrome, Hirschsprung megacolon, and Marcus Gunn ptosis. *Am. J. Med. Genet.*, 27, 683–686 (1987).

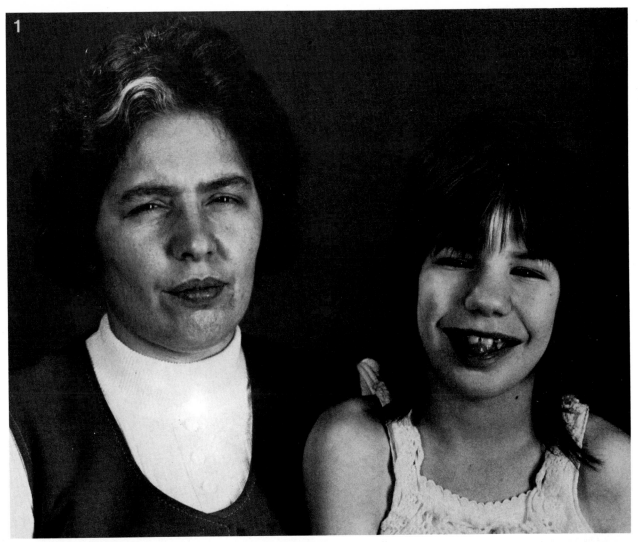

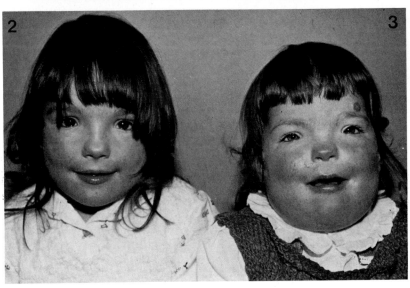

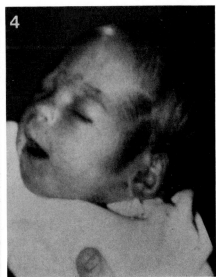

172. Piebaldness

Genetically determined, congenital, patchy localized hypopigmentation of the skin, found mostly on the ventral surfaces of head and trunk.

Main signs:
1. Circumscribed areas of skin devoid of pigmentation on the ventral surfaces of the head and trunk. White forelock; absent pigmentation medially of the eyebrows, eyelids, eyelashes, nose, and chin. Occasional pigmentation anomalies of the chest, abdomen, and ventral region of the arms and legs. Hands, wrists, feet, ankles, occipital region, back of the neck, and back are normally pigmented.
2. Hyperpigmented borders between the pigmented and unpigmented zones.

Supplementary findings: Islands of pigmentation within the hypopigmented areas; occasionally hypopigmentation of the gingiva, heterochromia of the iris. Histologically, melanocytes absent, but Langerhans cells present.

Manifestation: At birth or shortly thereafter.

Etiology: Incomplete migration of the melanocytes from the neural crest to the ventral midline or disorder of differentiation of ventrally lying melanoblasts. Autosomal dominant inheritance.

Frequency: Described worldwide, especially in the African population.

Course, prognosis: Normal life expectancy. No increased morbidity or mortality.

Treatment: Cosmetic.

Differential diagnosis: Clearly separate from Waardenburg syndromes I and II. Vitiligo (begins peripherally, progresses intermittently, and occurs anywhere on the body).

Illustrations:
1 Healthy 25-year-old, white forelock since birth.
2a–2c Diabetic 13-year-old with depigmentation of the forehead, extending to the left eyebrow, to the eyelid and eyelashes; also in the lateral eyebrow region and in front of the left ear (N.B. sides reversed in the pictures). Isolated islands of pigment. Remainder of skin normal.

J.K.

References:
Jahr, H.M. and McIntyre, M.S. Piebaldness, or familial white skin spotting (partial albinism). *Am. J. Dis. Child.*, 88, 481–484 (1954).
Comings, D.E. and Odland, G.F. Partial albinism. *JAMA*, 195, 510–523 (1966).
Taylor, D.R. Piebaldism, *Br. J. Dermatol.*, 95, 43–44 (1976).
Bonevandi, J.J., Baran, R., Breton, A. et al. Piebaldism. Clinical, pathological, and ultrastructural study of three cases. *Am. J. Dermatol. Venerol.*, 105, 67–72 (1978).
Hultén, M.A., Honeyman, M.M., Mayne, A.J. et al. Homozygosity in piebald trait. *J. Med. Genet.*, 24, 568–571 (1987).
Kaplan, P., de Chaderévian, J.-P. Piebaldism–Waardenburg syndrome . . . *Am. J. Med. Genet.*, 31, 679–688 (1988).

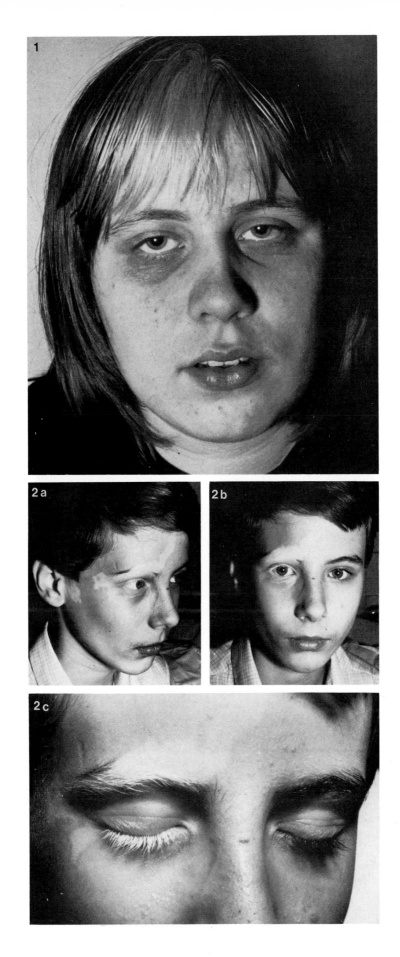

173. Oculocutaneous Albinism (Tyrosinase Negative Type)

The 'classic' form of albinism with total absence of pigment from all of the skin and hair and from the eyes and absent pigment formation in the tyrosinase test (see below).

Main signs:
1. Generalized absence of visible pigment in the skin and hair (1–4). No tanning of the skin. Absence of pigmented nevi and freckles. Light white hair.
2. Total pigment deficiency of the eyes. Unpigmented fundus, 'red pupils', translucent irides, appearing blue to grey-blue in oblique light. Marked nystagmus, pronounced photophobia, and poor vision. Incapable of binocular vision.
3. No pigment formation by hair roots incubated in L-tyrosine solution.

Supplementary findings: Possible additional anomalies of the eyes.

Manifestation: At birth.

Etiology: Hereditary defect with autosomal recessive inheritance.

Frequency: About 1:20,000 (1–2% of all persons are heterozygotes for albinism).

Course, prognosis: No change of the pigment deficiency, nor improvement in visual acuity during the course of life. Average life expectancy probably somewhat shortened by increased danger of accidents due to poor vision and increased disposition to develop skin cancer.

Differential diagnosis: Tyrosinase-positive oculocutaneous albinism (p.350) and other forms of albinism.

Treatment: Avoidance of exposure to sunlight (clothing, sun-ray filter cream). Tinted spectacles or contact lenses. Genetic counseling.

Illustrations:
1–3 Two people with this form of albinism.
4 Two affected brothers with their healthy sister.

H.-R.W.

References:

Witkop, C.J., Jr. et al. Oculocutaneous albinism. In: Nyhan, W.L. (ed.) *Heritable Disorders of Amino Acid Metabolism.* J. Wiley & Sons, New York, 1974.

Witkop, C.J., Jr., Jay, B. et al. Optic and otic neurologic abnormalities in oculocutaneous and ocular albinism. *Birth Defects,* 18, 6, 299–318 (1982).

van Dorp, D.B., Delleman, J.W. et al. Oculocutaneous albinism and anterior chamber cleavage malformations. *Clin. Genet.,* 26, 440–444 (1984).

King, R.A. Albinism. In: Gomez, M.R. (ed.) *Neurocutaneous Diseases.* Butterworths, Boston, 1987 (chapter 35).

Taylor, W.O.G. Prenatal diagnosis in albinism. *Lancet,* I, 1307–1308 (1987).

van Dorp, D.B. Albinism, or the NOACH syndrome. *Clin. Genet.,* 31, 228–242 (1987).

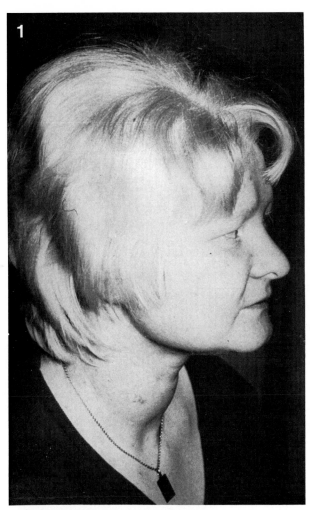

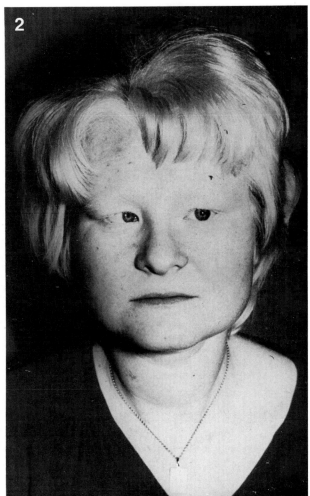

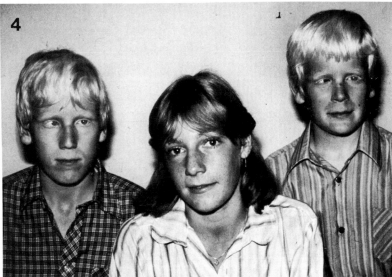

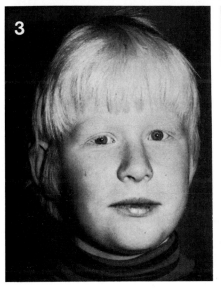

174. Oculocutaneous Albinism (Tyrosinase Positive Type)

('Albinism Type II')

Oculocutaneous albinism with decreased pigment in all of the skin, the hair, and the eyes, and evidence of pigment formation in the tyrosinase test (see below).

Main signs:
1. Generalized decrease of pigment of all skin and hair. (**1**, **2**). The degree of pigment deficiency depends on age (and race), and the clinical picture of this form varies from that of 'classic' albinism (p.348) to that of a normal pale complexion. Pigmented nevi and freckles may be present.
2. Pigment deficiency of the eyes. Unpigmented fundus and 'red pupils' in early childhood (possibly with some improvement later). Translucent irides. Distinct nystagmus and photophobia (but both less severe than in 'classic' albinism). Poor vision. Absence of binocular vision.
3. Pigment formation by hair roots incubated in L-tyrosine solution.

Supplementary findings: Possible additional eye anomalies.

Manifestation: At birth.

Etiology: Hereditary defect with autosomal recessive inheritance.

Frequency: About 1:20,000 (in American Negroes about 1:15,000, in Ibos about 1:1,000).

Course, prognosis: Increasing pigmentation over the years with corresponding darkening and changing of eye and hair color (in some cases to light brown) and improvement of vision. However, average life expectancy probably somewhat shortened as a result of increased danger of accidents due to poor vision and increased disposition to develop skin cancer.

Differential diagnosis: Oculocutaneous albinism tyrosinase negative type (p.348) and other forms of albinism.

Treatment: Avoidance of exposure to sunlight (clothing, sun-ray filter cream). Tinted spectacles or contact lenses. Genetic counseling.

Illustrations:
1 Affected siblings.
2 Dark-complexioned parents and their affected child.

H.-R.W.

References:

Witkop, C.J., Jr. et al. Oculocutaneous albinism. In: Nyhan, W.L. (ed.) *Heritable Disorders of Amino Acid Metabolism.* J. Wiley & Sons, New York, 1974.
King, R.A. Albinism. In: Gomez, M.R. (ed.) *Neurocutaneous Diseases.* Butterworths, Boston, 1987 (chapter 35).
Taylor, W.O.G. Prenatal diagnosis in albinism. *Lancet*, I, 1307–1308 (1987).
van Dorp, D.B. Albinism, or the NOACH syndrome. *Clin. Genet.*, 31, 228–242 (1987).

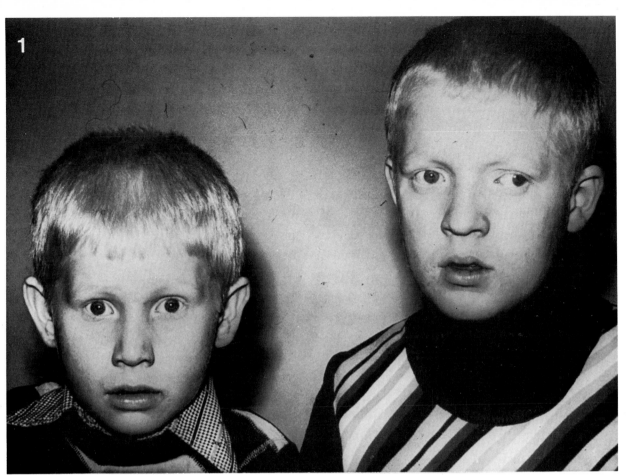

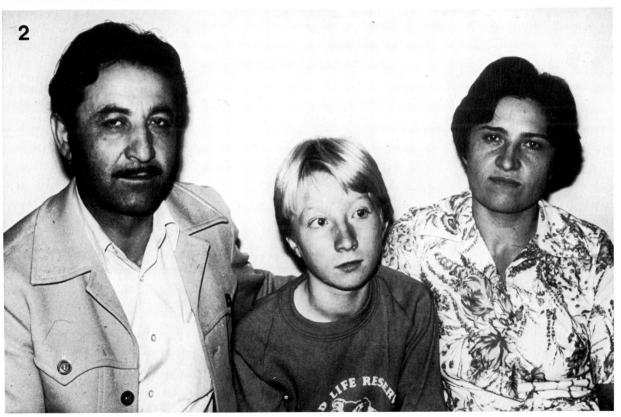

351

175. Proteus Syndrome

An exclusive, sporadically observed 'Proteus-like' polymorphic and variable dysplasia syndrome of the phakomatosis/hamartosis type, partly present at birth and partly later in childhood.

Main signs:
1. Partial, perhaps bizarre macrosomia involving the hands and/or feet (including metacarpals or metatarsals (1–3).
2. Hemiatrophy—partial or complete (1).
3. Cranial anomalies: macrocrania with prominent forehead, cranial asymmetry, *Buckelschädel* ('bumpy' skull) due to hyperostoses and/or exostoses (the latter also possibly in the auditory canal, alveolar process, and other locations).
4. Other anomalies of growth: sometimes generalized 'gigantism' with or without accelerated ossification—but also growth deficiency; abnormal length of the trunk and/or neck due to 'megaspondylodysplasia', which may lead to a gazelle-neck appearance. Distension of the ribs.
   Development of kyphoscoliosis, and many other abnormalities.
5. Pigmented and nonpigmented nevi, usually widespread, often generalized, and sometimes with raised, rough surfaces (1). Vascular nevi and venectasia also possible.
6. Subcutaneous tumors—lipomas, lymph- and hemangiomas or correspondingly 'mixed' tumors —especially on the trunk, in the axillae, on the flanks (1). Intra-abdominal development of tumors not infrequent, sometimes with protrusion of the abdominal wall, intestinal obstruction, etc.
7. Soft-tissue hypertrophy involving the soles, also possibly the palms, especially due to lipomatous deposits, nevus-like and possibly gyriform ('moccasin soles').

Supplementary findings: Possible atrophy of subcutaneous adipose tissue and muscle atrophy of variable severity; joint disorders.
   Dysplasia of the external ears in some cases; anomalies of the eyes (ptosis, strabismus), the palate, and/or the dentition.
   Occasional cysts of the lung, and others.
   According to experience to date, mental impairment is the exception, but may be severe when present, occasionally with CNS seizures.

Manifestation: At birth and later. The latter is true especially for subcutaneous tumors, but also for the appearance of nevi, exostoses, elongation of the neck, scoliosis, and 'moccasin soles'.

Etiology: Uncertain. Mosaicism for a somatic mutation (with lethal effect in the nonmosaic state) has been proposed and would fit with the exclusively sporadic occurrence observed. For practical purposes, there should be no risk of recurrence.

Frequency: Low. Since publication of the syndrome in 1983, at least 25 further cases have been reported and about the same number of fairly similar cases were found in the older literature.

Course, prognosis: Very uncertain. Possible progression for years, e.g., of giant growth of fingers or toes, of soft-tissue hypertrophy, or constant new manifestation of hamartomatous tumors; but standstill also possible, even spontaneous regression, e.g., of soft-tissue tumors. Intra-abdominal tumors may become dangerous, auditory canals may become closed by bony growths, the appearance of semimalignant or malignant growths must be anticipated. There are adults who—although sometimes after a multitude of operations—become independent, but also patients who die in early childhood. Crucial, of course, is whether cerebral function is impaired.

H.-R.W.

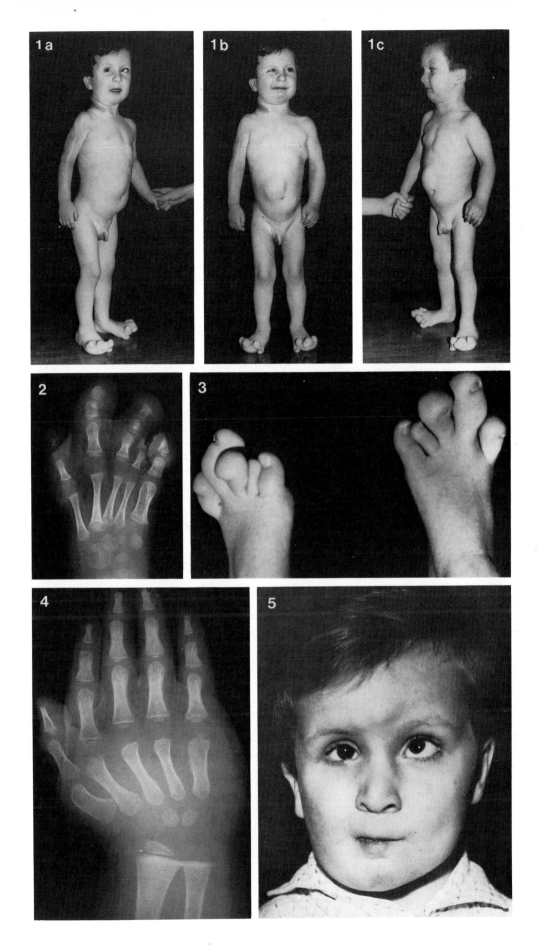

176. Proteus Syndrome (cont.)

Differential diagnosis: Bilateral macrosomia of fingers and toes, 'gazelle neck', soft-tissue tumors of the trunk, and 'moccasin soles' are so unusual that they can be considered diagnostic within the framework of the complete clinical picture. Incomplete or weak manifestations of this syndrome may not be infrequent and could cause diagnostic difficulties.

In the differential diagnosis: especially the Klippel–Trenaunay (p.358), possibly the Sturge–Weber (p.356) syndromes; furthermore, the Marfucci syndrome (p.410), von Recklinghausen disease (p.332), and the Schimmelpenning–Feuerstein–Mims syndrome (p.314) should be considered. Re: encephalocraniocutaneous lipomatosis, see p.318.

Treatment: Symptomatic. Amputation of severely oversized rays of the hands and feet may be indicated in consultation with a hand surgeon. Otherwise, restraint with operative measures is advised since triggering of a local increase of excess growth cannot be ruled out. Psychological guidance. Genetic counseling for the parents.

Illustrations:

1–5 (p.353) A 2-year-old, the first of four children of young, healthy, nonconsanguineous parents. Congenital, mostly symmetrical macrosomia of the third, fifth, and especially the fourth toes bilaterally. Distinctly greater development of the left side of the face, the left arm, and especially the left forearm with a short, stubby left hand. Over a great part of the right side of the throat, the right half of the trunk, and the right arm, epidermal nevoid dysplasia of the skin (grey-brown discoloration of variable intensity with a mostly coarse, rough surface) with sharp medial borders, also on the penis and scrotum. Within this pigmented nevus, several thin streaks of normal skin on the right arm. Subcutaneous 'tumors', some congenital, some appearing in early childhood: venous angioma on the right of the neck, lumpy swellings on the soles of both feet and on the left thenar and hypothenar eminences. Soft mobile cystic lymphangiomas (or lymphohemangiomas; lipomatous components could not be ruled out) on both sides of the chest, in the left epigastric and right paraumbilical areas. Asymmetric macrocranium (51 cm) with two bony protuberances on the forehead. Low-set, dysplastic right ear. Considerable left amblyopia with ipsilateral convergent strabismus. Normal height and mental development.

1–6 (p.355) A 4-year-old, the second child of healthy, nonconsanguineous parents. Congenital asymmetric macrosomia of fingers 2–4 bilaterally and of the feet and toes (1–5 left, 3–5 right). Hemihypertrophy of the whole left side of the body. Extensive left-sided epidermal nevoid dysplasia. Lipomas and lipolymphohemangiomas on both sides of the upper trunk. 'Moccasin soles', similar but less severe soft-tissue hypertrophy of the palms. Asymmetric *Buckelschädel* ('bumpy' skull). Convergent strabismus. General 'gigantism' (>98%); beginning development of gazelle-neck appearance. Normal mental development for age.

H.-R.W.

References:

Wiedemann, H.-R., Burgio, G.R. et al. The Proteus syndrome. *Eur. J. Pediatr.*, 140, 5–12 (1983).
Burgio, G.R. and Wiedemann, H.-R. Further and new details on the Proteus syndrome. *Eur. J. Pediatr.*, 143, 71–73 (1984).
Gorlin, R.J. Proteus syndrome. *J. Clin. Dysmorphol.*, 2, 8–9 (1984).
Lezama, D.B. and Buyse, M.L. The Proteus syndrome. The emergence of an entity. *J. Clin. Dysmorphol.*, 2, 10–13 (1984).
Costa, T., Fitch, N. et al. Proteus syndrome . . . *Pediatrics*, 76, 984–989 (1985).
Mücke, J., Willgerodt, H. et al. Variability in the Proteus syndrome . . . *Eur. J. Pediatr.*, 143, 320–323 (1985).
Azouz, E.M., Costa, T. et al. Radiologic findings in the Proteus syndrome. *Pediatr. Radiol.*, 17, 481–485 (1987).
Clark, R.D., Donnai, D. et al. Proteus syndrome: an expanded phenotype. *Am. J. Med. Genet.*, 27, 99–117 (1987).
Cremin, B.J., Viljoen, D.L. et al. The Proteus syndrome . . . *Pediatr. Radiol.*, 17, 486–488 (1987).
Malamitsi-Puchner, A., Kitsiou, S. et al. Severe Proteus syndrome . . . *Am. J. Med. Genet.*, 27, 119–125 (1987).
Viljoen, D.L., Nelson, M.M. et al. Proteus syndrome in Southern Africa . . . *Am. J. Med. Genet.*, 27, 87–89 (1987).

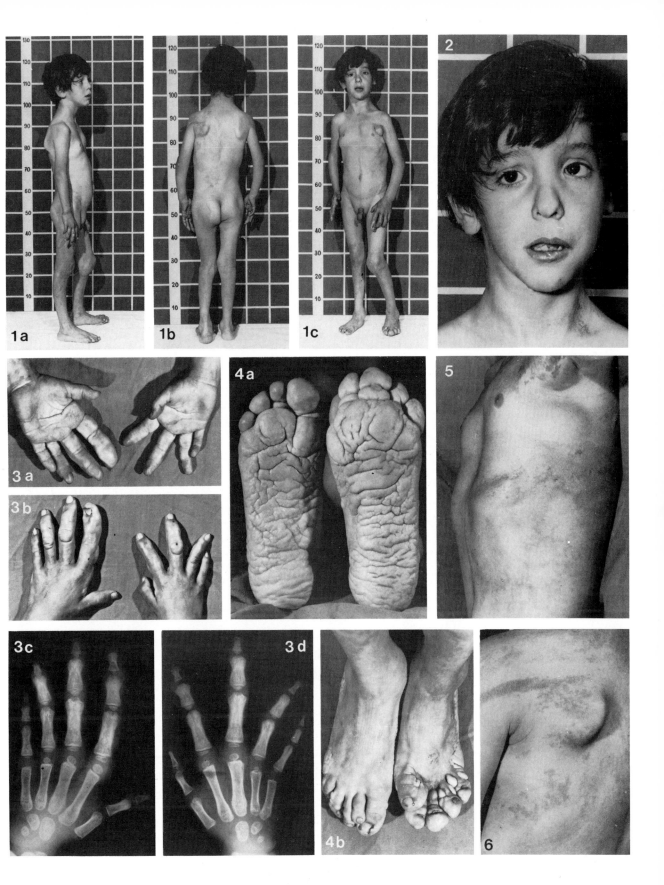

177. Sturge–Weber Syndrome

(Cerebrocutaneous Angiomatosis Syndrome; Angiomatosis Encephalofacialis)

A characteristic syndrome of macular hemangiomas especially of the face, signs of cerebral foci (due to ipsilateral meningeal angiomas), and usually mental retardation.

Main signs:
1. Port-wine stain nevus flammeus of the face and head, varying in extent, preferentially of the trigeminal area, mostly unilateral, often sharply outlined medially (possibly with corresponding involvement of the oral mucosa), less frequently bilateral, and sometimes involving the body (1–5).
2. Focal or generalized cerebral seizures. Spastic hemiparesis (contralateral to the side of the angioma). Secondary mental impairment, of varying severity.

Supplementary findings: In almost half of the cases, angiomatous changes of the ipsilateral choroid, possibly resulting in congenital glaucoma (buphthalmos) (7). Possible hemianopia contralateral to the facial angioma.

Macrocephaly. Skull X-ray: garland-like, double-contoured calcifications, varying in extent, especially over the posterior parietal and occipital regions on the side of the hemangioma (6, 8).

Occasionally, markedly asymmetrical development of the cranium.

Manifestation: Nevus flammeus usually present at birth. Possible congenital glaucoma (7). First signs of epileptic activity, spastic hemiparesis, and mental impairment usually in infancy. Calcifications within the cerebral cortex usually not demonstrable on a routine skull X-ray until the latter half of early childhood; demonstration of increased density possible much earlier by means of CT scan.

Etiology: In spite of almost invariable sporadic occurrence, inherited factors are probably of causal significance.

Frequency: Not particularly low; estimated one case of the fully expressed syndrome in about 230,000 of the general population.

Course, prognosis: Epileptic seizures often very difficult to control. Occurrence also of milder cases with fewer signs, some with undiminished intelligence. Although the intensity of the color of the angiomas tends to decrease with increasing age, the affected area of skin usually tends to become thicker and coarser.

Treatment: Prompt surgery for glaucoma when indicated; otherwise, conservative in principle. A neurosurgical procedure, possibly even hemispherectomy, should only be considered in cases with very widespread intracranial changes, and in which consistent appropriate antiepileptic treatment is ineffective in preventing relentless progressive intellectual and psychical deterioration. More recently, laser therapy has been recommended for the nevus flammeus; in older children the nevus can be cosmetically covered with Covermark products.

Illustrations:
1 Patient 1 at birth. Congenital glaucoma on the right, seizures since birth; early development of left-sided spasticity and of retardation; intracranial calcifications demonstrable since age 18 months.
2 and 7 Patient 2 at birth (**2**). Glaucoma on the left (**7**) with subsequent need for enucleation; right-sided focal findings on EEG, left-sided seizures.
3–6 and 8 Patients 3, 4, and 5 (6-year-old, 9½-year-old, and 14-year-old boys) all mentally retarded and epileptic; hemiparesis in patients 3 and 4; foci of calcification in patient 4 and also patient 5 (**6, 8**), who was operated on for glaucoma at age 3 months.

H.-R.W.

References:
Any neurology, pediatric, or internal medicine text book.
Noe, J., Barsky, S. et al. Portwine stains and the response to argon laser therapy . . . *Plast. Reconstr. Surg.*, 65, 130–136 (1980).
Enjolras, O., Riche, M.C. et al. Facial portwine stains and Sturge–Weber syndrome. *Pediatrics*, 76, 48–51 (1985).
Fritsch, G., Sacher, M. et al. Klinik und Verlauf des Sturge–Weber-Syndrom im Kindersalter. *Monatschr. Kinderheilkd.*, 134, 242–245 (1986).
Garden, J.M., Tan, O.T. et al. The pulsed dye laser: its use at 577 nm wavelength. *J. Dermatol. Surg. Oncol.*, 13, 134–138 (1987).
Gomez, M.R. and Bebin, E.M. Sturge–Weber syndrome. In: *Neurocutaneous Diseases*. Butterworths, Boston, 1987 (pp.356–367).

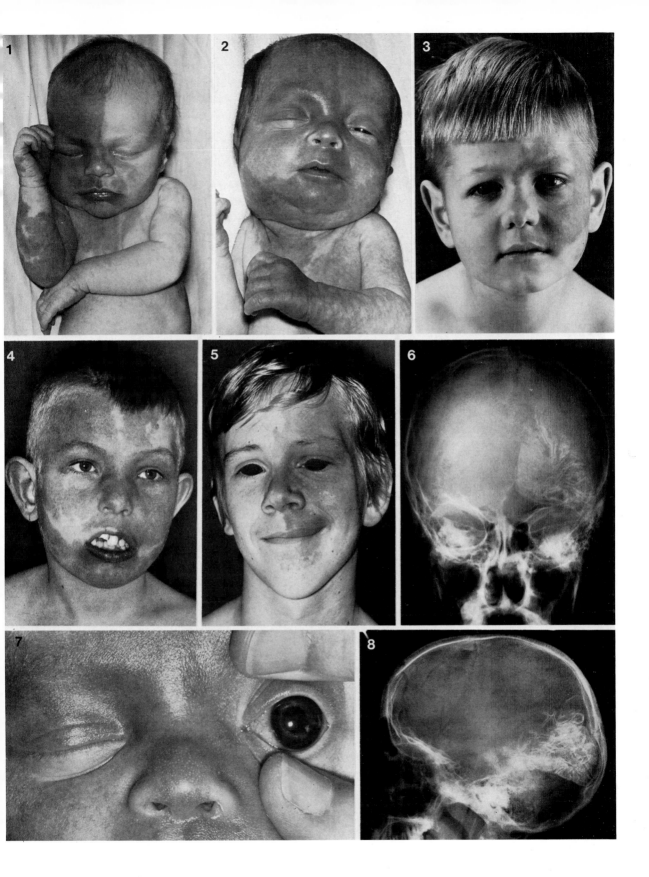

178. Klippel–Trenaunay Syndrome

(Angio-Osteohypertrophy; Nevus Varicosus Osteohypertrophicus Syndrome)

A dysplasia syndrome with localized, frequently disproportionate, macrosomia, nevi, and varicosities on the affected side.

Main signs:
1. As a rule, one extremity is completely or partially affected, the lower ones much more frequently than the upper.
2. Flat hemangiomas of the skin (nevus flammeus), bright red to dark violet, varying in extent, solitary or multiple, irregularly contoured, and when located on the trunk, not necessarily sharply outlined at the midline (1, 3, 4a, 6).
3. Partial macrosomia involving all tissues, usually in the region of the vascular nevus (1, 3, 4), but also occasionally contralaterally (6, 7), which is frequently also disproportionate.
4. Venous angiomas, varices may be readily apparent (5) or detectable on X-ray (phleboliths) or by phlebography (lymphangiectasis exclusively by lymphangiography).

Supplementary findings: Local anomalies of hair, sweating, etc.

Frequent secondary osteoarticular changes (4).

Numerous other anomalies may or may not occur, e.g., remotely situated vascular dysplasias, macrocrania, changes involving the skin, skeleton, eyes, oral cavity, urinary tract, etc. Thus, a highly variable clinical picture.

Manifestation: At birth and later. Vascular nevi usually congenital, but postnatal appearance and expansion possible. Variably rapid onset and progression of macrosomic development; skeletal involvement radiologically demonstrable only with time. Varicosities usually not clinically identifiable in young children.

Etiology: The great majority of cases are sporadic (somatic mutation?); perhaps exceptionally an autosomal dominant pleiotropic gene with relatively low penetrance or an autosomal recessive gene might be responsible.

Frequency: Not particularly low (well over 500 cases described).

Course, prognosis: At first often distinct progression of development of the macrosomia and handicap; after the child stops growing, the changes may remain stationary. Possible late complication: leg ulcers with tendency for poor healing.

Diagnosis: Phlebography to rule out an obstruction; dysplasia or aplasia of deep leg veins may be found. In some cases arteriography to rule out an arteriovenous fistula. Possible lymphangiography. The studies can be done once the child has reached an appropriate age. Ultrasonographic prenatal diagnosis in isolated cases.

Differential diagnosis: In some cases, Sturge–Weber syndrome (p.356), von Recklinghausen neurofibromatosis (p.332), F.P. Weber syndrome (p.400), Proteus syndrome (p.352).

Treatment: Symptomatic (compression, positioning, etc.). Orthopedic care, conservative and/or operative. In some cases, removal of a section causing venous stenosis. Procedures on superficial varices contraindicated.

Illustrations:
1–3 A patient at 3 and 14 months. Macrosomia of the right leg and generalized, mild hemihypertrophy. Flat hemangioma on the right, in part sharply bordered at the midline, in part extending onto the left side. Scoliosis.
4 and 5 A 3-year-old patient with an irregular flat hemangioma, varicosities, and excessive growth of the left leg (tilted pelvis, scoliosis), especially of second and third toes.
6 A 1¾-year-old patient; angioma especially of the right leg (and the left half of the trunk) with macrosomia of the left leg.
7 Lower extremity of an infant: macular vascular nevus vasculosus on the right, disproportionate macrosomia on the left.

H.-R.W.

References:

Weber, J. Der umschriebene Riesenwuchs, Typ Parkes Weber (Beitrag zur Diskussion des Klippel–Trenaunay–Weber-Syndroms). *Fortschr. Röntgenstr.*, 113, 734 (1970).

Servelle, M. Klippel and Trenaunay's syndrome: 768 operated cases. *Ann. Surg.*, 201, 365–373 (1985).

Stickler, G.B. Klippel–Trenaunay syndrome. In: Gomez, M.R. (ed.) *Neurocutaneous Diseases*. Butterworths, Boston, 1987 (pp.368–375).

Mahmoud, S.F., El-Benhawi, M.O. et al. Klippel–Trenaunay syndrome. *J. Am. Acad. Dermatol.*, 18, 5/2, 1170–1172 (1988).

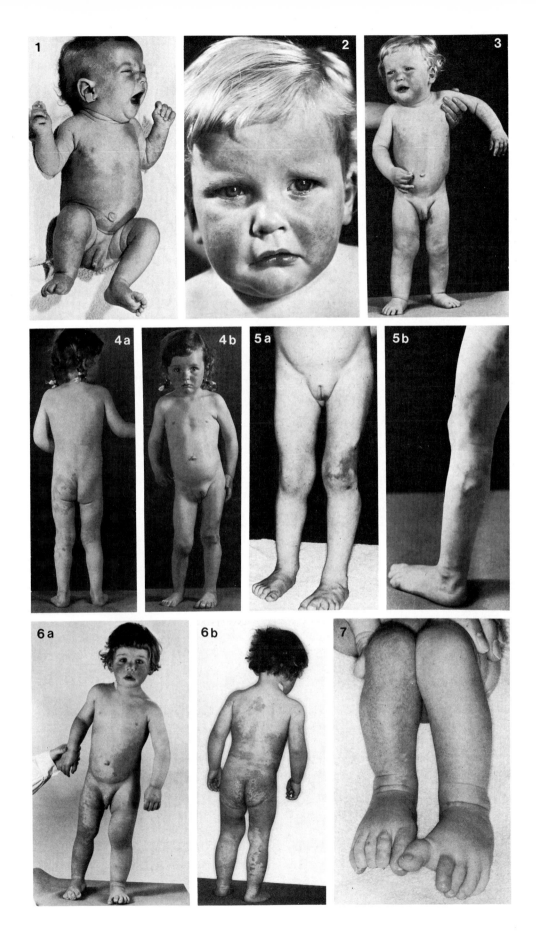

179. Bloom Syndrome

(Congenital Telangiectatic Erythema and Stunted Growth)

A recessive hereditary syndrome of primordial growth deficiency and telangiectatic erythema.

Main signs:
1. Marked pre- and postnatal growth deficiency (average birth weight of males about 2100 g, of females about 1850 g; adult height about 150 cm), with a distinctly slender body build (1).
2. Telangiectatic erythema, more marked after exposure to sun, most commonly in a butterfly distribution on the face, also on the dorsal surfaces of the forearms. Sometimes blistering and scarring of the lips and lower eyelids. Skin changes more pronounced in males than in females (1–3).
3. Long, narrow face with prominent nose; hypoplastic zygoma region; micrognathia; sometimes microcephaly (1, 2).

Supplementary findings: Small testicles, probable infertility in males (no data on married females).

Frequent infections, especially when younger.

Tendency to develop malignant tumors, especially leukemia in the younger age group.

Chromosome instability with typical chromosome breaks and increased rate of sister chromatid exchange (SCE), but not in heterozygotes.

Manifestation: At birth; however, erythema usually appears during the first summer after birth.

Etiology: Autosomal recessive disorder. The preponderance of males probably explained by easier diagnosis due to more marked skin involvement. In a few cases a DNA ligase I defect demonstrated.

Frequency: Low; since first described in 1954, over 130 cases have been reported.

Prognosis: Dubious. Early malignant tumors have occurred in about 20% of the patients to date. The rate is probably much higher, as the average age of living patients in 1987 was quite low, at 18.9 years, and so far all patients over 30 years have developed tumors (Wilms' tumor, carcinoma, lymphoma, leukemia, Hodgkin's disease).

Differential diagnosis: Rothmund–Thomson syndrome (p.328); in Bloom syndrome the reticular pigmentation of poikiloderma is not present, growth deficiency is more distinct, and the shape of the face is different.

Treatment: Regular check-ups for cancer, restricted exposure to sun, genetic counseling. In case of further pregnancies, prenatal diagnosis (ultrasonography; amniocentesis and chromosome analysis).

Illustrations:
1–3 A patient at age 7 years 11 months (1) and at 8½ years (2, 3). Birth measurements 2020 g and 45.5 cm. Moderately retarded development in early childhood. Erythema appeared in the first summer of life. Frequent infections during the first year of life. Body measurements at 7 years: height 116 cm (third to tenth percentile), weight 16.3 kg (< third percentile) and head circumference 47.1 cm (about third percentile). Typical chromosome findings.

H.-R.W./J.K.

References:

German, J., Bloom, D., Passarge, E. Bloom's syndrome. 7th progress report for 1978. *Clin. Genet.*, 15, 361 (1979).
Thomas, P. Das Bloom-Syndrom. *Pädiatr. Prax.*, 24, 283 (1980/81).
Mulcahy, M.T. and French, M. Pregnancy in Bloom's syndrome. *Clin. Genet.*, 19, 156 (1981).
German, J., Bloom, D. et al. Bloom's syndrome . . . *Clin. Genet.*, 25, 166–174 (1984).
Vanderschueren-Lodeweyckx, M., Fryns, J.-P. et al. Bloom's syndrome. *Am. J. Dis. Child.*, 138, 812–816 (1984).
Cahn, J.Y.H., Becker, F.F. et al. Altered DNA ligase I activity in Bloom's syndrome cells. *Nature*, 325, 357–359 (1987).
Cairney, A.E.L., Andrews, M. et al. Wilms tumor in three patients with Bloom syndrome. *J. Pediatr.*, 111, 414–416 (1987).
Takemiya, M., Shiraishi, S. et al. Bloom's syndrome with . . . multiple cancers . . . *Clin. Genet.*, 31, 35–44 (1987).
Willis, A.E. and Lindahl, T. DNA ligase I deficiency in Bloom's syndrome. *Nature*, 325, 355–357 (1987).
van Kerekhove, C.W., Ceuppens, J.L. et al. Bloom's syndrome . . . immunologic abnormalities of four patients. *Am. J. Dis. Child.*, 142, 1089–1093 (1988).
German, J. and Passarge, E. Bloom's syndrome. XIIth report from the registry for 1987. *Clin. Genet.*, 35, 57–69 (1988).

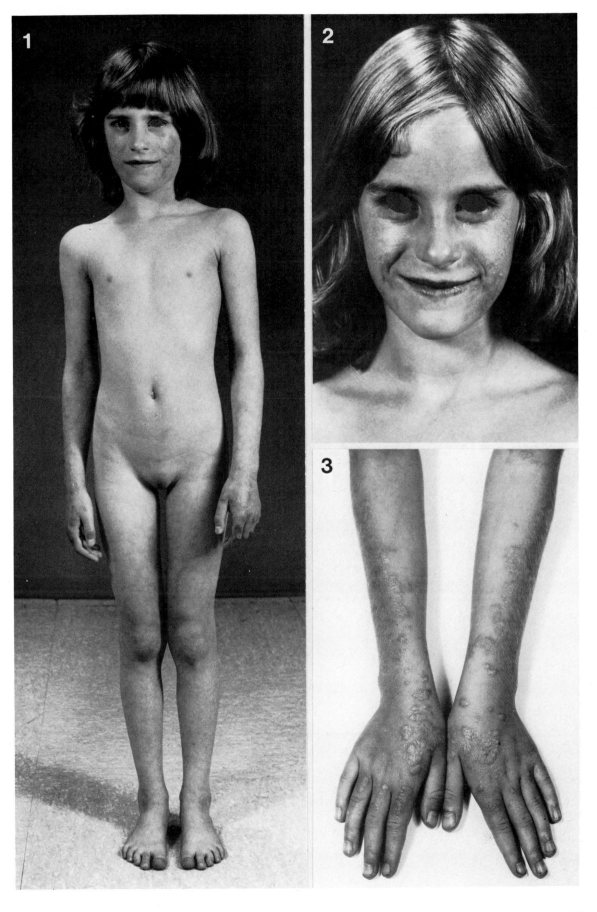

180. Simple Joint Hyperextensibility Syndrome

(Familial Simple Joint Laxity/Hypermobility Syndrome)

A familial hyperextensibility of all joints without further unusual phenotypic features.

Main signs: Generalized hyperextensibility of the joints, seldom dislocation of joints.

Supplementary findings: Only occasional further problems involving the connective tissue, such as inguinal hernia, etc.

Manifestation: At birth(?)

Etiology: Autosomal dominant inheritance with high penetrance. Basic defect unknown.

Frequency: Not rare, inasmuch as the spectrum blends smoothly into the normal. Great intrafamilial variability.

Course, prognosis: As a rule, no complications.

Differential diagnosis: Ehlers–Danlos syndrome types III and VII, familial joint instability syndrome with joint dislocations ('congenital or acquired dislocation of the hip'), Marfan syndrome, osteogenesis imperfecta, Larsen syndrome.

Treatment: None.

Illustrations:
1a–1c A 1-day-old female newborn, unusual spontaneous hyperextensibility of the large and small joints, large feet (marfanoid appearance).
2a and 2b The 24-year-old mother of the child.

J.K.

References:

Beighton, P.H. and Horan, F.T. Dominant inheritance in familial generalized articular hypermobility. *J. Bone Jt. Surg.*, 52B, 145–147 (1970).
Horton, W.A., Collins, D.L., DeSmet, A.A. et al. Familial joint instability syndrome. *Am. J. Med. Genet.*, 6, 221–228 (1980).
Child, A., Symmons, D., Light, N. et al. Joint hypermobility syndrome: an inherited collagen disorder? *J. Med. Genet.*, 21, 138 (1984).

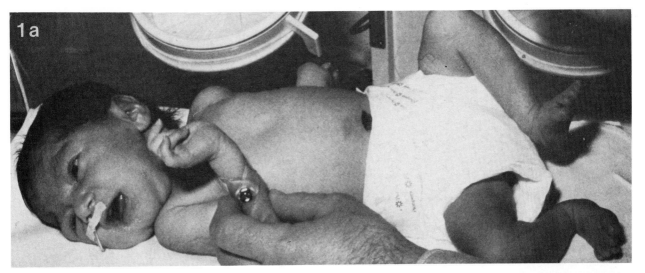

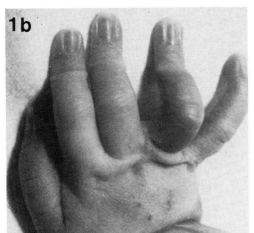

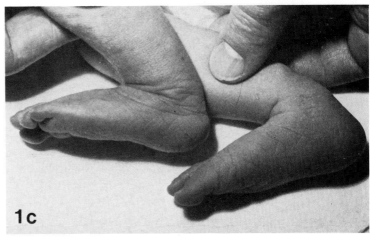

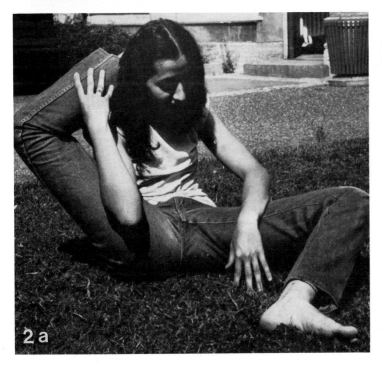

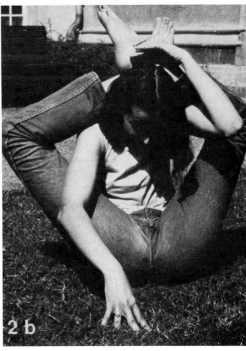

181. Ehlers–Danlos Syndrome

A group of diseases with connective-tissue weakness characterized by hyperelastic skin, hypermobility of the joints, tissue fragility, eye changes, and bleeding diathesis.

Main signs:
1. Hyperelastic, velvety in childhood, strikingly white, very fragile skin, with characteristic 'fish mouth' gaping following trauma. When injured, slow healing leaving a cigarette paper-like scar, e.g., on the forehead. Development of so-called molluscoid pseudotumors on exposed areas, e.g., knees, elbows, shins (3–5). Ears very elastic and pliable. Blood vessels easily damaged, thus skin and soft-tissue hemorrhages, which may calcify. Calcification of frequently occurring subcutaneous fatty cysts also.
2. Hypermobility of the joints (2, 6–8) with danger of dislocation, instability, and bleeding into the joints. Kyphoscoliosis (1). Spondylolisthesis; pes planus (2).
3. Epicanthus, blue sclera, strabismus; myopia; ectopic lenses, retinal detachment and bulbar tears following light trauma.

Supplementary findings: Raynaud's phenomenon, inguinal hernias, incisional hernias, diaphragmatic hernias.

Occasionally, small stature.

Rapid physical fatigability.

Diverticula and perforations of the gastrointestinal tract in some cases.

Haemorrhages from any possible site; dissecting aneurysms; heavy bleeding after dental extractions (frequent periodontitis, early loss of teeth). Rumpel–Leede sign often positive. Varicosities.

Possible demonstration of specific enzyme defects for certain types.

Pregnancy signifies a high risk for the affected mother due to further slackening of the connective tissues and heavy post partum bleeding; also for the affected child, subject to premature rupture of the dysplastic fetal membranes and subsequent premature birth.

Manifestation: At birth. The diagnosis is usually made later.

Etiology: This is a heterogeneous group of disorders with hereditary anomalies of connective tissue as their basis. About ten forms have been differentiated, based on severity of the clinical picture, various types of signs in individual organs, the genetics, and the specific enzyme defects; of the ten, the autosomal dominant type I (gravis) has probably been described the most. Type V follows an X-linked recessive mode of inheritance; further types (e.g., type IV, with a disorder of collagen III synthesis) are autosomal recessive.

Frequency: Relatively low.

Course, prognosis: Average life expectancy reduced due to the above-mentioned possible complications (e.g., in type IV about 25% mortality during pregnancy due to rupture of uterine or intestinal vessels).

Treatment: Avoidance of trauma. Surgery only if unavoidable. Since sutures do not hold well, tissue clamps preferable. Caution with angiography. Very thorough biochemical and genetic analysis, and genetic counseling. Prenatal diagnosis possible in some cases, e.g., with type IV.

Illustrations:
1–8 A girl at age 12 years, probably affected with autosomal recessive type VI. Myopia, keratoconus.

H.-R.W./J.K.

References:

McKusick, V.A. Multiple forms of the Ehlers–Danlos syndrome. *Arch. Surg.*, 109, 475 (1974).
McEntyre, R.L. and Raffensperger, J.G. Surgical complications of Ehlers–Danlos syndrome in children, *J. Pediatr. Surg.*, 12, 531 (1977).
Byers, P.H., Holbrook, K.A. et al. Ehlers–Danlos syndrome. In: Emery, A.E. and Rimoin, D.L. (eds.) *Principles and Practice of Medical Genetics*. Churchill Livingstone, Edinburgh, 1983 (pp.836–850).
Kozlova, S.I., Prytkov, A.N. et al. Presumed homozygous Ehlers–Danlos syndrome type I . . . *Am. J. Med. Genet.*, 18, 763–767 (1984).
Sartoris, D.J., Luzzatti, L. et al. Type IX Ehlers–Danlos syndrome. *Radiology*, 152, 665–670 (1984).
Sulh, H.M.B., Steinmann, B. et al. Ehlers–Danlos syndrome type IV D . . . *Clin. Genet.*, 25, 278–287 (1984).
Beighton, P. and Curtis, D. X-linked Ehlers–Danlos syndrome type V . . . *Clin. Genet.*, 27, 472–478 (1985).
Tsipouras, P., Byers, P.H. et al. Ehlers–Danlos syndrome type IV . . . *Hum. Genet.*, 74, 41–46 (1986).
Rizzo, R., Contri, M.B. et al. Familial Ehlers–Danlos syndrome type II . . . *Pediatr. Dermatol.*, 4, 197–204 (1987).
Pope, F.M., Narcisi, P. et al. Clinical presentation of Ehlers–Danlos syndrome type IV. *Arch. Dis. Child.*, 63, 1016–1025 (1988).
Editorial. Type III collagen deficiency. *Lancet*, I, 197–198 (1989).

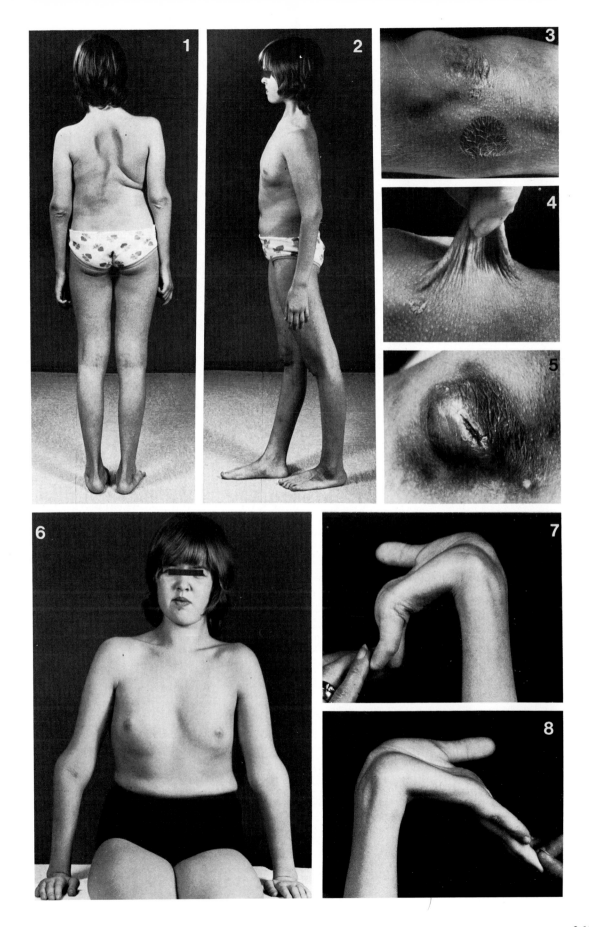

182. Osteogenesis Imperfecta

(Type seen most often in neonates)

A clinically and genetically heterogeneous hereditary disease of connective tissue (due to various collagen defects). Types II A, B, and C and type III present at birth and have a poor prognosis.

Main signs:

1. Congenitally abnormal proportions due to abnormally short, fractured, compressed, 'pseudomicromelic', bowed extremities, some possibly with pseudarthrosis; a trunk of approximately normal length (often with multiple broken ribs, 'beaded ribs'); large head with membranous calvaria (*Kautschukschädel*, or 'rubber' skull); and usually unremarkable hands and feet (**1**).
2. Radiologically: thick, short, fractured, bowed shafts of the long tubular bones, especially the legs ('accordian femora'), often with signs of prenatal callus formation; platyspondylisis; little calcification of the skull; generalized osteoporosis (**2–4**).

Supplementary findings: Frequent exophthalmos low nasal root, small nose.

Blue sclerae; lax ligaments, possible inguinal hernias; muscular hypotonia.

Often hypertrichosis (lanugo hair).

Manifestation: At birth.

Etiology: Types II A–C are thought to be autosomal recessive (IIA possibly also an autosomal dominant form); type III occurs in both dominant and recessive forms. In the future, with molecular-level collagen studies of a patient and his parents, it should be possible to make increasingly clear statements about the genetics.

Frequency: About 1:40,000 births.

Course, prognosis: Very unfavorable; death often perinatally, otherwise in early infancy.

Differential diagnosis: There are further forms of osteogenesis imperfecta with variable congenital manifestations (types IV A and B). These show variable, but as a whole less severe clinical pictures, better prognosis for survival; autosomal dominant inheritance.

Treatment: Symptomatic. Genetic counseling. In case of further pregnancy, prenatal diagnosis with ultrasonography.

Illustrations:

1 and 2 (N.B. A separate skull X-ray added.) A 4-day-old newborn with caput membranaceum, blue sclerae, right-sided inguinal hernia, lanugo hypertrichosis. Death at 17 days (subarachnoid bleeding, pulmonary bleeding).
3 and 4 X-rays of a further child, in the second month of life (serial rib fractures).

H.-R.W.

References:

Sillence, D.O., Senn, A., Danks, D.M. Genetic heterogeneity in osteogenesis imperfecta. *J. Med. Genet.*, 16, 101 (1979).
Sillence, D.O., Rimoin, D.L., Danks, D.M. Clinical variability in osteogenesis imperfecta . . . *Birth Defects*, XV, 5B, 113 (1979).
Spranger, J., Cremin, B., Beighton, P. Osteogenesis imperfecta congenita . . . *Pediatr. Radiol.*, 12, 21 (1982).
Shapiro, J.E., Phillips, J.A., Byers, P.H. et al. Prenatal diagnosis of lethal perinatal osteogenesis imperfecta . . . *J. Pediatr.*, 100, 127 (1982).
Gillerot, Y., Druart, J.M. et al. Lethal perinatal type II . . . in a family with a dominantly inherited type I. *Eur. J. Pediatr.*, 141, 119–122 (1983).
Byers, P.H. Bonadio, J.F. et al. Osteogenesis imperfecta: update . . . *Am. J. Med. Genet.*, 17, 429–435 (1984).
Maroteaux, P. and Cohen-Salal, L. L'ostéogenèse imparfaite létale. *Ann. Génét.*, 27, 11–15 (1984).
Sillence, D.O., Barlow, K.K. et al. Osteogenesis imperfecta type II: delineation of the phenotype with reference to genetic heterogeneity. *Am. J. Med. Genet.*, 17, 407–423 (1984).
Spranger, J. Osteogenesis imperfecta: a pasture for splitters and lumpers. *Am. J. Med. Genet.*, 17, 425–428 (1984).
Maroteaux, P., Frézal, J. et al. Les formes anténatales de l'ostéogenèse imparfaite. *Arch. Fr. Pédiatr.*, 43, 235–241 (1986).
Sillence, D.O., Barlow, K.K. et al. Osteogenesis imperfecta type III . . . *Am. J. Med. Genet.*, 23, 821–826 (1986).
Stöss, H., Pontz, B.F. et al. Heterogeneity of osteogenesis imperfecta . . . *Eur. J. Pediatr.*, 145, 34–39 (1986).
Ternes, M.L. and Pontz, B.F. Kinder mit Osteogenesis imperfecta. *Der Kinderarzt*, 16, 769–774 (1987).
Thompson. E.M., Young, I.D. et al. Recurrence risk and prognosis in severe sporadic osteogenesis imperfecta. *J. Med. Genet.*, 24, 390–405 (1987).
Young, I.D., Thompson, E.M. et al. Osteogenesis imperfecta type IIA: evidence for dominant inheritance. *J. Med. Genet.*, 24, 386–389 (1987).
Byers, P.H., Tsipouras, P. et al. Perinatal lethal osteogenesis imperfecta (OI type II) . . . *Am. J. Hum. Genet.*, 42, 237–248 (1988).
Williams, E.M., Nicholls, A.C. et al. Phenotypical features . . . Osteogenesis imperfecta. *Clin. Genet.*, 35, 181–190 (1989).

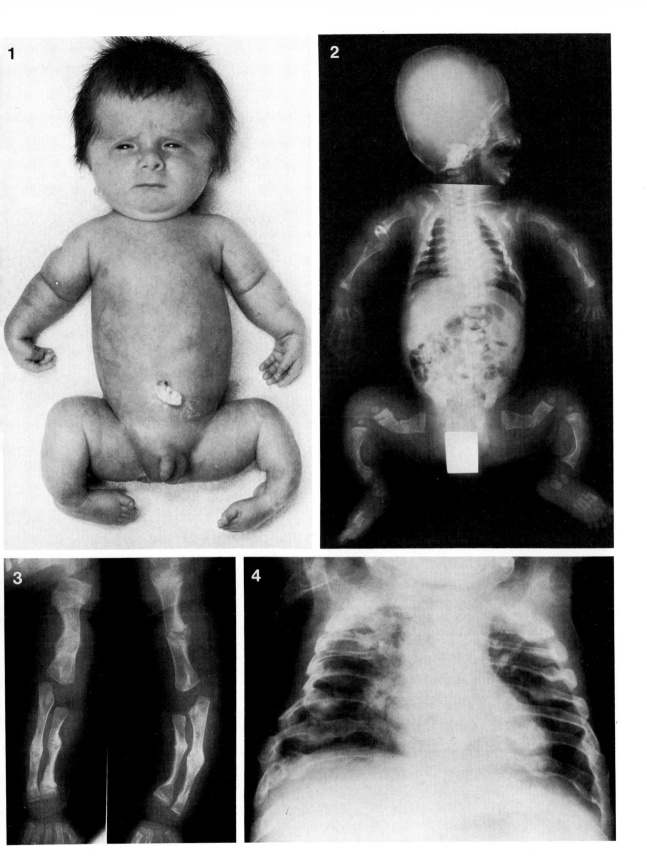

183. Osteogenesis Imperfecta (cont.)

(Further clinical pictures)

Hereditary disorders with abnormal fragility of bones (frequently with secondary deformities of extremities, spine, and thorax), small face with bulging forehead and temples, frequently small stature, laxity of joint capsules and ligaments, blue or—less frequently—bluewhite sclerae, hypoplasia of dentin and enamel in some cases, and hearing impairment (possibly late-onset).

Main signs:

1. Increased fragility of bones (commonly called 'brittle-bone disease'), often especially of the proximal extremities, with frequent secondary deformities of the limbs, spine, and thorax and correspondingly reduced height (**1–3, 6**).
2. Small 'triangular' face below a relatively large calvarium; bulging forehead and temples (**1, 2**).
3. Blue sclerae (not infrequently, also tympanic membrane); possible dentinogenesis imperfecta with increased disposition to caries, possible otosclerotic hearing impairment.
4. Laxity of joint capsules and ligaments, possible tendency to dislocate. Tendency to develop hernias. Genu valgus. Pes planus. Thin, translucent skin, possible bleeding diathesis. Formation of broad, hypertrophic scars.

Supplementary findings: Radiologically, mineral-deficient, narrow, frequently bowed, long bones with thin cortices (**4–6**), and flat to biconcave transparent vertebral bodies; delayed ossification of the calvaria with a Wormian bone mosaic-like picture.

In some cases, marginal corneal clouding (embryotoxon, with blue sclerae), farsightedness or other eye anomalies.

Manifestation: During childhood; occasionally at birth. Hearing impairment possibly not until adulthood.

Etiology: This is a group of hereditary disorders, of which at least four show autosomal dominant transmission (types I A, B; IV A, B) with variable expression. Often due to new mutations. Good prognosis for the first two types, variable for the latter two. Delineation of further types can be expected.

Frequency: About 1:25,000.

Course, prognosis: Dependent on the severity of the clinical picture (see above). With early presentation, increased mortality; but after survival of the first half of infancy, usually good life expectancy. As a rule, decrease in bone fragility after puberty. For the most part, good healing of fractures, but development of pseudarthroses not unusual.

Treatment: Multidisciplinary. Attempts at modification with medications are still in the experimental stage. Conservative and/or operative treatment of fractures and deformities, avoiding long immobilization as far as possible. Cesarean section may be indicated with pregnancies. Conservative and/or operative methods to improve hearing for otosclerotic hearing impairments. Genetic counseling.

Illustrations:

1 An 18-month-old patient with typically shaped head, blue sclerae, bowing and shortening of the extremities (subsequent successful osteotomies).

2, 4, and 5 A 5½-year-old patient with 'triangular' face, pseudarthroses of the right tibia and left humerus, small stature.

3–6 A 13½-year-old girl, severely deformed after extremely numerous fractures (recently, a decrease in the tendency to breaks); asymmetric thorax, extreme lumbar lordosis, scoliosis and gibbus of the thoracic spine with 'fish vertebrae'; normal hands and feet.

H.-R.W.

References:

Paterson, C.R., McAllion, S. et al. Heterogeneity of osteogenesis imperfecta type I. *J. Med. Genet.*, 20, 203–205 (1983).
Paterson, C.R., McAllion, S. et al. Osteogenesis imperfecta after the menopause. *N. Engl. J. Med.*, 310, 1694–1696 (1984).
Spranger, J. Osteogenesis imperfecta: a pasture for splitters and lumpers. *Am. J. Med. Genet.*, 17, 425–428 (1984).
Beighton, P., Winship, I. et al. The ocular form of osteogenesis imperfecta: a new autosomal recessive syndrome. *Clin. Genet.*, 28, 69–75 (1985).
Stefan, L.S., Wright, J.M. et al. Osteogenesis imperfecta . . . *Am. J. Med. Genet.*, 21, 257–269 (1985).
Shea-Landry, G. and Cole, D.E.C. Psychosocial aspects of osteogenesis imperfecta. *Can. Med. Assoc. J.*, 135, 977–981 (1986).
Wenstrup, R.J., Hunter, A.G.W. et al. Osteogenesis imperfecta type IV . . . *Hum. Genet.*, 74, 47–53 (1986).
Paterson, C.R., McAllion, S. et al. Clinical and radiological features of osteogenesis imperfecta type IV A. *Acta Pediatr. Scand.*, 76, 548–552 (1987).
Tsipouras, P., Schwartz, R.C. et al. Prenatal prediction of osteogenesis imperfecta . . . type IV . . . *J. Med. Genet.*, 24, 406–409 (1987).
Levin, L.S., Young, R.J. et al. Osteogenesis imperfecta type I . . . *Am. J. Med. Genet.*, 31, 921–932 (1988).
Ternes, M.L. and Pontz, B.F. Kinder mit osteogenesis imperfecta. *Der Kinderarzt*, 19, 769–774 (1988).

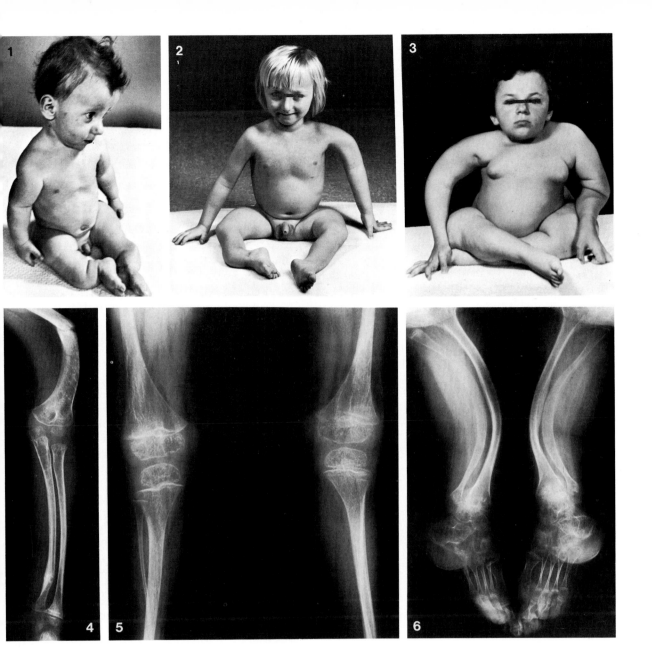

369

184. Thalidomide Embryopathy

A fairly extensive and characteristic malformation sequence due to maternal ingestion of thalidomide during early pregnancy.

Main signs:
1. Hypo- and agenesis of the extremities of all grades of severity. Ranges from minimal expression such as hypoplasia of the thumb or thenar eminence (or excessive growth in the form of triphalangeal thumb), to hypo- or aplasia of the radius, to intercalary phocomelia with absence of the marginal radial rays, or even finally amelia. Similar, but less frequent, involvement of the legs. In extreme cases, tetra-'phocomelia' or tetra-amelia (1, 2).
2. Malformations of the head region: ear abnormalities, microtia to anotia, frequently combined with deafness or with defects of the seventh, also of the third, fourth, and sixth cranial nerves, occasionally with malformation of the labyrinths. Malformations of the eyes: epiphora, coloboma, microphthalmos. Dental anomalies (2, 6).
3. Malformation of internal organs, especially of the heart, the great vessels and the lungs, the kidneys and the urogenital tract, the biliary tract, and the gastrointestinal tract (esophageal, duodenal-intestinal, or anal atresia).

Supplementary findings: Frequently broad, flat nasal root and nose; pronounced nevus flammeus of the midface area varying in extent (occasionally also isolated 'mustache' distribution) (1–5).

Intelligence normal as a rule.

Manifestation: At birth.

Etiology: Maternal ingestion of substances containing thalidomide (alpha-phthalimidoglutarimide), 34–50 days after the last menstrual period or between 25–27 and 44 days after conception.

Frequency: Between 1958 and 1963, thousands of children born with thalidomide embryopathy in Europe, Australia, America, and Japan.

Course, prognosis: High rate of early mortality. Further prognosis dependent on the extent of the individual defects and success of surgical correction.

Differential diagnosis: Holt–Oram syndrome (p.438), tetraphocomelia–cleft palate syndrome (p.372), Fanconi anemia syndrome (and conditions in its differential diagnosis) (p.440).

Treatment: Comprehensive rehabilitation.

Illustrations:

1–6 Children with thalidomide embryopathy, born between 1958 and 1962.

1 Neonate with bilateral 'phocomelia', each hand with three three-segmented fingers, nevus flammeus of the entire medial region of the face; kidney malformations; cardiac anomaly.

2 A 4-week-old infant. Hypoplasia of the radius with wrist-drop and absence of the first ray bilaterally; proximal radioulnar synostoses. Severe bilateral abnormalities of the ears with aplasia of the auditory canal. Peripheral paresis of the facial nerve. Capillary hemangioma of the face. Cardiac anomaly.

3–5 Three children with non-specific but so-called thalidomide facies; in **5** only the suggestion of a 'mustache' hemangioma remaining.

3 Neonate with radial aplasia and absence of the marginal rays; left dislocated hip; dysplasia of the right hip; possible cardiac anomaly.

4 A 3-month-old girl with 'phocomelia' and absence of the first ray bilaterally; possible cardiac defect.

5 A 2-year-old boy with radial aplasia or intercalary hemimelia bilaterally and absence of the marginal radial rays.

6 An 11-year-old, mentally normal girl. Severe bilateral abnormalities of the ears, hypoplastic external auditory canal on the left only. Severe hearing impairment. Disturbance of balance. Paresis of the right facial nerve; also paralysis of lateral conjugate gaze bilaterally. Left side of the face flatter than the right. Congenital facial capillary hemangioma, which has receded. Maternal intake of thalidomide preparation on the 27th day after conception.

H.-R.W.

References:

Wiedemann, H.-R. Klinische Bemerkungen zur pharmakogenen Teratogenese. In: *Teratogenesis*. Schwabe & Co, Basel, 1964.
Willert, H.-G. and Henkel, H.-L. *Klinik und Pathologie der Dysmelie*. Springer, Berlin, Heidelberg, New York, 1969.
Burgio, G.R. The thalidomide disaster briefly revisited. *Eur. J. Pediatr.*, 136, 229 (1981).
Lenz, W. Thalidomide embryopathy in Germany, 1959–1961. In: *Prevention of Physical and Mental Congenital Defects, Part C: Basic and Medical Science, Education and Future Strategies*. Alan Liss Inc., 1985 (pp.77–83).
Fraser, F.C. Thalidomide retrospective: what did we learn? *Teratology*, 38, 201–202 (1988).
Lenz, W. A short history of thalidomide embryopathy. *Teratology*, 38, 203–215 (1988).

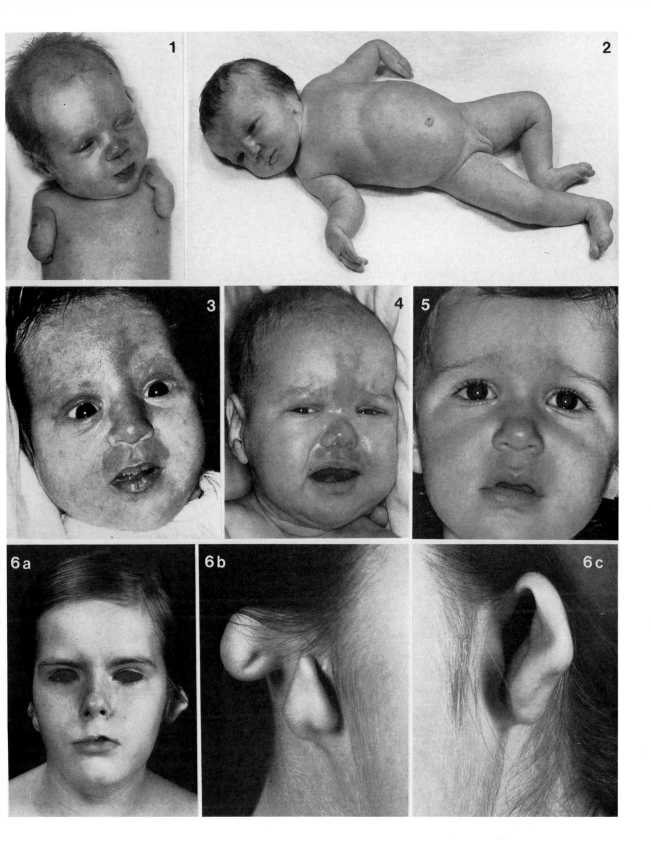

185. Roberts Syndrome

(Tetraphocomelia–Cleft Palate Syndrome; Pseudothalidomide Syndrome; SC Syndrome)

An autosomal recessive syndrome of tetraphocomelia, cleft lip and palate, and mental retardation.

Main signs:
1. Tetraphocomelia due to absence or shortening of the long bones of the extremities (1–6); usually reduction of the rays of the fingers, and occasionally toes, to four or less.

Syndactyly and fusion of metacarpals and metatarsals (5, 6).
2. Usually double-sided cleft lip and palate (1, 2); cleft palate alone or high palate also possible.
3. Mental retardation.

Supplementary findings: Primordial growth deficiency. Hypertelorism, hypoplastic alae nasi (4). Hemangioma of the face; fine, thin silver-blond hair.

Penis or clitoris relatively large; cryptorchidism. Possible horseshoe kidneys, polycystic kidneys.

Possible encephalocele, hydrocephalus.

Divided centromere region in C-banded metaphase chromosome preparations.

Manifestation: At birth.

Etiology: Monogenic disorder, autosomal recessive with variable expression.

Frequency: Very low; between first description in 1829 and 1980, about 50 cases described.

Prognosis: About 50% of cases are stillborn or die within the first weeks of life, frequently of pneumonia.

Differential diagnosis: Thalidomide syndrome.

Treatment: Operative correction of clefts and orthopedic care as indicated.

After birth of an index case, prenatal diagnosis in subsequent pregnancies (ultrasound; chromosome analysis—premature separation of the centromeres is suggestive of this syndrome).

Illustrations:
1 A 16-month-old, the second child of young, healthy, nonconsanguineous parents after a healthy girl. The proband was followed by two similarly affected fetuses (pregnancies terminated) and a further healthy child.
2 A male newborn: typical appearance with 'phocomelia' and bilateral cleft lip and palate; cytogenetically, 'fissured centromeres'.
3 and 4 A 4½-year-old child, only 64 cm tall, head circumference 46 cm. Mental retardation. Dermoid cyst of the anterior neck region; cleft palate.
5 and 6 X-rays of the child in 3 and 4 at 2 days and 4½ years, respectively. Absent radii, shortened ulnae, fusion of metacarpals one, two, four and five bilaterally; high, narrow pelvis with rudimentary ischial rami; the only long bone present in the legs is probably the tibia; fusion of metatarsals four and five; the bone age corresponds to that of a 2½-year-old girl.

H.-R.W.

References:

Freeman, M.V.R., Williams, O.W., Schimke, R.N., Temtamy, S.A., Vachier, E., German, J. The Roberts syndrome. *Clin. Genet.*, 5, 1 (1974).
Grosse, F.R., Pandel, C., Wiedemann, H.-R. The tetraphocomelia–cleft palate syndrome. *Humangenetik*, 28, 353 (1975).
Herrmann, J. and Opitz, J.M. The SC phocomelia and the Roberts syndrome: nosologic aspects. *Eur. J. Pediatr.*, 125, 117 (1977).
Quazi, Q.H., Kassner, E.G., Masakawa et al. The SC phocomelia syndrome: report of two cases with cytogenetic abnormality. *Am. J. Med. Genet.*, 4, 231 (1979).
Fryns, H., Goddeeris, P., Moerman, F. et al. The tetraphocomelia–cleft palate syndrome in identical twins. *Hum. Genet.*, 53, 279 (1980).
Leonard, P., Rendle-Short, J., Skardoon, L. Roberts–SC phocomelia syndrome with cytogenetic findings. *Hum. Genet.*, 60, 379 (1982).
Pfeiffer, R.A. and Zwerner, H. Das Roberts-Syndrom. *Monatschr. Kinderheilkd.*, 130, 296 (1982).
Zergollern, L. and Hitrec, V. Four siblings with Robert's syndrome. *Clin. Genet.*, 21, 1 (1982).
Römke, C., Froster-Iskenius, U., Heyne, K. et al. Roberts syndrome and SC phocomelia. A single genetic entity. *Clin. Genet.*, 31, 170–177 (1987).
Robins, D.B., Ladda, R.L. et al. Prenatal detection of Roberts–SC phocomelia syndrome. *Am. J. Med. Genet.*, 32, 390–394 (1989).

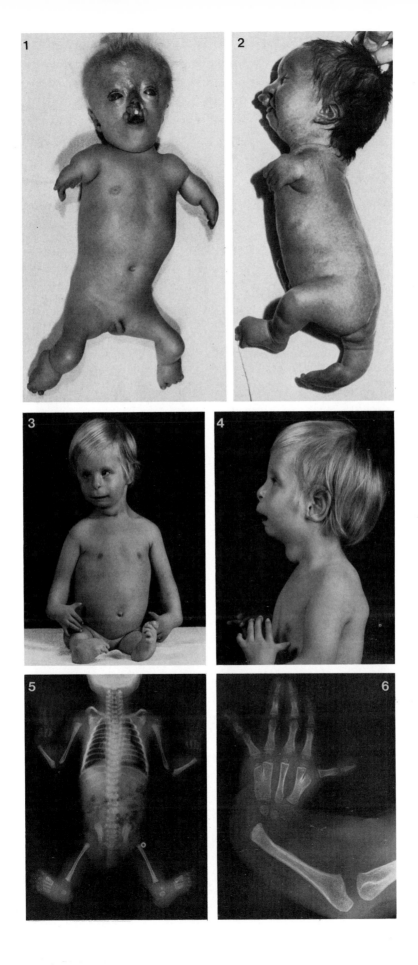

186. Thrombocytopenia-Absent Radius Syndrome

(TAR Syndrome)

A syndrome of bilateral aplasia of the radius with retention of the thumbs, thrombocytopenia, and other anomalies.

Main signs:
1. Bilateral aplasia of the radius with radial wrist-drop, thumbs always present (1–6). Frequently also hypoplasia of the humerus, aplasia in isolated cases ('phocomelia').
2. Thrombocytopenia, fluctuating and often severe, with megakaryocytopenia and frequent life-threatening episodes of bleeding or bleeding tendency (including cerebral hemorrhage). The platelet deficiency is episodic and severity is possibly aggravated by allergy to cow's milk, intercurrent infections, etc. Anemia due to bleeding and hemolysis possible in infancy. Often pronounced eosinophilia. Leukocytosis. Also frequent leukemoid reactions, possibly with hepatosplenomegaly, in infancy.
3. Cardiac defect in about one-third of cases (atrial septal defect, tetralogy of Fallot).
4. Short stature (around or below the tenth percentile).

Supplementary findings: Allergy to cow's milk not unusual, precipitating abrupt fall in platelet count and hemolysis; episodes of diarrhea with vomiting and dehydration during the first year of life.

Other skeletal anomalies common: hypoplasia of the lower jaw or midface with low nasal root (1, 2). Hypoplasia of the shoulder girdle, ribs, or vertebral column.

Hip dysplasia; limited movement at the knees, dislocation of the patellae; internal rotation of the tibiae; genu varus; club feet. Exceptionally, severe reduction defects of the lower extremities.

Possible extensive capillary hemangioma on the face, including 'mustache' location (2). Cutis laxa in the nuchal area (2); edema of the dorsum of the feet.

Radiologically, distinct hypoplasia and bowing of the ulnae possible (5, 6), occasionally aplasia; hypoplasia involving wrists or fingers. Hook formation on the lateral ends of the clavicles, and other signs.

Manifestation: At birth.

Etiology: Genetically determined syndrome. Severity of skeletal, hematological, and cardiac anomalies varies within and among families. The assumption of autosomal recessive inheritance does not fit all observed cases; different mutations at the same gene locus?

Frequency: Low; estimated 1 : 0.5–1 million newborns; by 1988, more than 100 published observations.

Course, prognosis: Tendency for platelet count to improve (normal values in adulthood). If the child survives the first year of life, during which mortality is very high, life expectancy is probably almost normal. Mental development dependent on the occurrence of intracranial hemorrhages during the first two years of life.

Differential diagnosis: Aase syndrome (p.436), Holt–Oram syndrome (p.438), Fanconi anemia (p.440), thalidomide embryopathy (p.370), pseudothalidomide syndrome (p.372), trisomy 18 (p.88).

Treatment: Intensive hematological support (platelet or whole blood transfusions). Conservative orthopedic care. Omission of cow's milk protein from the diet in some patients. Operative repair of cardiac defect if indicated. As far as possible, prevention of infections, operative procedures, and stress in the first year of life to safeguard against life-threatening episodes of thrombocytopenia and bleeding. Later possible operative orthopedic treatment (e.g., to correct malpositioned knees). Genetic counseling. Ultrasonographic prenatal diagnosis for further pregnancies. Cases diagnosed prenatally should be delivered by cesarean section.

Illustrations:

1–6 A newborn, the first child of healthy, young parents. Fully expressed syndrome; thrombocytopenia, hypereosinophilia, anemia. Hypoplasia of the distal humeri and of the shoulder girdles; bilateral hip dysplasia, mild talipes calcaneus; clinodactyly of both little fingers (5, 6). Pronounced allergy to cow's milk, exposure being followed by diarrhea, vomiting, and decreased weight and platelet count, making a cow's milk-free diet mandatory. Persistent low nasal root; development of pronounced bowed legs.

H.-R.W.

References:

Ward, R.E., Bixler, D. et al. Parent to child transmission of the thrombocytopenia absent radius (TAR) syndrome. *Am. J. Med. Genet.*, Suppl, 2, 207–214 (1986).

Hall, J.G. Thrombocytopenia and absent radius . . . *J. Med. Genet.*, 24, 79–83 (1987).

Sehbur, R.E., Eunpu, D.L. et al. Thrombocytopenia with absent radius in a boy and his uncle. *Am. J. Med. Genet.*, 28, 117–123 (1987).

Giuffré, L., Cammarata, M. et al. Two new cases of . . . TAR syndrome . . . *Klin. Pädiatr.*, 200, 10–14 (1988).

Marec, B.L., Odent, S. et al. Genetic counselling in a case of TAR . . . *Clin. Genet.*, 34, 104–108 (1988).

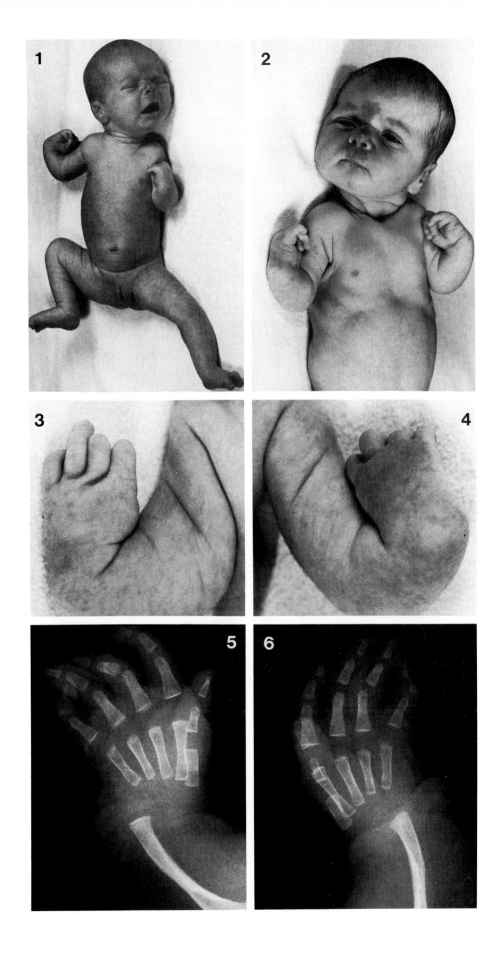

187. Syndrome of Deafness, Radial Hypoplasia, and Psychomotor Retardation

A syndrome of congenital deafness, marked psychomotor retardation, mild bilateral hypoplasia of the radius, and other anomalies.

Main signs:
1. Congenital bilateral deafness.
2. Mild bilateral hypoplasia of the radius with radial abduction of the hands, hypoplasia of the thenar musculature and of the thumbs (left side more severely affected radiologically and clinically) (**1, 7–9**).
3. Considerable mental and motor retardation (still unable to stand without support at almost 2 years old) (**1–3**).

Supplementary findings: High, short cranium with broad forehead (**1, 3**). Low-set, prominent, dysplastic ears (**4–6**).

Hypoplasia of the first ribs. Slightly retarded bone age.

Ocular fundi normal; heart normal; i.v. pyelogram normal; blood count, including thrombocytes, normal.

Manifestation: At birth.

Etiology: Unknown.

Diagnosis, differential diagnosis: The clinical picture described here does not appear to be one of the many recognized syndromes with either hearing impairment or radial hypoplasia.

Treatment: Symptomatic.

Illustrations:
1–9 The proband at almost 2 years of age. The first child of young, healthy parents. Consanguinity not known. No family history of hearing impairment. Pregnancy unremarkable, birth at term. Normal development of height and weight.

H.-R.W.

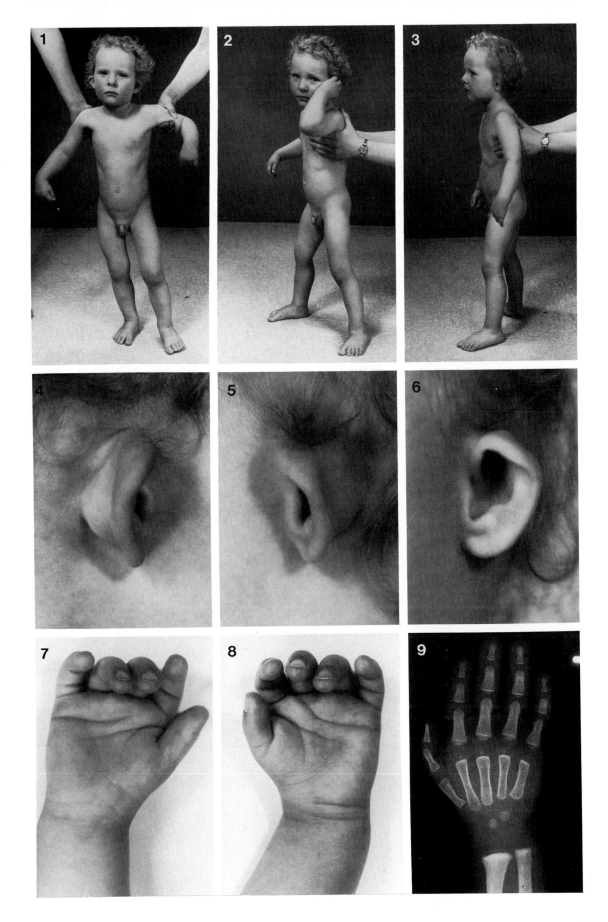

188. Lacrimo-Auriculo-Dento-Digital Syndrome

(LADD Syndrome)

A syndrome of hypoplasia, aplasia, or atresia involving the lacrimal system, ear anomalies and hearing impairment, aplasia or atresia within the salivary system, and anomalies of teeth and fingers.

Main signs:
1. Epiphora or deficiency of tears as a result of atresia, hypoplasia, or aplasia of the lacrimal apparatus (e.g., absence of the lacrimal puncta, atresia of the tear ducts, aplasia of the lacrimal glands).
2. Malformed external ears; possible hearing impairment (different types).
3. Dryness of the mouth with eating difficulties due to hypo- or aplasia of the large salivary glands or absence of the duct openings.
4. Possibly hypo- or aplasia of the teeth or other anomalies of dentition.
5. Diverse anomalies of the fingers, usually of the preaxial rays (e.g., hypoplasia of the thumbs).

Supplementary findings: Irritation of ocular and oral mucous membranes; possible candidiasis. Early development of dental caries, possibly severe leading to total loss of teeth. Additional minor anomalies optional (see also **1–4**).

Manifestation: Infancy and later.

Etiology: Autosomal dominant disorder with very variable expression.

Frequency: Low; to date only about 15 published cases that appear certain.

Course, prognosis: No decrease in life expectancy. Early recognition important because of possible hearing impairment and for the early institution of oral hygiene.

Diagnosis, differential diagnosis: In spite of unremarkable facial outline, hypo- or aplasia of the parotids may be present (CT scan, scintiscan). Hypohydrotic ectodermal dysplasia, the EEC syndrome, oculo-dento-osseus dysplasia, and many other clinical pictures can be easily ruled out.

Treatment: Ophthalmological surgical measures (e.g., for stenosis or atresia of the nasolacrimal ducts). Hearing and speech aids may be indicated. Intensive oral hygiene and dental care.

Illustrations:
1–4 A 2½-year-old boy with LADD: deficient tears, anomalies of the external ears, dental decay (**3**) with deficient salivation. Note also the short neck and form of the nose; in addition, short stature (third percentile).

H.-R.W.

Reference:
Wiedemann, H.-R. and Drescher, J. LADD syndrome: report of new cases and review of the clinical spectrum. *Eur. J. Pediatr.*, 144, 579–582 (1986).

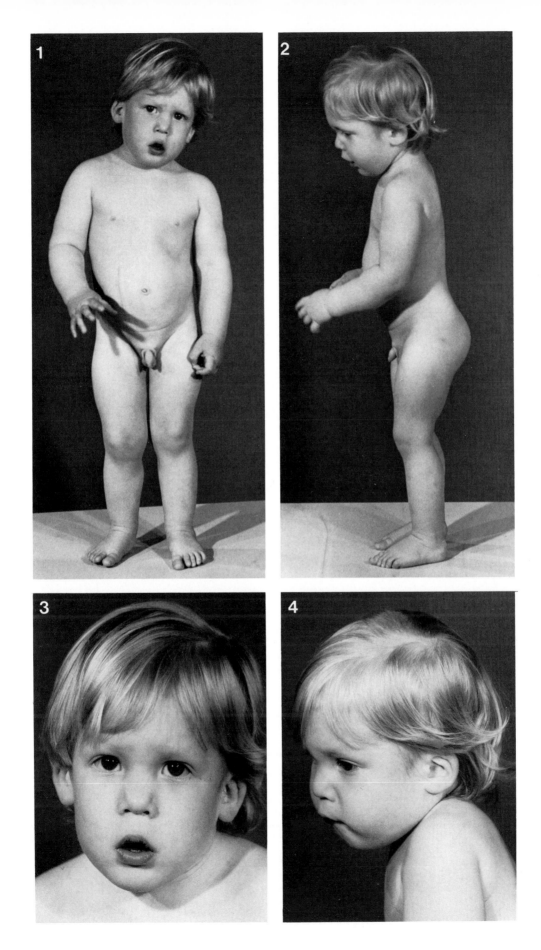

189. Oro-Acral 'Syndrome'

(Aglossia–Adactyly Syndrome, Ankyloglossia Superior Syndrome, Glossopalantine Ankylosis Syndrome, Hanhart Syndrome, Hypoglossia–Hypodactyly Syndrome, Oromandibular–Limb Hypogenesis Syndrome)

A spectrum of malformations of the oral cavity region and reduction anomalies of the extremities.

Main signs:

1. Micro-to aglossia; cleft palate.
2. Adhesion of the tongue to the upper jaw; fibrous bands between the upper and lower jaws, also bony adhesions; micrognathia (**1–3**).
3. Transverse reduction anomalies of the extremities, ranging from stump-like hands/feet to upper arm/upper leg stumps. Also usually pronounced right–left and upper–lower asymmetry (**1, 3**).
4. Syndactyly.

Supplementary findings: Low birth weight (average in 21 cases is 2572 g). Cranial nerve palsies (see Möbius sequence). Absence of the dental germs. Exceptionally, mental retardation.

(Possible splenogonadal fusion, anal atresia.)

Manifestation: At birth.

Etiology: Unknown. Developmental field defect. No increased risk of recurrence.

Frequency: Low; about 80 cases reported up to 1985.

Course, prognosis: Good, except for the danger of aspiration as a result of oral malformations. Speech development amazingly good, with the exception of 'tongue-teeth consonants', even with aglossia. Full development of the mandible is usual.

Treatment: Surgery for oral malformations. Prostheses.

Differential diagnosis: Möbius sequence (p.492), in which cranial nerve palsy is always present, while malformations of the extremities are rare except for frequent club feet. Whenever malformations of the extremities of the type described here are associated with micrognathia, oro-acral 'syndrome' should be considered.

Comment: This spectrum includes the above-mentioned 'syndromes', some of which were previously regarded as independent entities.

Illustrations:

1–3 Two newborns. Note the extreme micrognathia in **2** (same patient as in **1**). Unfortunately, clinical records on these children were not available, so that the oral anomalies are not known.

H.-R.W./J.K.

References:

Hermann, J., Pallister, P.D., Gilbert, E.F. et al. Nosologic studies in the Hanhart and the Möbius syndrome. *Eur. J. Pediatr.*, 122, 19 (1976).

Grosse, F.R. and Wiedemann, H.-R. Syndromes with reduction and surplus anomalies of the hand. *Birth Defects*, XIII, 1, 301 (1977).

Johnson, G.F. and Robinow, M. Aglossia-adactylia. *Radiology*, 128, 127 (1978).

Schmitt, K., Fries, R. et al. Das oro-akrale Syndrom. *Monatschr. Kinderheilkd.*, 129, 245–247 (1981).

Pauli, R.M. and Greenlaw, A. Limb deficiency and splenogonadal fusion. *Am. J. Med. Genet.*, 13, 81–89 (1982).

Bökesoy, I., Aksüyek, C. et al. Oromandibular limb hypogenesis/Hanhart's syndrome... *Clin. Genet.*, 24, 47–49 (1983).

Ikeda, T., Ohdo, S. et al. Syndromes associated with microglossia and ectrodactyly... *Cong. Anom.*, 23, 195–205 (1983).

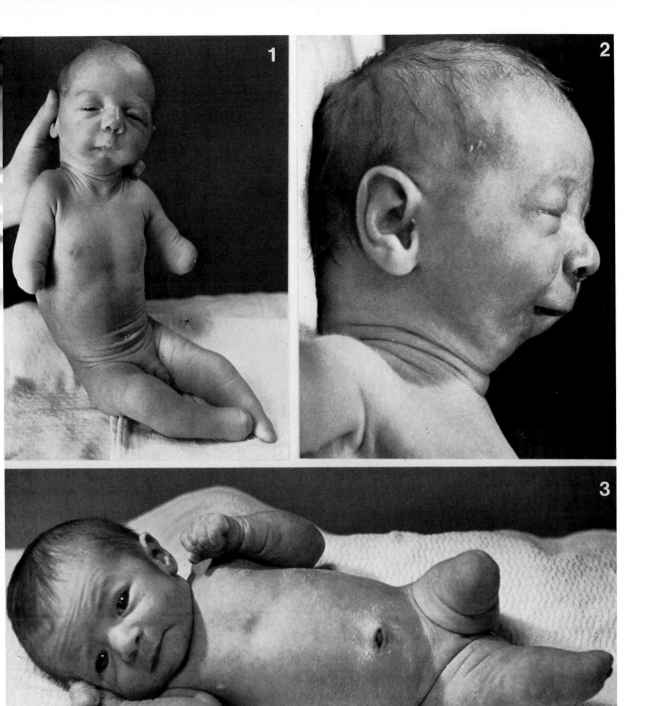

190. Syndrome of Symmetrical Tetraperomelia with Anal Atresia, Microphallus with Hypospadias, and Accessory Lacrimal Puncta

A malformation complex comprising peromelia of the upper and lower extremities associated with multiple other internal and external anomalies.

Main signs:
1. Symmetrical peromelia of the arms directly below the elbows (with congenital lateral scars), and of the legs just below the knees (**1–3, 7, 8**).
2. Anal atresia. Hypoplasia of the external genitalia (**6**) with glandular hypospadias; bilateral undescended testicles.
3. Bilateral dislocated hips.
4. Accessory lacrimal puncta (below the lower lacrimal puncta; **4**) with occasional secretion.

Supplementary findings: Mild micrognathia (present at birth) (**1–3**); tongue, oral mucosa, and palate unremarkable. However, hypoplasia of the left processus muscularis mandibulae and (at 2½ years) absence of the germs of the first and second left lower deciduous molars. Dissimilar auricles with preauricular pit on the left (**5**).

Bilateral cervical ribs. Right convex lumbar scoliosis. Asacria. Marked bilateral hydronephrosis and hydroureter; dystopia of the bladder superiorly and to the right; multiple diverticula of the urinary bladder.

Normal mental development for age.

Manifestation: At birth.

Etiology: Unknown.

Course, prognosis: With appropriate physical rehabilitation, favorable.

Comment: The clinical picture of this child is close to that of the oro–acral, or Hanhart, syndrome (p.380). Whether it can be classified under that syndrome or — in view of atypically minimal oral manifestations, atypically symmetrical limb defects, the 'extended spectrum', and other peculiarities — whether it is a separate entity cannot be resolved at this time.

Treatment: Symptomatic: surgery for anal atresia; treatment of the hip; prostheses; orthodontic dental care; appropriate handicap aids.

Illustrations:
1–6 The proband at 5½ years. The second child of young, healthy, nonconsanguineous parents (first- and third-born children healthy). Birth after an unremarkable pregnancy, 3 weeks before term at 2500 g. No problems with early care.
7 and 8 X-rays taken at 2 years.

H.-R.W.

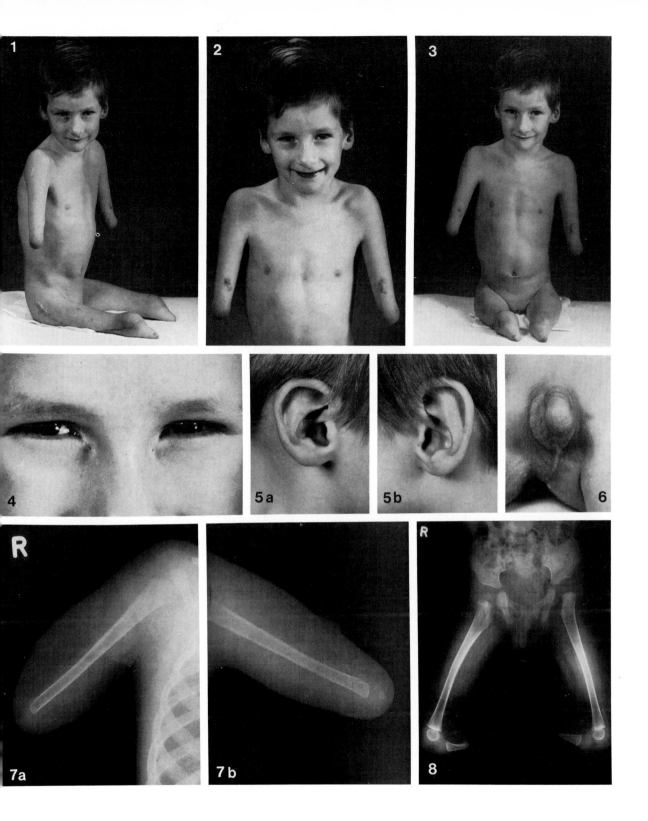

191. Femur–Fibula–Ulna Complex

A usually asymmetrically occurring combination of femoral and fibular defects with contralateral malformation of the ulna (FFU Complex).

Main signs:
1. Unilateral proximal defect of the femur.
2. Ipsilateral agenesis of the fibula with defect of the fibular ray of the corresponding foot (fourth and fifth).
3. Contralateral ulnar malformation of the upper extremity (hypoplasia of the ulna, peromelia, amelia, humero-radial dysostoses, ulnar ray defects of fourth and fifth fingers).

There is no correlation between the severity of the malformations in the two extremities. There is no single clinical sign that is found in all FFU patients (not a syndrome – see Lenz).

Supplementary findings: Growth of cranium and trunk not retarded. In 123 cases, the left arm was affected; in 121, the right; the left leg was affected 57 times, the right 59 times. The arm deformities were more severe on the left (42 times) than on the right (9 times).

Manifestation: At birth.

Etiology: No familial occurrence, no parental consanguinity, no paternal-age effect. Neither geographic nor temporal clustering; occurrence all over the world. No precipitating prenatal factors known. One observation in siblings.

Frequency: Up to 1977, documented in 321 cases; 106 of these in Germany. Of 178 cases, 109 were boys and 69 were girls.

Course, prognosis: Dependent on the severity and possibility of correction of the individual defects.

Treatment: Orthopedic measures; any appropriate handicap aids.

Differential diagnosis:
1. Atypical cleft hand.
2. Amniotic-bands.
3. Oro-acral syndrome.
4. Femoral hypoplasia with unusual facies syndrome.

Illustrations:
1–6 A female newborn.
1 Shortening of the right thigh, malformations of the right foot and left hand.
2 Asymmetry of the ilial wings; no acetabulum on the right; hypoplasia of the caudal portion of the os ilium; severe hypoplasia of the right femur; ipsilateral tibial hypoplasia and absence of the fibula.
3a and 3b The left hand with complete cutaneous syndactyly of rays I and II, partial syndactyly of rays II and III, normal ray IV, and absent ray V.
6a and 6b Corresponding X-rays: Only three rays in the metacarpal region; the broad ray in the middle may represent a fusion of rays II and III, to which the partially fused proximal phalanges of rays II and III are adjoined; ray V is absent.
4 and 5 The child's right foot: absence of both fibular marginal rays.

J.K.

References:

Lenz, W. and Feldmann, U. Unilateral and asymmetric limb defects in man: delineation of the femur–fibula–ulna complex. *Birth Defects*, XIII, 1, 269–285 (1977).

Zlotogora, J., Rosenmann, E., Menashe, M. et al. The femur, fibula, ulna (FFU) complex in siblings. *Clin. Genet.*, 24, 449–452 (1983).

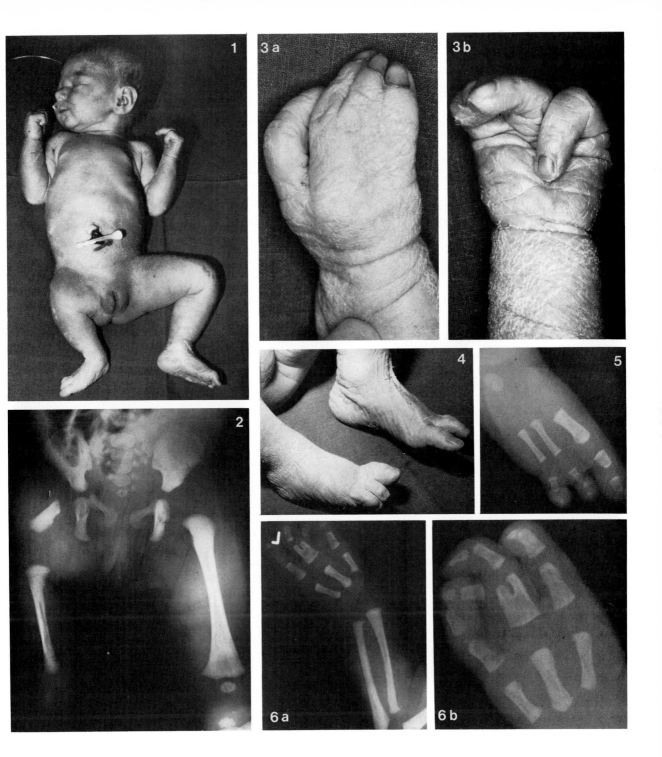

385

192. 'EEC' Syndrome

(Ectrodactyly–Ectodermal Dysplasia–Clefting Syndrome)

A syndrome comprising ectrodactyly of the hands and feet, signs of ectodermal dysplasia, and facial clefts (usually of the lips).

Main signs:
1. Variably severe anomalies of the midportion of the hands and feet, ranging from syndactyly to clefting of the hands and feet (**1, 3–5**).
2. Cleft lip, palate, or both. High palate, hypoplastic maxilla.
3. Sparse, thin, light scalp hair; sparse eyebrows and eyelashes (**2b**). Thin, light, dry, and possibly hyperkeratotic skin; inability to sweat. Possible mamillary hypoplasia, nail anomalies, small pigmented nevi.
4. Stenosis or atresia of the nasolacrimal canals, blepharitis, keratoconjunctivitis (possible dacryocystitis, corneal scars), blepharophimosis, photophobia (**2b**).
5. Dysodontiasis (small carious teeth with hypoplastic enamel; also, missing teeth). Possible xerostomia.

Supplementary findings: Conductive hearing impairment may be a feature, also anomalies of the kidneys, urinary tract, and genitalia.

Mental development usually normal; however retardation, sometimes with microcephaly, occasionally reported.

Manifestations: At birth.

Etiology: Genetically determined syndrome. Frequently sporadic occurrence, probably due to new mutations. Autosomal dominant inheritance with reduced penetrance and quite variable expression (no one sign is obligatory). Heterogeneity or multiple alleles are possible. Basic defect unknown.

Frequency: Low (about 100–150 cases in the literature).

Course, prognosis: Dependent on the severity of the features and on the success of efforts toward 'rehabilitation' and social adjustment.

Diagnosis, differential diagnosis: In case of doubt, other syndromes in which facial clefts may occur should be considered.

Treatment: Early correction of stenosis of the nasolacrimal canals; continuous ophthalmologic care for this problem may be very important in some cases. In addition, care by an orthopedic surgeon, oral surgeon, and orthodontist. A wig may be beneficial. Genetic counseling.

Illustrations:
1–6 A patient at ages 10 weeks (**2a, 4b, 5**), 3 years (**1, 2b, 3a, 3b, 4a, 6**), and 4 years (**3c**). Psychomotor retardation, microcephaly. High palate, mild mamillary hypoplasia, left renal agenesis and right hydronephrosis, cryptorchidism.
3 The left hand.
4 The right hand.
5 The feet.

In addition to the familiar signs of EEC, the child shows the following: bilateral microphthalmos with coloboma of the iris, the choroid membrane, the retina, and the optic nerve (**2a**); bifid clavicle on the right (**6**); and ventricular septal defect with pulmonary hypertension. Height below the third percentile.

H.-R.W.

References:

Gehler, J. and Grosse, R. Fehlbildungs-Syndrom mit Spalthänden-Spaltfüßen, Iriskolobom, Nierenagenesie und Ventrikelseptumdefekt. *Klin. Pädiatr.*, 184, 389 (1972).
Pashayan, H.M. et al. The EEC syndrome. *Birth Defects*, 10, 105–127 (1974).
Schmidt, R. and Nitowsky, H.M. Split hand and foot deformity . . . (EEC). *Hum. Genet.*, 39, 15–25 (1977).
Mücke, J. and Sandig, K.-R. Zur Expressivität des EEC-Syndroms. *Kinderärztl. Praxis*, 48, 198–203 (1980).
Predine-Hug, F., le Merrer, M. et al. Dysplasie ectodermique et ectrodactylie familiale. *Arch. Fr. Pëdiatr.*, 41, 49–50 (1984).
Küster, W., Majewski, F. et al. EEC syndrome without ectrodactyly? *Clin. Genet.*, 28, 130–135 (1985).
London, R., Heredia, R.M. et al. Urinary tract involvement in EEC syndrome. *Am. J. Dis. Child.*, 139, 1191–1193 (1985).
Majewski, F. and Küster, W. EEC syndrome sine sine? *Clin. Genet*, 33, 69–72 (1988).

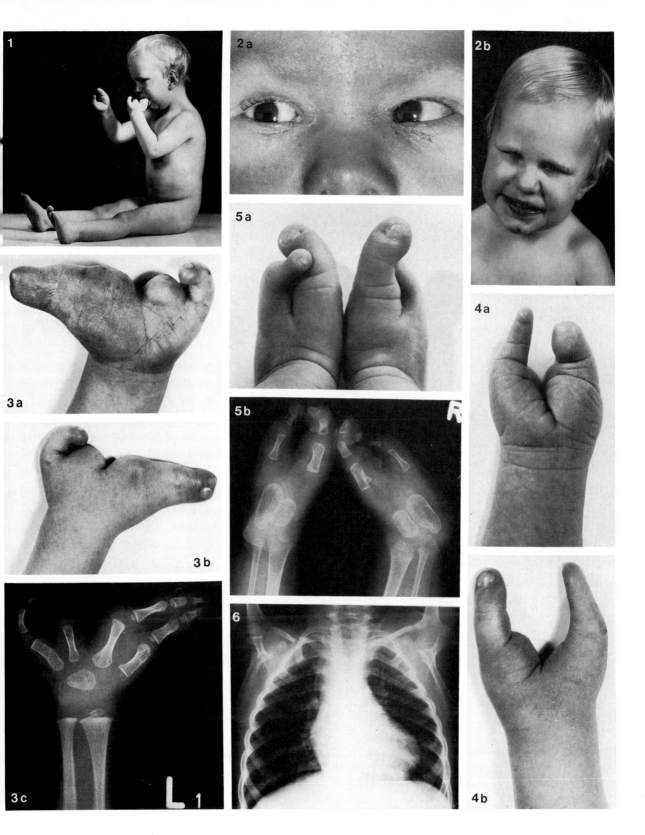

193. Amniotic Constriction Grooves

(ABS: Amniotic Band Sequence; ADAM Complex: Amniotic Deformity, Adhesions, Mutilations; Amniotic Band Disruption Complex/Sequence; Amniotic Bands; Amniotic Constriction Bands; Congenital Amputations; Early Amnion Rupture Sequence; Ring Constrictions; Streeter Anomaly/Dysplasia)

A syndrome of usually multiple malformations resulting from grooves, constrictions, and adhesions caused by amniotic bands *in utero*.

Main signs:
1. Circular grooves – mainly involving the extremities – usually with swelling, hypoplasia, or even amputation of the distal structures (**3, 5, 6**).
2. Peripheral syndactyly, frequently with grooves from the amniotic bands encircling the fused rays (**2**). Adhesions of the cranium to the placenta. Defects of the cranium with or without herniation of the brain or other brain anomalies (**1, 4**).
3. Cleft lip and palate (or its individual components) or facial clefts, which frequently do not correspond with temporal physiological intrauterine development (**1, 4**).
4. Clefts and adhesions of the eyelids; microphthalmos to anophthalmos. Anomalies of the nose and auricles (**1, 4**).
5. Ectopia cordis, abdominal clefts, focal skin defects (**4**).
6. Not infrequently evidence of amnion in the grooves (**2, 5, 6**).

The anomalies may occur alone or in quite varied combinations – independent of the time of amniotic rupture.

Supplementary findings: Scoliosis, dislocated hips, club feet and club hands are regarded as the results of the above-mentioned malformations. Very rarely, 'birth' of an amputated limb. Occurrence also of associated malformations that are not etiologically related (e.g., holoprosencephaly).

Manifestation: At birth.

Etiology: Controversial. The prevailing theory is that fibrous strands that are formed after amniotic rupture cause the anomalies by constriction and adhesion. Almost always sporadic occurrence; practically no risk of recurrence. Familial occurrence as an exception (genetic factors here?).

Frequency: About 1:3,000 newborns.

Course, prognosis: Decreased life expectancy only in those cases with brain malformations or deep facial clefts.

Differential diagnosis: The multiple deep, benign transverse grooves of the skin, especially of the extremities, that occur in some individuals as an autosomal dominant trait (p.308) should not be confused with those of the amniotic band syndrome. The same holds true for the congenital scalp defects occurring with amniotic band-like changes of the extremities (Adams–Oliver syndrome), which is also autosomal dominant.

Treatment: Symptomatic (possibly plastic surgery, prostheses). Genetic counseling (see above). Prenatal diagnosis by ultrasonography in some cases.

Illustrations:
1–3 Case 1 on the first day of life; death on the second day due to respiratory insufficiency, Dysplasia of the left pinna, internal hydrocephalus, left club foot.
4–6 Case 2 at age 5 days. Death at 3 months from pneumonia. Aplasia of the corpus callosum.
In both cases, pregnancy uneventful.

H.-R.W./J.K.

References:

Torpin, R. Amniochorionic mesoblastic fibrous strings and amniotic bands: associated constricting fetal malformations or fetal death. *Am. J. Obstet, Gynecol.*, 91, 65 (1965).

Heege, K. *Amniogene Fehlbildungen der Gliedmaßen mit Beteiligung von Kopf und Gesicht.* Med. Inaugural Dissertation. Westfälische Wilhelms-Universität zu Münster, 1971.

Keller, H., Neuhäuser, G. et al. 'ADAM' complex (Amniotic Deformity, Adhesions, Mutilations) a pattern of craniofacial and limb defects. *Am. J. Med. Genet.*, 2, 81 (1978).

Higgenbottom, M.C., Jones, K.L., Hall, B.D. et al. The amniotic band disruption complex: timing of amniotic rupture and variable spectra of consequent defects. *J. Pediatr.*, 85, 544 (1979).

Etches, P.C., Stewart, A.R. et al. Familial congenital amputations. *J. Pediatr.*, 101, 448–449 (1982).

Lubinsky, M., Sujansky, E. et al. Familial amniotic bands. *Am. J. Med. Genet.*, 14, 81–87 (1983).

Donnenfeld, A.E. and Dunn, L.K. Discordant amniotic band sequence in monozygotic twins. *Am. J. Med. Genet.*, 20, 685–694 (1985).

Hunter, A.G.W. and Carpenter, B.F. Implications of malformations not due to amniotic bands in the amniotic band sequence. *Am. J. Med. Genet.*, 24, 691–700 (1986).

Küster, W., Lenz, W. et al. Congenital scalp defects with distal limb anomalies (Adams–Oliver syndrome) . . . *Am. J. Med. Genet.*, 31, 99–115 (1988).

Garza, A., Cordero, J.F. et al. Epidemiology of the early amnion rupture spectrum of defects. *Am. J. Dis. Child.*, 142, 541–544 (1988).

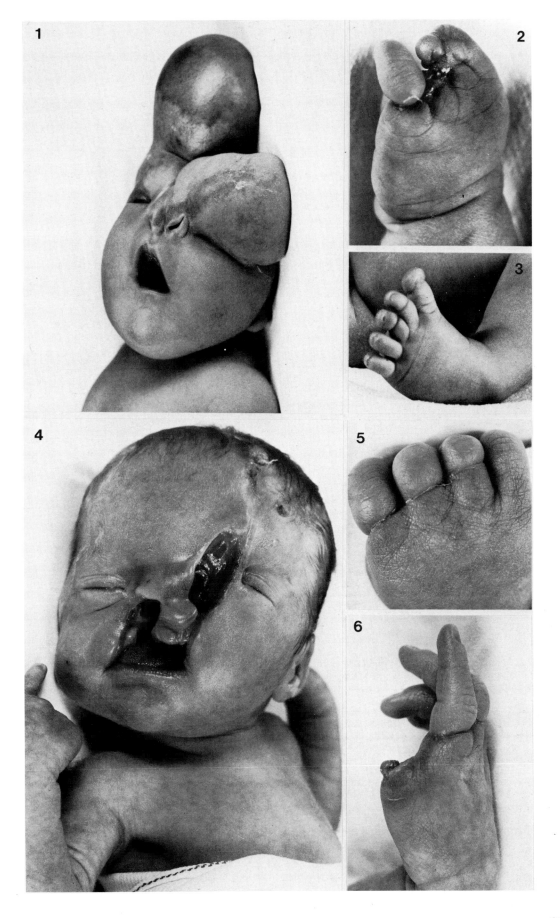

194. Poland Anomaly

(Poland Complex, Poland Sequence, Poland's Syndactyly, Poland Syndrome)

Unilateral aplasia of the pectoral muscle and ipsilateral hand anomalies.

Main signs:
1. Aplasia of pectoralis major muscle (usually only the sternocostal portion) and also pectoralis minor, with frequent hypoplasia, and occasionally aplasia, of the ipsilateral mamilla and mamillary gland (1). Not infrequently, flattening of the ipsilateral thoracic skeleton; rarely bony defects.
2. Ipsilateral anomalies of the upper extremity, mainly in the form of synbrachydactyly, but also with absent rays, ankylosis of finger joints. Hypoplasia of the forearm and very rarely of the arm (2–6).

Supplementary findings: Very occasionally, ipsilateral hypoplasia of the kidneys and hemivertebrae.
Defect on the right side in 75% of cases.
Sex ratio (boys:girls) 3–4:1.

Manifestation: At birth.

Etiology: Sporadic occurrence in the great majority of cases; autosomal dominant inheritance has been assumed in occasional cases. No increased risk of recurrence for the affected family when neither parent is affected. Developmental field defect. Presumed to be a disruption sequence resulting from embryonal interruption of the subclavian artery.

Frequency: About 1 in 30,000 of the general population. Over 500 cases reported by 1985.

Course, prognosis: Normal life expectancy.

Differential diagnosis: The Poland anomaly may occur as part of the Möbius sequence (p.492).

Treatment: Plastic surgery may be indicated. Genetic counseling.

Illustrations:
1–3 and 6 Patient 1: Synbrachydactyly, rudimentary index finger.
4 Patient 2: Aplasia of first to fourth finger on the right, rudimentary fifth finger, ipsilateral absence of pectoralis major muscle.
5 Patient 3: Synbrachydactyly on the right with hypoplastic middle phalanges, short right arm, aplasia of the right pectoralis major muscle.

H.-R.W./J.K.

References:

Ireland, D.C.R., Takayama, N., Flatt, A.E. Poland's syndrome. A review of forty-three cases. *J. Bone Jt. Surg.*, 58-A, 52 (1976).
Sujansky, E., Riccardi, V.M., Matthew, A.L. The familial occurrence of Poland syndrome. *Birth Defects*, 13/3A, 117 (1977).
Castilla, E.E., Paz, J.E., Orioli, I.M. Pectoralis major muscle defect and Poland complex. *Am. J. Med. Genet.*, 4, 263 (1979).
Parker, D.L., Mitchell, P.R., Holmes, G.L. Poland–Möbius syndrome. *J. Med. Genet.*, 18, 317 (1981).
David, T.J. Familial Poland anomaly. *J. Med. Genet.*, 19, 293–296 (1982).
Hegde, H.R. and Shokeir, M.H.K. Posterior shoulder girdle abnormalities with absence of pectoralis major muscle. *Am. J. Med. Genet.*, 13, 285–293 (1982).
Hester, T.R. and Bostwick, J. Poland's syndrome: correction with latissimus muscle transposition. *Plast. Reconstruct. Surg.*, 69, 226–233 (1982).
König, R. and Lenz, W. Pektoralis-Handdefekte. *Z. Orthop.*, 121, 244–254 (1983).
Lowry, R.B. and Bouvet, J.-P. Familial Poland anomaly. *J. Med. Genet.*, 20, 152–154 (1983).
Oppolzer, A. and Sacher, M. Poland-Syndrom. *Klin. Pädiatr.*, 185, 135–137 (1983).
Bosch-Banyeras, J.M., Zuasnabar, A. et al. Poland–Möbius syndrome... *J. Med. Genet.*, 21, 70–71 (1984).
Gausewitz, S.H., Meals, R.A. et al. Severe limb deficiency in Poland's syndrome. *Clin. Orthopaed.*, 185, 9–13 (1984).
David, T.J. and Winter, R.M. Familial absence of the pectoralis major, serratus anterior, and latissimus dorsi muscles. *J. Med. Genet.*, 22, 390–392 (1985).
Bavinck, J.N.B. and Weaver, D.D. Subclavian artery supply disruption sequence... *Am. J. Med. Genet.*, 23, 903–918 (1986).
Esquembre, C., Ferris, J. et al. Poland syndrome and leukemia. *Eur. J. Pediatr.*, 146, 444 (1987).

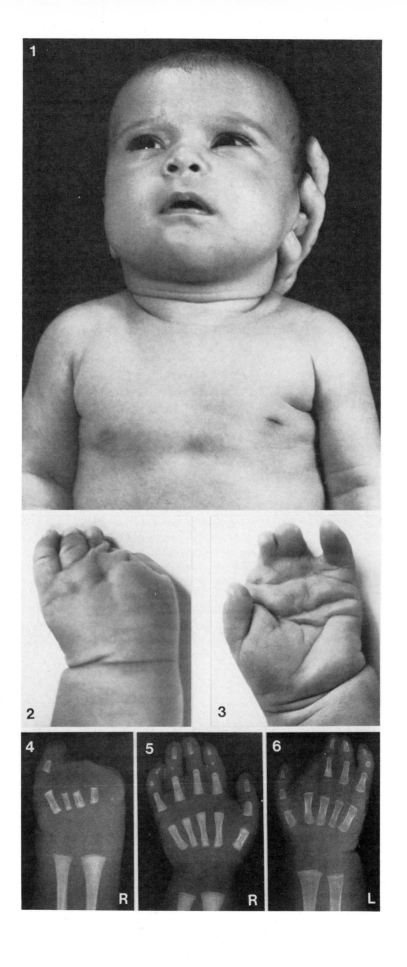

195. Tibial Aplasia or Hypoplasia with Cleft Hand/Cleft Foot

A relatively rare, autosomal dominant anomaly of extreme variability.

Main signs:
1. Ectrodactyly (in about 75% of observed familial cases).
2. Tibial defects of different grades of severity (in up to 60%); club feet.
3. Ulnar defects, variously manifest (in about 12%).
4. Femoral defects of varied severity (in about 8%); bifurcation of the distal end of the femur, among other anomalies.

Supplementary findings: Contractures of the knee joints, occasionally absent patellae, hypoplasia of the big toes, polydactyly, malformation of the external ears.

Manifestation: At birth.

Etiology: Although heterogeneity cannot be excluded with certainty, an autosomal dominant gene with extraordinarily variable expression, decreased penetrance, and low 'specificity' appears likely.

The variability of expression of anomalies extends from cleft hands and feet to monodactyly; bilateral tibial aplasia and contractures of the knee joints to mere syndactyly of two fingers or even only hypoplasia of one or both big toes.

Frequency: Relatively low; up to 1985 there were known to be about 30 sporadic cases and about the same number of families with affected members.

Course, prognosis: Dependent on the degree of expression. Since mental development and internal organs are unaffected, the outlook for even severely affected patients, when optimally treated, is relatively favorable.

Diagnosis, differential diagnosis: Tibial aplasia or hypoplasia with preaxial polydactyly (q.v.).

Treatment: Orthopedic care and appropriate handicap aids. Genetic counseling. Ultrasonographic prenatal diagnosis in some cases.

Illustrations:
1–3 A male newborn with right-sided cleft hand (**1**, **2**) and ipsilateral tibial aplasia, shortening of the lower leg, and club foot with toe anomalies. Sporadic case.
4 and 5 A female newborn, the first child of a similarly affected father, with bilateral cleft hand (with a postminimus on the left hand). Bilateral tibial aplasia with club feet. Hypoplasia of the right foot with tibial deviation of the big toe, complete cutaneous syndactyly of the third and fourth toes, absence of the second, and a somewhat enlarged fifth toe. On the left, a broadened big toe, absence of the second and third toes.

H.-R.W.

References:

Lenz, W. Genetische Ursachen von Fehlbildungen beim Menschen. *Verh. Dtsch. Ges. Path.*, 66, 16–24 (1982).
Majewski, F., Küster, W., ter Haar, B. et al. Aplasia of tibia with split-hand/split-foot deformity. Report of six families with 35 cases and considerations about variability and penetrance. *Hum. Genet.*, 70, 136–147 (1985).
Richieri-Costa, A., Ferrareto, I., Masiero, D. et al. Tibial hemimelia: Report on 37 new cases, clinical and genetic considerations. *Am. J. Med. Genet.*, 27, 867–884 (1987).
Richieri-Costa, A., Brunoni, D., Filho, J.L. et al. Tibial aplasia-ectrodactyly as variant expression of the Gollop–Wolfgang complex: report of a Brazilian family. *Am. J. Med. Genet.*, 28, 971–980 (1987).
Sener, R.N., Isikan, E. et al. Bilateral split-hand with bilateral tibial aplasia. *Pediatr. Radiol.*, 19, 258–260 (1989).

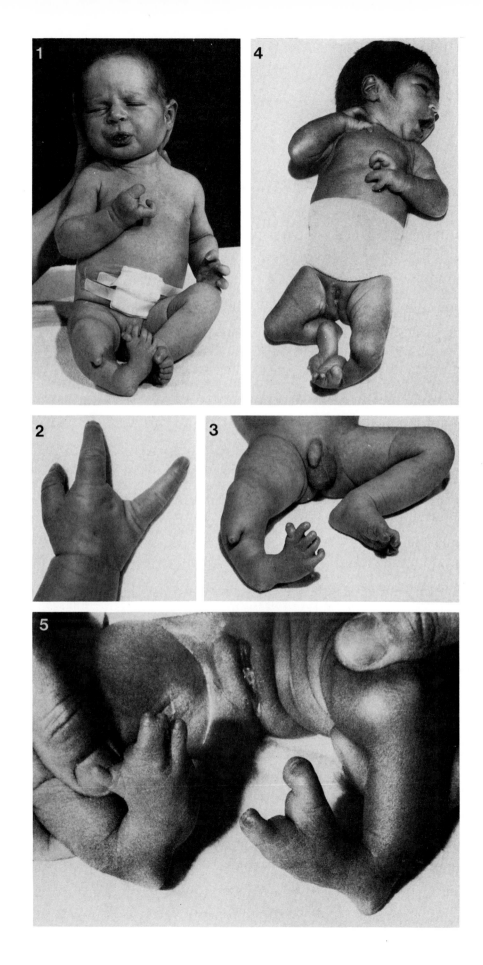

196. Tibial Aplasia or Hypoplasia with Preaxial Polydactyly and Triphalangeal 'Thumbs'

(Werner Syndrome)

A relatively rare autosomal dominant anomaly with very variable expression.

Main signs:
1. Absence or hypoplasia of the tibiae bilaterally.
2. Bowed and thickened fibulae.
3. Club feet with preaxial octa- to nonodactyly.
4. Five- to six-fingered hands without thumbs; the first ray is not operable, the thenar musculature is absent.

Supplementary findings: Occasional syndactyly and/or camptodactyly of fingers and toes. The first metacarpal is long and has a distal epiphysis.

Rarely, also postaxial polydactyly of the hands. Radioulnar synostosis in isolated cases.

Manifestation: At birth.

Etiology: An autosomal dominant gene is responsible for the anomaly, with the two sexes equally frequently and equally severely affected.

Penetrance usually high, but occasionally reduced and, rarely, even absent. Variable expression. The variability extends from the full picture, through preaxial polydactyly of the feet without tibial defect, to a unilateral five-fingered (thumbless) hand without tibial hypoplasia.

Frequency: Relatively low; about 10 sporadic cases and 10 families with the syndrome are known to date – however, numerous cases have probably remained unpublished.

Course, prognosis: Dependent on the degree manifest; but even when fully manifest, relatively favorable with 'rehabilitation'.

Diagnosis, differential diagnosis: Cf. syndrome no. 197 (p.396). In addition, tibial aplasia or hypoplasia with cleft hand (p.392).

Treatment: Orthopedic care and appropriate handicap aids. Genetic counseling. In future pregnancy, or pregnancy in an affected individual, prenatal diagnosis with ultrasonography.

Illustrations:
1–3 A 5-month-old boy, the first child of young, healthy, nonconsanguineous parents. No patellae palpable; skin retracted over the knee joints. Shortened lower legs with radiologically bowed and thickened fibulae and absent tibiae. Club feet. Bilaterally, six metatarsals and eight toes; of these, three preaxial supernumerary; the hypoplastic first toe is syndactylous with the second toe. A triphalangeal finger instead of a thumb bilaterally; on the left, five rays, on the right, six plus an additional preaxial rudimentary appendage. On the right, bony syndactyly of rays III and IV with V-shaped forking, up to 80% cutaneous syndactyly; rays IV and V show complete cutaneous syndactyly. In addition, camptodactyly of rays I and II on the right, III and IV on the left.

Internal organs of the child unremarkable, but somewhat large testes (3–4 ml). Short penis. Epicanthus.

H.-R.W.

References:

Werner, P. Über einen seltenen Fall von Zwergwuchs. *Arch. Gynäkol.*, 104, 278–300 (1915).

Lamb, S.W., Wynne-Davis, R., Whitmore, J.M. Five-fingered hand associated with partial or complete tibial absence and pre-axial polydactyly. *J. Bone Jt. Surg.*, 65-B, 60–63 (1983).

Canún, S., Lomeli, R.M., Martinez, R. et al. Absent tibiae, triphalangeal thumbs and polydactyly: description of a family and prenatal diagnosis. *Clin. Genet.*, 25, 182–186 (1984).

Canún, S: Absent tibiae, triphalangeal thumbs, polydactyly and non-penetrance. *Clin. Genet.*, 29, 347 (1986).

Cordeiro, I., Santos, H., Maroteaux, P. Congenital absence of the tibiae and thumbs with polydactyly. A rare genetic disease (Werner's syndrome). *Ann. Génét.*, 29, 275–277 (1986).

Majewski, F. Personal communication, 1986.

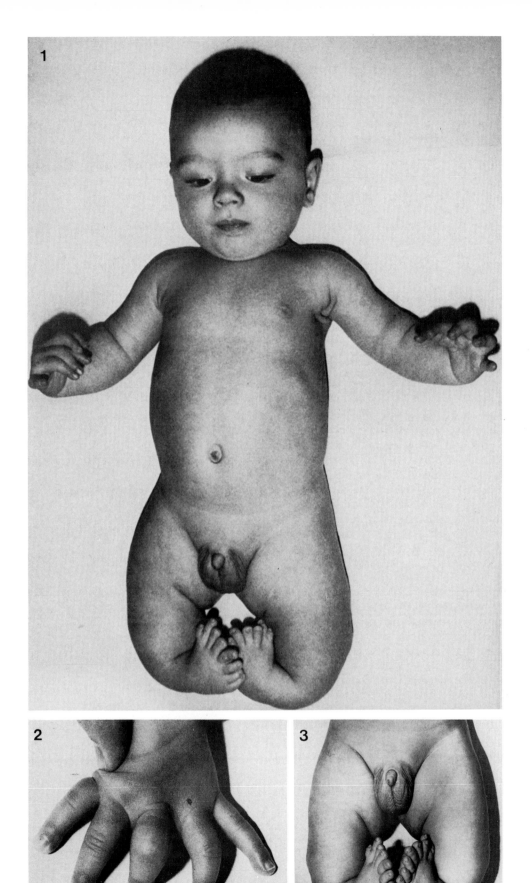

197. An Unknown Syndrome of Dysplastic Extremities–Polydactyly–Dyscrania

A syndrome of partial tibial defect, preaxial polydactyly, generalized micromelia, and macrotrigonocephaly.

Main signs:
1. Unilateral partial tibial defect (1a, 2, 5). Ipsilateral preaxial polydactyly (clinically, nonodactyly, 3; radiologically, octodactyly). Generalized micromelia (1).
2. Macrotrigonocephaly with prominent medial ridge of the forehead (1a). Low nasal root. Initially slight antimongoloid slant of the palpebral fissures. Bluish sclera.
3. Short neck. Thickset trunk with low-lying umbilicus (1a). Dislocation of the left hip, limited extension of the left knee joint. Dislocation of the right knee joint.

Supplementary findings: Unremarkable hands and fingers.

Left inguinal hernia, left cryptorchidism, undescended testicle on the right. Muscular hypotonia.

On X-ray: Large cranium with relatively small facial part of the skull; convex curvature of the base of the skull; delayed closure of the fontanelles (anterior fontanelle still open at age 3 years). High, narrow pelvis with steep ischia. Dislocation of the left hip, dysplasia of the right. Strikingly narrow femora, with the left shorter than the right. Half-moon-shaped dysplastic, shortened tibia on the right; short crudely formed dislocated fibula. Short left tibia with relatively elongated fibula. Seven metatarsals on the right. The four toes on the fibular side correspond to four three-membered toes; two additional three-membered toes preaxially (and the rudimentary third preaxial toe also later showed three bony phalanges); abnormally broad proximal phalanx of the big toe, duplicated second phalanx (clinically: double nail). Duplication of the right talus was also recognizable later. Bilateral ureteral dilatation and blunting without evidence of gross renal malformation.

Manifestation: At birth.

Etiology: Genetic basis likely. Mother macrocephalic with flat orbits and mild exophthalmos (very marked facial resemblance of the proband with his mother); the mother's grandfather had had a congenital malformation of the right foot, perhaps with shortening since he 'limped' (further medical details not available).

Course, prognosis: Favorable, with 'rehabilitation'.

Comment: The typical picture of the tibial defect and the accompanying formation of *pre*axial polydactyly is presented here within the framework of a clinical picture of generalized dysplasia, which we have not been able to identify as a previously described syndrome. Not Werner syndrome (cf. p.394).

Illustrations:
1–5 The child discussed here, at age 3 months. The boy is the second child of young, healthy parents (first child healthy); no parental consanguinity. Birth at term with normal weight but length (of 47 cm) below average.

Head circumference: at 5 months, 44.5 cm; at 2½ years, 52.5 cm; at 5 years, 54 cm. Mental development normal for age.

H.-R.W.

Reference:
Wiedemann, H.-R. and Opitz, J.M. Unilateral partial tibia defect... *Am. J. Med. Genet.*, 14, 467–471 (1983).

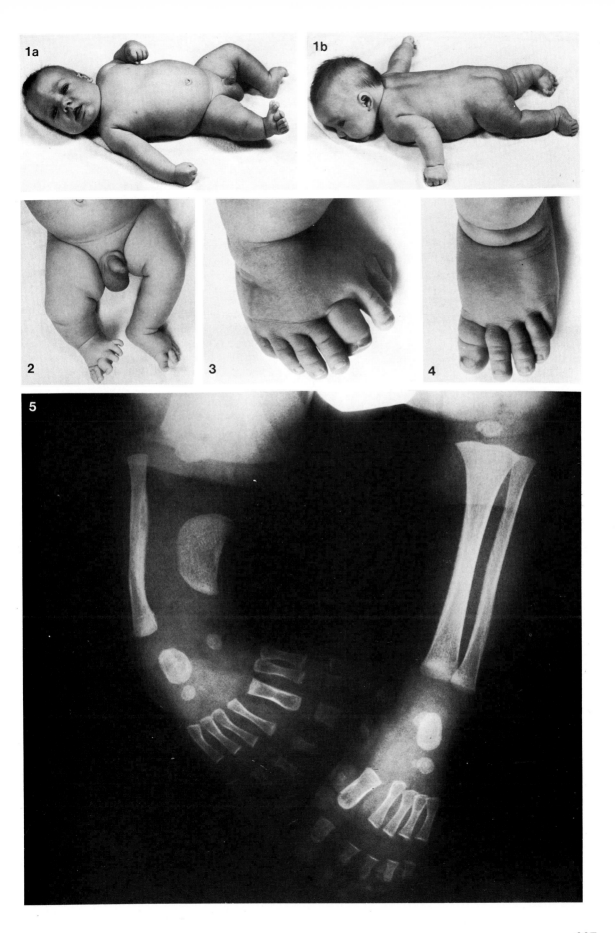

198. Dysplasia Epiphysealis Hemimelica

(Trevor Disease, 'Tarsomegaly')

Osteochondromatous outgrowth and overgrowth usually at one, but possibly several, joints of a lower extremity, with consequent disability, deformity, and possibly pain.

Main signs:
1. Usually unilateral swelling (more frequently medially than laterally) or limited motion at an ankle or knee joint. Occasionally, other joints, such as the hip or wrist, are involved. In addition, deformity of the affected joint in the form of pes valgo-planus or equinus, genu valgum or varum, or occasionally unequal length of the legs, usually due to shortening rather than to lengthening of the affected extremity (1–4). Pain usually occurs later, particularly in the ankle region.
2. Radiologically, usually evidence of accelerated development of the ossification center in the affected area and of an irregular, frequently multicentric opacity adjacent to the affected epiphysis or to the affected carpal or tarsal bone (5), later fusing with it and giving the appearance of irregular enlargement or of a protuberance (5, 7).

Supplementary findings: The dysplasia affects principally epiphyses of tarsal bones; only exceptionally is the analogous region of an upper extremity affected instead. Usually localized medially, less frequently laterally, involvement of the whole epiphysis is an exception (5, 6). Not infrequently, several epiphyses in one extremity are affected. Involvement of more than one limb very unusual; systemic involvement (see caption to illustrations) has been reported only in isolated cases.

Manifestation: The disorder is usually discovered sometime during childhood (or later), exceptionally, in the first year of life or even at birth.

Etiology: Unclear. Sporadic occurrence; boys:girls = about 3:1. (The formal pathogenesis involves asymmetrical cartilaginous overgrowth and extension of one or several epiphyses – or of a carpal or tarsal bone – with subsequent endochondral ossification.)

Frequency: Low; up to 1985, about 140 observations in the literature.

Course, prognosis: Good with early and adequate orthopedic care.

Differential diagnosis: Differentiation from enchondromatosis (p.410), multiple cartilaginous exostoses (p.406), and chondrodysplasia punctata (p.220) should not be difficult.

Treatment: Prompt orthopedic care of a conservative or, if indicated, operative nature (excision or partial resection of the osteochondromatous growths).

Illustrations:
1–7 The first child of young, healthy, nonconsanguineous parents. Contractures of all large joints of the right lower limb noted at birth, and increasing overgrowth of the extremity after the second month of life.
1–4 The severely physically handicapped boy as a 3-year-old; the left lateral malleolus is also enlarged and lower than normal; limited pro- and supination of both hands and limited motion of the fingers bilaterally.
5 Overgrowth of the right pelvis and proximal femur with epiphyseal dysplasia from age 10 months.
6 and 7 Similar coarse changes in the right knee and foot ('tarsomegaly' with severe deformity of the talus) at age 3 years.

Milder epiphyseal changes in the left lower extremity and subtle changes in both of the upper extremities, as in a systemic disorder.

H.-R.W.

References:

Kettelkamp, D.B., Campbell, C.J., Benfiglio, M. Dysplasia epiphysealis hemimelica. A report of fifteen cases. *J. Bone Jt. Surg.*, 48-A, 746.
Spranger, J.W., Langer, L.O., Jr., Wiedemann, H.-R. *Bone Dysplasias. An Atlas of Constitutional Disorders of Skeletal Development.* G. Fischer and W.B. Saunders, Stuttgart and Philadelphia, 1974.
Fasting, O.J. and Bjerkreim, I. Dysplasia epiphysealis hemimelica. *Acta Orthop. Scand.*, 47, 217 (1976).
Carlson, D.H. and Wilkinson, R.H. Variability of unilateral epiphyseal dysplasia. *Radiology*, 133, 369 (1979).
Wiedemann, H.-R., Mann, M., Spreter, V., Kreudenstein, P. Dysplasia epiphysealis hemimelica. *Eur. J. Pediatr.*, 136, 311 (1981).
Lamesch, A.J. Dysplasia epiphysealis hemimelica of the carpal bones. *J. Bone Jt. Surg.*, 65-A, 398–400 (1983).
Azouz, E.M., Slomic, A.M. et al. The variable manifestations of dysplasia epiphysealis hemimelica. *Pediatr. Radiol.*, 15, 44–49 (1985).
Hoeffel, J.C., Capron, F. et al. Dysplasia epiphysealis hemimelica of the ulna. *Eur. J. Pediatr.*, 145, 450 (1986).
Hinkel, G.K. and Rupprecht, E. Hemihypertrophie als Leitsymptom einer Dysplasia epiphysealis hemimelica. *Klin. Pädiatr.*, 201, 58–62 (1989).

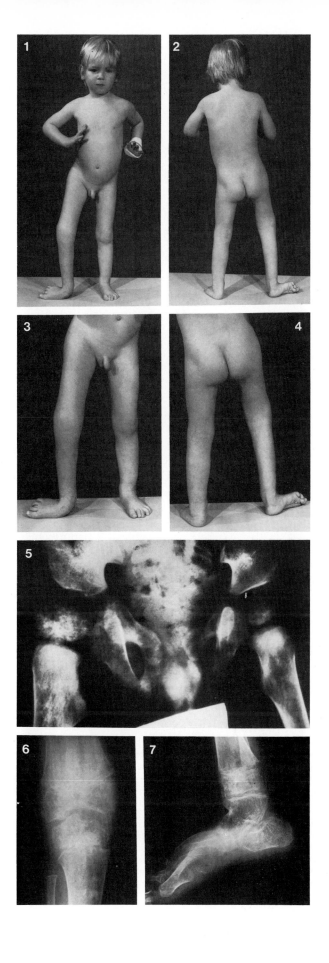

199. F.P. Weber Syndrome

(Angiomatous Dysplasia F.P. Weber Type; Partially Macrosomic Limb with a Hemodynamically Significant Arteriovenous Fistula)

A dysplasia syndrome comprising partial macrosomia, usually proportional in itself and usually of a lower extremity, due to hemodynamically active, usually multiple, congenital arteriovenous (A-V) fistulas.

Main signs:
1. Partial macrosomia of an extremity or part of a limb. As a rule, a lower extremity is affected and the enlarged region usually remains more or less proportional in itself (**1–4**).
2. Evidence of an A-V shunt: dilatation of arteries and veins; prominent vascular pulsations, continuing into the veins; vascular thrills; and hyperthermic skin.
3. Arteriographic evidence of congenital A-V fistulas, usually multiple, in soft tissue or bone.

Supplementary findings: Large A-V shunts lead to signs of cardiac overload, possibly to severe cardiac failure, with no signs of cardiac malformation.

Possibly secondary osteoarticular changes such as tilted pelvis, scoliosis, etc.

Nevus flammeus may occur over the affected region, or in other areas.

Manifestation: In childhood.

Etiology: Unexplained. Genetic factors may be assumed. Usually sporadic occurrence. Cf. Klippel–Trenaunay syndrome (p.358).

Frequency: Relatively low.

Course, prognosis: Tendency to continue to progress after the child has stopped growing. The affected extremity and the patient's life may be seriously threatened.

Diagnosis: Careful angiographic analysis essential.

Differential diagnosis: Simple partial macrosomia without vascular malformations. Klippel–Trenaunay syndrome (p.358), which may be extremely difficult to differentiate, if, in fact, this is a different entity (opinions vary).

Treatment: Urgent measures to decrease the shunt volume by vascular surgery, if possible. If unsuccessful or impossible, amputation may need to be considered as a last resort.

Illustrations:
1–4 A 10-year-old girl with 'gigantism' of the entire right lower extremity, especially of the lower leg and foot. Equinus position of the foot, flexion contracture of the knee, tilted pelvis and scoliosis. No nevus flammeus of the skin. Hyperthermia of the affected leg. Dilated veins, pulsations. Multiple A-V fistulas on angiogram.

H.-R.W.

References:

Vollmar, J. Zur Geschichte und Terminologie der Syndrome nach F.P. Weber und Klippel–Trenaunay. *VASA*, 3, 231 (1974).

Vollmar, J. Die Chirurgie kongenitaler arteriovenöser Fisteln der Gliedmaßen. In: Vollner, J.F. and Nobbe, F.P. (eds.) *Arteriovenöse Fisteln – Dilatierende Arteriopathien.* Thieme, Stuttgart, 1976, (p.66 ff).

Leipner, N., Janson, R. et al. Angiomatöse Dysplasie (Typ F.P. Weber). *Fortschr. Röntgenstr.*, 137, 73–77 (1982).

Leipner, N., Lackner, K. et al. Röntgenbefunde bei einer angiomatösen Dysplasie (Typ Weber). *Fortschr. Röntgenstr.*, 142, 571–573 (1985).

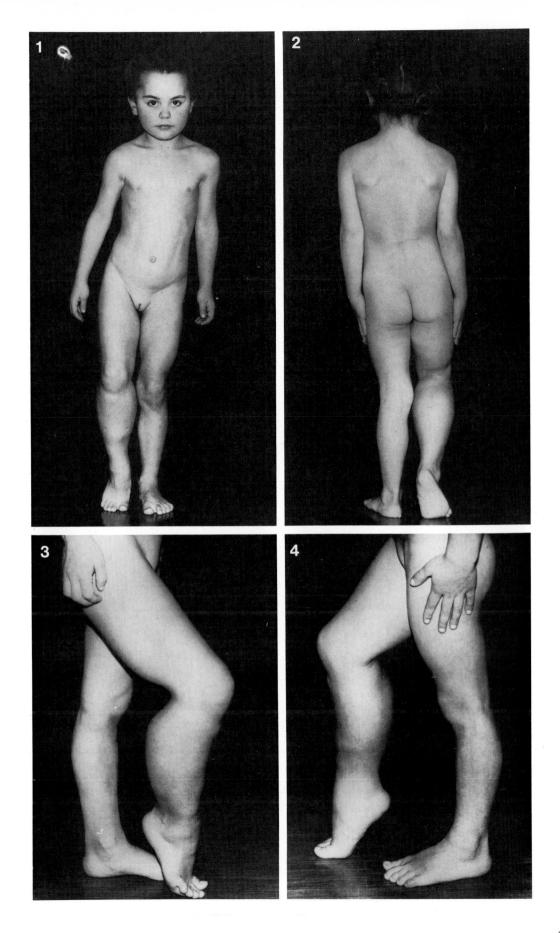

200. Classic Arthrogryposis: Amyoplasia

A sporadically occurring 'classic' clinical picture of congenital nonprogressive joint contractures (due to impaired muscle development) with characteristic positioning of the extremities, and round face.

Main signs:
1. Multiple congenital contractures (with taut connective and adipose tissue replacing muscle) and typical positioning of the extremities: usually, shoulders internally rotated; elbows in extension; wrists flexed; severe talipes equinovarus (1, 4). Knee and hip joint contractures in various positions; fingers flexed.
2. Frequent absence of normal flexion creases over the joints; presence of abnormal skin dimples or of soft-tissue folds in the joint regions (3–5).
3. Typical round face with capillary angioma in the upper midline and micrognathia (2).
4. Normal intelligence.

Supplementary findings: Although usually all extremities are fairly symmetrically affected, in some cases contractions may occur mainly in the legs, and even less frequently, mainly in the arms. Hypoplasia of the fingers, hypoplasia of the labia or scrotum, cryptorchidism, and other anomalies possible.

History of decreased fetal movements during pregnancy; breech presentation frequent.

Manifestation: At birth.

Etiology: Unknown. Sporadic occurrence. No monozygotic twin concordance.

Frequency: Not particularly low.

Course, prognosis: Delayed motor development due to limitation of movements. Otherwise dependent on the severity of the disorder and on the quality and intensity of treatment.

Differential diagnosis: Other causes of arthrogryposis.

Treatment: Intensive physiotherapeutic and multiple orthopedic measures are required, and not infrequently orthopedic surgery. Genetic counseling.

Illustrations:
1–5 A newborn with arthrogryposis.

H.-R.W.

References:

Hall, J. G., Reed, S.D. et al. Amyoplasia: a common sporadic condition with congenital contractures. *Am. J. Med. Genet.*, 15, 571–590 (1983).

Hall, J.G., Reed, S.D. et al. Amyoplasia: twinning... *Am. J. Med. Genet.*, 15, 591–599 (1983).

Hageman, G., Ippel, E.P.F. et al. The diagnostic management of newborns with congenital contractures: a nosologic study of 75 cases. *Am. J. Med. Genet.*, 30, 883–904 (1988).

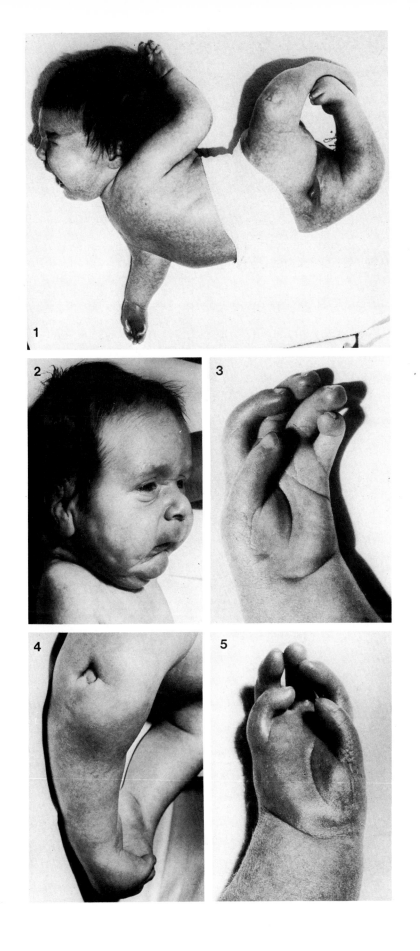

201. Larsen Syndrome

A quite characteristic inherited disorder with multiple congenital joint dislocations, facial dysmorphism, and anomalies of the hands, fingers, and feet.

Main signs:
1. Dislocations especially of the hips, knees, and elbows (**1, 3**). Flat, rectangular face with low nasal root, prominent forehead, and hypertelorism (**2, 3, 5**).
2. 'Spatula-like' thumbs and in general cylindrically shaped fingers with broad ends and short nails (**4**). Short arms. Talipes equinovarus or -valgus with torsion of the anterior part of the foot (**3**).

Supplementary findings: Cleft palate not uncommon. Frequent development of progressive curvature of the spine. Decreased adult height.

On X-ray, distal phalanx of the thumb triangular; further distal phalanges short and broad, shortened metacarpals (especially II), accessory ossification centers in the wrist bones and an accessory ossification center in the calcaneus. Frequent segmentation anomalies especially in the upper spine.

Possible cardiovascular anomalies, e.g., aortic lesions.

Manifestation: At birth.

Etiology: Monogenic disorder; heterogeneity; clinically, an autosomal dominant and a more severe autosomal recessive form, which to date cannot be differentiated with certainty. More girls than boys affected. Basic defect unknown, probable collagen defect.

Frequency: Relatively low, although it is likely that many cases are not recognized; well over a hundred case reports in the literature.

Course, prognosis: Respiration may be impaired in early infancy due to softness of thoracic cartilage, especially in the laryngotracheal airway (and especially in the recessive form?). Variable, frequently severe physical disability due to the dislocations. In the absence of appropriate measures to prevent severe deformity of the vertebral column, danger of developing spinal cord compression. As a rule, mental development within normal limits.

Differential diagnosis: Differentiation from the oto-palato-digital syndrome is often difficult. Numerous dislocated joints, including the knee joint, multiple carpal ossicles, and an additional ossification center in the calcaneus would suggest Larsen syndrome. The two syndromes may be closely associated genetically. Ehlers–Danlos syndrome, the Marfan syndrome, and arthrogryposis are easily excluded by their characteristic features.

Treatment: Early application of various orthopedic measures (for the feet and hips and the particularly problematic knee dislocations; careful observation of the vertebral column, etc.) and comprehensive, continuous, multidisciplinary care for the physical handicaps. Genetic counseling. Ultrasonographic prenatal diagnosis should be feasible (dislocations).

Illustrations:
1 A characteristically affected newborn; severe genu recurvatum.
2–5 A 6-year-old, typically affected boy. Height when supported by orthopedic appliances, at the third percentile. Kyphoscoliosis; spina bifida at two cervicothoracic vertebrae; 13 pairs of ribs. Slight pectus excavatum. Bifid uvula.

H.-R.W.

References:

Spranger, J.W., Langer, L.O., Jr., Wiedemann, H.-R. *Bone Dysplasias. An Atlas of Constitutional Disorders of Skeletal Development.* G. Fischer and W.B. Saunders, Stuttgart and Philadelphia, 1974.
Micheli, L.J., Hall, J.E., Watts, H.G. Spinal instability in Larsen's syndrome. *J. Bone Jt. Surg.,* 58-A, 562 (1976).
Galanski, M. and Statz, A. Radiologische Befunde beim Larsen-Syndrom. *Fortschr. Röntgenstr.,* 128, 534 (1978).
Kiel, E.A., Frias, J.L., Victorica, B.E. Cardiovascular manifestations in the Larsen syndrome. *Pediatrics,* 71, 942–946 (1983).
Stanley, D. and Seymour, N. The Larsen syndrome occurring in four generations of one family. *Int. Orthoped.,* 8, 267–272 (1985).

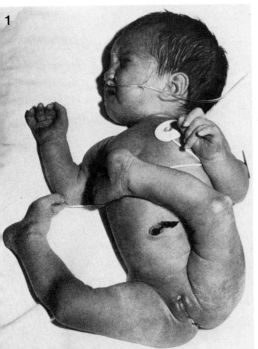

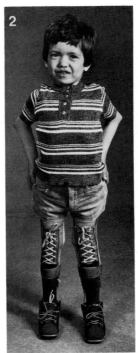

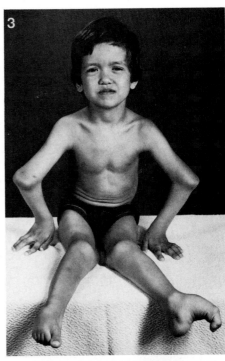

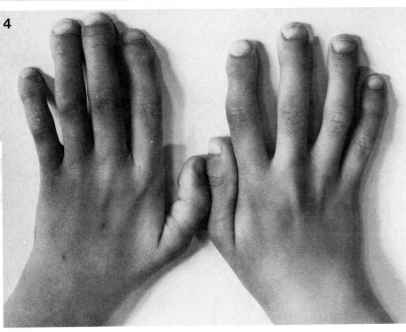

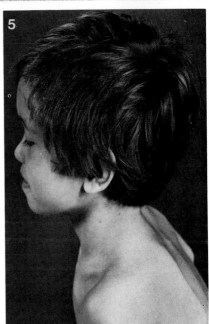

202. Multiple Cartilaginous Exostoses

A hereditary syndrome, which is very characteristic in its severe form, with variable numbers of bony outgrowths and protuberances, usually at the ends of the long bones, resulting in deformity and limited movement of the extremities.

Main signs:
1. Multiple bony excrescences (covered by hyaline cartilage) especially on the ends of the long bones (**1b, 2, 3**), usually in the knee region, but also often on the ribs, the medial edges of the scapulae, the iliac crest, and other areas.
2. Secondary deformity of the long bones such as shortening and bowing; most frequently of the ulna, with shortening of the forearm (**1a, 1b**) and with ulnar deviation of the hand; radioulnar synostosis in some cases. Also shortening of the fibula, tibiofibular synostosis, genu valgum and/or pes valgus.

Supplementary findings: Possible moderate short stature.

X-rays show exostoses in addition to those which are palpable.

Manifestation: Variable; usually early childhood and into the first decade of life. (The exostoses originating in the metaphyseal areas move to the diaphyses as the child grows.)

Etiology: Autosomal dominant disorder with complete penetrance in males, incomplete in females. Definite sporadic cases should be considered new mutations.

Frequency: Not low (by 1964 over 1,000 cases had been reported in the literature).

Course, prognosis: During adolescence, slowing of growth of the exostoses (with occasional exceptions); after puberty, no further growth of excrescences. Impaired function due to resulting disproportion of parts of the skeleton (see above) and possibly also impairment from pressure on the tendons, vessels, or nerves. Neoplastic degeneration of the exostoses in adulthood possible (about 10% of cases).

Differential diagnosis: The Langer–Giedion syndrome (p.408) should not be difficult to rule out. Some newly described syndromes should be considered – exostoses combined with anetodermia and brachydactyly; exostoses associated with hypochondroplasia.

Treatment: Surgery in cases of markedly impaired function (e.g., to prevent dislocation of a radial head) with excision of exostoses together with osteotomies for suspected development of malignancy. Regular follow-up. Genetic counseling.

Illustrations:

1a and **1b** A 6-year-old boy with deformity of the left forearm, typical X-ray findings (bowing of the radius, which alone articulates with the wrist, and especially of the markedly shortened ulna with distal exostoses), bilateral pes valgus, and multiple further palpable and/or radiologically demonstrable exostoses.

2 Large, sharply demarcated exostosis originating from the proximal humeral metaphysis in a 7-year-old boy with multiple bony excrescences.

3 X-ray of the right knee of a 3½-year-old boy with exostoses on all long tubular bones and on several ribs, a scapula, and the hands and feet.

H.-R.W.

References:

Spranger, J.W., Langer, L.O., Jr., Wiedemann, H.-R. *Bone Dysplasias. An Atlas of Constitutional Disorders of Skeletal Development.* G. Fischer and W.B. Saunders, Stuttgart and Philadelphia, 1974.

Ochsner, P.E. Zum Problem der neoplastischen Entartung bei multiplen kartilagenären Exostosen. *Z. Orthopäd.*, 116, 369 (1978).

Shapiro, F., Simon, S., Glimcher, M.J. Hereditary multiple exostoses. *J. Bone Jt. Surg.*, Ser. A61/6, 815 (1979).

Gordon, S.L., Buchanan, J.R. et al. Hereditary multiple exostoses . . . *J. Med. Genet.*, 18, 428–430 (1981).

Finidori, G., Allard de Grandmaison, P. et al. Anomalies de croissance osseuse de la maladie exostosante. *Ann. Pédiatr.*, 30, 657–662 (1983).

Hudson, T.M., Chew, F.S. et al. Scintigraphy of benign exostoses . . . *AJR*, 140, 581–586 (1983).

Dominguez, R., Young, L.W. et al. Multiple exostotic hypochondroplasia . . . *Pediatr. Radiol.*, 14, 356–359 (1984).

Fogel, G.R., McElfresh, E. et al. Management of deformities of the forearm in multiple hereditary osteochondromas. *J. Bone Jt. Surg.*, 66-A, 670–680 (1984).

Mollica, F., Li Volti, S. et al. Exostoses, anetodermia, brachydactyly. *Am. J. Med. Genet.*, 19, 665–667 (1984).

Hall, J.G., Wilson, R.X. et al. Familial multiple exostoses – no chromosome 8 deletion observed. *Am. J. Med. Genet.*, 22, 639–640 (1985).

Pritchett, J.W. Lengthening the ulna in patients with hereditary multiple exostoses. *J. Bone Jt. Surg.*, 68-B, 561–565 (1986).

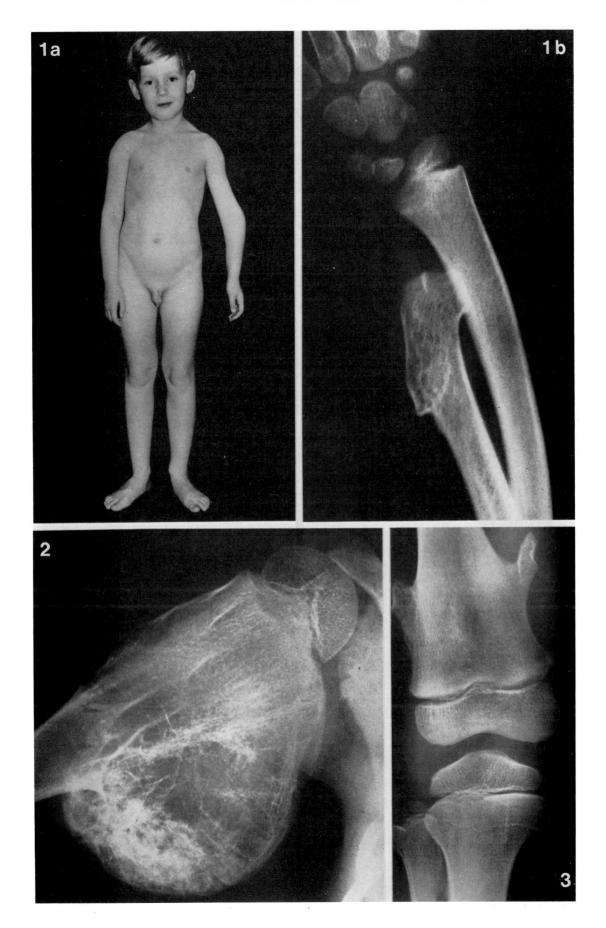

407

203. Langer–Giedion Syndrome

(Giedion–Langer Syndrome, Trichorhinophalangeal Syndrome Type II, Syndrome of Acrodysplasia with Exostoses)

A malformation–retardation syndrome of short stature; unusual facies; sparse, fragile scalp hair; multiple exostoses; mild microcephaly; and mental retardation.

Main signs:

1. Typical facial dysmorphism: large, prominent, poorly differentiated ears; broad eyebrows rising craniolaterally; deep-set eyes; bulbous nose with a broad septum and simple alae; prominent philtrum; long, narrow upper lip; high palate; malocclusion; receding chin (1).

2. Short stature. Mild microcephaly and mild to moderate mental retardation.

3. Fine scalp hair (1). Early features include flaccid or loose-wrinkled skin and muscular hypotonia. Later, maculopapular pigmented nevi especially on the upper half of the body.

4. Multiple cartilaginous exostoses of the long tubular bones (also possibly on the short tubular bones, the shoulder blades, ribs, and pelvis). X-rays show cone-shaped epiphyses of the hands and feet (2).

Supplementary findings: Optic defects, sensorineural hearing impairment and delayed speech development may occur. Also, winged scalpulae and generalized hyperextensibility of the joints, Perthes-like dysplasia of the femoral head, and increased tendency to fractures; clinobrachydactyly, abnormal nails. In early childhood, possible difficulties with rearing, increased susceptibility to infections.

Manifestation: At birth and in early childhood. Radiologically, the combination of exostoses/cone-shaped epiphyses usually becomes apparent by age 3–4 years.

Etiology: Initially, all reported cases were sporadic, with both sexes affected; subsequently a case report of transmission from father to daughter. Thus autosomal dominant inheritance, possibly with new mutations in the majority of previously published observations. There have recently been repeated observations of a chromosomal abnormality (8q-deletion) with various breakpoints.

Frequency: Very low (up to 1986, only about 50 cases in the literature).

Course, prognosis: The loose, wrinkled skin tends to improve in infancy; the susceptibility to infections disappears by about school age. The extent to which the patient is handicapped depends principally on the severity of a mental and/or hearing impairment, then on the exostoses and their effect on joint mobility and bony growth. General health and life expectancy are not necessarily reduced.

Differential diagnosis: In mutiple cartilaginous exostoses (p.406) only exostoses and possible short stature are seen. In trichorhinophalangeal syndrome type I (p.420): absence of exostoses and no microcephalic mental retardation, short stature, or other features.

Treatment: Symptomatic. Genetic counseling.

Illustrations:

1a and 1b A 15-year-old with the typical syndrome, but unimpaired mental development. Exostoses at both ends of the long bones toward the end of the first year of life. Head circumference 48.5 cm; height, 133.5 cm, below the third percentile. Delayed speech development; considerable hearing impairment (first noted at 4 years old). Normal sexual development.

2a and 2b X-rays of the same child at different ages.

H.-R.W.

References:

Spranger, J.W., Langer, L.O., Jr., Wiedemann, H.-R. *Bone Dysplasias. An Atlas of Constitutional Disorders of Skeletal Development.* G. Fischer and W.B. Saunders, Stuttgart and Philadelphia, 1974.

Oorthuys, J.W.E. and Beemer, F.A. The Langer–Giedion syndrome or trichorhino-phalangeal syndrome, type II. *Eur. J. Pediatr.*, 132, 55 (1979).

Bühler, E.M., Bühler, U.K., Stalder, G.R. et al. Chromosome deletion and mutiple cartilaginous exostoses. *Eur. J. Pediatr.*, 133, 163 (1980).

Murachi, S., Nogami, H., Oki, T. et al. Familial trichorhinophalangeal syndrome type II. *Clin. Med.*, 19, 149 (1981).

Fryns, J.P., Logghe, N., van Eggen, M. et al. Langer–Giedion syndrome and deletion of the long arm of chromosome 8. *Hum. Genet.*, 58, 231 (1981).

Zabel, B.U. and Baumann, W.A. Langer–Giedion syndrome with interstitial 8q-deletion. *Am. J. Med. Genet.*, 11, 353 (1982).

Bühler, E.M. Editorial comment: Langer–Giedion syndrome and 8q-deletion. *Am. J. Med. Genet.*, 11, 359 (1982).

Fryns, J.P., Heremans, G. et al. Langer–Giedion syndrome and deletion of the long arm of chromosome 8 . . . *Hum. Genet.*, 64, 194–195 (1983).

Bühler, E.M., Malik, N.J. The tricho-rhino-phalangeal syndrome(s) . . . *Am. J. Med. Genet.*, 19, 113–119 (1984).

Langer, L.O., Jr., Krassikoff, N. et al. The tricho-rhino-phalangeal syndrome with exostoses (or Langer–Giedion syndrome): four additional patients . . . review . . . *Am. J. Med. Genet.*, 19, 81–111 (1984).

Okuno, T., Inoue, A. et al. Langer–Giedion syndrome with del 8 (q24.13–q24.22). *Clin. Genet.*, 32, 40–45 (1987).

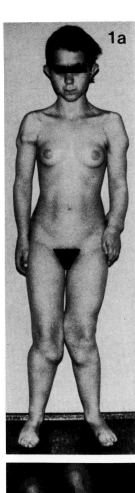

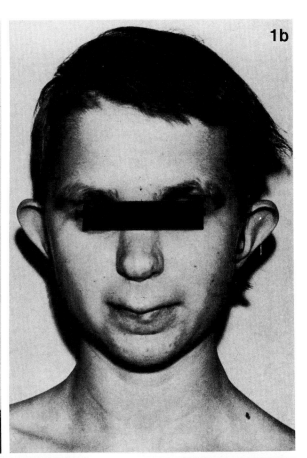

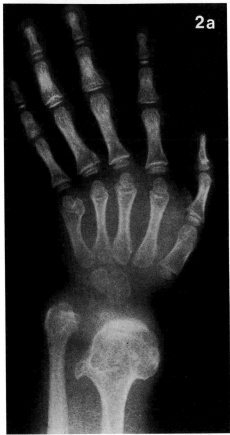

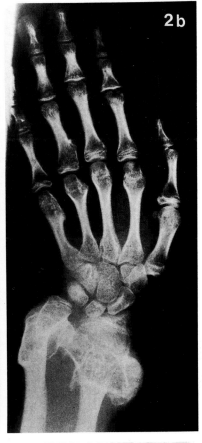

204. Enchondromatosis

(Dyschondroplasia, Multiple Enchondromas, Ollier Syndrome, Osteochondromatosis)

A syndrome of firm, localized, asymmetrical swellings of the fingers and/or toes combined with asymmetrical shortening of the extremities.

Main signs:
1. Tautly elastic, firm, indolent, rounded swellings or outgrowths continuous with the bone on one or more fingers or toes (1, 2).
2. Shortening and possibly bowing of parts of the extremities, most frequently the forearm and/or lower leg (1, 4).
3. Marked asymmetry of the swellings (unilateral involvement possible).

Supplementary findings: Possible secondary impairment of mobility of one or several joints; occasional compression effects.

Occasional spontaneous fracture in an affected area.

On X-ray, characteristic ovoid, pyramid-shaped, and linear translucent defects in the metaphyses of affected long bones and in flat bones (with sparing of the calvarium); often considerable swelling and cortical thinning of the affected area (3, 4).

Manifestation: Usually after the second year of life.

Etiology: Not known (somatic mutation?). Isolated reports of familial occurrence should be viewed sceptically. Sporadic occurrence. No increased risk of recurrence for the affected family.

Frequency: Relatively low.

Course, prognosis: Guarded. Further lesions may appear and grow until sexual maturity; impairment of growth and mobility of all or part of extremities may be substantial and thus cause considerable handicap. As a rule, no new lesions after adolescence; rather, replacement of old lesions by bony substance. Malignant degeneration of enchondromas may occur in adulthood (perhaps in about 5% of cases); renewed growth of a lesion should suggest this possibility.

Comment: Multiple enchondromas combined with multiple cavernous hemangiomas (tending to form phleboliths) and capillary hemangiomas in the same area represent a special form, the so-called Maffucci syndrome. This is associated with a high risk of degeneration (about 15%).

Treatment: Surgical resection in cases of marked impairment of function, considerable disfigurement, or suspected malignant transformation. Orthopedic management of leg length discrepancy (either surgical or conservative).

Illustrations:
1–4 A 6½-year-old boy, normal psychological development; endochondromatosis since the third year of life. Only unilateral involvement. Left extremities, especially the leg, shorter than the right. Secondary tilting of the pelvis. Considerable impairment and disfiguration of the left hand. Carpal bones, radius, humerus, ilium, os pubis, tarsal bones, and toes also show enchondromatous changes.

H.-R.W.

References:

Spranger, J.W., Langer, L.O., Jr., Wiedemann, H.-R. *Bone Dysplasias. An Atlas of Constitutional Disorders of Skeletal Development.* G. Fischer and W.B. Saunders, Stuttgart and Philadelphia, 1974.
Shapiro, F. Ollier's disease. *J. Bone Jt. Surg.,* 64-A, 95 (1982).
Sun, T.-C., Swee, R.G. et al. Chondrosarcoma in Maffucci's Syndrome. *J. Bone Jt. Surg.,* 67-A, 1214–1219 (1985).
Blauth, W. and Sönnichsen, S. Enchondromatosen der Hand. *Z. Orthop.,* 124, 165–172 (1986).
Urist, M.R. A 37-year follow-up evaluation of multiple-stage femur and tibia lengthening in dyschondroplasia … with a net gain of 23.3 centimetres. *Clin. Orthop. Rel. Res.,* 242, 137 (1989).

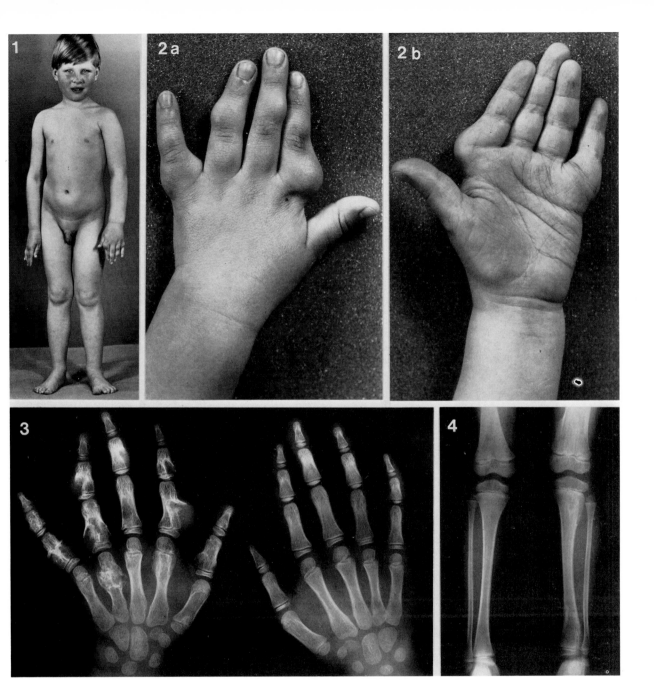

205. Cenani–Lenz Syndactyly Syndrome

An autosomal recessive syndrome with Apert-like spoon hands (syndactyly) and dysphalangism of the toes but an otherwise unremarkable phenotype.

Main signs:
1. Almost complete syndactyly of all fingers, but occasionally only partial syndactyly. Fixation of the metacarpophalangeal and interphalangeal joints in flexion.
2. Dysphalangism of the toes, occasionally syndactyly.
3. On X-ray, synostosis of the metacarpals, occasionally radio-ulnar synostosis.

Supplementary findings: Occasionally, shortened forearms with radio-ulnar synostosis, increase in the number of carpal ossification centers (in our sibling cases, to 11 and 12), three-part nail bed. Otherwise unremarkable phenotype, normal intelligence.

Manifestation: At birth.

Etiology: Autosomal recessive disorder.

Frequency: To date about 20 cases have been reported; of these, sibling observations in five different families.

Course, prognosis: Normal life expectancy.

Treatment: The patient's manual dexterity with buttoning, writing, etc., is quite impressive; a specialist hand surgeon should be consulted.

Differential diagnosis: Variants of Cenani–Lenz syndactyly?

Note: The patients presented here apparently show a variant of the syndrome.

Illustrations:
1 A 15-year-old.
2 His 20-year-old sister.
1c–1f The patient's hands; on the right: first, second and fifth fingers single; third and fourth, syndactylous; tripartite nail; on the left: corresponding situation with syndactyly of third and fourth fingers, but only one nail.
1g Dysphalangism of the feet.
2c–2f Similar changes in the sister: first finger, one phalangeal bone present; second and fifth fingers, two phalanges; the syndactylous third and fourth fingers show the same numbers of nails on the right and the left hands respectively as those of the brother.
   X-ray: no radio-ulnar synothoses; 11 and 12 carpal bones.

J.K.

References:

Cenani, A. and Lenz, W. Totale Syndaktylie und totale radioulnare Synostose bei zwei Brüdern. Ein Beitrag zur Genetik der Syndaktylien. *Z. Kinderheilkd.*, 101, 181–190 (1967).

Drohm, D., Lenz, W., Yang, T.S. Totale Syndaktylie mit mesomeler Armverkürzung, radioulnären und metacarpalen Synostosen und Disorganisation der Phalangen ('Cenani-Syndaktylie'). *Klin. Pädiatr.*, 188, 359–365 (1976).

Verma, I.C., Joseph, R., Bhargava, S. et al. Split-hand and split-foot deformity inherited as an autosomal recessive trait. *Clin. Genet.*, 9, 8–14 (1976).

Dodinval, P. Oligodactyly and multiple synostoses of the extremities: two cases in sibs. A variant of Cenani–Lenz syndactyly. *Hum. Genet.*, 48, 183–189 (1979).

Pfeiffer, R.A. and Meisel-Stosiek, M. Present nosology of the Cenani–Lenz type of syndactyly. *Clin. Genet.*, 21, 74–79 (1982).

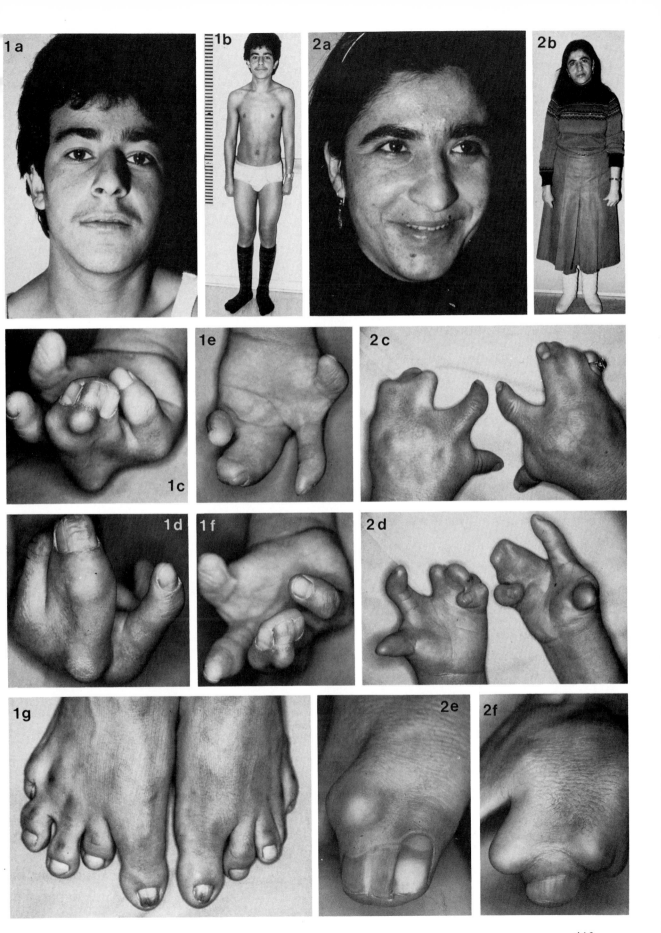

413

206. Greig's Polysyndactyly–Cranial Dysmorphism Syndrome

(Greig's Cephalopolysyndactyly Syndrome = GCPS)

A syndrome of polydactyly and syndactyly of the hands and feet with an unusually shaped skull.

Main signs:
1. Broad thumbs and halluces or preaxial polydactyly of the feet and, occasionally, the hands and postaxial polydactyly of the hands, less frequently also of the feet. Usually significant syndactyly of second to fourth (fifth) fingers and of various toes (3–6).
2. Macro- and brachycephaly with high, prominent forehead with a median ridge (1, 2). Broad nasal root, hypertelorism, possible slight antimongoloid slant of the palpebral fissures, and wide nares.

Supplementary findings: Radiological picture of the thumbs and big toes varies from minor abnormalities of shape to complete duplication of the ray.

Manifestation: At birth.

Etiology: Autosomal hereditary defect with complete penetrance but variable expression. Gene localized to the short arm of chromosome 7 (7p13).

Frequency: Low (to date, at least 100 cases reported).

Course, prognosis: Favorable.

Diagnosis, differential diagnosis: Delineation from Carpenter syndrome (p.22) should not be difficult. The acrocallosal syndrome (Schinzel) shows agenesis of the corpus callosum (cranial ultrasound useful), psychomotor retardation, and autosomal recessive inheritance as differentiating features.

Treatment: Surgical correction of the extremities should be begun sufficiently early, at a time determined with the hand surgeon and suited to the individual case. Genetic counseling.

Illustrations:
1 A 4-month-old boy.
2 His twin brother.
3 and 5 Polysyndactyly, clinically and radiologically, of the right hand of the boy in 1.
4 The right forefoot of the same boy.
6 Unusually severe polysyndactyly of the right foot of the twin in 2.

H.-R.W./J.K.

References:
Hootnick, D. and Holmes, L.B. Familial polysyndactyly and craniofacial anomalies. *Clin. Genet.*, 3, 124 (1972).
Fryns, J.P., van Noyen, G., van den Berghe, H. The Greig polysyndactyly craniofacial dysmorphism syndrome. *Eur. J. Pediatr.*, 136, 217 (1981).
Chudley, A.E. and Houston, C.S. The Greig cephalopolysyndactyly syndrome . . . *Am. J. Med. Genet.*, 13, 269–276 (1982).
Fryns, J.P. Le syndrome de Greig . . . *J. Génét. Hum.* 30, (Suppl. 5), 403–408 (1982).
Baraitser, M., Winter, R.M. et al. Greig cephalopolysyndactyly: report of 13 affected individuals . . . *Clin. Genet.*, 24, 257–265 (1983).
Tommerup, M. and Nielsen, F. A familial reciprocal translocation t(3;7)(p21.1;p13) associated with the Greig . . . syndrome. *Am. J. Med. Genet.*, 16, 313–321 (1983).
Gollop, T.R. and Fontes, L.R. The Greig cephalopolysyndactyly syndrome . . . *Am. J. Med. Genet.*, 22, 59–68 (1985).
Kunze, J. and Kaufmann, H.J. Greig cephalopolysyndactyly syndrome. *Helv. Ped. Acta.*, 40, 489–495 (1985).
Legius, E., Fryns, J.P. et al. Schinzel acrocallosal syndrome: a variant example of the Greig syndrome? *Ann. Génét.*, 28, 239–240 (1985).
Brueton, L., Huson, S.M. et al. Chromosomal localisation of a developmental gene in man . . . *Am. J. Med. Genet.*, 31, 799–804 (1988).
Philip, N., Apicella, N. et al. The acrocallosal syndrome. *Eur. J. Pediatr.*, 147, 206–208 (1988).
Krüger, G., Götz, J. et al. Greig syndrome in a large kindred due to reciprocal chromosome translocation t(6;7)(q27;p13). *Am. J. Med. Genet.*, 32, 411–416 (1989).

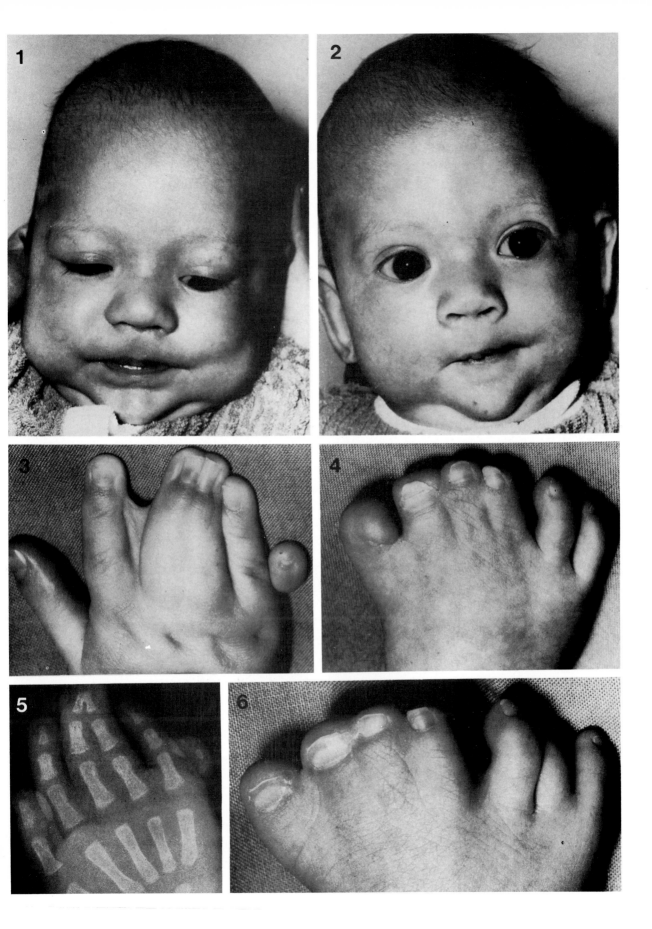

207. Orofaciodigital Syndrome Type II

(OFD Syndrome II, Mohr Syndrome)

A hereditary disorder occurring in both sexes and comprising bilateral postaxial polydactyly of the hands, polysyndactyly of the big toes, lobulation of the tongue, hyperplastic frenula, and unusual facies.

Main signs:
1. Postaxial and in some cases also preaxial, polydactyly of the hands, as well as brachy-, syn-, and clinodactyly (**1**).
2. Duplication of the big toes; possibly also postaxial polydactyly of the feet (**2**).
3. Clefting or lobulation of the tongue (into two or more lobes) with nodules at the base of the lobular clefts; hyperplastic oral frenula.
4. Unusual facies: hypertelorism or telecanthus; broad nasal root and broad nasal tip, which may show a median groove; possible median cleft of the upper lip; mandibular and maxillary hypoplasia; frequent absence of the central incisors; high palate or cleft palate.

Supplementary findings: X-rays of the feet show broad, short (or possibly duplicated) first metatarsals, cuneiform, and navicular bones.

Possible conductive hearing impairment with malformation of the incus. Mental development normal as a rule. Occasionally, brain malformations, short stature.

Manifestation: At birth.

Etiology: Autosomal recessive disorder.

Frequency: Low.

Course, prognosis: Usually normal life expectancy.

Differential diagnosis: Orofaciodigital syndrome I occurs only in females (X-chromosomal dominant inheritance); for differentiating characteristics see p.62; see also 'Comment' there.

Treatment: Surgical correction of clefts and hypertrophic frenula; early evaluation of hearing with treatment when indicated; orthodontic and dental care; removal of additional big toes and correction of the hands in some cases. Genetic counseling.

Illustration:
1 and 2 A girl with Mohr syndrome, the second child of healthy parents. Broad nasal root, median notch of the upper lip, cleft tip of the tongue with small fibromas bilaterally; high palate, notched alveolar ridges and thick frenula. Polydactyly of the hands and feet with duplication of the rays of the big toes.

H.-R.W.

References:

Pfeiffer, R. A., Majewski, F., Mannkopf, H. Das Syndrom von Mohr und Claussen. *Klin. Pädiatr.*, 184, 224 (1972).
Levy, E.P., Fletcher, B.D., Fraser, C. Mohr syndrome with subclinical expression of the bifid great toe. *Am. J. Dis. Child.*, 128, 531 (1974).
Anneren, G., Arvidson, B. et al. Oro-facio-digital syndromes I and II ... *Clin. Genet.*, 26, 178–186 (1984).
Baraitser, M. The orofaciodigital (OFD) syndromes. *J. Med. Genet.*, 23, 116–119 (1986).
Silengo, M.C., Bell, G.L. et al. Oro-facio-digital syndrome II ... *Clin. Genet.*, 31, 331–336 (1987).
Toriello, H.V. Heterogeneity and variability in the oral-facial-digital syndromes. *Am. J. Med. Genet.*, (Suppl.), 4, 149–159 (1988).

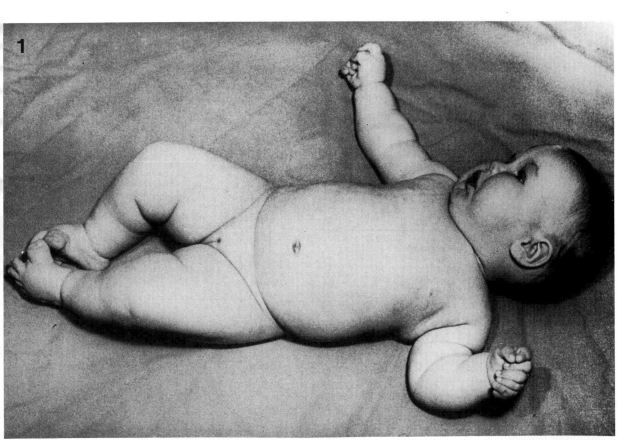

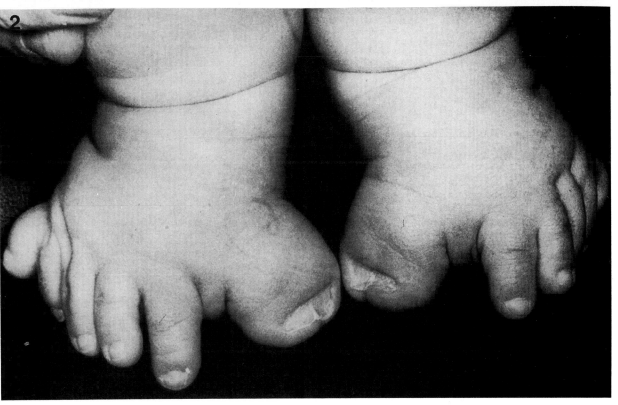

208. Acrofacial Dysostosis of the Predominantly Postaxial Type

(Acrofacial Dysostosis Genée–Wiedemann Type, Genée–Wiedemann Syndrome, Postaxial Acrofacial Dysostosis Syndrome [POADS]

A hereditary disorder with oligodactyly due to absence of the fifth rays as the main sign, and including cleft palate, micrognathia, dysplastic ears and eyelids, and in some cases, a characteristic large-eyed appearance.

Main signs:
1. Bilateral absence (or rudimentary appendage in isolated cases) of the fifth fingers and toes with abnormally short forearms (particularly the ulnae) and tendency to club-hand position with ulnar deviation. (1–4, 6–7).
2. Receding chin; cleft lip and/or palate; deformity of the external ears (5); anomalies of the eyelids (short palpebral fissures with antimongoloid slant; usually distinct lateral coloboma of the lower lids; deficient eyelashes; inability to completely close the eyes; and in some cases characteristically large-appearing eyes).

Supplementary findings: Accessory nipples frequently found.

Psychomotor retardation in a few cases.

X-rays show absence of the fifth ray, carpal anomalies, and in some cases radioulnar synostosis.

Various other clinical and/or radiological skeletal anomalies—including mild, preaxial limb defects—or anomalies of the internal organs (heart, kidneys, genitalia) may occur.

Possible conjunctivitis, inflammation of the middle ear; possible hearing impairment.

Manifestation: At birth.

Etiology: Probably autosomal recessive disorder; heterogeneity not excluded.

Frequency: Low (at least 20 documented observations).

Differential diagnosis: Nager's acrofacial dysostosis presents almost an 'opposite' clinical picture, with marked preaxial involvement of the extremities. Mandibulofacial dysostosis can likewise be excluded, in spite of a variety of similar facial signs.

Treatment: Symptomatic. Closure of clefts. Orthopedic or limb surgery, cosmetic surgery, or orthodontic correction may be indicated. Early assessment of hearing. Speech therapy when indicated. Genetic counseling.

Illustrations:
1–8 The same patient, as an infant (1, 5), at 3 years (6, 8), at 4½ years (2, 3, 7), and at 15 years (4a–c). Brachycephaly. Eyelid anomalies with notching of the lateral lower lids; incomplete closure of the eyelids, large-appearing eyes. Cleft palate, micrognathia. Congenital heart defect (VSD). Cryptorchidism. Pes planus. Mental retardation. Radiologically (6, 8), apart from aplasia of the fifth ray, hypoplasia of the ulna with proximal broadening; delayed ossification; anomalies of the metacarpals and phalanges and of metatarsals and toe bones.

H.-R.W.

References:
Genée, E. Une forme extensive de dysostose mandibulofaciale. *J. Génét. Hum.*, 17, 45–52 (1969).
Wiedemann, H.-R. Missbildungs-Retardierungs-Syndrom mit Fehlen des 5. Strahls an Händen und Füßen, Gaumenspalte, dysplastischen Ohren und Augenlidern und radioulnarer Synostose. *Klin. Pädiatr.*, 185, 181–186 (1973).
Miller, M., Fineman, R., Smith, D. Postaxial acrofacial dysostosis syndrome. *J. Pediatr.*, 95, 970–975 (1979).
Lewin, S.O. and Opitz, J.M. Fibular A/hypoplasia: review and documentation of the fibular developmental field. *Am. J. Med. Genet.*, (Suppl.), 2, 215 (1986).
Donnai, D., Hughes, H.E., Winter, R.M. Postaxial acrofacial dysostosis (Miller) syndrome. *J. Med. Genet.*, 24, 422 (1987).
Meinecke, P. and Wiedemann, H.-R. Robin sequence and oligodactyly in mother and son ... *Am. J. Med. Genet.*, 27, 953 (1987).
Opitz, J.M. and Stickler, G.B. The Genée–Wiedemann syndrome ... *Am. J. Med. Genet.*, 27, 971 (1987).
Hauss-Albert, H. and Passarge, E. Postaxial acrofacial dysostosis syndrome ... *Am. J. Med. Genet.*, 31, 701–703 (1988).
Chrzanowska, K.H., Fryns, J.P. et al. Phenotype variability in ... acrofacial dysostosis syndrome ... *Clin. Genet.*, 35, 157–160 (1989).

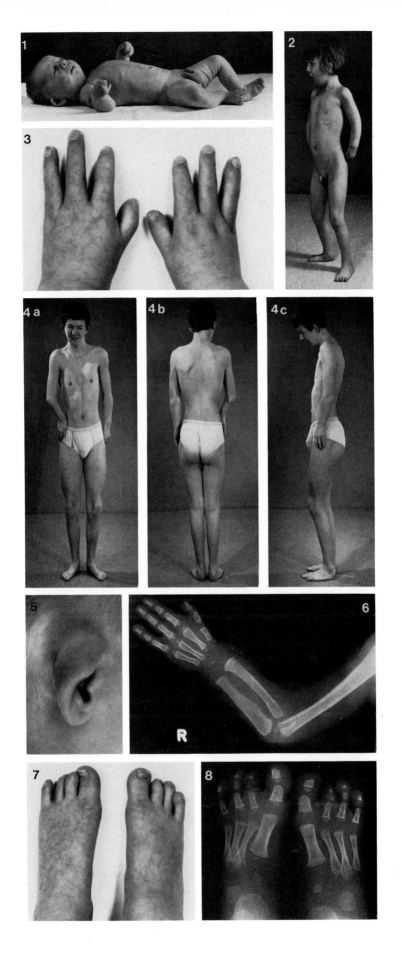

419

209. Trichorhinophalangeal Syndrome Type I

A syndrome of unusual facies; sparse, fragile scalp hair; clinical and radiological abnormalities of the hands; and not infrequently, short stature.

Main signs:

1. Facial dysmorphism with more or less 'bulbous' or 'pear-shaped' nose, large and sometimes prominent ears, long broad philtrum, and thin upper lip. Eyebrows poorly developed laterally (**1**).

2. Sparse, fine, brittle, and usually light-colored scalp hair (**1**).

3. Short hands and feet with finger deformities due to broadening of the proximal interphalangeal joints, and sometimes deviation of the phalangeal axis, with little or no limitation of motion. Thumbs and big toes short and broad (**2, 3**). 'Cone-shaped' epiphyses on X-ray; shortening of some metacarpals and metatarsals (**5, 6**).

Supplementary findings: Not infrequently, moderate short stature.

Fragile, brittle finger- and toenails. Possible dysodontiasis.

Perthes-type dysplasia of the head of the femur, kyphosis, scoliosis, winging of the scapulae alatae, thoracic deformity, and cardiovascular anomalies may occur.

Manifestation: Facial characteristics and sparse hair growth may be apparent from birth, but as a rule the children are first brought to medical attention later in childhood because of 'swelling' over the proximal interphalangeal joints.

Etiology: Hereditary defect. Usually autosomal dominant transmission; variable penetrance, very variable expression. Apparently there is an autosomal recessive form too. Presumably also heterogeneity. Recent demonstrations of small chromosomal (8q-) deletions.

Frequency: Low; up to 1985 about 200 cases reported in the literature.

Course, prognosis: Normal life expectancy. The osteoarticular changes are usually progressive; in some cases early arthritis in the hands, vertebral column, and other areas. Sparse scalp hair and the poor self-image because of the shape of the nose, deformed fingers, and in some cases short stature, may cause problems, especially in girls and women.

Differential diagnosis: Trichorhinophalangeal syndrome type II (Langer–Giedion syndrome, p.408).

Treatment: Orthopedic and orthodontic care, plastic surgery (nose), and a wig may be indicated. Psychological guidance. Genetic counseling.

Illustrations:

1–6 A 15-year-old, 167.5-cm-tall (= ±0) school boy showing the typical syndrome, apparently inherited from his father. Scalp hair, lateral eyebrows, and body hair sparse. Narrowly spaced teeth with relatively small lower jaw. Nails thin and extremely brittle; skin of the fingertips very fragile and sensitive. Nails of the big toes ingrown, with inflammation. Painless enlargement and slight flexion of the proximal interphalangeal joints, but good mobility. Thumbs and big toes especially short and broad.

H.-R.W.

References:

Spranger, J.W., Langer, L.O., Jr., Wiedemann, H.-R. *Bone Dysplasias. An Atlas of Constitutional Disorders of Skeletal Development.* G. Fischer and W.B. Saunders, Stuttgart and Philadelphia, 1974.

Frias, J.L., Felmann, A.H., Garnica, A.D. et al. Variable expessivity in the trichorhinophalangeal syndrome type I. *Birth Defects*, 15/5B, 361 (1979).

Ranke, M.B. and Heitkamp, H.-C. Tricho-rhino-phalangeales Syndrom. *Monatschr. Kinderheilkd.*, 128, 208 (1980).

Goodman, R.M., Trilling, R., Hertz, M. et al. New clinical observations in the trichorhinophalangeal syndrome. *J. Craniofacial Genet. Develop. Biol.*, 1, 15, (1981).

Gaardsted, C., Madsen, E.H., Friedrich, U. A Danish kindred with tricho-rhino-phalangeal syndrome type I. *Eur. J. Pediatr.*, 139, 84–87 (1982).

Fryns, J.P. and van Berghe, H. 8q24.12 Interstitial deletion in trichorhinophalangeal syndrome type I. *Hum. Genet.*, 74, 188–189 (1986).

Goldblatt, J. and Smart, R.D. Tricho-rhino-phalangeal syndrome without exostoses, with an interstitial deletion of 8q23. *Clin. Genet.*, 29, 434–438 (1986).

Howell, C.J. and Wynne-Davies, R. The tricho-rhino-phalangeal syndrome … 14 cases in 7 kindreds. *J. Bone Jt. Surg.*, 68 B, 311–314 (1986).

Schlesinger, A.E. and Poznanski, A.K. Flattening of the distal femoral epiphyses in the trichorhinophalangeal syndrome. *Pediatr. Radiol.*, 16, 498–500 (1986).

Bühler, E.M., Bühler, U.K. et al. A final word on the tricho-rhino-phalangeal syndromes. *Clin. Genet.*, 31, 273–275 (1987).

Yamamoto, Y., Oguro, N. et al. Prometaphase chromosomes in the tricho-rhino-phalangeal syndrome type I. *Am. J. Med. Genet.*, 32, 524–527 (1989).

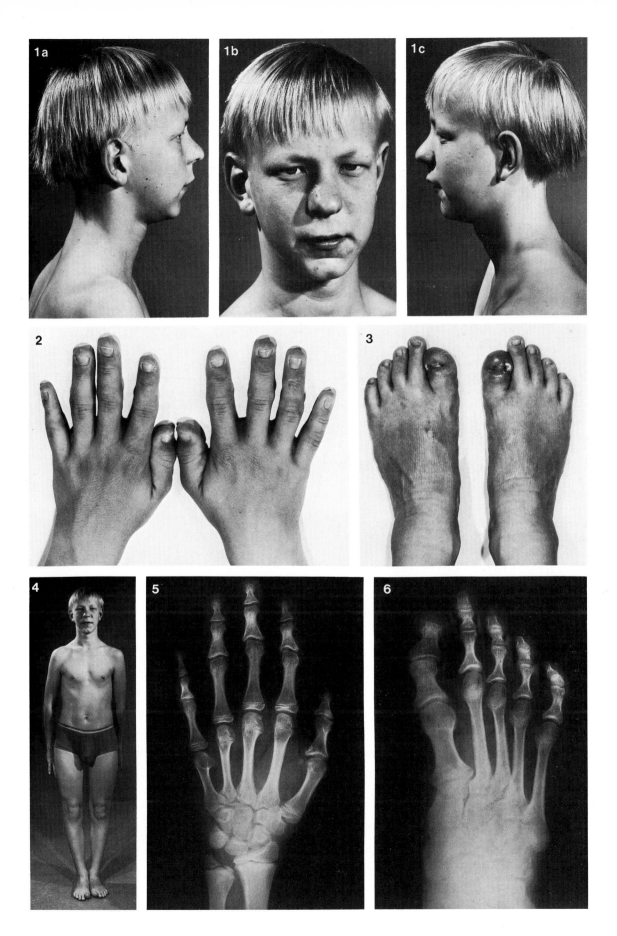

210. Oculo-Dento-Osseus Dysplasia

(Oculodentodigital Dysplasia, Meyer–Schwickerath Syndrome, Osteodentodigital Dysplasia)

A characteristic syndrome with microcornea, hypoplastic alae nasi, enamel hypoplasia, bilateral syndactyly of the fourth/fifth fingers, and hypo- to aplasia of the phalanges of the toes.

Main signs:
1. Microcornea with normal-sized eyeball.
2. Long, thin nose with pronounced nasal columella, hypoplastic alae nasi, and narrow nostrils.
3. Enamel hypoplasia or dysplasia.
4. Syndactyly of the fourth/fifth fingers bilaterally; dys-, hypo-, or aplasia of one or more middle phalanges of the toes (seen on X-ray).

Supplementary findings: Narrow palpebral fissures, medial epicanthus, refraction anomalies, strabismus, glaucoma.

Clinodactyly, camptodactyly, cranial hyperostosis, thickened mandible, broad clavicles, thickened ribs, deficient tubulation of the long bones.

Generalized anomaly of hair growth, including eyebrows and eyelashes; hypotrichosis, trichorrhexis; lusterless, brittle hair.

Rarely, conductive hearing impairment and neurological signs: hyperreflexia, ataxia, dysarthria.

Manifestation: At birth; other features, such as glaucoma, later.

Etiology: Usually autosomal dominant disorder with variable expression; but also sporadic cases (dominant new mutations, increased paternal age). Single cases due to autosomal recessive inheritance? Possible heterogeneity.

Frequency: 53 cases reported up to 1983.

Course, prognosis: As a rule normal psychomotor development; about 10% of patients show mild mental retardation. Impaired vision.

Differential diagnosis: Craniotubular hyperostoses, sclerosteosis, Pyle disease.

Treatment: Ophthalmological (glaucoma). Hand surgery? Genetic counseling.

Illustrations:
1a and 1b Female neonate; hypoplastic alae nasi, symmetrical syndactyly of the fourth/fifth fingers.
2a–2f A 6-month-old boy; thin, sparse eyebrows and eyelashes. Microcornea, medial epicanthi, pronounced nasal columella with hypoplastic alae nasi; syndactyly of the fourth/fifth digits bilaterally; absent middle phalanges of the toes and hypoplastic distal phalanges.
3a and 3b A 3-day-old female newborn; depressed nasal root, hypoplastic alae nasi, syndactyly of third to fifth digits bilaterally.

J.K.

References:

Beighton, P., Hamersma, H., Raad, M. Oculodento-osseus dysplasia: heterogeneity or variable expression. *Clin. Genet.*, 16, 169–177 (1979).

Judisch, G.F., Martin-Casals, A., Hanson, J.W. et al. Oculodentodigital dysplasia. Four new reports and a literature review. *Arch. Ophthalmol.*, 97, 878–884 (1979).

Patton, M.A. and Laurence, K.M. Three new cases of oculodentodigital (ODD) syndrome: development of the facial phenotype. *J. Med. Genet.*, 22, 386–389 (1985).

Traboulsi, E.I., Faris, B.M., Der Kaloustian, V.M. Persistent hyperplastic primary vitreous and recessive oculo-dento-osseus dysplasia. *Am. J. Med. Genet.*, 24, 95–100 (1986).

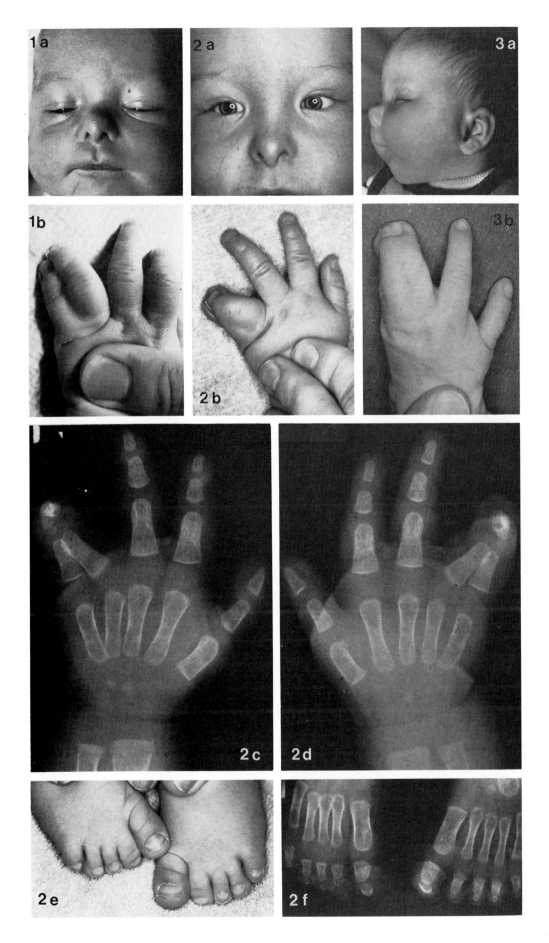

211. Symphalangism–Brachydactyly Syndrome with Conductive Hearing Impairment

(Facioaudiosymphalangism Syndrome, Syndrome of Multiple Synostoses with Conductive Hearing Impairment)

A syndrome of malformations of the hands and feet, characteristic facies, and defective hearing.

Main signs:

1. Congenital limitation of movement at the proximal interphalangeal joints of the second to fifth fingers (radiologically, phalangeal fusion may not be seen until later) with absence of the normal articular creases; possible limited motion at the elbow joints and, later, at the wrist and ankle joints, in some cases with abnormal gait.

2. Brachydactyly, possible absence of distal segments of fingers (and/or toes), cutaneous syndactylies (**1**, **2**).

3. Unusual facies: long and rather narrow face with long, quite prominent nose, broad nasal bridge, asymmetrical mouth with thin upper lip (**1**).

4. Conductive hearing impairment, possibly first apparent in adolescence (ankylosis of the auditory ossicles).

Supplementary findings: Normal height but possible abnormal proportions due to short arms.

Radiologically, abnormally short first metacarpals/metatarsals; gradual development of symphalangism of the proximal phalanges of second to fifth fingers (**3**, **4**); later, ankylosis also of the carpals (**4**) and tarsals; various anomalies of the elbow region, even radio-humeral synostosis (**5**).

Manifestation: At birth and thereafter.

Etiology: Hereditary disorder, autosomal dominant. Considerable intrafamilial variability.

Frequency: Very low (up to 1985, only about 20 documented observations).

Course, prognosis: Symphalangism, ankylosis in the wrist and ankle region, and hearing impairment tend to progress.

Treatment: Corrective surgical measures for the extremities usually not indicated. Early evaluation of hearing; treatment as indicated. Genetic counseling.

Illustrations:

1–3 and 5 A 2-year-old boy.
4 An X-ray of his father's hand.

H.-R.W.

References:

Maroteaux, P., Bouvet, J.P. et al. La maladie des synostoses multiples. *Nouv. Presse Méd.*, 1, 3041–3047 (1972).
Herrmann, J. Symphalangism and brachydactyly syndrome ... *Birth Defects.*, X, 5, 23–53 (1974).
Königsmark, B.W. and Gorlin, R.J. Dominant symphalangism and conduction deafness. In: *Genetic and Metabolic Deafness.* W.B. Saunders, Philadelphia, 1976.
Poisson, D., Zerbib, M. et al. Maladies des synostoses multiples. *Arch. Fr. Pédiatr.*, 40, 35–37 (1983).
da Silva, E.O., Filho, S.M. et al. Multiple synostosis syndrome ... *Am. J. Med. Genet.*, 18, 237–247 (1984).
Hurvitz, S.A., Goodman, R.M. et al. The facio-audio-symphalangism syndrome ... review of the literature. *Clin. Genet.*, 28, 61–68 (1985).

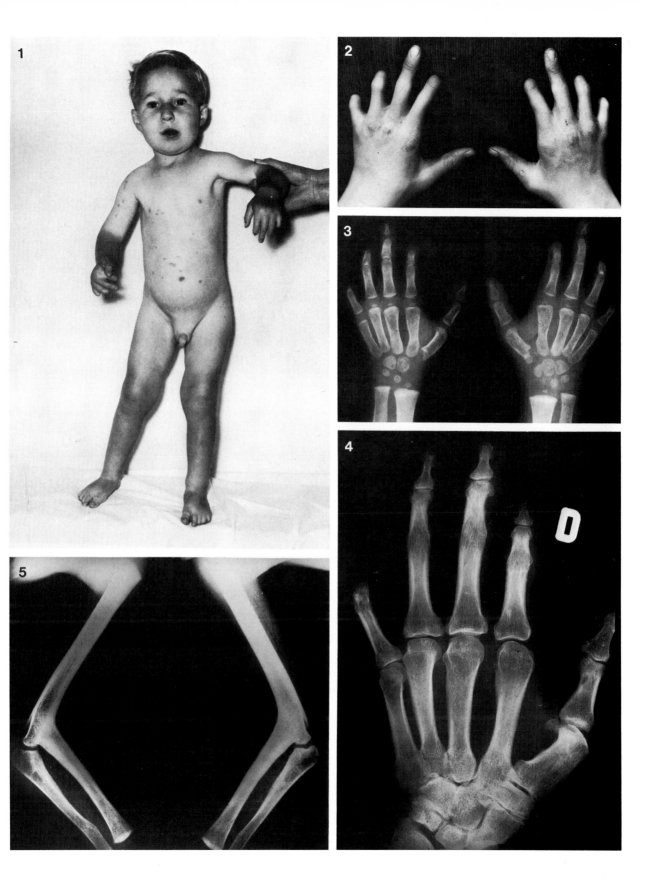

212. An Unknown Malformation–Retardation Syndrome

A syndrome of psychomotor retardation with micro-cephaly, unusual facies, and other diverse anomalies.

Main signs:

1. Primary psychomotor retardation; (brachy-) micro-cephaly.
2. Facies: slight antimongoloid slant of the palpebral fissures, left more than right; right epicanthus; relatively narrow palpebral fissures; thin alae nasi; and large mouth. Low-set, prominent, simple ears (**1, 2**). Microretrognathia. High-arched palate.
3. Broad wrists, barely distinguishable from the forearms (**4**) and shapeless pillar-like lower legs (**1, 3**). Progressive right-convex scoliosis of the thoracic spine (**3c**). Short hands with proximal cutaneous syndactyly between second to fifth fingers bilaterally, clinodactyly of the left index finger and short tapering fingers with hypoplastic terminal phalanges (**4**). Limited motion at the ankles. Recurrent dislocation of the left patella. Short feet in club-foot position with dysdactyly; elongated halluces (**6, 7**).

Supplementary findings: Short stature (below the tenth percentile). Suggestion of pterygium colli. Relatively sparse hair growth. Bilateral undescended testes (at 4 years) and left cryptorchidism (at 12¾ years); small penis.

Small atrial septal defect; possible small ventricular septal defect.

Radiologically, poorly modelled clavicles, high narrow pelvis, marked coxa valga. Clubbing of the proximal ends of the metacarpals, especially fifth, bilaterally. Slender fingers with strikingly short terminal phalanges (**5**).

Manifestation: At birth and later.

Etiology: Not clear.

Treatment: Symptomatic.

Illustrations:

1–7 The patient at 12¾ and 15½ years, the third child of healthy, nonconsanguineous parents (father 43 and mother 33 years old at the patient's birth). Unremarkable pregnancy; normal birth 3 weeks before term with weight 2500 g and length 49 cm. Endocrinological and laboratory examinations negative; repeated chromosome analyses unremarkable (including banded preparations).

H.-R.W.

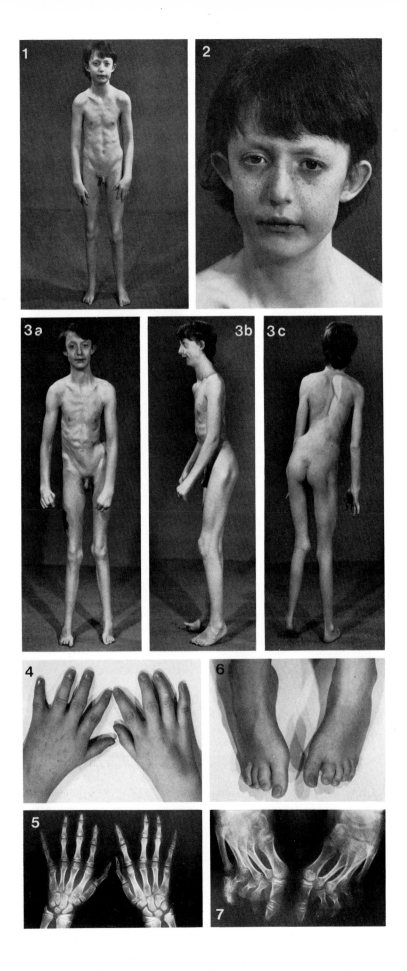

427

213. Hereditary Carpotarsal Osteolysis with Nephropathy

(Idiopathic Multicentric Osteolysis)

A hereditary disorder with progressive carpotarsal osteolysis and chronic progressive nephropathy.

Main signs:
1. Gradual shortening of wrists, ankles, metacarpus, and metatarsus bilaterally—and usually symmetrically—as a result of progressive osteolysis starting in the carpals and tarsals (**1, 3, 5–10**). Possibly preceded or accompanied by soft-tissue swelling, tenderness, limited mobility, and warming of the affected region. Increasing deformity with ulnar deviation or volar subluxation of the shortened hands and eventual formation of claw hands or short pes cavus with overlapping toes (**7**).
2. Progressive nephropathy (proteinuria, possible hematuria; development of arterial hypertension, etc.).

Supplementary findings: Kyphoscoliosis not infrequent; development of muscular atrophy, especially in the distal extremities, and of flexion contractures of the large joints.

Unusual facies with mild exophthalmos, hypoplasia of the upper jaw and micrognathia has been noted; furthermore, mental retardation and short adult stature in isolated cases.

Manifestation: Osteolysis apparent in the first decade of life, generally in the toddler, rarely as early as the first year of life. Nephropathy toward the end of the first decade or during the second.

Etiology: Autosomal dominant disorder with basic defect unknown. Also autosomal recessive inheritance reported. Heterogeneity.

Frequency: Low.

Course, prognosis: Usually slow progression of the osteolysis on to complete dissolution of the carpal and tarsal bones and 'licked candy-stick' appearance of the shortened and narrowed ends of the adjacent long bones (**9**). Thus, gradual shortening of the forearms and sometimes of the lower legs; possible analogous involvement of the elbow regions and other joints, with corresponding limitation of motion. Skeletal changes may stabilize toward the end of the second decade of life. However, the nephropathy runs a protracted course, with possibly poor prognosis.

Differential diagnosis: Other osteolysis syndromes (see also pp.430, 432). Rheumatoid arthritis may be considered at the onset of the illness, but is easily excluded.

Treatment: Symptomatic. Career guidance. Genetic counseling. Kidney transplantation may be indicated.

Illustrations:
1, 2, 5, 7, 9 A 39-year-old woman.
3, 4, 6, 8, 10 Her 9-year-old, mildly mentally retarded son.

Two older children healthy. Mother and son of normal height; both show a slightly receding chin; the mother finds her son's broad nasal bridge unusual ('not at all in the family'). In both, onset of symptoms in the left hand in early school years, subsequently less severe involvement of the right hand; feet more severely affected (left > right). The mother's narrowed, shortened left hand, with markedly limited mobility—as in the son—shows a Dupuytren-like picture; similar development of connective tissue nodules and cords on the plantar fascia bilaterally. Proteinuria in both mother and son (in the former, fluctuating hypertension) varying between 1 and 3 g/day.

H.-R.W.

References:
Erickson, C.M., Hirschberger, M., Stickler, G.B. Carpal-tarsal osteolysis. *J. Pediatr.*, 93, 779 (1978).
Fryns, J.P. Ostéolyse essentielle à début carpien et tarsien. *J. Génét. Hum.*, 30, Suppl. 5, 423–428 (1982).
Carnevale, A., Canún, S. et al. Idiopathic multicentric osteolysis with facial anomalies and nephropathy. *Am. J. Med. Genet.*, 26, 877–886 (1987).
Turner, M.C., Gonzalez, O.R. et al. Multicentric osteolysis: report of the second successful renal transplant. *Pediatr. Nephrol.*, 1, 42–45 (1987).
Pai, G.S. and Macpherson, R.I. Idiopathic multicentric osteolysis . . . review of the literature. *Am. J. Med. Genet.*, 29, 929–936 (1988).
Barr, R.J., Hughes, A.E. et al. Idiopathic multicentric osteolysis . . . *Am. J. Med. Genet.*, 32, 556 (1989).

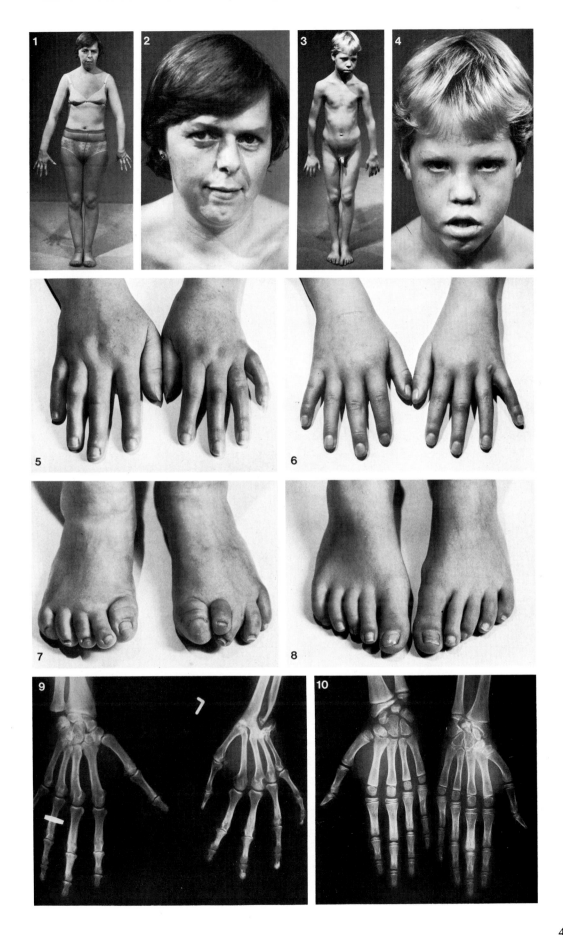

214. Idiopathic Carpotarsal Osteolysis François Type

(Dystrophia Dermo-Chondro-Cornealis Familiaris)

A hereditary syndrome of progressive carpotarsal osteolysis with skin and corneal changes.

Main signs:
1. Gradual shortening of the wrist, ankle, metatarsus and metacarpus bilaterally (with preceding tenderness, warming, and soft-tissue swelling) as a result of progressive osteolysis starting in the wrists and ankles (3–5). Increasing deformity (ulnar deviation of the shortened hands, eventual claw-hand [1, 2]; short pes cavus).
2. In some cases, decreased vision from school age on.
3. Xanthomatous nodules on, e.g., the hands, elbows, face.

Supplementary findings: Subepithelial and central corneal clouding, possibly only seen on slit-lamp examination).
   Idiopathic nephropathy with proteinuria in some cases.

Manifestation: Usually at a pre-school or school age.

Etiology: Monogenic disorder, autosomal recessive.

Frequency: Very low.

Course, prognosis: Slow progression of osteolysis with corresponding physical handicap. Life expectancy, without nephropathy, probably unaffected; with nephropathy, possibly unfavorable.

Differential diagnosis: Other osteolysis syndromes (see also pp. 428, 432). Rheumatoid arthritis may be considered early in the disease, but is easily excluded.

Treatment: Symptomatic. Renal transplantation may be indicated. Genetic counseling.

Illustrations:
1–5 a 16-year-old girl; bone changes manifest in early childhood; xanthomatous nodules; corneal clouding noted at age 14 years with slit-lamp examination; nephropathy since an early school age; death at 22 years from nephrosclerosis.

H.-R.W.

References:
Wiedemann, H.-R. Zur François'schen Krankheit. *Ärztl. Wochenschr.*, 13, 905 (1958).
Spranger, J.W., Langer, L.O., Jr., Wiedemann, H.-R. *Bone Dysplasias. An Atlas of Constitutional Disorders of Skeletal Development.* G. Fischer and W.B. Saunders, Stuttgart and Philadelphia, 1974.

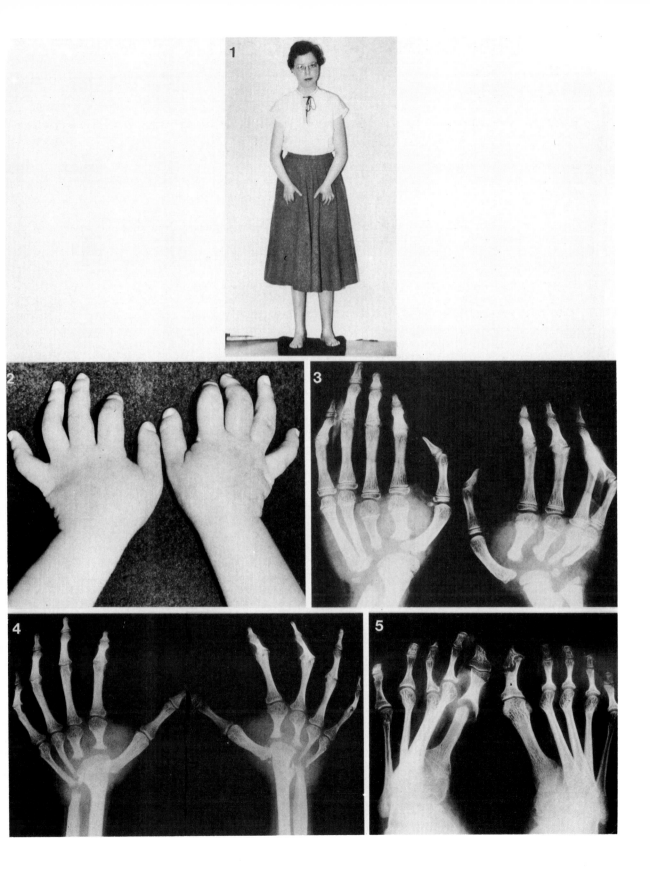

215. Hajdu–Cheney Syndrome

(Idiopathic Osteolysis Hajdu–Cheney Type)

A syndrome of characteristic facies, persistence of cranial sutures and fontanelles, hyperextensible joints, increased tendency to fractures, premature loss of teeth, and acro-osteolysis on X-ray.

Main signs:
1. Characteristic facies: broad and strikingly heavy eyebrows; maxillary and mandibular hypoplasia; broad philtrum; and broad, thin-lipped mouth (1). Coarse, thick scalp hair.
2. Cranial anomalies: persistence of the fontanelles and sutures; eventual development of dolichocephaly with protruding occiput.
3. Joint laxity; usually short stature with short neck; tendency to pathologic fractures; carious teeth.
4. Short, broad tips of the fingers and sometimes of the toes, which may be tender or painful and may be associated with nail deformities (2).

Supplementary findings: Coarse skin in some patients, often with hypertrichosis. Hoarse voice common. Possible conductive hearing impairment; possible defective vision or other eye anomalies.
  Radiologically: Persistence of fontanelles and sutures with numerous wormian bones especially within the lambdoid suture (5, 6); later, in addition, dolichocephaly with protruding occiput, platybasia, elongation of the sella (6); small jaw, deficient pneumatization of the sinuses.
  Osteolysis, in particular acro-osteolysis with formation of typical transverse clefts of the distal phalanges of the fingers (3, 4).
  Generalized osteoporosis in some cases, with corresponding changes in shape of the vertebral bodies, with secondary kyphoscoliosis in some cases; multiple fractures; also abnormal modeling, or deformity of the long tubular bones.

Manifestation: The characteristic facies, abundant body hair, and hoarse voice may come to attention in the newborn. Changes in the ends of the fingers with radiologically demonstrable osteolysis and generalized osteoporosis, sometimes with compression fractures, may be apparent in early childhood, but also may not come to medical attention until much later. The diagnosis has often not been made until adolescence or even adulthood.

Etiology: An autosomal dominant gene is apparently responsible. Predominantly sporadic occurrence (as new mutations).

Frequency: Low; to date, only about 30 cases are described in the literature.

Course, prognosis: Progressive increase in extent and severity of changes, including secondary changes, is usual.

Differential diagnosis: Other types of osteolysis (see also pp.428, 430) as well as pyknodysostosis (p.200) and cleidocranial dysplasia (p.32) are usually easy to rule out. Normal mental development immediately excludes the Brachmann–de Lange syndrome (p.182), which may be suggested by the facies.

Treatment: Early audiological and ophthalmological assessment; adequate care as needed. Dental attention. Orthopedic care and treatment of secondary complications. Genetic counseling.

Illustrations:
1–6 A girl, the third child of nonconsanguineous parents, at ages 7 years (1, 2, 4) and 2¼ years (3, 5, 6). At 7 years: short stature (around the third percentile), short neck, pectus excavatum, and scoliosis; general laxity of the joints and muscular hypotonia. Coarse skin with abundant hair, bristly scalp hair; defective dentition; hearing impairment, hoarse voice; normal intellect. X-rays show early dolichocephaly, widened sutures with wormian bones; generalized osteoporosis, platyspondyly; multiple fractures (since age 5 years); short terminal phalanges of the feet, acro-osteolysis of the terminal phalanges of first, second and fifth fingers now more pronounced.

H.-R.W.

References:
Weleber, R.G. and Beals, R.K. The Hajdu–Cheney syndrome. *J. Pediatr.*, 88, 243 (1976).
Wendel, U. and Kemperdick, H. Idiopathische Osteolyse vom Typ Hajdu–Cheney. *Monatschr. Kinderheilkd.*, 127, 581 (1979).
Udell, J., Schumacher, H.R. et al. Idiopathic familial acroosteolysis . . . review of the Hajdu–Cheney syndrome. *Arthritis Rheumatism*, 29, 1032–1038 (1986).

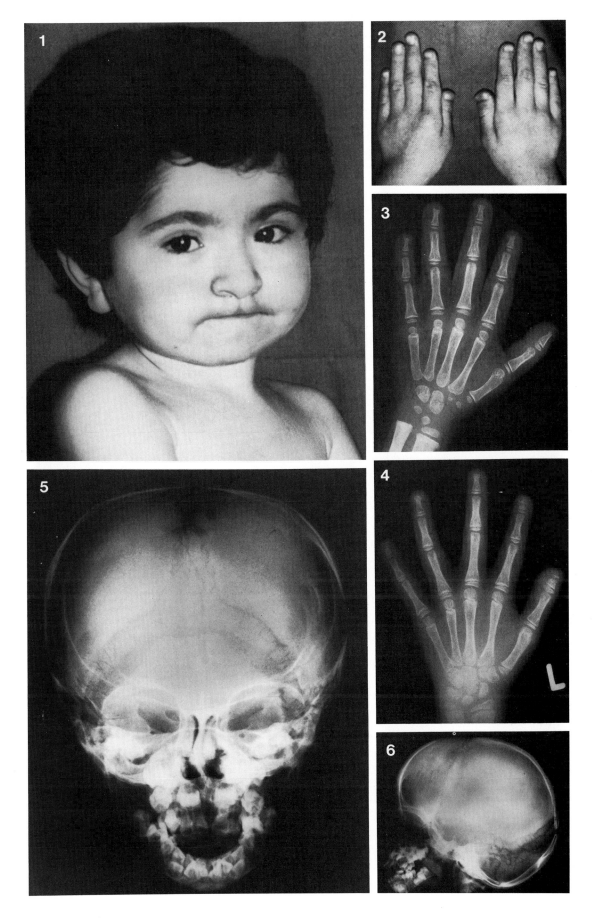

216. Syndrome of Triphalangism of the First Rays of the Hands, Thrombasthenia, and Sensorineural Hearing Impairment

A syndrome comprising triphalangeal digits instead of thumbs, a thrombasthenic bleeding diathesis, and sensorineural hearing impairment.

Main signs:
1. Well-developed or hypoplastic triphalangeal digits instead of thumbs (4–6), possibly with hypoplasia of the forearm (1a, 1b) or of the radius, and with radiological anomalies of the wrist.

2. Bleeding diathesis with episodes of skin and mucous membrane bleeding.
3. Sensorineural hearing impairment.

Supplementary findings: Facial dysmorphism (hypertelorism, broad nasal root, prognathism).

Normal platelet count. Pathologically, prolonged bleeding time and further findings of Glanzmann's thrombasthenia.

Manifestation: At birth and early in life.

Etiology: Probable monogenic disorder, presumably autosomal recessive transmission in view of the thrombasthenia.

Frequency: Probably very low.

Course, prognosis: As far as can be determined, relatively favorable.

Differential diagnosis: Fanconi anemia (p.440), Aase syndrome (p.436), TAR syndrome (p.374), Holt–Oram syndrome (p.438), Blackfan–Diamond syndrome, and IVIC syndrome.

Treatment: Symptomatic (transfusions of fresh blood or platelet concentrate for bleeding episodes; surgical correction of finger contractures).

Illustrations:
1–6 A 13¼-year-old girl, normal birth, robust development and normal height; recurrent, sometimes severe, skin and mucous membrane bleeding from 12 months of age. Repeated hospital admissions and transfusions required. No bleeding into the joints; heavy menstrual bleeding. Probably congenital sensorineural hearing impairment. Triphalangeal, strong, non-opposable digit in the thumb position on the right with broad, thenar-like bridge of soft tissue to the second ray; hypoplastic, triphalangeal digit contracted in flexion in the thumb position of the left hand (which as a whole is somewhat smaller than the right). Various asymmetrical anomalies of the wrist (4–6).

Relatively coarse facies with hypertelorism, broad nose, and prognathism (1a, 1c). Large area of alopecia on the scalp (2). Pigmented nevus on the right side of the back (1b, 3). Multiple hematomas (e.g., on the inner surfaces of the left arm and left lower leg (1a). Pelvic kidney on the right. Normal platelet count, extremely prolonged bleeding time, detailed hematological findings as in Glanzmann's thrombasthenia. Chromosome analysis unremarkable.

H.-R.W.

References:
Schlegelberger, B., Grote, W., Wiedemann, H.-R. Probable autosomal recessive syndrome with triphalangia of the thumbs, thrombasthenia Glanzmann and deafness of internal ear. *Klin. Pediatr.*, 198, 337–339 (1986).
Quazi, Q. and Kassner, E.G. Triphalangeal thumb. *J. Med. Genet.*, 25, 505–520 (1988).

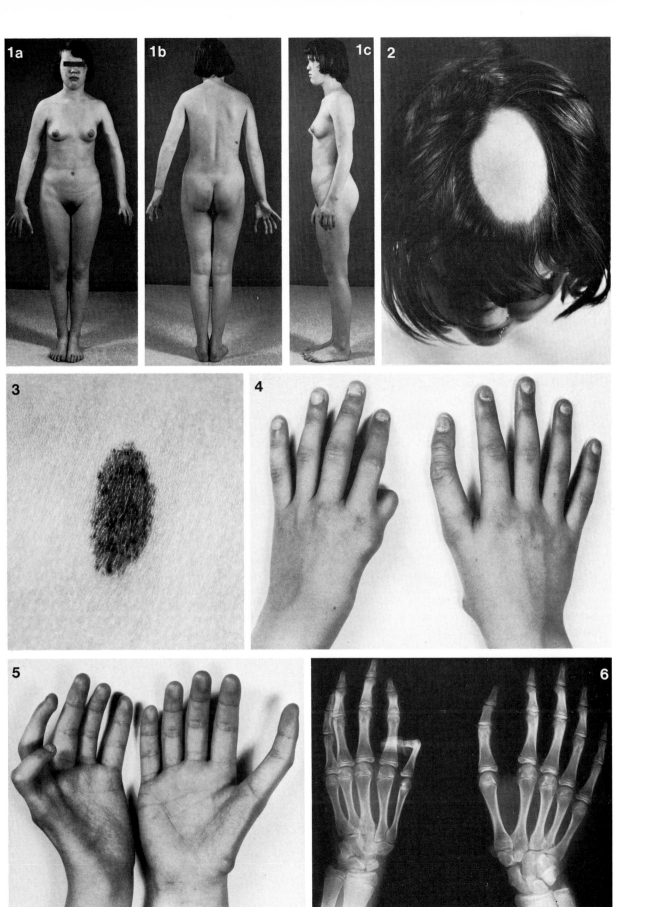

217. Hypoplastic Anemia with Triphalangeal Thumbs Syndrome

(Aase Syndrome, Aase–Smith Syndrome)

A characteristic syndrome with triphalangeal thumbs, early manifested hypoplastic anemia, and short stature.

Main signs:
1. Intrauterine growth retardation and decreased postnatal growth (with some degree of catch-up growth eventually).
2. Triphalangeal thumb (with possible hypoplasia of the thenar eminence and radius); possible unilateral occurrence.
3. Normochromic normocytic anemia manifest from infancy (low reticulocyte count, decreased erythropoiesis in the marrow).
4. Possible mild mental retardation.

Supplementary findings: Unusual appearance, antimongoloid slant of the palpebral fissures, cleft lip or palate, low nuchal hairline, unusual skin pigmentation, ventricular septal defect, anomalies of clavicles and ribs have been noted in some cases.

Normal values for leukocytes and platelets and their precursors. Possibly increased fetal hemoglobin. No increase of chromosome breakage.

Manifestation: At birth (anemia may also be present during the first year of life, usually in the first 6 months).

Etiology: Probable monogenic disorder with recessive transmission.

Frequency: Very low (up to 1986, only about a dozen documented cases).

Course, prognosis: On the whole, favorable.

Differential diagnosis: Fanconi anemia (p.440), in which however, the blood disorder is usually manifest much later, initially with thrombocytopenia, then pancytopenia; hypoplasia or aplasia of the thumbs in the great majority; increased chromosome breakage. Blackfan–Diamond anemia: see 'comment' below. Compare also with the preceding syndrome.

Treatment: Blood transfusion, corticosteroids may be indicated. (Iron medication contraindicated.) Surgical correction of the hands in some cases. Genetic counseling.

Comment: Some authors consider that this syndrome falls within the spectrum of Diamond–Blackfan hypoplastic anemia. However, in the latter the dysmorphic features are absent (especially triphalangeal thumbs), in the great majority of cases. And the disorder does not appear to be genetically consistent.

Illustrations:
1–4 A 12½-year-old boy. Hypoplastic anemia since early infancy. On admission to the hospital, Hb 8.3 g%; 2.5 million erythrocytes; 0.6% reticulocytes; leuko- and thrombopoiesis normal. Shortly after increasing corticosteroids: Hb 10.3 g%; 2.8 million erythrocytes; 7.8% reticulocytes. Short stature (height of a 9½-year-old). Triphalangeal thumbs, low nuchal hairline, pigmented moles. IQ 77. Ocular fundi normal, no clefts, no organomegaly, testicles normally descended. Hb electrophoresis unremarkable. X-rays: no radial dysplasia; in the right wrist, absence of the navicular, fusion of the carpal bones (3).

H.-R.W.

References:

Aase, J.M. and Smith, D.W. Congenital anemia and triphalangeal thumbs: a new syndrome. *J. Pediatr.*, 74, 471 (1969).
Terheggen, F.C. Hypoplastische Anämie mit dreigliedrigem Daumen. *Z. Kinderheilkd.*, 118, 71 (1974).
Wood, V.E. Treatment of the triphalangeal thumb. *Clin. Orthop.*, 120, 188 (1976).
Alter, B.P. Thumbs and anemia. *Pediatrics*, 62, 613 (1978).
Pfeiffer, R.A. and Ambs, E. Das Aase-Syndrom... *Monatschr. Kinderheilkd.*, 131, 235–237 (1983).
Patton, M.A., Sharma, A. et al. The Aase–Smith syndrome. *Clin. Genet.*, 28, 521–525 (1985).
Muis, N., Beemer, F.A. et al. The Aase syndrome... review of the literature. *Eur. J. Pediatr.*, 145, 153–157 (1986).
Quazi, Q. and Kassner, E.G. Triphalangeal thumb. *J. Med. Genet.*, 25, 505–520 (1988).

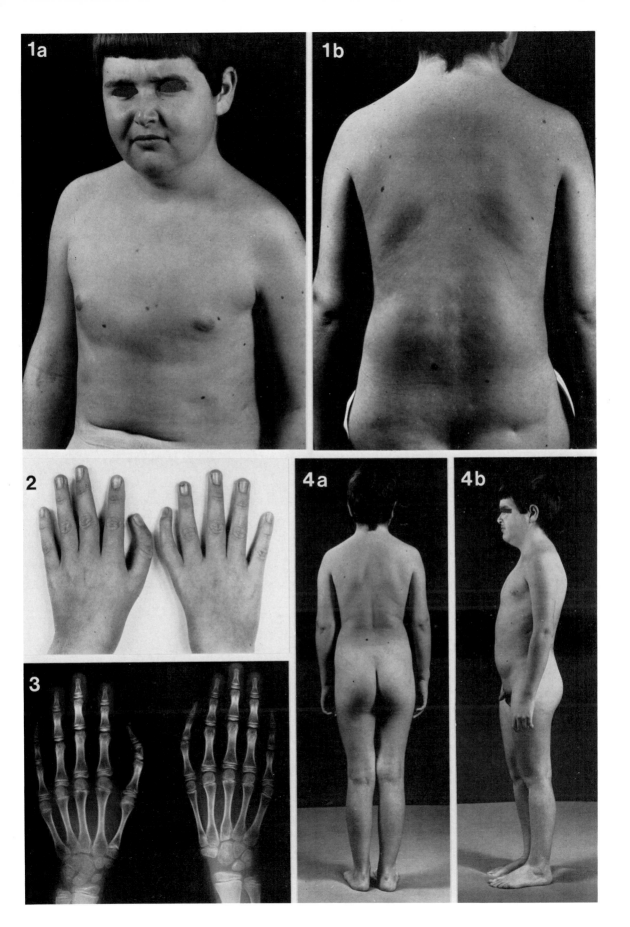

437

218. Holt–Oram Syndrome

(Heart–Hand Syndrome; Cardio-Digital Syndrome)

A hereditary disorder with malformations of the heart and upper extremities.

Main signs:
1. Malformations of the upper extremities, which may be symmetrical or asymmetrical. Triphalangism (**3a; 2c** *left*), hypoplasia (**1a, 1b**), or even aplasia of the thumbs; more extensive defects of the first ray in some cases (dys- or aplasia of the radius; dysplasia of the arm).
2. Congenital heart defect (**2d, 3**) in the form of septal defects (frequent atrial septal defect, secundum type; possibly with dysrhythmia) or other malformation.

Supplementary findings: Possible dysplasia of the little fingers (note clinodactyly: **1, 1a, 1b**), of the wrist (**3a** *right*), of the elbow joints, and of the shoulder girdles (clavicles, scapulae, and other; **3**). On X-ray, spur formation on the lateral ends of the clavicles as a characteristic (but non-specific) finding.

Manifestation: At birth (malformations of the upper extremities) and later, depending on the severity of the cardiac malformation.

Etiology: Monogenic disorder, autosomal dominant. Variable expression, often more severe in females. About 40% of the cases represent new mutations.

Frequency: Relatively low; however, a series of affected sibships and several hundred cases have been reported.

Course, prognosis: Dependent in each case on the severity of the cardiac defect and on the possibility for surgical correction.

Differential diagnosis: TAR syndrome (p.374), Fanconi anemia (p.440), thalidomide syndrome (p.370).

Treatment: Adequate care of the specific anomalies. Genetic counseling.

Illustrations:
1 and **2** Mother and daughter.
1a and **1b** Hands of the mother.
2a, 2b, 2c Hands of the daughter. X-ray of the daughter's hands (**2c**) shows triphalangeal thumb on the left with hypoplasia of the first metacarpal, of the wrist, and of the radius.
2d Chest X-ray of the daughter.
3, 3a X-rays from another girl; note shoulder anomalies (os acromiale on the left, among others) and the almost symmetrical triphalangeal thumbs with asymmetry of the wrists.

H.-R.W./J.K.

References:

Holt, M. and Oram, S. Familial heart disease with skeletal malformations. *Br. Heart. J.*, 22, 236 (1960).
Kaufmann, R.L., Rimoin, D.L., McAlister, W.H., Hartmann, A.F. Variable expression of the Holt–Oram syndrome. *Am. J. Dis. Child.*, 127, 21 (1974).
Capek-Schnachner, E., May, L., Schwarzbach, E. Holt–Oram-Syndrom. *Pädiatr. Prax.*, 21, 607 (1979).
Smith, A.T., Sack, G.H., Taylor, G.J. Holt–Oram syndrome. *J. Pediatr.*, 95, 538 (1979).
Gladstone, I., Jr. and Sybert, V.P. Holt–Oram syndrome: penetrance of the gene and lack of maternal effect. *Clin. Genet.*, 21, 98–103 (1982).
van Regemorter, N., Haumont, D. et al. Holt–Oram syndrome mistaken for thalidomide embryopathy . . . *Eur. J. Pediatr.*, 138, 77–80 (1982).
Najjar, H., Mardini, M. et al. Variability of the Holt–Oram syndrome . . . *Am. J. Med. Genet.*, 29, 851–855 (1988).
Cox, H., Viljoen, D. et al. Radial ray defects . . . *Clin. Genet.*, 35, 322–330 (1989).
Pfeiffer, R.A., Böwing, B., Deeg, K.H. Varianten der radialen Hemimelie mit und ohne Vitium cordis (Holt–Oram-Syndrom) in zwei Familien. *Monatschr. Kinderheilkd.*, 137, 275–279 (1989).

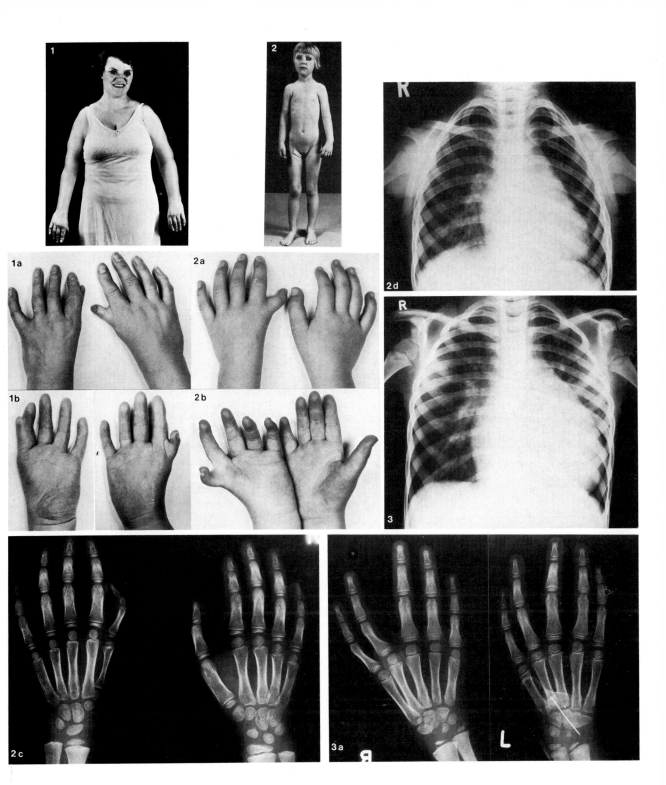

219. Fanconi Anemia

(Fanconi Pancytopenia Syndrome)

A characteristic syndrome of reduction malformations of the thumbs and radii, small stature, hyperpigmentation, and signs of aplastic anemia.

Main signs:
1. Pronounced pre- and postnatal growth deficiency; hypo- or aplasia of the thumbs (also, duplication or triphalangism), short or absent radii (4, 5, 7, 8). Extensive or patchy dirty-brown skin pigmentation, mainly truncal and in skin creases.
2. Unusual facies (3, 6). Possible microphthalmos, strabismus, nystagmus, coloboma.
3. Microcephaly, even relative to body size; moderate mental retardation in about 20%.

Supplementary findings: Hypoplastic male genitalia, undescended testes, hypospadias. Ear deformities, possible deafness. Hyperreflexia. Renal malformations. Occasional cardiac defects. Increased infections.

Pancytopenia (also lymphocytopenia); aplastic anemia. Increased fetal hemoglobin. Increased chromosome breakage with exchange figures in heterologous chromosome pairs. Increased frequency of malignant tumors, especially leukemia. Retarded bone age on X-ray (5, 7).

Comment: There are several patients without dysmorphic features.

Manifestation: Malformations and chromosome breakage present at birth. Increasing pigmentation from birth or later. Signs of pancytopenia usually between 5 and 10 years of age; rarely, as early as infancy, or as late as the third decade. Initially, reduced numbers of platelets, then of leuko- and erythrocytes. Chromosome findings are of particular importance, as other signs may be only partially expressed.

Etiology: Autosomal recessive disorder with extremely variable picture; heterogeneity. Increased chromosome breakage, small stature, thrombocytopenia, or other signs possible in heterozygotes. DNA repair defect.

Frequency: About 1:40,000 newborns.

Course, prognosis: Chronic, progressive. Untreated patients survive about 2 years after onset of hematological signs; survival has increased significantly since the introduction of therapy. Death from bone marrow failure or malignancy, especially leukemia (about 10%).

Treatment: Testosterone, in some cases with corticosteroids; bone marrow transplantation. Genetic counseling. Prenatal diagnosis possible.

Differential diagnosis:
1. Holt–Oram syndrome (p.438): shows only similar thumb and arm malformations and cardiac anomalies, the latter rarely present in Fanconi anemia.
2. Thrombocytopenia–radial aplasia (TAR) syndrome (p.374): always shows radial aplasia with thumbs present; thrombocytopenia alone, beginning in the first year of life; good prognosis once thrombocytopenic episodes have been overcome.
3. Hypoplastic anemia with triphalangial thumbs syndrome (p.436): shows only the signs of the name.
4. Syndrome of triphalangism of the first ray of the hands, thrombasthenia, and labyrinthine hearing impairment (p.434): normal platelet count.

Illustrations:
1–5 A 3¼-year-old patient; mother only 1.52 m tall. Birth measurements 2250 g, 45 cm. Presently, 79 cm (= ∼ 16 months), 8.8 kg (= ∼ 8 months), head circumference 48 cm (= normal for body size). Bone age 4–5 months. Mental age 2½ years. Isolated areas of hyperpigmentation. Bilateral microphthalmos with coloboma on the right. Hypoplastic genitalia. Hematologically, only mild thrombocytopenia to date.
6–8 2-year-old patient. Birth measurements 2640 g, 48 cm. Presently, 80 cm (= ∼ 17 months); 8.8 kg (= ∼ 8 months); head circumference, 43 cm (= 5 months). Bone age 3 months. Psychomotor development about normal for age. Generalized hyperpigmentation. Persistent foramen ovale. Genital hypoplasia. Elevated fetal hemoglobin. Thrombocytopenia and anemia since age 13 months.

H.-R.W.

References:

Voss, R., Kohn, G., Shaham, M. et al. Prenatal diagnosis of Fanconi anemia. *Clin. Genet.*, 20, 185 (1981).
Druckworth-Rysiecki, G., Hultén, M. et al. Clinical and cytogenetic diversity in Fanconi's anemia. *J. Med. Genet.*, 21, 197–203 (1984).
Schindler, D., Kubbies, M. et al. Presymptomatic diagnosis of Fanconi's anemia. *Lancet*, I, 937 (1985).
Rosendorff, R., Bernstein, R. et al. Fanconi's anemia . . . *Am. J. Med. Genet.*, 27, 793–797 (1987).
Digweed, M., Zakrezewski, S. et al. Fanconi's anemia . . . *Hum. Genet.*, 78, 51–54 (1988).

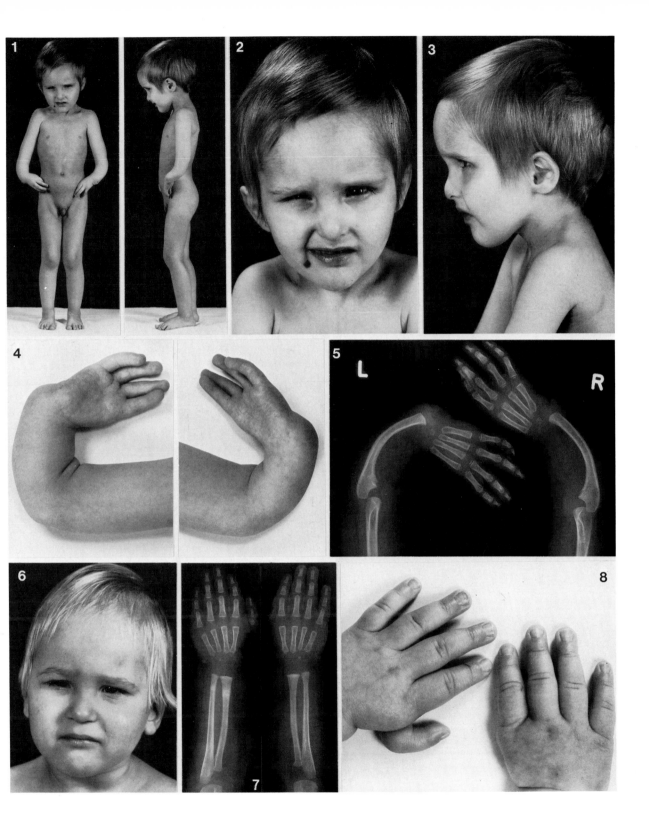

441

220. Acro-Renal Complex

A combination of acral and renal malformations of variable etiology.

Main signs:
1. Morphological anomalies of the radial rays: preaxial polydactyly, triphalangeal thumbs, mild to severe hypoplasia of the thumbs, syndactyly.
2. Malrotation of the kidneys, renal ectopia, ureteral anomalies, vesicoureteral reflux, diverticulum of the bladder.

Supplementary findings: In view of the various etiologies, eye anomalies, dysplasia of the pinnae, congenital deafness, facial weakness, cardiac defects, musculoskeletal anomalies, and many other anomalies may occur.

Manifestation: At birth. Disorders of renal function may occur later.

Etiology: Developmental field defect. Sporadic occurrence, not infrequently autosomal dominant. A complex of signs of at least 25 etiologically different congenital anomalies: e.g., Fanconi anemia, Sorsby syndrome, acro–renal–mandibular syndrome, acro–renal–ocular syndrome, etc. (see Temtamy–McKusick).

Frequency: The complex has only been diagnosed in numbers in the last few years.

Course, prognosis: Depends on the anomalies of the specific organs, e.g., of the kidneys.

Treatment: Symptomatic and in some cases surgical.

Differential diagnosis: Acro–renal–mandibular syndrome, acro–renal–ocular syndrome, Fanconi anemia, Sorsby syndrome, etc.

Illustrations:
1 An infant with hypospadias and bilateral vesicoureteral reflux, grade IV.
1a Bilaterally hypoplastic thumbs, absence of nail anlagen.
1b In addition, bilateral hypoplasia of the big toe.
2a, 2b The father of the child. Small, slender thumbs (compared with his large hands and fingers, and tall stature); short big toes with hypoplastic nails.

J.K.

References:
Halal, F., Homsy, M., Perreault, G. Acro–renal–ocular syndrome: autosomal dominant thumb hypoplasia, renal ectopia, and eye defect. *Am. J. Med. Genet.*, 17, 753–762 (1984).
Temtamy, S. and McKusick, V. The genetics of hand malformations. *Birth Defects*, XIV, 3, 171–172 (1984).

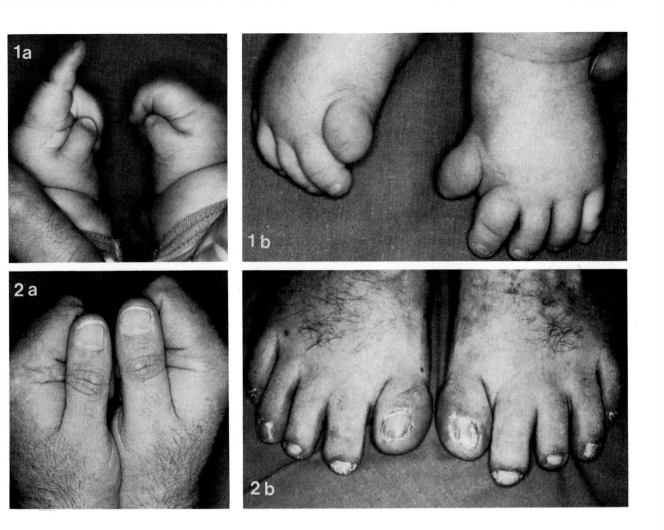

443

221. Fibrodysplasia Ossificans Progressiva

(Münchmeyer Syndrome, 'Myositis' Ossificans Progressiva)

A syndrome of congenital microdactyly of the big toes, also often of the thumbs, and—usually not until later—dysplastic connective-tissue swellings with subsequent ossification intra- and extramuscularly.

Main signs:
1. Congenital shortening and valgus position of the big toes (**8, 11, 12**) due to dysplasia of the first metatarsal; less often, analogous shortening of the thumbs (**5, 6, 9, 10**) and inward curving of the little finger (clinodactyly, **5, 6, 9**) or reduction defects of all fingers.
2. Soft-tissue swellings (occasionally with pain and fever), which may be noted perinatally, but usually appear during the first two years of life and on into the first decade; preferentially located in the occipito-nuchal region, neck, and shoulder girdle ('torticollis', **1, 2**). Risk of subsequent ossification. Intermittent progressive course with new episodes of ossification affecting further body and muscle regions in a craniocaudal direction and causing increasing limitation of motion (**3, 4**), in some cases on to almost complete mechanical 'freezing'.

Supplementary findings: Hearing impairment or deafness not infrequent. Possible mental retardation, loss of scalp hair, dental anomalies (frequent), and disorders of sexual maturation.

Etiology: Monogenic disorder, autosomal dominant with complete penetrance but variable expression. Most cases represent new mutations, often associated with above-average paternal age. Basic defect unknown.

Frequency: Not so very low. Up to 1958, over 300 cases reported in the literature; the great majority of subsequent observations have not come to publication.

Prognosis: In patients with the typical dysplastic connective-tissue swellings: subsequent progressive ectopic ossifications from infancy and early childhood are unfavorable for life expectancy; not infrequently, death before the end of the second decade of life from pulmonary disease or heart failure after the thorax has become immobile. After completion of the growth period, slowing or cessation of the ossification process.

Diagnosis, differential diagnosis: Soft-tissue swellings appearing in an individual with anomalies of the extremities should suggest the diagnosis and thus the avoidance of active procedures. Minor trauma can provoke new swelling and ossification. Thus, refrainment from incisions (for suspected inflammation) or biopsy (for suspected tumor).

Treatment: Although 'diphosphonate' (EHDP) administered during exacerbations seemed to limit further calcification and ossification in a few cases, this trial of therapy has also proved disappointing. Psychological guidance.

Illustrations:
1 and 2 A 2-year-old boy with an acute attack of occipito–nuchal–dorsal soft-tissue swelling with torticollis and marked limitation of movement—still without calcifications.
3 and 4 A 6½-year-old boy with typical stiff posture, numerous sites of ossification in the musculature of the back, bizarre, clasp-like new-bone formation on X-ray.
5 and 7 X-rays of the hands and feet of the child in 2.
6 and 9; 8 and 11 Hands and feet of the boy in 4.
10 and 12 Hands and feet of a 13-year-old girl with Münchmeyer syndrome.

H.-R.W./J.K.

References:

Becke, P.E. and v, Knorre, G. Myositis ossificans progressiva. *Ergeb. Inn. Med. Kinderheilkd. N.F.*, 27, 1 (1968).
Schnakenburg, K., Groß-Selbeck, G., Wiedemann, H.-R. Zur Behandlung der Fibrodysplasia ossificans progressiva mit 'Diphosphonat' (EHDP). *Dtsch. Med. Wochenschr.*, 97, 1873 (1972).
Azmy, A., Bensted, J.P.M., Eckstein, H.B. Myositis ossificans progressiva. *Z. Kinderchir.*, 26, 252 (1979).
Holmsen, H., Ljunghall, S., Hierton, T. Myositis ossificans progressiva. *Acta Orthop. Scand.*, 50, 33 (1979).
Connor, J.M. and Evans, D.A. Fibrodysplasia ossificans progressiva . . . 34 patients. *J. Bone Jt. Surg.*, 64-B, 76–83 (1982).
Connor, J.M. and Evans, D.A. Genetic aspects of fibrodysplasia ossificans progressiva. *J. Med. Genet.*, 19, 35–39 (1982).
Schulze-Solce, N. and Lanser, K. Fibrodysplasia ossificans progressiva. *Medwelt*, 1984, 407–410.
Lindhout, D., Golding, R.P. et al. Fibrodysplasia ossificans progressiva . . . *Pediatr. Radiol.*, 15, 211–213 (1985).
Carter, S.R., Davies, A.M., Evans, N. et al. Value of bone scanning . . . in fibrodysplasia ossificans progressiva. *Brit. J. Radiol.*, 62, 735: 269 (1989).

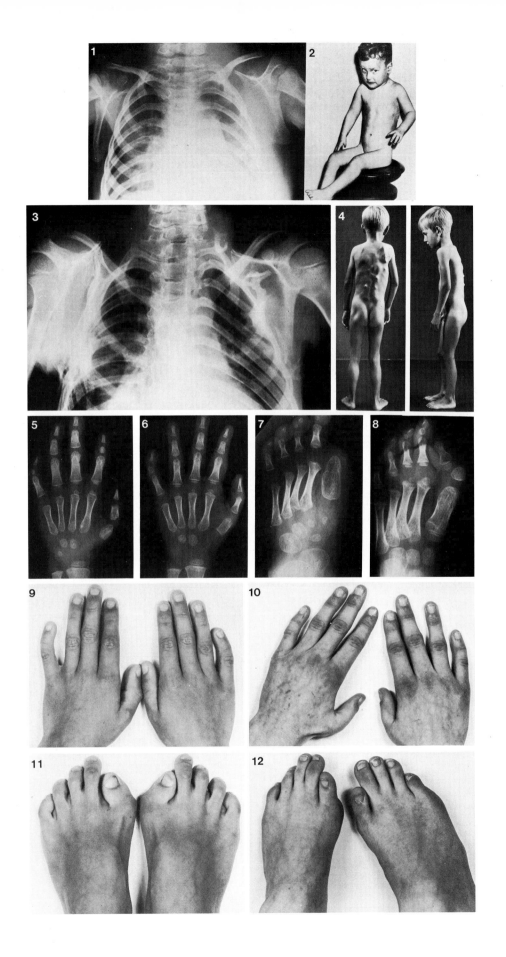

445

222. Rigid Spine Syndrome

A characteristic, slowly progressive syndrome with impaired flexion, stiffness, and hyperextension of the entire spinal column ('reverse Bekhterev'); decrease in subcutaneous fatty tissue; reduced muscle mass; and joint contractures.

Main signs:
1. Markedly limited flexion of the whole vertebral column with hyperextension of the cervical, thoracic, and lumbar regions ('reverse Bekhterev'), contracture of the extensor muscles.
2. Generalized muscular hypotonia and weakness, permanently elevated shoulders, decrease of muscle mass.
3. Decrease of adipose tissue.

Supplementary findings: Not consistent. Depending on the etiology: absent or normal tendon reflexes; decreased nerve conduction velocity and normal biochemistry in some cases, but pathologic electromyogram and elevated creatine kinase in other cases; possible cardiomyopathy with sudden death, but normal cardiac findings also possible; different muscle biopsy findings with normal structure, or muscle fiber type 1 or 2 atrophy with or without connective tissue changes.

Manifestation: From birth on into adulthood, peak between the second and twelfth years of life.

Etiology: Genetic heterogeneity: X-linked recessive (the most frequent), autosomal recessive, and autosomal dominant inheritance have all been observed, but also sporadic cases (cf. also under Differential diagnosis).

Frequency: Low; about 50 patients have been described.

Prognosis, course: Depending on etiology, minimal, slow, or rapid progression with sudden cardiac death in all age groups.

Differential diagnosis:
1. X-linked recessive benign Emery–Dreifuss muscular dystrophy (also called Cestan–LeJonne disease).
2. Scapuloperoneal atrophies and myopathies.
3. Mitochondrial myopathies.
4. Congenital muscular dystrophies; Fukuyama muscular dystrophy.
5. Autosomal dominant fibrodysplasia ossificans progressiva.
6. Hypertrophic cardiomyopathy in children of diabetic mothers, Pompe glycogen storage disease, Friedreich ataxia.

Treatment: Symptomatic. Surgical intervention for joint contractures; physiotherapy. Cardiac pacemaker, e.g., for Emery–Dreifuss muscular dystrophy.

Illustrations:
1a–1c, 2a–2c Young men with shoulders permanently elevated in the typical manner, hyperextension in the cervical, thoracic, and lumbar regions ('reverse Bekhterev').

J.K.

References:
Colver, A.F., Steer, C.R., Godman, M.J. et al. Rigid spine syndrome and fatal cardiomyopathy. *Arch. Dis. Child.*, 56, 148–151 (1981).
Echenne, B., Astruc, J., Brunel, D. et al. Congenital muscular dystrophy and rigid spine syndrome. *Neuropediatrics*, 14, 97–101 (1983).
Pavonne, L., Gullotta, F., La Rosa, M. et al. Rigid spine syndrome. Some evidence of varying pathological patterns. *Helv. Pediatr. Acta*, 38, 367–372 (1983).
Rowland, L.P. and Layzer, R.B. Emery–Dreifuss muscular dystrophy. In: Vinkin, P.J. and Bruyn, G.W. (eds.) Handbook for Clinical Neurology, vol. 40. *Disease of muscle*, part I. North-Holland Publishing Co., Amsterdam, New York, Oxford, pp.389–392 (1979).
Hanefeld, F., von Maltzan, V., Stoltenburg, G. Mitochondriale Myopathie bei Rigid-Spine-Syndrom. *Monatschr. Kinderheilkd.*, 130, 648 (1982).

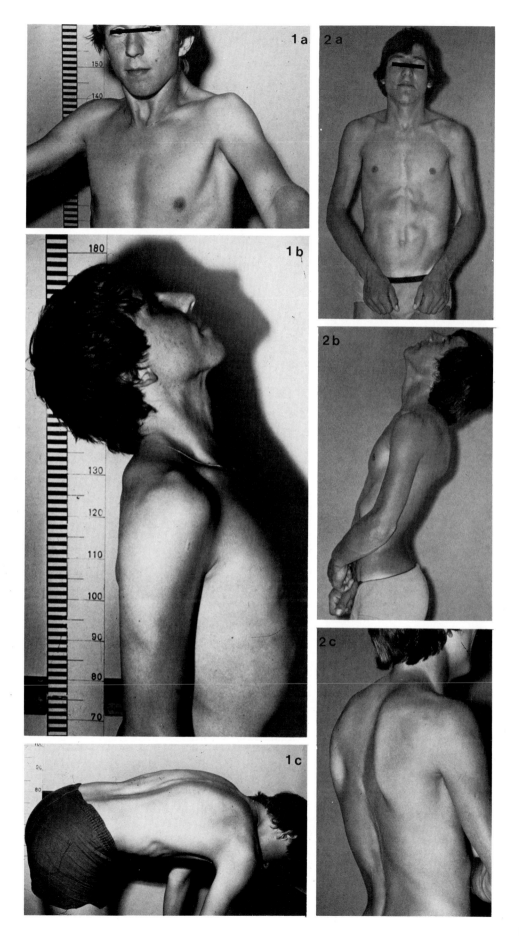

223. Nail–Patella Syndrome

(Nail–Patella–Elbow Syndrome with Iliac Horns, Osteo–Onycho Dysplasia, [Österreicher–] Turner–Kieser Syndrome)

A characteristic syndrome particularly of skeletal anomalies, dysplasia of nails, and frequently renal disease.

Main signs:
1. Hypo- and dysplasia of the nails (softness, discoloration, longitudinal ridging, abnormal splitting), preferentially involving the thumb and index fingers (**1, 2**).
2. Hypoplasia of the patellae (**5**) with frequent lateral dislocation; occasionally aplasia.
3. Hypoplasia of the radial head with frequent dorsal dislocation and impaired mobility (**6**).
4. 'Iliac horns' (symmetrically located pyramidal outgrowths of the dorsal surfaces of the iliac wings [**4**]—usually readily palpable, or seen on X-ray or CT scan).

Supplementary findings: Hypoplasia of the scapulae; radiologically, hypoplasia of the lateral femoral condyle, coxa valga, and other findings.

Poorly defined, darkly pigmented pupillary margin of the iris.

Proteinuria/nephropathy in some cases, not infrequently beginning in childhood.

Possible development of cords or webbing over the elbow joints (**3**); also muscle aplasias.

Manifestation: Although diagnosis is possible in the newborn, the child usually first comes to attention because of difficulties in walking, related to the patellar abnormality.

Etiology: Monogenic disorder, autosomal dominant, with considerably variable expressivity. Gene localized to the distal long arm of chromosome 9, linked to the ABO blood group locus.

Frequency: Not particularly low. Well over 500 cases in the literature; estimation (1965) of 22 carriers of the trait in 1 million of the general population.

Prognosis: Dependent on the development and course of renal disease, which occurs in over 50% of cases (unusual slowly progressive nephropathy, with unfavorable outcome in at least 10%).

For a patient with nail-patella syndrome and nephropathy, the risk for nephropathy in a child is about 1:4.

Treatment: Orthopedic care; renal follow-up. Genetic counseling.

Illustrations:
1–6 A 14-year-old affected boy with nephropathy.
1 and 2 Dysplasia of the nails (fingers > > toes).
3 Firm 'web' formation at both elbow joints.
4 Iliac horns.
5 Patellar hypoplasia; angular appearance of the flexed knees.
6 Elbow joint with distinct dorsal dislocation of the radial head.

H.-R.W./J.K.

References:

Caliebe, M.-R., Rohwedder, H.-J., Wiedemann, H.-R. Über das Mißbildungs-Erbsyndrom Osteo-Onycho-Dysplasie mit Nierenbeteiligung. *Arch. Kinderheilkd.*, 169, 149 (1963).

Spranger, J.W., Langer, L.O., Jr., Wiedemann, H.-R. *Bone Dysplasias. An Atlas of Constitutional Disorders of Skeletal Development.* G. Fischer and W.B. Saunders, Stuttgart and Philadelphia, 1974.

Sabnis, S.G., Antonovych, T.T. et al. Nail–patella syndrome. *Clin. Nephrol.*, 14, 148–153 (1980).

Reed, D. and Nichols, D.M. Computed tomography of 'iliac horns' in hereditary osteo-onychodysplasia... *Pediatr. Radiol.*, 17, 168–169 (1987).

Looij, B.J., Teslaa, B.L. et al. Genetic counseling in... nail–patella syndrome with nephropathy. *J. Med. Genet.*, 25, 682–686 (1988).

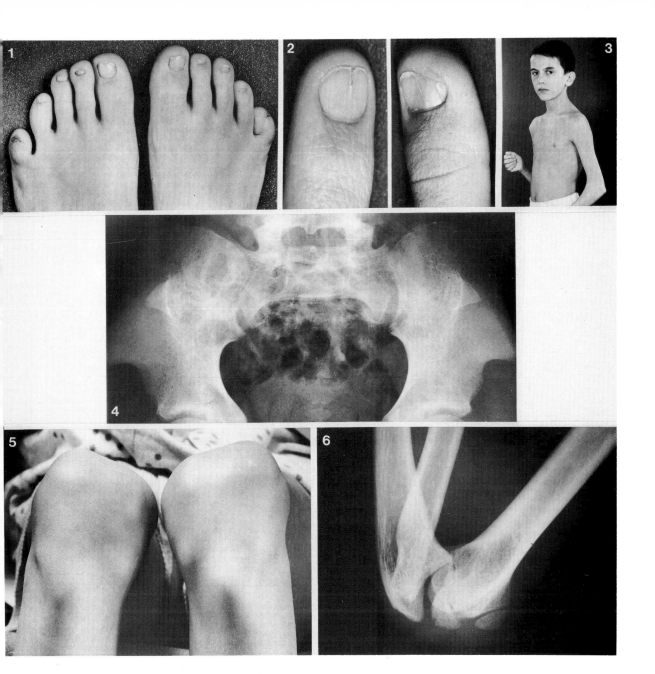

449

224. Hydantoin–Barbiturate Embryopathy

(Embryofetal Hydantoin Syndrome, Phenytoin Syndrome)

A syndrome of mostly minor malformations regarded as being due to antiepileptic medication with hydantoin, phenobarbital, or carbamazepine.

Main signs:
1. Hypoplasia of the distal phalanges of the fingers; shortening of the distal phalanges and hypo- to aplasia of the nails (5, 6). Possible simian creases.
2. Facial dysmorphism, mainly involving the midface: short, broad nose with anteverted nostrils; broad, low nasal root; hypertelorism; possible epicanthic folds; low-set, poorly modeled ears (1–4).
3. Treatment of the child's mother with anticonvulsant medication in early pregnancy (hydantoin and/or phenobarbital or carbamazepine).

Supplementary findings:
1. Not infrequently, pre- and postnatal growth retardation—but with compensation possible.
2. Major malformations also possible: for example cardiac defects.
3. Possible psychomotor retardation.

Comment: Independent of anticonvulsant medication, children of epileptic mothers have a higher risk of major malformations, primarily cleft lip or palate, and cardiac anomaly.

Manifestation: At birth.

Frequency: Not particularly low.

Illustrations:
1–6 A series of typically affected children of various ages.

H.-R.W.

References:
Dieterich, E. Antiepileptika-Embryopathien. *Ergeb. Inn. Med. Kinderheilkd. N.F.*, 43, 93 (1979).
Dieterich, E., Lukas, A., Steveling, A. et al. Art und Ausmaß von Fehlbildungen bzw. Fehlbildungsmustern bei Kindern antiepileptisch behandelter Väter und Mütter. In: Doose, H. et al. (eds.) *Epilepsie 1979*. Thieme, Stuttgart and New York, 1980 (p.47).
Van Dyke, D.C., Hodge, S. et al. Family studies in fetal phenytoin exposure. *J. Pediatr.*, 113, 301–306 (1988).
Karpathios, T., Zervoudakis, A., Venieris, F. et al. Genetics and fetal hydantoin syndrome. *Acta Pediatr. Scand.*, 78, 125–126 (1989).
Jones, K.L., Lacro, R.V., Johnson, K.A., Adams, J. Pattern of malformations in the children of women treated with carbamazepine during pregnancy. *N. Engl. J. Med.*, 320, 1661–1666 (1989).

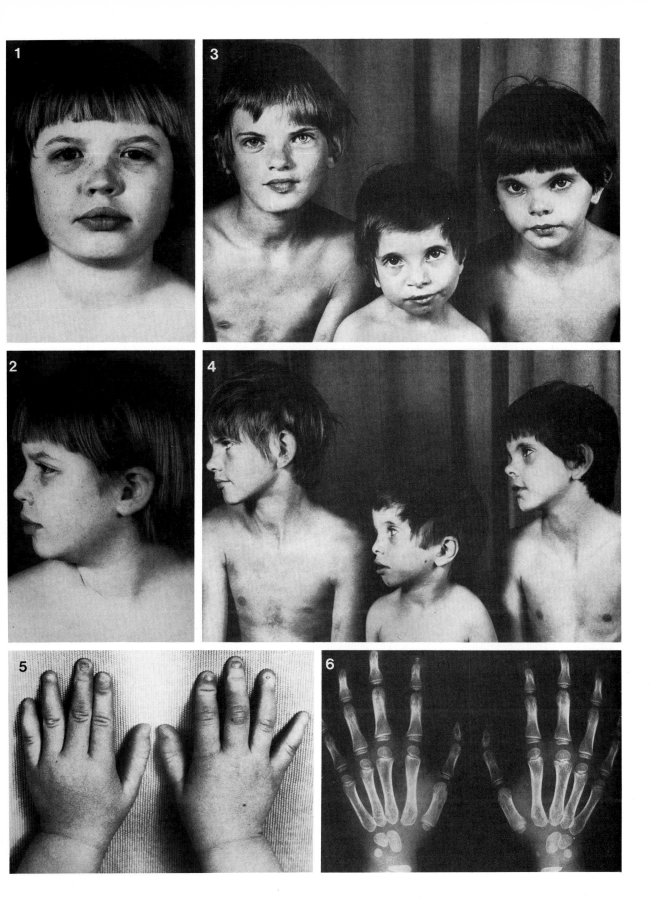

451

225. Fetal Valproic Acid Syndrome

(Fetal Valproate Syndrome, Valproic Acid Embryopathy)

A syndrome of characteristic craniofacial abnormalities, frequent developmental delay, and in some cases, serious malformations after valproate treatment of the mother in the first trimester of pregnancy.

Main signs:

1. Facial phenotype: metopic ridge, prominent glabella, or trigonocephaly due to early closure of the metopic suture. Unusually narrow forehead, poorly developed outer orbital ridges. Hypoplasia of the midface. Epicanthic folds. Short pug nose with broad or flat root. Long and/or flat philtrum and long, narrow upper lip. Small mouth. Retrognathia. Slight deformity of the external ears in some cases.

2. Developmental retardation, usually mild to moderate, or neurological abnormalities in (as far as can be judged at present) over half of the children.

3. Possible lumbrosacral spina bifida aperta (myelomeningo- or meningocele); club feet. Long fingers and toes.

4. Valproate treatment of the child's mother in the first trimester of pregnancy.

Supplementary findings:

1. Frequent hyperexcitability in the early postnatal period as part of a withdrawal syndrome (especially pronounced when the mother required additional anticonvulsants). Possible hypotonia, delayed motor and, not infrequently, speech development.

2. Possible cardiac or urogenital anomalies (e.g., hypospadias, cryptorchidism), hernias, and peculiarities of the hands and feet, or fingers and toes.

3. Combinations of valproic acid with other anticonvulsant treatment of an expectant mother may lead to further defects—microcephaly, postnatal growth delay, and others.

Manifestation: At birth and later.

Etiology: Valproate treatment of the expectant mother, especially in the first trimester.

Frequency: Not particularly low.

Course, prognosis: Dependent on the extent of expression of the syndrome (e.g., myelocele).

Diagnosis, differential diagnosis: Despite many similar features, the syndrome differs from hydantoin–barbiturate embryopathy (p.450).

Treatment: As indicated: symptomatic. Prenatal diagnosis using amniocentesis and ultrasonography, especially of the lower vertebral column.

Illustrations:

1 and 2 The fairly characteristic facies of an infant with fetal valproate acid syndrome: narrow prominent forehead, slight mongoloid slant of the palpebral fissures, epicanthic folds, short pug nose with low root, flat bridge, long flat philtrum, thin upper lip, and retrognathia.

H.-R.W.

References:

Di Liberti, J.H., Farndon, P.A., Dennis, N.R. et al. The fetal valproate syndrome. *Am. J. Med. Genet.*, 19, 473–481 (1984).

Jäger-Roman, E., Deichl, A., Jakob, S. et al. Fetal growth, major malformations, and minor anomalies in infants born to mothers receiving valproic acid. *J. Pediatr.*, 108, 997–1004 (1986).

Winter, R.M., Donnai, D., Burn, J. et al. Fetal valproate syndrome: is there a recognisable phenotype? *J. Med. Genet.*, 24, 692–695 (1987).

Ardinger, H.A., Atkin, J.F., Blackston, R.D. et al. Verification of the fetal valproate syndrome phenotype. *Am. J. Med. Genet.*, 29, 171–185 (1988).

Chitayat, S., Farrell, K. et al. Congenital abnormalities in two sibs exposed to valproic acid in utero. *Am. J. Med. Genet.*, 31, 369–373 (1988).

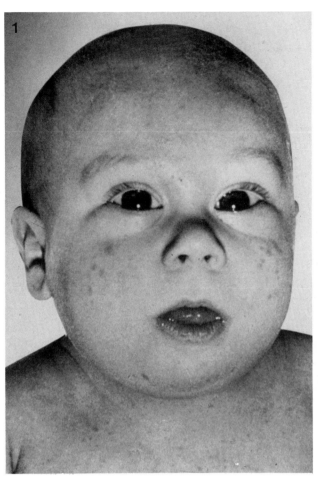
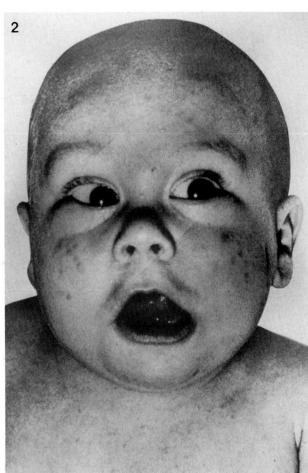

226. Dyskeratosis Congenita

(Zinsser–Cole–Engman Syndrome)

A hereditary disorder of poikiloderma, nail dystrophy, leukoplakia, and possibly pancytopenia.

Main signs:
1. *Skin:* Formation of subepidermal blisters (clinically usually not very prominent), reticular hyper- and depigmentation, atrophy, and telangiectasia, which result in a 'mottled skin' appearance (poikiloderma) (1).
2. *Mucous membranes* (especially those bordering on the external integument): blisters, ulcers, scars, stenoses and strictures, and also hyperkeratoses and leukoplakia or leukokeratoses (3).
3. *Nails:* Dystrophic (longitudinal ridges, splitting, shortness, atrophy) (2, 4–6).
4. *Eyes:* Blepharitis, lacrimal conjunctivitis with obliteration of the lacrimal puncta and disturbance of the flow of tears; possible ectropion and loss of eyelashes.

Supplementary findings: Development of pancytopenia (panmyelophthisis) in about 50% of cases.

'Connective tissue weakness' with hyperextensible joints (2), tendency to hernias, etc. Sparse, thin hair growth or alopecia. Dental anomalies.

Manifestation: Usually between the third and tenth years of life (pancytopenia usually develops during the second or third decade).

Etiology: Hereditary disorder; definite preponderance of males. Autosomal recessive, X-linked recessive, and also, in isolated cases, autosomal dominant transmission reported. Basic defect unknown.

Frequency: Low; up to 1980 only 60 cases described.

Course, prognosis: Shortened life expectancy for patients with pancytopenia, and from possible malignant transformation of precancerous hyperkeratoses of the mucous membranes.

Diagnosis: Apart from the facial poikiloderma, the lacrimal conjunctivitis and nail changes are the most important signs. Differentiate from Franconi anemia.

Treatment: Symptomatic. Close hematological and oncological follow-up; excision of leukoplakia patches. Genetic counseling.

Illustrations:
1, 3, 5, and 6 A 10-year-old affected boy. Hyperpigmentation of the lower eyelids, reticular hyperpigmentation paranasally; lacrimal conjunctivitis, blepharitis, obliteration of the lacrimal puncta. Pancytopenia.
2 and 4 A 13-year-old boy.

H.-R.W./J.K.

References:

Reich, H. Zinsser–Cole–Engman-Syndrom. *Med. Klin.*, 68, 283 (1973).
Trowbridge, A.A., Sirinavin, C.H., Linman, J.W. Dyskeratosis congenita: Hematologic evaluation of a sibship and review of the literature. *Am. J. Hematol.*, 3, 143 (1977).
Rodermund, O.E., Hausmann, G., Hausmann, D. Zinsser–Cole–Engman-Syndrom. *Z. Hautkr.*, 54, 273 (1979).
De Boeck, K., Degreef, H., Verwilghen, R. et al. Thrombocytopenia: first symptom in a patient with dyskeratosis congenita. *Pediatrics*, 67, 898 (1981).
Kelly, T.E. and Stelling, C.B. Dyskeratosis congenita: radiologic features. *Pediatr. Radiol.*, 12, 31 (1982).
Womer, R., Clark, J.E. et al. Dyskeratosis congenita: two examples of this multisystem disorder. *Pediatrics*, 71, 603–607 (1983).
Shashidhar Pai, G., Morgan, S., Whetsell, C. Etiologic heterogeneity in dyskeratosis congenita. *Am. J. Med. Genet.*, 32, 63–66 (1989).

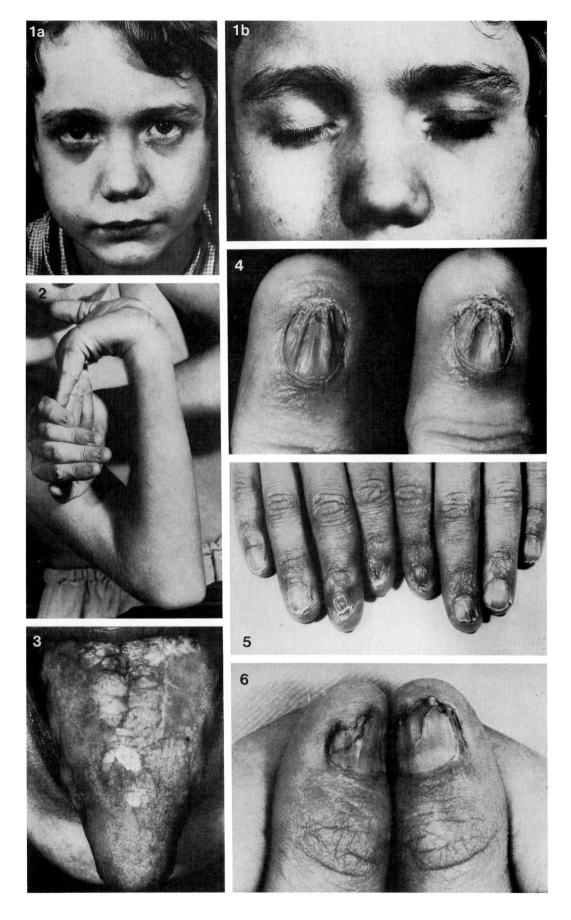

227. Hypohidrotic Ectodermal Dysplasia

A highly characteristic hereditary disorder of 'anhidrosis' with the danger of recurrent hyperthermia, hypotrichosis, hypo- or anodontia, and typical facies.

Main signs:
1. Characteristic facies with bulging forehead, prominent supraorbital ridges, hypertelorism, low nasal root and short nose with hypoplastic alae nasi, maxillary hypoplasia, full pouting lips, prognathism, and possible prominent ears pointed at the top ('satyr ears') (1, 2, 6).
2. Sparse, light scalp hair; short, fine, and dry. Eyebrows and eyelashes absent or extremely sparse. Fine wrinkling of the periocular and sometimes perioral skin, often heavily pigmented (1–4). Premature baldness.
3. Alveolar ridges almost absent, with anodontia or hypodontia (5).
4. Skin is hypoplastic, translucent, soft and very dry, almost no sweat formation. Possible papular changes on the face and axillae; frequent depigmentation of the nuchal and genital regions. Possible hyperkeratosis of the palms and soles. No lanugo hair in the neonate. Later, little or no body hair.
5. Rise in body temperature even with minimal physical exertion (especially in early childhood and infancy) or increased environmental temperature; heat intolerance; failure to thrive.

Supplementary findings: Dry, sensitive mucous membranes with tendency to atrophy. Possible deficiency of tears, conjunctivitis. Frequent photophobia. Tendency to chronic atrophic rhinitis. Possible hyposmia; hoarseness. Not infrequently, eczema. Possible mild dystrophy of the nails. Possible hypo- or aplasia of the mamillary glands and/or nipples.

Mental retardation in some cases, presumably as the result of cerebral damage from repeated severe hyperthermia. Possible sensorineural hearing impairment.

On biopsy, hypo- or aplasia of the exocrine sweat glands and sebaceous glands of the skin and hypoplasia to absence of mucous glands in the mucous membranes.

Manifestation: At birth.

Etiology: Hereditary disorder. Heterogeneity. X-linked recessive type most common: males affected; in females only minor features (see below); identification of female carriers important. Autosomal recessive type far less common.

Frequency: About 1:100,000 newborns; hundreds of cases in the literature.

Course, prognosis: Initially, survival or cerebral function endangered by episodes of hyperthermia. Mortality in childhood about 30%. In adults, life expectancy and functioning usually no longer appreciably affected.

Diagnosis: Ectodermal dysplasia should be ruled out in all cases of unexplained fever in small infants, even when other signs are minimal. Caution with sweat tests in suspected cases. Female carriers of the X-linked recessive form may show only mild dental dysplasia, decreased ability to sweat (regional aplasia of sweat glands; linear distribution of hypohidrotic areas along the V-shaped lines of Blaschko over the back), minimal breast development.

Differential diagnosis: Other ectodermal dysplasia syndromes.

Treatment: Immediate cooling for hyperthermia; prevention of convulsions/brain damage. Protection against overheating and sunstroke; possible move to cooler climate. Eyedrops may be required. Otological care. Dentures, possibly from early childhood. A wig may be indicated. Skin care. Genetic counseling.

Illustrations:
1 Infant with hypotrichosis, 'satyr ears', prominent forehead, fine creases in eyelids, full lips. Deficient tears; rhinitis sicca; dysphonia and hoarseness. Aplasia of the dental germs. Dry scaly skin. History of life-threatening episodes of hyperthermia.
2–6 A 2-year-old cousin of the patient in 1, also with the full clinical picture. Hypoplastic nipples. Skin biopsy showed aplasia of sweat and sebaceous glands.

H.-R.W./J.K.

References:

Freire-Maia, N. and Pinheiro, M. *Ectodermal dysplasias: a clinical and genetic study.* Alan Liss, New York, 1984.

Happle, R. and Frosch, P.J. Manifestation of the lines of Blaschko in women heterozygous for X-linked hypohidrotic ectodermal dysplasia. *Clin. Genet.*, 27, 468–471 (1985).

Zonana, J., Clarke, A. et al. X-linked hypohidrotic ectodermal dysplasia: localization within the region Xq11-21.1 by linkage analysis and implications for carrier detection and prenatal diagnosis. *Am. J. Hum. Genet.*, 43, 75–85 (1988).

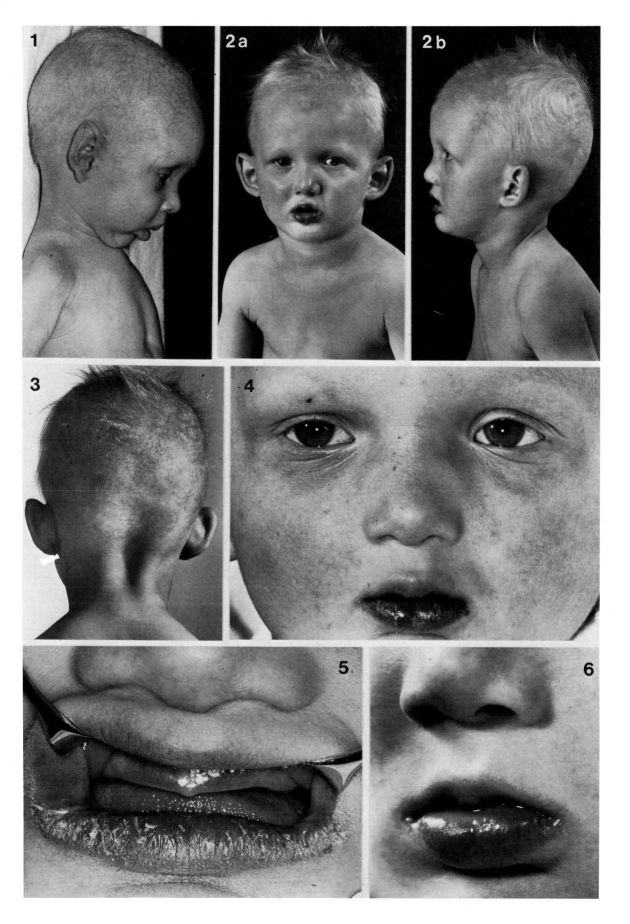

228. Ectodermal Dysplasia with Hair Anomalies and Syndactyly

A syndrome of hypotrichosis with pili torti, dental hypoplasia, ichthyosiform skin changes, and cutaneous syndactyly of the hands and feet.

Main signs:

1. Hypotrichosis of the scalp, eyebrows, and eyelashes (1, 4–9). Helical twisting of the hair (pili torti).
2. Generalized dryness of the skin, with hyperkeratosis especially on the lower trunk, lower extremities, palms, and soles, with sparing of the axillae and elbows (10c, 10d).
3. Variable cutaneous syndactyly of various grades on the hands (III/IV > II/III; 10a–10d, 12) and feet (II/III > III/IV; 11a–11c).
4. Marked hypoplasia of the crowns of the teeth with normal number of teeth and dental germs. (Slight delay in loss of milk teeth and eruption of permanent dentitions and atypical order of eruption.) Hyperlordosis.

Supplementary findings: No hyperthermia. A dermatological sweat test (using 1,4-dehydroxy anthrachinon powder and an electric cradle) is positive (axillae, elbows, soles of the feet, anterior sweat grooves, anogenital area, thighs, popliteal areas).

Thickening and yellow discoloration of some of the toenails.

Bilateral simian creases.

Absence of hypertelorism, of low nasal root and short nose, of full lips, of periocular or perioral wrinkling of the skin, and of 'satyr' (pointed) ears.

High palate, normal alveolar processes. Unremarkable mucous membranes.

Very fine lens opacities on ophthalmoscopic examination. No photophobia. Slight hyperopia.

Normal mental development. Normal audiometric results. Normal height and skeletal maturity. Normally formed nipples.

Unusual familial resemblance of the affected persons.

Manifestation: At birth.

Etiology: Hereditary disorder; probably autosomal recessive transmission as a result of close parental consanguinity.

Frequency: Unknown; presumably low.

Course, prognosis: Favorable.

Differential diagnosis: Other ectodermal dysplasias (a great variety of types described in the literature).

Treatment: Dental care. A wig may be indicated for both cosmetic and psychological reasons. Genetic counseling.

Illustrations:

1–12 Three siblings aged 12, 6, and 3 years (two other siblings healthy). Pili torti; other parts of hair smooth or wavy; hair mostly white-blond, fine and soft, other parts darker, stronger, and firm; very variable length due to easy breakage. Eyebrows merely suggested; very scanty eyelashes. Bilateral simian creases in all three children.

Patient 1 (1, 2, 4, 7, 10a, 11c) shows additionally a blind fistula below the tragus of each ear. On ophthalmological examination, very tiny peripheral punctate lens opacities.

Patient 2 (3, 5, 8, 10b, 10c, 11b) has had surgical correction of syndactyly of the left hand. Ophthalmologically, small subcapsular opacities of the right lens at the dorsal pole.

Patient 3 (3, 6, 9, 10d, 11a, 12) was allegedly 'hairless' at birth. Both hands surgically corrected for syndactyly.

H.-R.W.

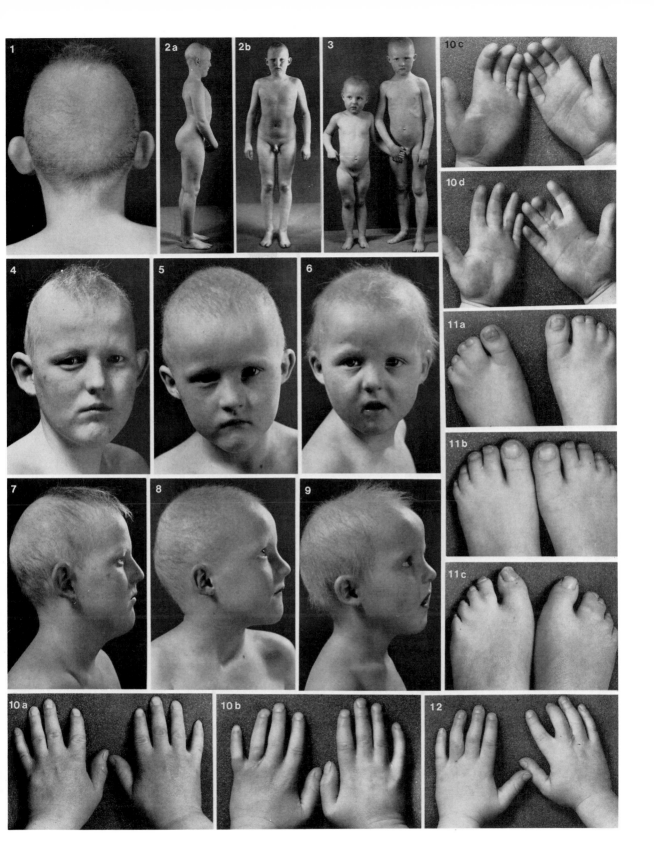

459

229. Lymphedema–Distichiasis Syndrome

A hereditary disorder of late-onset lymphedema of the lower extremities combined with double rows of eyelashes on the eyelids (distichiasis) and other anomalies.

Main signs:
1. Lymphedema of the legs (2), especially from the knees downward, in males also possibly with considerable scrotal swelling.
2. Double rows of eyelashes on the upper and lower lids (3).

Supplementary findings: Ectropion of the lower lids; uni- or bilateral ptosis; webbed neck (1); dilatation of the spinal canal; formation of arachnoidal and extradural spinal cysts, in some cases with neurological signs; and diverse anomalies of the vertebral column have been repeatedly observed.

Manifestation: Lymphedema usually present from the second half of the first decade of life, but possibly not until the second decade or later. One side may be affected many years before the other.

Etiology: Autosomal dominant disorder with incomplete penetrance and variable expression.

Frequency: Low; about 85 cases reported up to 1980.

Course, prognosis: For the most part dependent on the extent and severity of edema and on development of spinal column complications.

Differential diagnosis: Other forms of late-onset lymphedema, Meige type.

Treatment: Symptomatic. Removal of annoying lid hair (irritating the conjunctiva or even cornea). Surgical treatment of edematous regions not very successful. Genetic counseling.

Illustrations:
1 and 2 A 31-year-old woman, 1.60 m tall, with extensive edema of the lower legs: of the right, since age 13 years; of the left, increasing since her third pregnancy. Double rows of eyelashes on all four eyelids; ptosis of the right upper eyelid. A dysplastic left auricle and neck webbing have been surgically corrected. Aneurysm of the ascending aorta, tilted kidneys. Two sons of the proband, aged 11 and 9½ years, also show distichiasis; no edema to date. Further affected persons in the family.
3 The lower lid of one of the sons: double row of lashes, some have been removed.

H.-R.W.

References:

Holmes, L.G., Fields, J.P., Zabriskie, J.B. Hereditary late-onset lymphedema. *Pediatrics*, 61, 575 (1978).
Fuhrmann-Rieger, A. Familiäres Distichiasis-Lymphödem-Syndrom. In: Tolksdorf, M. and Spranger, J. (eds.) *Klinische Genetik in der Pädiatrie.* I. Symposium in Kiel. Thieme, Stuttgart, 1979.
Schwartz, J.F., O'Brien, M.S., Hoffmann, J.C., Jr. Hereditary spinal arachnoid cysts, distichiasis, and lymphedema. *Ann. Neurol.,* 7, 340 (1980).
Pap, Z., Biró, T. et al. Syndrome of lymphoedema and distichiasis. *Hum. Genet.,* 53, 309–310 (1980).
Dale, R.F. Primary lymphoedema when found with distichiasis of the type defined as bilateral hyperplasia by lymphography. *J. Med. Genet.,* 24, 170–171 (1987).

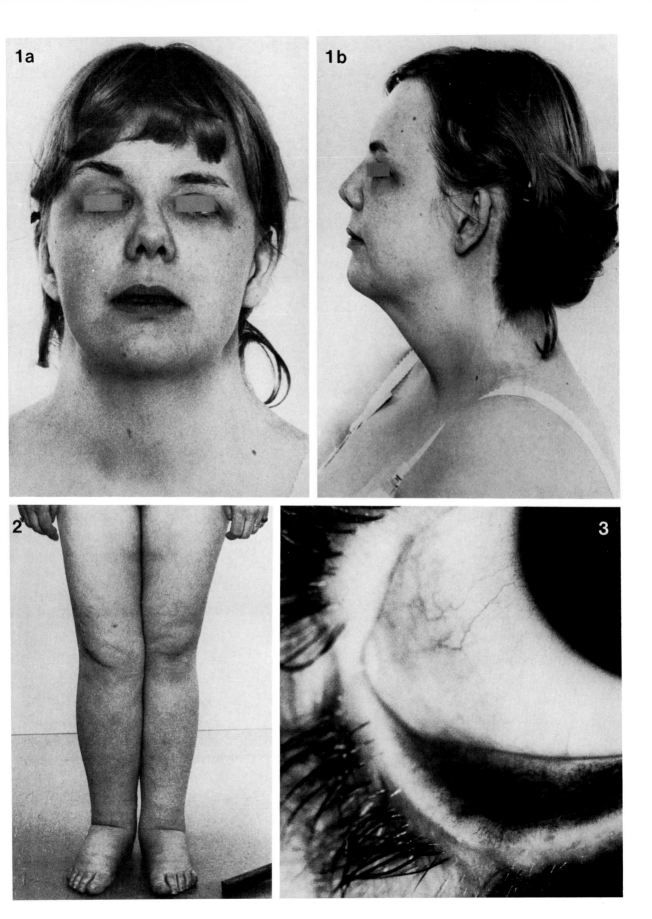

230. Acrodermatitis Enteropathica

A hereditary disorder, frequently with an intermittent course, of peri-orificial and acral skin changes, alopecia, and diarrhea, due to a disorder of zinc metabolism.

Main signs:
1. A distinctive skin disorder usually with initial vesicobullous eruptions, which later become dry-crusted and scaly-lamellar (to psoriatic), at first distributed in symmetrical groups around the body orifices (especially the anogenital region) and eyes (1), then the back of the head and neck, elbows, knees, hands, and feet. Nails and interdigital spaces between the fingers and toes are often significantly involved (3, 4). Frequent secondary bacterial or parasitic infections.
2. Alopecia (possibly even total loss of scalp hair, eyebrows, and eyelashes) (1).
3. Possible diarrhea (various grades of severity).

Supplementary findings: In addition to failure to thrive, poor growth, and severe psychological problems: frequent secondary glossitis (2) and stomatitis, conjunctivitis, blepharitis, and photophobia (1) as well as severe nail dystrophies (3b) and even loss of nails.

Increased susceptibility to infections.

Low serum and urinary zinc levels (and low serum alkaline phosphatase).

Manifestation: Usually presents during the first year of life; often after weaning from breast milk; occasionally not until later.

Etiology: Autosomal recessive disorder (disorder of zinc metabolism with zinc malabsorption, and its sequelae).

Frequency: Low.

Course, prognosis: Without therapy, intermittent but relentlessly progressive course usually leading to early death. With adequate treatment, usually normal life expectancy.

Treatment: Oral zinc substitution (usually with zinc sulfate) brings about dramatic improvement and healing of all lesions within a few weeks. Follow-up and specific treatment, if necessary, of accompanying secondary infections. Genetic counseling.

Illustrations:
1 and 3 An 8-year-old boy with the fully developed clinical picture.
2, 3b, 4 A 3-year-old girl.

H.-R.W.

References:

Lombeck, I., Schnippering, H.G., Kasperek, K. et al. Akrodermatitis enteropathica—eine Zinkstoffwechselstörungmit Zinkmalabsorption. *Z. Kinderheilkd.*, 120, 181 (1975).
Chandra, R.K. Acrodermatitis enteropathica: zinc levels and cell-mediated immunity. *Pediatrics*, 66, 789 (1980).
Brenton, D.P., Jackson, M.J. et al. Two pregnancies in a patient with acrodermatitis enteropathica treated with zinc sulphate. *Lancet*, II, 500–502 (1981).
Gordon, E.F., Gordon, R.C. et al. Zinc metabolism: basic, clinical, and behavioral aspects. *J. Pediatr.*, 99, 341–349 (1981).
Ohlsson, A. Acrodermatitis enteropathica: reversibility of cerebral atrophy with zinc therapy. *Acta Pediatr. Scand.*, 70, 269–273 (1981).

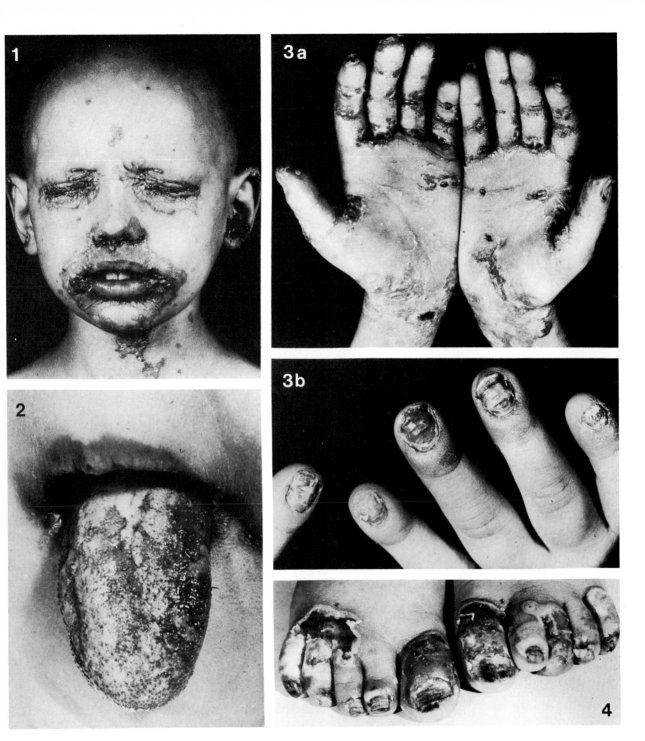

463

231. Ichthyosis Congenita

('Fish Skin' Disease)

Ichthyosis congenita is a heterogeneous group of diseases with at least six different genotypes.

Main signs:
Depending on the genotype, considerable clinical variability but usually marked intrafamilial constancy, the clinical picture being dominated either by a markedly inflammatory component ('erythrodermie congénitale ichthyosiforme séche') or by dry scaling ('lamellar ichthyosis'). Particular involvement of flexion surfaces and the trunk. Newborns usually come into the world as 'collodion' babies: the children are enveloped by a taut membrane with the appearance of oiled parchment or collodion. Frequent ectropion of the eyelids; the ears are flattened, the mouth is fixed in an 'O' shape. Hair may be absent or may perforate the stratum corneum. Shortly after birth, desquamation begins in large sheet-like patches. Complete desquamation takes several weeks. Occasionally, fingers and toes are 'encased' in a fixed position.

Manifestation: At birth.

Etiology: All six clinical types of ichthyosis congenita are probably inherited as autosomal recessive traits.

Frequency: Gene frequencies of 1:20,000 are given.

Course, prognosis: Dependent on the type. Ichthyosis congenita gravis (Riecke type I, 'harlequin fetus', see p.466) is lethal. Ichthyosis congenita Riecke type II takes many forms, and thus a variable course. Lamellar ichthyosis may occasionally be limited to the newborn period and clear completely after desquamation. Further subtypes are the Sjögren–Larsson syndrome, the Rud syndrome, ichthyosis linearis circumflexa Comel, and the Netherton syndrome.

Differential diagnosis: Ichthyosis vulgaris (three subtypes) and ichthyosis hystrix (at least three subtypes).

Treatment: High humidity in an incubator, a non-occlusive lubricant (oil). Skin care after desquamation with salicyl vaseline or retinoic acid cream. Special attention to skin infections during desquamation. Later a maritime climate is favorable. A hot climate helps improve the rash. Genetic counseling. Prenatal diagnosis with electron microscopy after fetal skin biopsy.

Illustrations:
1a–1c A 4-day-old boy. 'Collodion baby' with a taut shiny skin 'armor'; desquamation in process.
2 A 5-day-old girl, sister of the patient in 1; identical picture.
3 A further 'collodion child'. **3a**, at 10 days; **3b**, at 3 weeks with sheet-like desquamation.
4a and 4b A brother of the child in 3, at age 2 days: O-shaped mouth; fingers and toes firmly enclosed by a shiny layer of skin; deep cracks in the sheets of skin on the trunk.
5a and 5b A further patient. Fingers and toes enveloped in an armor-like covering.

J.K.

References:
Anton-Lamprecht, I. Hereditäre Icthyosen. In: Herzberg, J.J. and Korting, G.W. (eds.) *Pädiatrische Dermatologie*. Schattauer, Stuttgart, 1978, (pp.161–182).
Anton-Lamprecht, I. Prenatal diagnosis of genetic disorders of the skin by means of electron microscopy. *Hum. Genet.*, 59, 392–405 (1981).

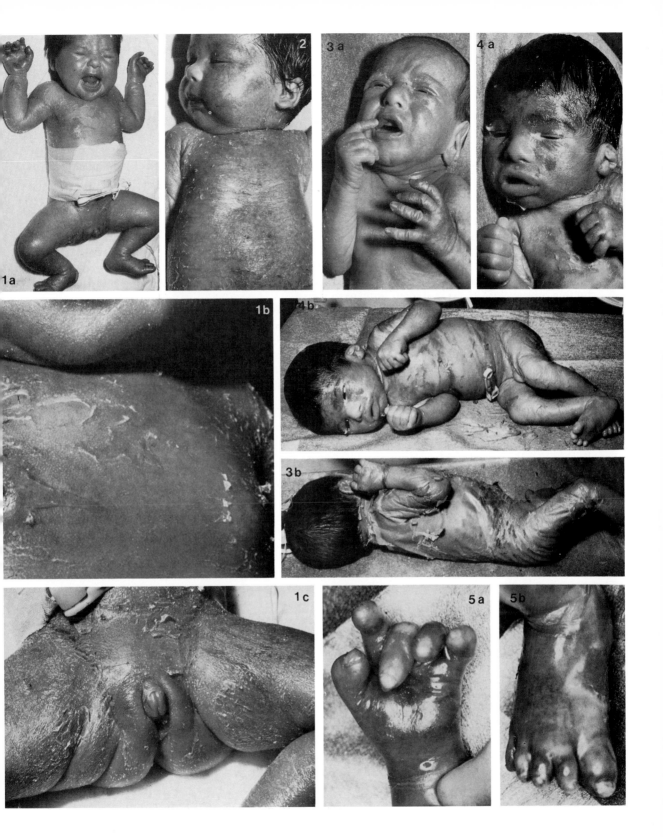

465

232. Ichthyosis Congenita Gravis or Fetalis

(Keratoma Malignum Riecke Type I, Harlequin Fetus)

An extreme, lethal form of ichthyosis congenita with a severe disorder of skin keratinization. Since the horny skin masses split or tear in a rhomboidal pattern *post partum*, such children have also been called 'harlequin' fetuses.

Main signs:
1. Postnatally, the infant appears to be constricted in a yellow-white thick armor of skin. Shortly after birth, cracks up to a centimeter deep appear in the skin: the hyperkeratotic epidermis takes on polygonal, rhomboidal forms (resembling a harlequin costume). Dark red cutis is visible at the base of the clefts (1–3).
2. The face is altered past recognition with ectropion of the mouth and eyes (2). The ears appear packed in armor (1, 3).
3. Hands and feet are also firmly constricted and the fingers and toes immobilized. Clawlike position (1, 3).

Supplementary findings: Histologically, a markedly thickened lamellar horny layer with absence of the stratum granulosum in some areas.

Manifestation: Prenatally, from the sixth month of pregnancy; post partum.

Etiology: Autosomal recessive inheritance very likely. Several affected siblings observed. In one child, the horny mass showed beta, instead of alpha, keratin and a pathologic amino acid composition.

Frequency: Low.

Course, prognosis: Death in the newborn period due to infection, sepsis, respiratory disorders.

Differential diagnosis: Ichthyosis congenita Riecke type II and other forms of 'collodion babies'.

Treatment: Attempt to peel off the horny plates in a humid incubator environment and with acetyl vaseline (?), oil. Prenatal diagnosis may be possible.

Illustrations:
1–3 A characteristically affected newborn; immediate death *post partum*.

J.K.

References:
Anton-Lamprecht, I. Hereditäre Ichthyosen. In: Herzberg, J.J. and Korting, G.W. (eds.) *Pädiatrische Dermatologie*. Schattauer, Stuttgart, New York, 1978, (pp.161–183).
Brenndorff, A.I. v. Ichthyosis congenita. *Pädiatr. Prax.*, 28, 499–506 (1983).
Blanchet-Bardon, C., Dumez, Y., Luzner, M.A. et al. Prenatal diagnosis of harlequin fetus. *Lancet*, I, 132 only (1983).

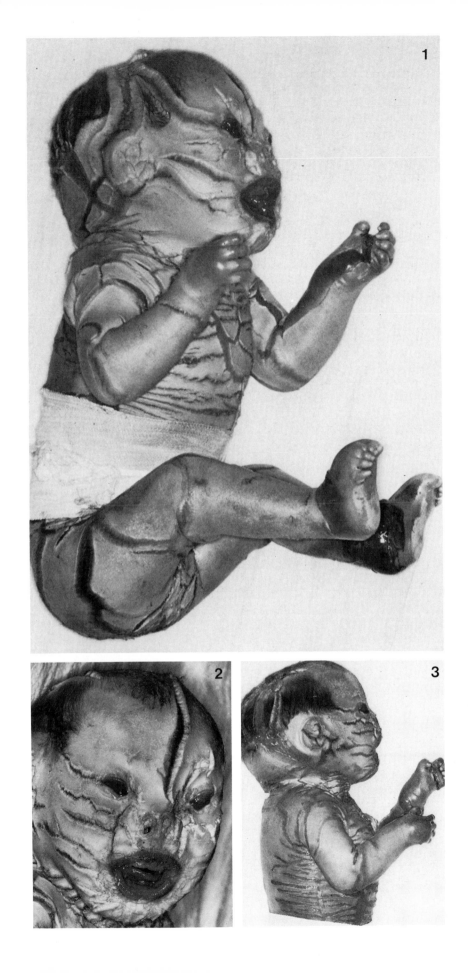

233. Sjögren–Larsson Syndrome

A hereditary disorder of ichthyosis, spastic paraparesis, mental retardation, and short stature.

Main signs:
1. Ichthyosis, especially of the nuchal, axillary, and other flexion areas; the face may remain clear. Possible hyperkeratoses of the hands and feet.
2. Spastic para- (to tetra-) plegia.
3. Considerable mental retardation (IQ usually between 30 and 60); usually a speech disorder of variable severity.
4. Short stature (often below the tenth percentile).

Supplementary findings: Seizures in about one-third of cases.

Pigmentary degeneration of the retina, possibly with macular involvement (seen as small reflecting spots), in about a quarter to a third of cases.

Decreased ability to sweat. Hypoplasia of teeth and enamel. Scalp hair may be sparse.

Manifestation: Ichthyosis, scaling, and hyperkeratosis from birth. The central nervous system manifestations become apparent in the first three years of life. Small size may be apparent at birth.

Etiology: Autosomal recessive disorder.

Frequency: Varies regionally, increased in areas where inbreeding is common; otherwise rare. Over 200 cases documented in the literature.

Course, prognosis: Very dependent on the severity of mental retardation, diplegia, and possible visual impairment.

Differential diagnosis: Rud syndrome (p.470) and others.

Treatment: Symptomatic. Genetic counseling. Prenatal diagnosis.

Illustrations: 1 and 2 A mentally retarded boy with spastic diplegia and congenital ichthyosis with hyperkeratosis.

H.-R.W.

References:

Theile, U. Sjögren–Larsson syndrome. Oligophrenia-Ichthyosis-Di/Tetraplegia. *Humangenetik*, 22, 91 (1974).
Jagell, S. and Lidén, S. Ichthyosis in the Sjögren–Larsson syndrome. *Clin. Genet.*, 21, 243 (1982).
Jagell, S. and Heijbel, J. Sjögren–Larsson syndrome: physical and neurological findings. *Helv. Paediatr. Acta*, 37, 519–530 (1982).
Kousseff, B.G., Matsuoka, L.Y. et al. Prenatal diagnosis of Sjögren–Larsson syndrome. *J. Pediatr.*, 101, 998–1001 (1982).
Gedde-Dahl, T., Jr., Rajka, G. et al. Autosomal recessive ichthyosis in Norway: II. Sjögren–Larsson-like ichthyosis without CNS or eye involvement. *Clin. Genet.*, 26, 242–244 (1984).
Chaves-Carballo, E. Sjögren–Larsson syndrome. In: Gomez, M.R. (ed.) *Neurocutaneous Diseases*. Butterworths, Boston, 1987, (pp.219–224).
Iselius, L. and Jågell, S. Sjögren–Larsson syndrome in Sweden: distribution of the gene. *Clin. Genet.*, 35, 272–275 (1989).

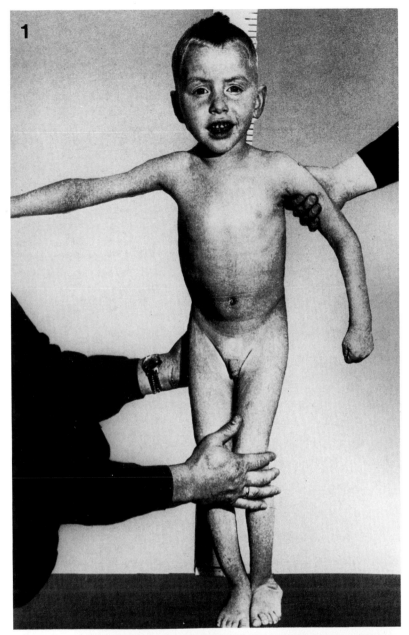

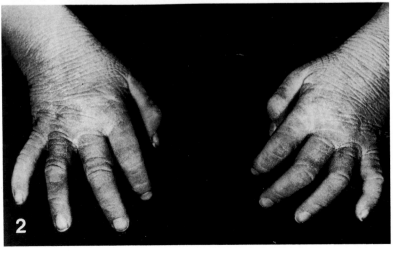

234. Rud Syndrome

(Ichthyosis-Hypogonadism-Mental Retardation-Epilepsy Syndrome)

A hereditary disorder comprising ichthyosis, mental retardation, epilepsy, and almost invariably hypogonadism.

Main signs:
1. Ichthyosis, usually from early infancy.
2. Psychomotor retardation of variable severity (IQ about 30–80).
3. Seizure disorder (time of onset variable).

Supplementary findings: Hypogonadism with eunuchoid habitus and in some cases fairly distinct sexual infantilism.

Short stature, possible hypoplastic teeth and nails, possible eye or hearing disorders.

Manifestation: At birth and/or later.

Etiology: Uniformity of this syndrome questionable. No doubt of a genetic basis. Autosomal recessive transmission has been presumed. An X-linked recessive type may also occur.

Frequency: Low.

Course, prognosis: Very dependent on the degree of mental retardation and severity of epilepsy.

Differential diagnosis: Sjögren–Larsson syndrome (p.468).

Treatment: Symptomatic. Genetic counseling.

Illustrations:
1–9 Three brothers, the children of healthy parents; one brother of the mother has ichthyosis congenita.
5 and 8 The oldest boy at 16¼ years: moderate ichthyosis since birth. Developmental retardation, low intelligence; no seizures (to date); genitalia in 8.
4 and 7 The 'middle' brother at 10 (4) and 13½ (1–3) years: ichthyosis since birth (see 7); mental retardation; seizure disorder; hypogenitalism (7).
6 and 9 The youngest brother at 10 years. Moderately severe ichthyosis since birth; low-normal mental development; no seizures (to date); genitalia in 9 (undescended testis on the right).

Chromosome analyses of the three brothers unremarkable (with banding). A 14½-year-old sister healthy and normally developed for her age.

H.-R.W.

References:

Maldonaldo, R.R. et al. Neuroichthyosis with hypogonadism (Rud's syndrome). *Int. J. Dermatol.*, 14, 347 (1975).
Larbrisseau, A. and Carpenter, S. Rud syndrome... *Neuropediatrics*, 13, 95 (1982).
Münke, M., Kruse, K. et al. Genetic heterogeneity of the ichthyosis, hypogonadism, mental retardation, and epilepsy syndrome... *Eur. J. Pediatr.*, 141, 8–13 (1983).
Traupe, H., Müller-Migi, C.R. et al. Ichthyosis vulgaris with hypogenitalism and hypogonadism: evidence for different genotypes... *Clin. Genet.*, 25, 41–51 (1984).
Scribanis, R., Buoncompagni, A. et al. La sindrome di Rud. *Min. Pediatr.*, 37, 823–826 (1985).
Marxmiller, J., Trenkle, I. et al. Rud syndrome revisited... *Develop. Med. Child Neurol.*, 27, 335–343 (1985).

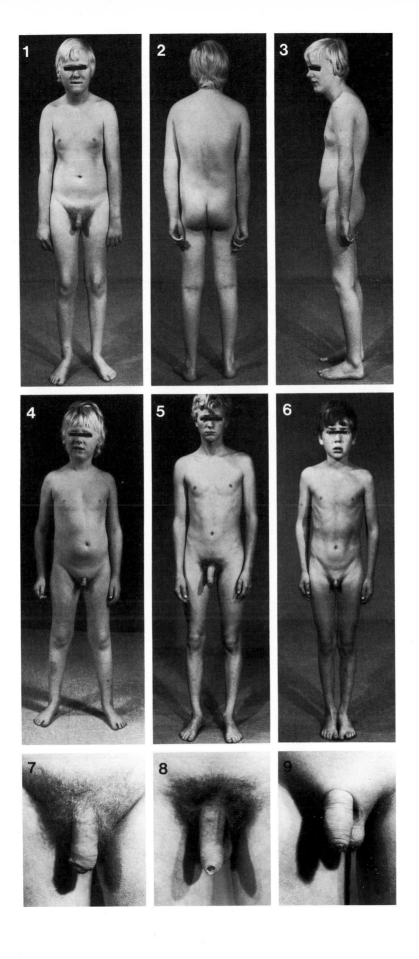

235. Hyperkeratosis Palmoplantaris with Periodontoclasia

(Papillon–Lefèvre Syndrome)

A syndrome of plantopalmar hyperkeratoses, periodontopathy, and loss of teeth.

Main signs:

1. Hyperkeratosis of the soles of the feet and the palms of the hands, the latter usually being less severely affected (**2, 3**).

2. Severe periodontal destruction of the deciduous and subsequent teeth with loosening and loss of all teeth (**1**).

Supplementary findings: Severe secondary periodontitis and gingivostomatitis.

Possible mental retardation, intracranial calcification, nail dysplasia, and increased susceptibility to infections.

Manifestation: Reddening and/or hyperkeratosis of the palms and soles may be apparent from birth and, when an older sibling is typically affected, makes early diagnosis possible. Otherwise the diagnosis can not be made until eruption of the primary dentition and the immediate onset of dental problems.

Etiology: Autosomal recessive disorder.

Frequency: Low. Estimated one per million of the general population; 126 cases known in the literature up to 1979.

Course, prognosis: Severe periodontosis (and secondary periodontitis) affects the primary and later the secondary dentition with loss of all teeth. The deciduous teeth are lost at age 5–6, and the permanent teeth at 13–14 years. No occupational difficulties from the palmar skin disorder of the palms.

Treatment: Symptomatic. Special oral hygiene. Dental care. Dental prostheses—upper and lower—at the appropriate time. Genetic counseling.

Illustrations:

1–4 A 3¾-year-old Turkish boy, family history not available. Dyskeratotic–hyperkeratotic changes of the palms and soles with garland-like, sharply delineated border to the healthy skin at the level of the malleoli and the heels. Reddening of the volar and plantar skin. Bilateral hyperkeratoses of the patellar regions. Early loss of deciduous teeth in both jaws; a few remaining, loose teeth with the necks extensively exposed; periodontosis.

H.-R.W.

References:

Giasanti, J.S. et al. Palmar-plantar hyperkeratosis and concomitant periodontal destruction (Papillon–Lefèvre syndrome). *Oral Surg.*, 36, 40 (1973).

Hacham-Zadeh, S., Schaap, T. et al. A genetic analysis of the Papillon–Lefèvre syndrome . . . *Am. J. Med. Genet.*, 2, 153–157 (1978).

Haneke, E. The Papillon–Lefèvre syndrome . . . report of a case and review . . . *Hum. Genet.*, 51, 1–35 (1979).

Geormaneanu, M., Ciofu, C. et al. Maladie de Papillon–Lefèvre . . . *Ann. Génét.*, 25, 189–192 (1982).

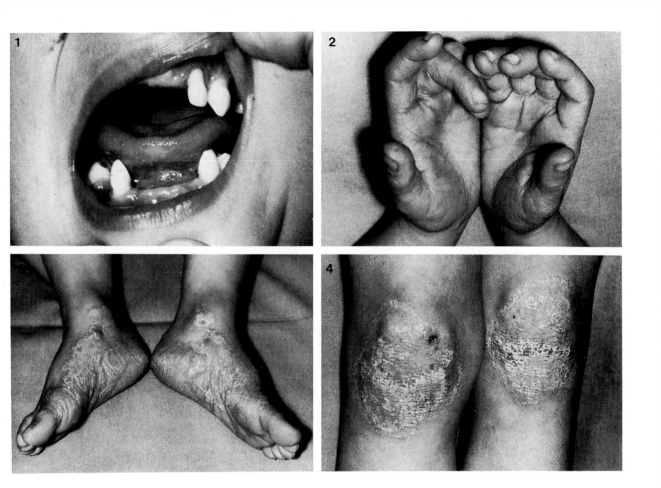

473

236. Epidermolysis Bullosa Hereditaria

A collective term for a group of hereditary dermatoses in which very mild trauma or mechanical or other factors lead to blistering of the skin.

Main signs:
Depending on the individual genotype (see below), formation of blisters on regions of the body subject to pressure or rubbing, but also in other areas and possibly 'spontaneously'. The precise characteristics of the blisters are also dependent on type, as are a positive or negative Nikolsky phenomenon; healing of the lesions with or without scarring and even, in extreme cases, adhesions ('mutilations') on the hands and feet, esophageal stenosis, and threat of carcinoma in scar tissue; involvement or noninvolvement of the mucous membranes; presence of palmoplantar hyperhidrosis; development of hyperkeratoses, of nail dystrophy and disorders of tooth enamel or other dental problems; dystrophy of the hair and alopecia; and numerous other features.

Manifestation: Often at birth or during the course of the first year of life, rarely later.

Etiology: Monogenic disorder. At present, about 16 types, on 9 gene loci, have been differentiated, with about equal numbers of autosomal dominant and autosomal recessive genotypes in addition to an X-linked recessive type.

Frequency: Taken as a group of diseases, epidermolysis bullosa hereditaria is not very rare. Many hundreds of cases in the literature.

Course, prognosis: Dependent on the type. There are early lethal and potentially early lethal types (especially with those that are autosomal recessive), but also types with a tendency to improve in or around puberty, and types with no effect on life expectancy.

Differential diagnosis: Epidermolysis bullosa (e.b.) simplex, e.b. atrophicans, and e.b. dystrophica are differentiated by light microscopy; the subtypes, by immunofluorescence, biochemistry, and electron microscopy. Acute exogenous conditions such as staphylogenic pemphigoid of infants or newborns, Ritter exfoliative dermatitis, toxic or allergic epidermal necrolysis Lyell's disease, erythema multiforme bullosum, or just scalding are easily differentiated. Even acrodermatitis enteropathica (p.462), congenital porphyria, dermatitis herpetiformis, and pemphigus should not cause diagnostic difficulties.

Treatment: Depending on the severity of the case, from intensive care to mere avoidance of precipitating trauma. Vocational counseling in some cases. Genetic counseling. Prenatal diagnosis possible by means of fetal skin biopsy.

Illustrations:
1a and **1b** A 2-day-old newborn.
2a–2d A 3-year-old girl with alopecia, lesions of the lips and teeth, nail dystrophy. Both **1** and **2** show autosomal recessive forms of the disorder.
3a and **3b** The lower leg of a newborn and the hand of his father with an autosomal dominant form of the disease.

H.-R.W.

References:
Voigtländer, V., Schnyder, U.W., Anton-Lamprecht, I. Hereditäre Epidermolysen. In: Korting, G.W. (ed.) *Dermatologie in Praxis und Klinik*, vol. III. Thieme, Stuttgart, 1979.
Rodeck, C.H., Eady, R.A.J., Gosden, C.M. Prenatal diagnosis of epidermolysis bullosa letalis. *Lancet*, I, 979 (1980).
Anton-Lamprecht, I. Prenatal diagnosis of genetic disorders of the skin by means of electron microscopy. *Hum. Genet.*, 59, 392–405 (1981).
Anton-Lamprecht, I., Rauskolb, R. et al. Prenatal diagnosis of epidermolysis bullosa dystrophica... *Lancet*, II, 1077 (1981).
Gedde-Dahl, T., Jr. and Anton-Lamprecht, I. Epidermolysis bullosa. In: Emery, A.E.H. and Rimoin, D.L. (eds.) *Principles and Practice of Medical Genetics*. Churchill Livingstone, Edinburgh, 1983 (pp. 672–687).

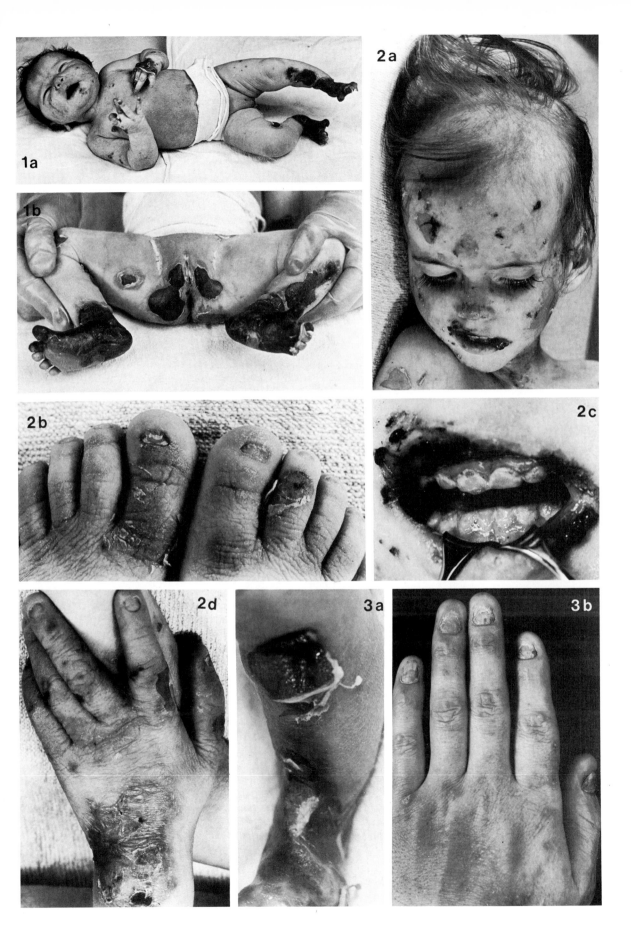

237. Wiskott–Aldrich Syndrome

An X-linked recessive disorder with the following triad of signs: eczema, thrombocytopenia with bleeding tendency, and recurrent infections.

Main signs:
1. Clinical onset frequently with eczema (T-cell defect).
2. Thrombocytopenia, bleeding tendency.
3. Recurrent infections.

Supplementary findings:
1. Disorder of humoral immunity with dysgammaglobulinemia, selective disorders of B- and T-lymphocytes, qualitative changes of the thrombocytes and their accelerated removal by the reticuloendothelial system, deficient formation of blood-group isoantibodies, and cutaneous anergy.
2. Markedly elevated IgE.

Manifestation: Eczema and irreversible thrombocytopenia frequently in the first weeks and months of life.

Etiology: X-linked recessive disease; a disorder of cell metabolism of the hematopoietic system.

Frequency: Four new cases in a million live-born boys.

Course, prognosis: Survival without therapy, 8 months; with therapy, 6.5 years for those born from before 1935 to after 1964. Currently, 25% of 301 patients have lived for 10 years (total life span of up to 36 years in isolated cases). Development of lymphoreticular tumors and leukemias in 12% of patients (100 times increased risk of tumors than the general population). The most frequent cause of death is from infections (e.g., pneumonia, sepsis; in 59%), followed by generalized bleeding (e.g., CNS, intestinal; in 27%), malignancies (in 5%), and various other problems (e.g., asphyxia, shock, aplastic anemia, vascular occlusion, pulmonary edema with cardiac failure—altogether 9%).

Differential diagnosis: Can be differentiated easily from congenital and acquired thrombocytopenias.

Treatment: Allogenic bone marrow transplantation. Administration of transfer factor. Splenectomy? Genetic counseling. Prenatal diagnosis?

Illustrations:
1 A male patient, aged 9 months, generalized eczematous skin changes with sharply delineated, round to oval erythematous foci, which coalesce into larger honeycombed and multicentric areas.
2 A boy, aged 1 year and 11 months, with generalized thrombocytopenic bleeding of the skin, particularly around the mouth.

J.K.

References:

Perry, G.S., Spector, B.D., Schuman, L.M. et al. The Wiskott–Aldrich syndrome in the United States and Canada (1892–1979). *J. Pediatr.*, 97, 72–78 (1980).

Erttmann, R., Thöne, I., Landbeck, G. Wiskott–Aldrich Syndrom. *Monatschr. Kinderheilkd.*, 131, 524–527 (1983).

Holmberg, L., Gustavii, B., Jönsson, A. A prenatal study of platelet count and size with application to the fetus at risk for Wiskott–Aldrich syndrome. *J. Pediatr.*, 102, 773–776 (1983).

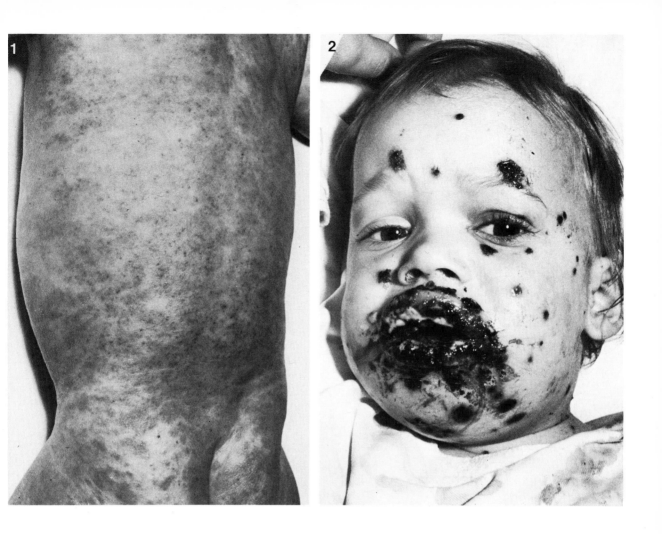

238. Abt–Letterer–Siwe Disease

(Acute Disseminated Histiocytosis X, Letterer–Siwe Disease)

A generalized malignant form of histiocytosis X in infants and children with seborrheic, macular, or petechial skin rash; generalized lymphadenopathy; hepatosplenomegaly; and pulmonary involvement.

Main signs:
1. Seborrheic dermatitis, maculopapular yellow-brown skin rash with petechial bleeding.
2. Hepatosplenomegaly.
3. Generalized lymphadenopathy.
4. Pulmonary infiltration with repiratory distress and coughing.
5. Hematological disorder: anemia, leukopenia, thrombocytopenia.

Supplementary findings: Sepsis-like clinical picture with recurrent fever. Histologically, demonstration of atypical histiocytes in the upper dermis. Electron microscopic demonstration of 'Langerhans cell granules'.

Manifestation: Infancy and childhood.

Etiology: Autosomal recessive inheritance. An affected sibling in many cases.

Frequency: About 1:100,000 for the first year of life; 0.2:100,000 for children under 15 years.

Course, prognosis: Lethal in about 30% of cases. Untreated, always a fatal outcome. Dramatic clinical picture in infants and toddlers.

Differential diagnosis: Initially, diaper rash, fungal infections, and scabies. Later, Hand–Schüller–Christian disease and eosinophilic granuloma.

Treatment: Chemotherapy using vinca alkaloids, antimetabolites, alkylating agents, and glucocorticoids. Splenectomy?

Illustrations:
1 and 2 Maculopapular, petechial skin rash mainly affecting the trunk; enlarged lymph nodes.

J.K.

References:
Any pediatric textbook.
Frisell, E., Björksten, B., Holmgren, G. et al. Familial occurrence of histiocytosis. *Clin. Genet.*, 11, 163–170 (1977).
Wolff, H.H. and Janka, G.E. Morbus Abt–Letterer–Siwe. Zur Diagnostik und Therapie. *Monatschr. Kinderheilkd.*, 126, 425–430 (1978).

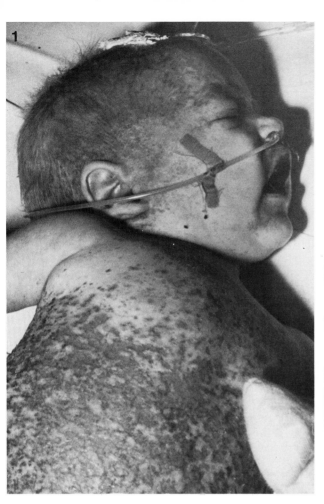

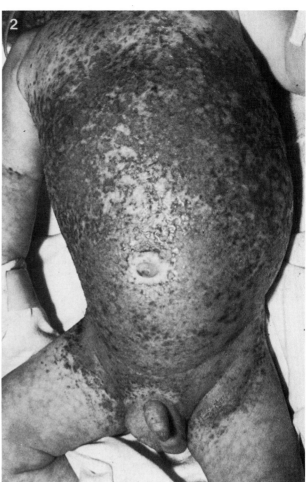

239. Alcohol Embryopathy

(Fetal Alcohol Syndrome)

A teratogenic disorder of mental and motor development, typical facies with microcephaly and growth deficiency, multiple further gross and subtle anomalies, and behavioral signs in children of chronic alcoholic mothers.

Main signs:
1. Marked prenatal and postnatal growth retardation, disproportionate small stature, and microcephaly.
2. Craniofacial dysmorphism: short palpebral fissures (blepharophimosis); epicanthus; ptosis; short, flat nasal root; hypoplastic philtrum; thin upper lip with narrow prolabium; micrognathia; frequent minor ear anomalies.
3. Delayed motor development with muscular hypotonia; marked postnatal irritability; transition to marked hyperactivity possible.
4. CNS disorder: mild to severe mental retardation, psychological disorders, unusual behavior, impaired concentration and learning.

Supplementary findings: Gross anomalies: cardiac defect in 30%, renal malformation in 10%, cleft palate, minor anomalies of the genitalia (hypoplasia of the labia majora, glandular hypospadias, cryptorchidism). Lesser anomalies: abnormal hand creases, clinodactyly, camptodactyly, limited supination, hypoplasia of the distal phalanges and nails, dislocation of the hips, coccygeal pits, hernias, hemangiomas, pectus excavatum.

Classification of Alcohol Embryopathy (AE) According to Three Grades of Severity:
AE III. Complete expression of the syndrome with typical facies (*primavista* diagnosis), microcephaly, gross malformations, and usually severe mental retardation. (About 20% of cases.)
AE II: Typical facies, pre- and postnatal growth retardation, microcephaly, isolated additional anomalies. Usually mild to moderate mental retardation. (About 30% of cases.)
AE I: Abortive form of the syndrome (fetal alcohol effects); no typical facies, only mild indications of craniofacial dysmorphism; small stature; microcephaly; hyperactivity and behavioral signs; mild mental retardation or learning disorders. (About 40–50% of cases.)

Manifestation: At birth.

Etiology: The teratogenicity of alcohol in itself *in utero* is still unknown. This embryopathy has only been observed in children of chronic alcoholic women. Whether ethyl alcohol and/or acetaldehyde plus additional secondary deficiencies of the mother are pathogenetically responsible remains unclear. A third of all children of chronic alcoholic mothers show diagnosable AE. About 60–70% show partial teratogenic effects. Individual genetic factors are probably responsible for the differences in vulnerability.

Frequency: Next to Down's syndrome and myelocele, AE is the most frequent congenital cause of mental retardation. The frequency varies markedly and is dependent on the drinking habits of women in different cultural groups (e.g., 1 in 100 in some Indian reservations in America). The frequency comes to 1/750 in the USA, 1/600 in Sweden, and with the registration also of milder cases, 1/212 in France. In the Federal Republic of Germany, probably 1,000–1,500 children with AE have been born per year, with a large, unknown number of mild or abortive cases.

Illustrations:
1–3 A 3-month-old child. Mother a chronic alcoholic. Birth weight 1590 g after unknown length of gestation. Measurements at 9 months: length 68.5 cm; weight 5700 g; head circumference 42 cm. Typical facies. Premature synostosis of the frontal suture, cardiac defect, psychomotor retardation.
4 and 5 Two more typically affected young children.

H.L. Spohr/H.-R.W.

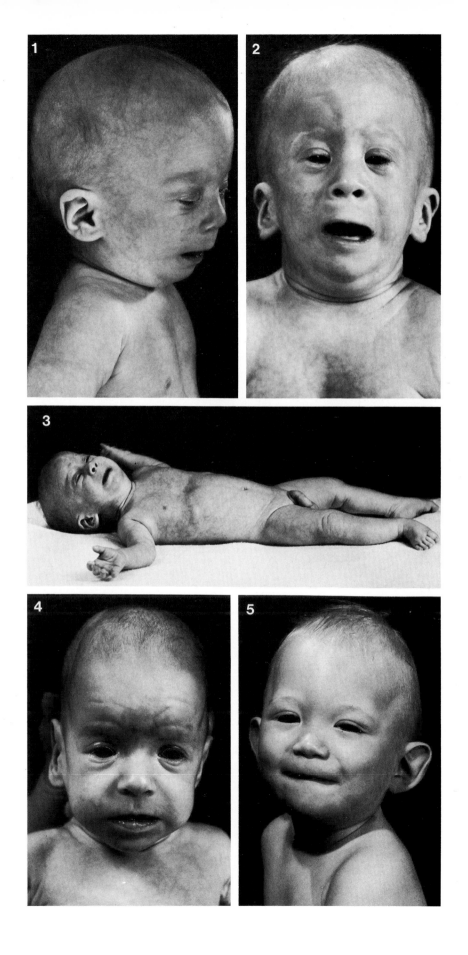

481

(Fetal Alcohol Syndrome)

Course, prognosis: Perinatal mortality is not increased. Frequent infections in the first two years of life, failure to thrive, and need for surgery are responsible for numerous hospital admissions. The extent of permanent mental retardation is of decisive importance for the patient's life. Even when all mild cases are included, only 20% can attend a normal school. About half of the children are suitable for special schools for learning disability or for the mentally retarded. About one-third of patients are severely retarded. The frequency of alcohol embryopathy is growing with increasing maternal alcoholism.

Differential diagnosis: Trisomy 18 syndrome, which shows extremely severe mental impairment, death almost always within the first year of life, characteristic chromosome findings. Dubowitz syndrome and Noonan syndrome should also not be difficult to rule out (especially considering the absence of the corresponding social history).

Treatment: Symptomatic; initial prolonged hospital admissions frequently necessary, operative correction of cleft palate, cardiac defects, hernias. All appropriate measures to help the handicapped. Only a third of the children live with one of their biological parents. Residential care or referral to special therapy centers is often necessary. Most importantly: AE is a preventable form of mental retardation, so measures to prevent chronic maternal alcoholism are imperative.

Illustrations: Infants and young children with alcohol embryopathy. Horizontally, 1st row: children in the first 3 months of life; 2nd row: children from 4 to 11 months; 3rd row: 1- to 2-year old children; 4th row: children of 2¼, 2½, and 5¼ years.

H.L. Spohr/H.-R.W.

References:

Lemoine, P., Harousseau, H., Boteyru, J.P. et al. Les enfants de parents alcooliques; anomalies observées. Apropos de 127 cas. *Quest. Med.*, 25, 477 (1968).

Jones, K.L., Smith, D.W., Ulleland, C. et al. Pattern of malformation in offspring of chronic alcoholic mothers. *Lancet*, I, 1267 (1973).

Hanson, J.W., Jones, K.L., Smith, D.W. Fetal alcohol syndrome. Experience with 41 patients. *J. Am. Med. Ass.*, 235, 1458 (1976).

Majewski, F., Bierich, J.R., Löser, H. et al. Zur Klinik und Pathogenese der Alkoholembryopathie (Bericht über 68 Patienten). *Münch. Med. Wochenschr.*, 118, 1635 (1976).

Clarren, S.K. and Smith, D.W. The fetal alcohol syndrome. Experience with 65 patients and a review of the world literature. *N. Engl. J. Med.*, 298, 1063 (1978).

Hanson, J.W., Streissguth, A.P., Smith, D.W. The effects of moderate alcohol consumption during pregnancy on fetal growth and morphogenesis. *J. Pediatr.*, 92, 457 (1978).

Streissguth, A.P., Herman, S., Smith, D.W. Intelligence, behavior, and dysmorphogenesis in the fetal alcohol syndrome: a report on 20 patients. *J. Pediatr.*, 92, 363 (1978).

Nestler, V.M., Spohr, H.L., Steinhausen, H.C. *Die Alkoholembryopathie*. Stuttgart, 1981.

Little, R.E., Young, A., Streissguth, A.P. et al. Preventing fetal alcohol effects: effectiveness of a demonstration project. In: *Mechanisms of Alcohol Damage In Utero*. London, 1984 (p.254).

Streissguth, A.P., Clarren, S.K., Jones, K.L. Natural history of the fetal alcohol syndrome: a 10-year follow-up of 11 patients. *Lancet*, II, 85 (1985).

Spohr, H.L. and Steinhausen, H.C. Follow-up studies of children with fetal alcohol syndrome. *Neuropediatrics*, 18, 13–17 (1987).

Sokolowski, F., Sokolowski, A., Majewski, F. Risiken für die Nachkommen alkoholkranker Frauen. *Pädiatr. Prax.*, 38, 373–387 (1989).

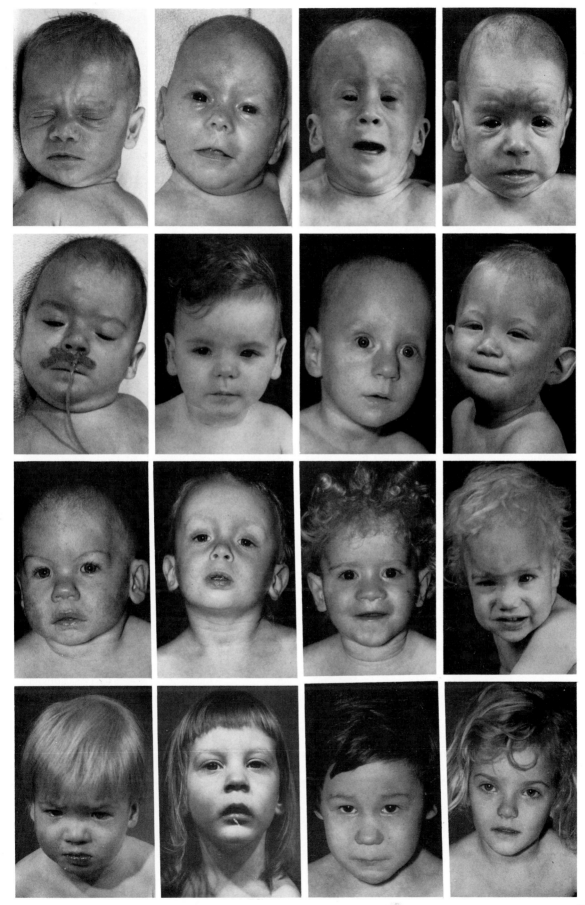

483

241. Williams–Beuren Syndrome

(Williams Syndrome, Fanconi–Schlesinger Syndrome, Williams' Elfin Face Syndrome)

A malformation–retardation syndrome with characteristic facial dysmorphism, small stature, mental retardation, vascular stenosis, and—infrequently—hypercalcemia.

Main signs:
1. So-called elfin facies, essentially characterized by a broad forehead, suprapalpebral fullness, short palpebral fissures, hyper- or hypotelorism, epicanthus, low nasal root, hypoplasia of the midface, slightly anteverted nostrils, long philtrum, full cheeks, large mouth, and occasionally drooping lips (1, 2, 6–8).
2. Internal strabismus (6). Mild microcephaly.
3. Hypoplastic teeth (5), occasionally hypodontia. Malpositioned teeth.
4. Pre- and especially postnatal growth retardation (reasonable catch-up growth possible later).
5. Moderate to severe mental retardation (mean IQ to 55), but normal intellectual development also occurs. Friendly, lively disposition; deep voice.

Supplementary findings: Vascular stenosis, especially supravalvular aortic stenosis, peripheral pulmonary stenoses, stenosis of the renal and mesenteric arteries and other vascular defects.

Ventricular and atrial septal defects. Prolapse of the mitral valve.

Hypercalcemia infrequent, usually limited to early infancy and, if present, associated with the related clinical signs (anorexia, constipation, failure to thrive, etc.), metastatic calcification, especially of the kidneys.

Osteosclerosis (especially of the skull, metaphyses; 3, 4). Possible craniosynostosis, kyphoscoliosis.

Short, hypoplastic nails; hallux valgus; radial deviation of the fifth finger.

Stellate pattern of the iris.

Manifestation: From birth; the typical facies cannot usually be recognized until the second year of life.

Etiology: Disorder of vitamin D metabolism with hypersensitivity to vitamin D or calcitonin deficiency assumed. Usually sporadic occurrence. An autosomal dominant gene with incomplete penetrance and very variable expression has been postulated.

Frequency: Not low (at least 1 in 10,000 newborns?); several hundred cases in the literature.

Prognosis: Infrequently death as a result of hypercalcemia or later, from nephrocalcinosis. Course otherwise dependent on the significance of the stenosed vessels, on the severity of the stenosis and its operability. Arterial hypertension and gastrointestinal and urogenital problems in adolescence or adulthood.

Treatment: Operative relief of vascular stenoses. Treatment of hypercalcemia in all cases.

Comment: Presumably, isolated supravalvular aortic stenosis could be due to the same pathogenetic mechanism. Williams–Beuren syndrome, like isolated supravalvular aortic stenosis, has been observed repeatedly in siblings.

Illustrations:
1–5 Patient 1 at 2¾ years (1 and 3); and at 4¾ years (2, 4, 5). Severe psychomotor retardation. On initial examination at 2¾ years, height 79 cm (50th percentile for a 14-month-old girl); under-weight by 1 kg in relation to height; head circumference 46 cm (normal for height); persistent hypercalcemia, up to 15 mg% (3.75 mmol/l). At 4¾ years, calcium still as high as 13.2 mg% (3.3 mmol/l). Death from uremia at 5¼ years. On autopsy: nephrocalcinosis; calcium deposits in the heart muscle, thyroid gland, and bronchial cartilages; left ventricular hypertrophy; stenosis of the aortic root.
6–8 Patient 2 at 15 months (6 and 7) and at 9 years (8). Since the second half-year of life: anorexia, insufficient weight gain. On initial examination at 15 months, height within normal limits, underweight by 1.5 kg for height. Head circumference normal. Calcium values as high as 17.4 mg% (4.35 mmol/l); supravalvular aortic stenosis with hypoplastic aorta; hypoplastic pulmonary vascular tree, two superior venae cavae. Mental impairment first recognized at 9 years. Height at this time (124 cm) in the low normal range.

H.-R.W./J.K.

References:
Beuren, A.J. Supravalvular aortic stenosis: a complex syndrome with and without mental retardation. *Birth Defects*, VIII/5, 45 (1972).
Jones, K.L. and Smith, D.W. The Williams elfin facies syndrome ... *J. Pediatr.*, 86, 718 (1975).
Preus, M. The Williams syndrome ... *Clin. Genet.*, 25, 422–434 (1984).
Burn, J. Williams syndrome. *J. Med. Genet.*, 23, 389–395 (1986).
Editorial: Williams syndrome—the enigma continues. *Lancet*, II, 490 (1988).
Morris, C.A., Demsey, S.A. et al. Natural history of Williams syndrome ... *J. Pediatr.*, 113, 318–326 (1988).

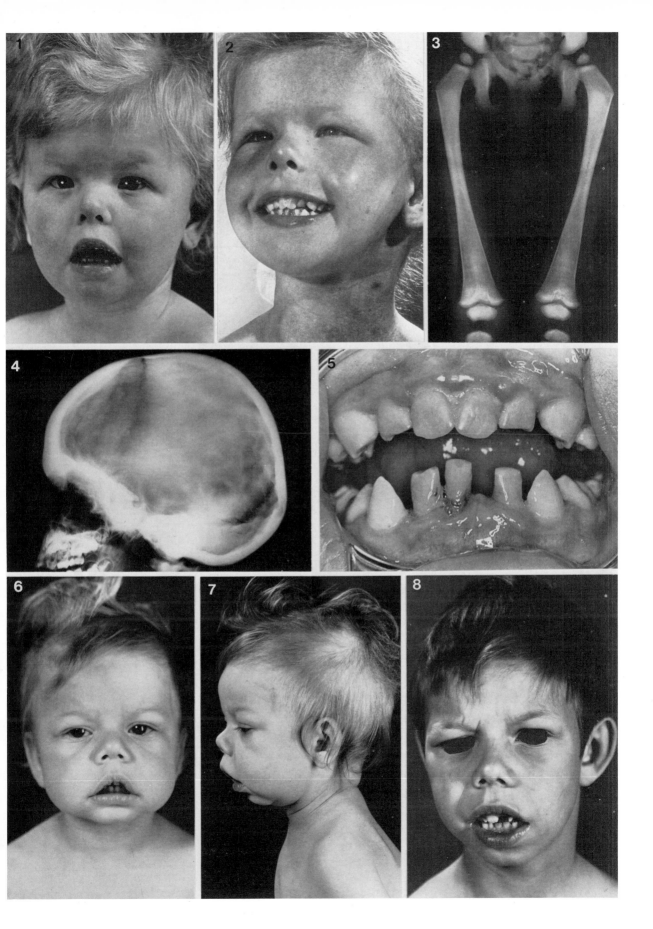

485

242. A Dysplasia Syndrome of Minor External Signs and Cardiovascular Anomalies

A syndrome of somewhat unusual appearance, goiter (familial), peculiarities of the hands and body proportions, and cardiovascular anomalies.

Main signs:
1. Facies: Pronounced supraorbital ridges; almond-shaped eyes; small nose with narrow root; hypoplasia of the zygomatic arches; large, prominent, simply modeled ears; microstomia, prognathism (**1, 2**). Whorl of hair at the back of the neck.
2. Goiter (familial).
3. Short, unusual hands with approximately equal lengths of second and fourth digits bilaterally; clinodactyly of second and fifth digits bilaterally (**3**). Short toes (**5**).
4. Lanky appearance (height around 75th percentile) with excessively long extremities and an almost feminine-appearing pelvic region. Winging of the scapulae with elevation of the left shoulder (**7–9**).
5. Cardiologically: partial transposition of the pulmonary veins with drainage into the left innominate vein; small atrial septal defect.

Supplementary findings: Radiologically, brachymesophalangism of the little fingers and of second to fifth toes bilaterally (**4, 6**).

Manifestation: At birth and later.

Etiology: Not known.

Treatment: Symptomatic.

Illustrations:
1–9 An 11-year-old boy with normal mental development, the second child of nonconsanguineous parents, Father 46 years, mother 36 years at the patient's birth. (Patient has had diffuse euthyrotic goiter since age 6 years. Mother of the boy and five of her siblings are similarly affected, as is the older sister of the proband.)

H.-R.W.

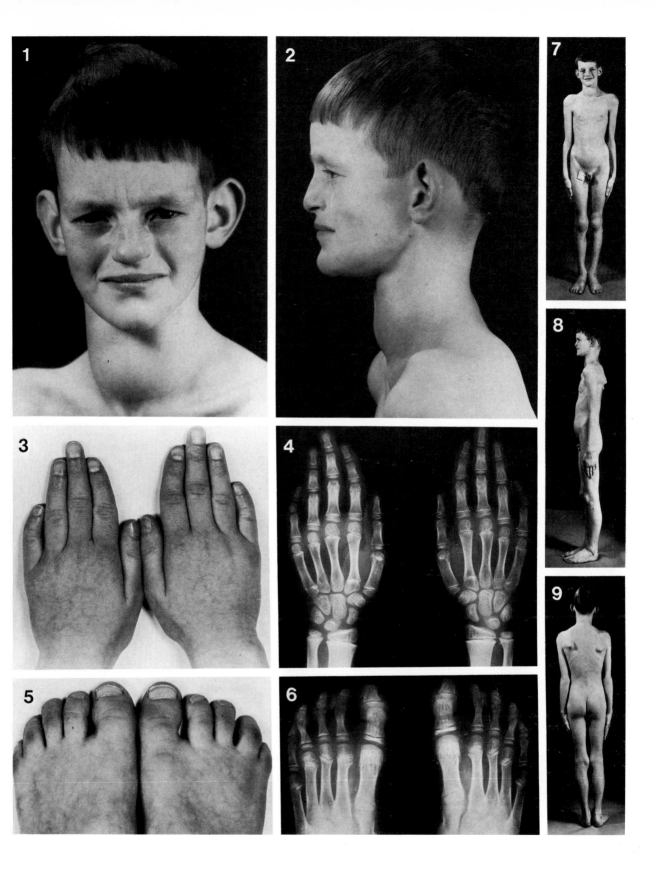

243. Velo-Cardio-Facial Syndrome

(Shprintzen Syndrome)

A malformation–retardation syndrome of characteristic facies, usually moderate mental retardation, cleft palate, and cardiovascular anomalies.

Main signs:
1. Typical appearance: long, narrow face with micrognathia (and malocclusion), prominent nose with broad bridge and hypoplastic alae nasi, slightly deformed ears. Frequently, abundant scalp hair (1–6).
2. Mild to moderate mental retardation with learning disability.
3. Cleft palate (open or submucous); hypernasal speech.
4. Cardiovascular anomalies such as ventricular septal defect, tetralogy of Fallot, or other.

Supplementary findings: Possible microcephaly; eye anomalies. Growth deficiency; narrow hands and fingers; possible scoliosis. Hernias. Secondary hearing and possible speech problems.

Manifestation: At birth and later.

Etiology: An autosomal dominant disorder with very variable expression; family members of the index case should be examined carefully. Heterogeneity cannot be excluded with certainty.

Frequency: Probably not very low.

Course, prognosis: Essentially dependent on the type and severity of cardiac defect.

Diagnosis, differential diagnosis: Early recognition important, not least to prevent secondary handicaps.

Treatment: Surgery for cardiac defects; in some cases hearing-, speech-, and other aids.

Illustrations:
1–4 Four boys (7 years, 5 years, 7 months, 6 years) with Shprintzen syndrome, from different families.
5 An affected 25-year-old with her 8-month-old daughter.
6 On the right, the girl shown as an infant in **5**, now 9 years old; on the left, her similarly affected 7¾-year-old sister.

H.-R.W.

References:

Shprintzen, R.J., Goldberg, R.B., Lewin, H.L. et al. A new syndrome involving cleft palate, cardiac anomalies, typical facies, and learning disabilities: velo-cardio-facial syndrome. *Cleft Palate J.*, 15, 56–62 (1978).
Meinecke, P., Beemer, F.A., Schinzel, A. et al. The velo-cardio-facial (Shprintzen) syndrome. *Eur. J. Pediatr.*, 145, 539–544 (1986).
Pagon, R.A., Shprintzen, R.J., Beemer, F.A. et al. Letters to the editor re. CHARGE versus velo-cardio-facial syndrome. *Am. J. Med. Genet.*, 28, 751–758 (1987).

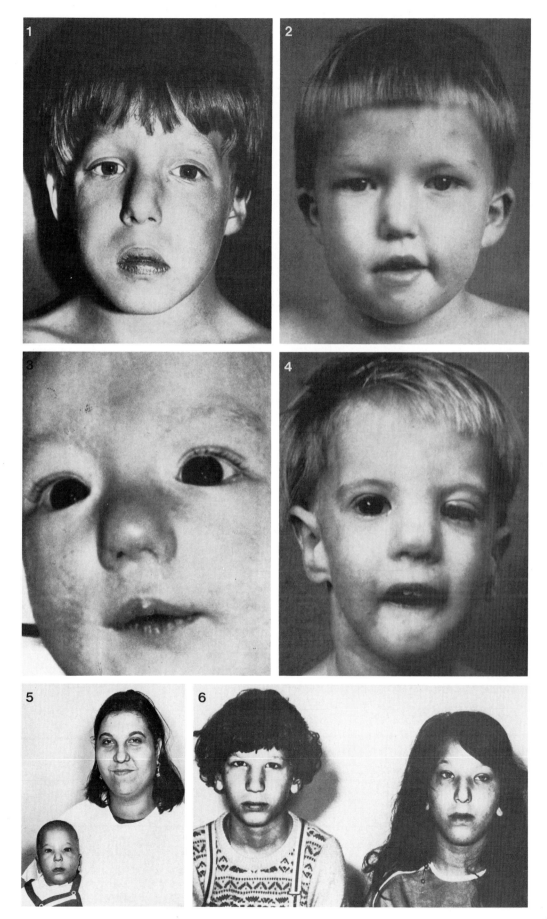

244. Rabenhorst Syndrome

A syndrome of typical facial dysmorphism, cardiac defect, and multiple lesser anomalies.

Main signs:
1. Narrow face with high narrow nose, slight mongoloid slant of the palpebral fissures, microstomia, prognathism, adherent ear lobes. High palate. Dolichocephaly (**1, 2**).
2. Markedly asthenic physique (**3**).
3. Limited mobility of the distal interphalangeal joints with hypoplasia of the corresponding articular creases. Simian crease. Syndactyly of the second and third toes.

Supplementary findings: Ventricular septal defect with pulmonary stenosis.

Manifestation: At birth.

Etiology: Probable autosomal dominant disorder.

Frequency: Two cases described to date.

Prognosis: As far as can be determined from the small number of cases, relatively good.

Treatment: Correction of the cardiac defect.

Illustrations:
1–4 A father and his 4-year-old daughter (**2–4**). Both had ventricular septal defect with pulmonary stenosis. In the meantime the girl has undergone successful surgery.

H.-R.W.

References:
Grosse, F.R. Rabenhorst syndrome. A cardio-acro-facial syndrome. *Z. Kinderheilkd.*, 117, 109 (1974).

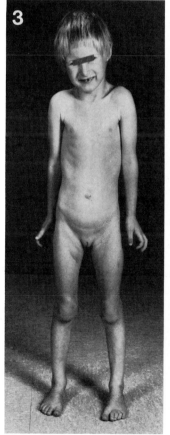
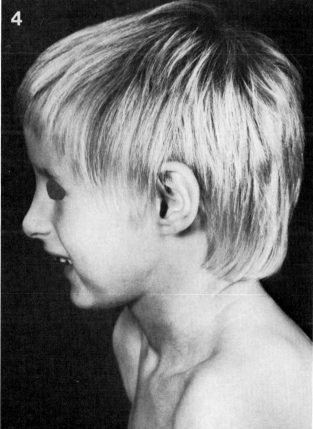
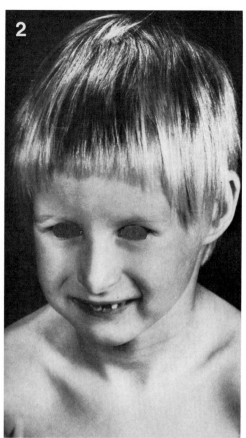
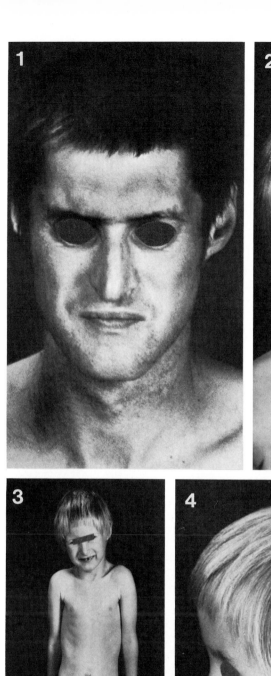

245. Möbius Sequence

A clinical picture comprising congenital, generally bilateral, cranial nerve (usually facial-abducent) paralysis with other anomalies.

Main signs:
1. Expressionless face; disorders of drinking, swallowing, and speech; strabismus and ptosis of the lids (1–3) due to congenital defect of the following cranial nerves: most frequently, the facial (usually with preservation of the oral branch) and abducent nerves; less frequently, the oculomotor (usually partial defect with no internal paralysis) and hypoglossal nerves; very seldom, the motor portion of the trigeminal or trochlear nerves.
2. Nerve involvement usually bilateral.
3. Club feet in about a fifth of cases (1).

Supplementary findings: Various hand anomalies, usually symbrachydactyly, also with ipsilateral aplasia of the pectoralis muscle.

Ear anomalies; occasionally deafness.

Aplasia of the lacrimal puncta.

Occasionally, mild mental retardation (about 10% of cases).

Manifestation: At birth.

Etiology: Hereditary occurrence has been described with autosomal dominant and autosomal recessive transmission. Heterogeneity, pleiotropism; inter- and intrafamilial variability. Most cases are sporadic and of unknown etiology; risk of recurrence then around 2%.

Frequency: Low (from 1888 to 1980 about 180 observations were reported in the literature).

Course, prognosis: Feeding problems in the newborn period and early infancy, danger of aspiration. Tendency for the paralysis to improve in some cases.

Differential diagnosis: Oral-acral 'syndrome' (p.380), of which Möbius syndrome can be considered a partial manifestation; Poland anomaly (p.390).

Treatment: Nurse prone and tube feedings for the young infant. Speech therapy. Multidisciplinary care and support. Genetic counseling.

Illustrations:
1–3 A 10-year-old girl with paralysis of the facial and abducent nerves; surgically corrected club feet.

H.-R.W./J.K.

References:

Henderson, J.L. The congenital facial diplegia syndrome: clinical features, pathology, and aetiology. A review of 61 cases. *Brain*, 62, 381 (1939).

Szabo, L. Möbius-Syndrom und Polandsche Anomalie. *Z. Orthop. Grenzgeb.*, 114, 211 (1976).

Herrmann, J., Pallister, P.D., Gilbert, E.F. et al. Nosologic studies in the Hanhart and the Möbius syndrome. *Eur. J. Pediatr.*, 122, 19 (1976).

Meyerson, M.D. and Foushee, D.R. Speech, language and hearing in Moebius syndrome: a study of 22 patients. *Develop. Med. Child. Neurol.*, 20, 357 (1978).

Legum, C., Godel, V., Nemet, P. Heterogeneity and pleiotropism in the Moebius syndrome. *Clin. Genet.*, 20, 254 (1981); ibid. 21, 290 (1982).

Benney, H. and Kinzinger, W. Kinder mit Moebius-syndrom . . . *Pädiatr. Prax.*, 26, 237 (1978).

Legum, C., Godel, V. et al. Heterogeneity and pleiotropism in the Moebius syndrome. *Clin. Genet.*, 20, 254–259 (1981).

Collins, D.L. and Schimke, R.N. Moebius syndrome in a child and extremity defect in her father. *Clin. Genet.*, 22, 312–314 (1982).

Stabile, M., Cavaliere, M.L. et al. Abnormal B.A.E.P. in a family with Moebius syndrome . . . *Clin. Genet.*, 25, 459–463 (1984).

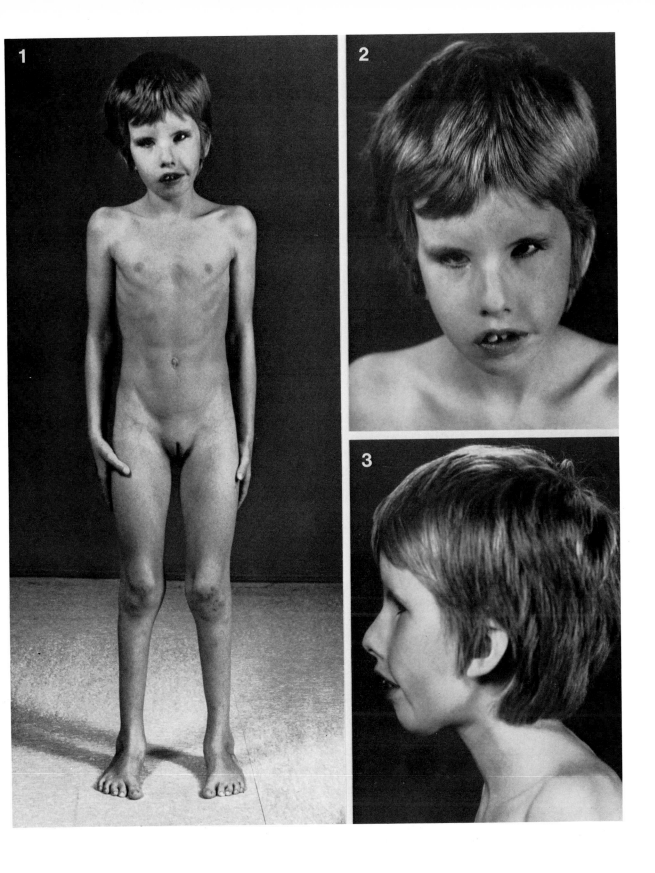

246. Smith–Lemli–Opitz Syndrome

A very variable hereditary disorder of primordial growth deficiency, mental retardation with microcephaly, unusual facies, genital anomalies in males, and other abnormalities.

Main signs:
1. Primordial growth deficiency (with failure to thrive and frequent vomiting in infancy).
2. Microcephaly (with metopic ridge in some cases).
3. Facies: ptosis, epicanthi, possible strabismus; posteriorly rotated or low-set ears; pug nose with broad tip; small tongue; broad alveolar ridge; micrognathia (3, 4).
4. Hypospadias (9), small penis, possible cryptorchidism or even a clinical appearance of pseudohermaphroditism in males.
5. Syndactyly of the second and third toes (8); abnormal palmar creases (6) and dermatoglyphics. Possible postaxial hexadactyly.
6. Psychomotor retardation of various grades of severity, often considerable, with abnormal muscle tone (2).

Supplementary findings: Possible cataract, prominent lateral palatine ridges (5) or cleft palate (5), abnormally positioned fingers (7), hip dysplasia, cardiac defect, and other severe internal malformations.

Hyperexcitability. Low resistance to infections.

Manifestation: At birth (predominantly breech presentation).

Etiology: Autosomal recessive disorder; very variable interfamilial (not intrafamilial) expression of the gene.

Frequency: Not so very low (1:40,000 has been estimated; about 130 cases known to date).

Comment: The spectrum of the syndrome is very broad. Apparently, especially those cases with hexadactyly, marked genital anomalies, cleft palate, cataract, and severe internal malformations may also show: diverse cardiac anomalies and/or incomplete lobulation of the lungs, gastrointestinal defects such as malrotation, agangliosis of the colon, hypoplasia of the kidneys, or other anomalies.

Course, prognosis: Unfavorable, especially in view of the severity of mental retardation. In severe cases, death in the neonatal period or the first years of life.

Treatment: Symptomatic. Genetic counseling of the parents.

Differential diagnosis: In severe cases, Meckel–Gruber syndrome (p.82) or hydrolethalus syndrome (p.554) should be considered.

Illustrations:
1–9 A 2-year-old child of young healthy parents; pregnancy unremarkable with birth at term, breech presentation (birth measurements unknown). Present measurements: 76 cm; 6.4 kg; 43.5 cm head circumference; all far below the second percentile. Typical facies. Cleft palate. Asymmetry of the nipples. Short first metacarpals; clinodactyly of the second and third fingers with ulnar deviation; cutaneous syndactyly of the second and third toes to the middle phalanges bilaterally, dysplasia of the third toes. Very severe psychomotor impairment, considerable muscular hypotonia and hyperirritability with attacks of dystonia (2). Severe failure to thrive; frequent vomiting. Abnormal EEG. Chromosomal analysis (including banded preparations) normal.

H.-R.W.

References:

Garcia, C.A., McGarry, P.A., Voirol, M. et al. Neurological involvement in the Smith–Lemli–Optiz syndrome . . . *Develop. Med. Child Neurol.*, 15, 48 (1973).

Johnson, V.P. Smith–Lemli–Opitz syndrome: Review . . . *Z. Kinderheilkd.*, 119, 221 (1975).

Fierro, M., Martinez, A.J., Harbison, J.W. et al. Smith–Lemli–Opitz syndrome . . . *Develop. Med. Child Neurol.*, 19, 57 (1977).

Kretzer, F.L., Hittner, H.M., Mehta, R.S. Ocular manifestations of the Smith–Lemli–Opitz syndrome. *Arch. Ophthalmol.*, 99, 2000 (1981).

Lowry, R.B. Variability in the Smith–Lemli–Opitz syndrome . . . *Am. J. Med. Genet.*, 14, 429–433 (1983).

Curry, C.J.R., Carey, J.C. et al. Smith–Lemli–Opitz syndrome, type II . . . *Am. J. Med. Genet.*, 26, 45–47 (1987).

Meinecke, P., Blunck, W. et al. Smith–Lemli–Opitz syndrome. *Am. J. Med. Genet.*, 28, 735–739 (1987).

Optiz, J.M., Penchaszadeh, V.B. et al. Smith–Lemli–Optiz (RSH) syndrome bibliography. *Am. J. Med. Genet.*, 28, 745–750 (1987).

Penchaszadeh, V.B. Thenosology of the Smith–Lemli–Opitz syndrome. *Am. J. Med. Genet.*, 28, 719–721 (1987).

Singer, L.P., Marion, R.W. et al. Limb deficiency in an infant with Smith–Lemli–Opitz syndrome. *Am. J. Med. Genet.*, 32, 380–383 (1989).

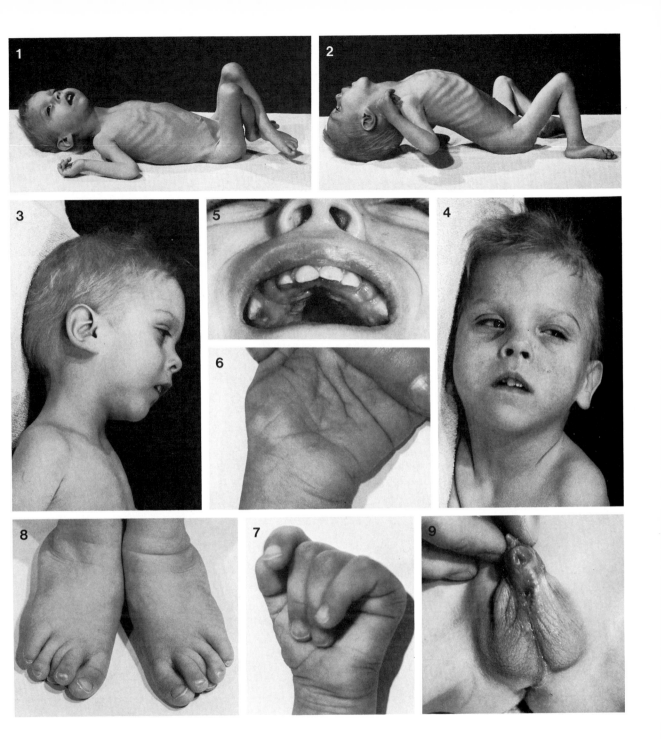

247. Myotubular (Centronuclear) Myopathy

A characteristic syndrome of ophthalmoplegia, ptosis, expressionless face, decrease in muscle mass, moderate to severe muscular hypotonia, severe respiratory disorder, and disorders of swallowing.

Main signs:
1. Ophthalmoplegia, ptosis.
2. Expressionless, 'sleepy' face (myopathic facies).
3. Decreased muscle mass, moderate to severe muscular hypotonia, waddling gait, absent deep-tendon reflexes.
4. Severe postnatal respiratory disorder, hypoplastic lungs, disorder of swallowing. Polyhydramnios.

Supplementary findings: Proptosis, strabismus, mild cataracts. Joint contractures; slender, fragile bones; 'excess skin'. Cryptorchidism. Abnormal type 1 muscle fibers with atrophy, central nucleus, formation of rows of nuclei and perinuclear myofibril-free haloes. Hypertrophy of type 2 muscle fibers. Pathologic electromyogram.

Manifestation: Variable. Postnatal asphyxia is a frequent cause of death. Otherwise onset in childhood. Mild signs and symptoms are often not noted until adulthood (see also under Course, prognosis).

Etiology: Heterogeneity. Autosomal dominant, autosomal recessive, and X-linked recessive inheritance have all been observed. Identification of female carriers by muscle biopsy and electron microscopy?

Frequency: First description in 1960; an increasing number of cases now being recognized.

Course, prognosis: Apparently dependent on the hereditary type. In adult cases, autosomal recessive heterozygotes with ptosis and typical muscle findings may be difficult to differentiate from autosomal dominant cases with variable expression and mild signs and symptoms. X-linked recessive disease is usually manifest at birth with severe asphyxia.

Differential diagnosis: Myotonic dystrophy, mitochondrial myopathy.

Treatment: Physical measures. Genetic counseling.

Illustrations:
1 A 12-year-old male patient. Ptosis, myopathic facies, extreme ophthalmoplegia, muscular hypotonia.

J.K.

References:

Mortier, W.E., Michaelis, E., Becker, J. et al. Centronucleäre Myopathie mit autosomal-dominantem Erbgang. *Humangenetik*, 27, 199–215 (1975).

Pavone, L., Mollica, F., Grasso, A. et al. Familial centronuclear myopathy. *Acta Neurol. Scand.*, 62, 33–40 (1980).

Sarnat, H.B., Roth, S.J., Yimenez, J.F. Neonatal myotubular myopathy: neuropathy and failure of postnatal maturation of fetal muscle. *Can. J. Neurol. Sci.*, 8, 313–320 (1981).

Heckmatt, J.Z., Sewry, C.A., Hodes, D. et al. Congenital centronuclear (myotubular) myopathy. A clinical, pathological, and genetic study in eight children. *Brain*, 108, 941–964 (1985).

Breningstall, G. and Marks, H. Maternal muscle biopsy in severe neonatal centronuclear (myotubular) myopathy. *Am. J. Med. Genet.*, 25, 722–723 (1986).

Bucher, H.U., Boltshauser, E., Briner, J. et al. Severe neonatal centronuclear (myotubular) myopathy: an X-linked recessive disorder. *Helv. Pediatr. Acta*, 41, 291–300 (1986).

Keppen, L.D., Husain, M.M., Woody, R.C. X-linked myotubular myopathy: intrafamilial variability and normal muscle biopsy in a heterozygous female. *Clin. Genet.*, 32, 95–99 (1987).

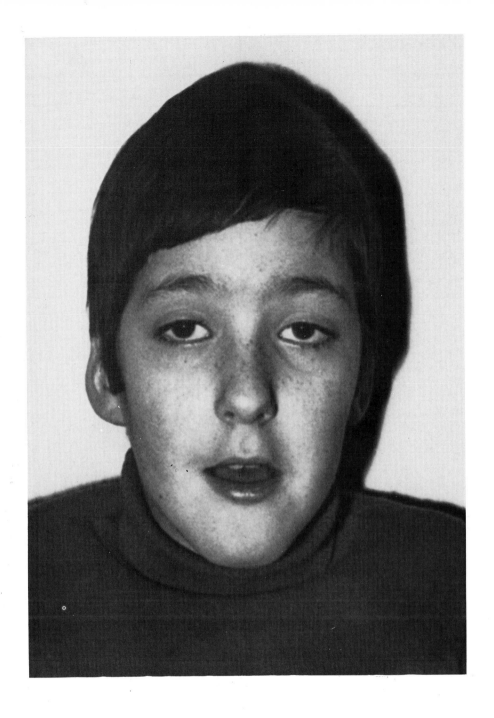

248. Mitochondrial Myopathy

A group of diseases with the characteristics of a primary dysfunction of the central nervous system and/or the musculature as a result of a disorder of oxidative metabolism in the mitochondria.

Main signs:
1. Disorder of CNS function: spinocerebellar degeneration, corticol blindness. Sensorineural hearing loss. Seizures. Psychomotor retardation. Ataxia, choreoathetosis. Hemiparesis. Respiratory disorder, somnolence, apathy. Confusion.
2. External ophthalmoplegia. Pigmented retinopathy, hemianopia, optic atrophy. Peripheral sensory neuropathy.
3. Muscle weakness, muscular hypotonia, fatigability with slow proximal to distal progression. Cardiomyopathy. Macroglossia.
4. Small stature. Microcephaly. Vomiting, headaches.

Supplementary findings: On EEG, generalized, slowing with foci of hypersynchronic activity. EMG with myopathic and neurogenic lesions, but often normal findings. Computerized axial tomography of the skull shows cerebral atrophy, cerebellar atrophy, decreased density of the silent area, dysmyelinization, multiple infarcts, calcification of the basal ganglia.

Muscle biopsy: accumulation of mitochondria at the periphery of the muscle fibers (ragged-red fibers) and/or abnormal mitochondria (abnormal size, unusual structure, paracrystalline inclusions).

In the oral glucose tolerance test, abnormal increase in serum lactate and pyruvate. Similar findings after a 24-hour fasting test.

Manifestation: Onset in childhood of progressive muscular hypotonia and initially obscure central nervous disorders.

Etiology: Biochemical defect of abnormal mitochondria. Usually sporadic cases. Familial cases may be autosomal dominant, autosomal recessive, or X-linked recessive. Since mitochondrial DNA can only be maternally transmitted, a non-hereditary pattern of transmission must be expected. In 30 examined families, maternal transmission occurred 27 times.

Frequency: An increasing number of diagnosed cases.

Course, prognosis: Progressive course; depending on the enzyme defect, lethal outcome possible as early as the newborn period. Also possible that the first manifestations may not occur until adulthood.

Differential diagnosis: Chronic progressive external ophthalmoplegia; Kearns–Sayre syndrome; familial myoclonus epilepsy syndrome with 'ragged-red fibers' (MERRF); mitochondrial myopathy, encephalopathy, lactic acidosis and stroke-like episodes (MELAS); Alpers progressive poliodystrophy; Canavan spongy degeneration of the white matter; Leigh's subacute necrotizing encephalomyopathy; Menkes kinky hair syndrome; and Zellweger cerebro-hepato-renal syndrome.

Treatment: No effective treatment known. With enzyme defects in the pyruvate dehydrogenase complex, a controlled ketogenic diet in isolated cases.

Illustrations:

1a–1c A 15-year-old male patient, progressive external ophthalmoplegia, bilateral abducent weakness, ptosis (tapetoretinal degeneration).

2a and 2b A 14½-year-old male patient, progressive external ophthalmoplegia, ptosis, (pigmented retinopathy).

J.K.

References:

Egger, J. and Wilson, J. Mitochondrial inheritance in a mitochondrially mediated disease. *N. Engl. J. Med.*, 309, 142–146 (1983).
Sengers, R.C.A., Stadhouders, A.M., Trijbels, J.M.F. Mitochondrial myopathies. Clinical, morphological, and biochemical aspects. *Eur. J. Pediatr.*, 141, 192–207 (1984).
Siemes, H. Mitochondriale Myopathien und Encephalomyopathien. Neuromuskuläre und zentralnervöse Erkrankungen infolge von Defekten des mitochondrialen oxydativen Stoffwechsels. *Monatschr. Kinderheilkd.*, 133, 798–805 (1985).
Reichmann, H., Rohkamm, R., Ricker, K. et al. Mitochondriale Myopathien. *Dtsch. Med. Wochenschr.*, 113, 106–113 (1988).
Smeitink, J.A.M., Sengers, R.C.A. et al. Fatal neonatal cardiomyopathy associated with cataract and mitochondrial myopathy. *Eur. J. Pediatr.*, 148, 656–659 (1989).

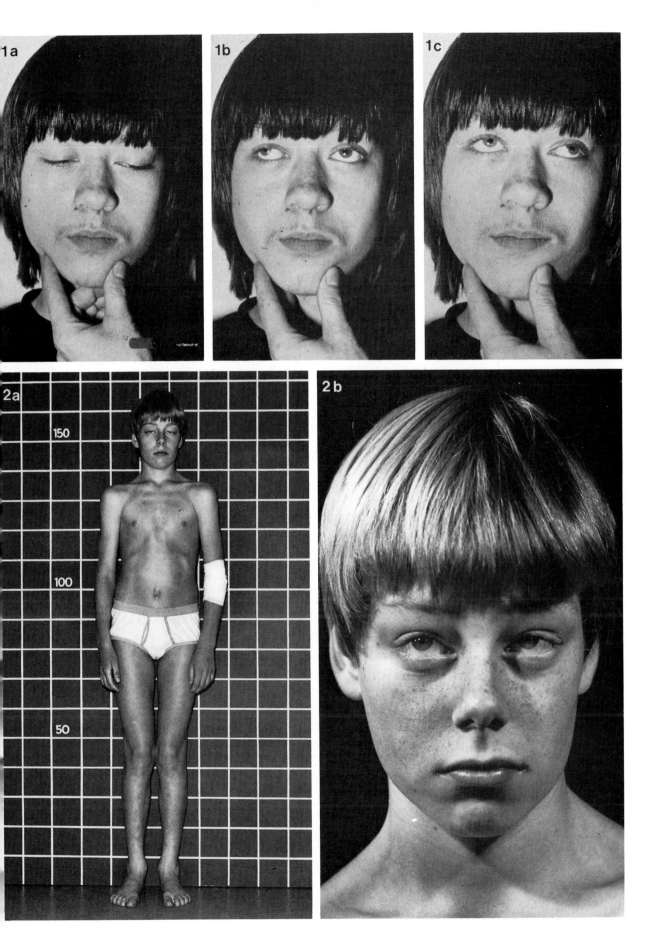

499

249. Kearns–Sayre Syndrome

('Progressive External Ophthalmoplegia Plus')

A mitochondrial encephalomyopathy with chronic, progressive external ophthalmoplegia and further neuromuscular defects, intracardiac conduction defect, tapetoretinal degeneration, and characteristic appearance.

Main signs:

1. Chronic, progressive external ophthalmoplegia (1, 2).
2. Disorders of intracardiac conduction or bundle branch block.
3. Pigmentary degeneration of the retina.
4. Characteristic appearance, especially typical facies (1, 2).

Supplementary findings: Many different defects of the central and peripheral nervous systems: optic atrophy, hearing impairment and vestibular defect, cerebellar ataxia, pareses, and pyramidal signs; myopathy of the proximal skeletal musculature; increased protein and sometimes cell count in the spinal fluid; EEG changes. In some cases, signs of spongy degeneration of the brain on computerized axial tomography.

Not infrequently, poor intellectual development or mental deterioration.

Possible hypogonadism and/or hypoparathyroidism, diabetes mellitus.

Electromyographic evidence of a generalized myopathy; on muscle biopsy characteristic (but non-specific) 'ragged-red fibers' (= special mitochondrial changes with paracrystalline inclusions, which may also be demonstrable in other organs).

Often considerable short stature. This and the lax posture, scant musculature, frequent secondary kyphoscoliosis and/or hyperlordosis, frequent wasting, and typical facies, all contribute to the characteristic general appearance (1, 2).

Manifestation: Possibly as early as the first year of life (ptosis), but onset more frequently toward the end of the first decade of life or later. Progressive external ophthalmoplegia, in some cases facial paresis, high-tone deafness, dysphonia, dysphagia, ataxia, spasticity, mental decline, congestive cardiomyopathy, and other signs.

Etiology: Still not established with certainty. Predominantly sporadic cases have been described, although familial occurrence has also been demonstrated and autosomal dominant inheritance with very variable expression has been suggested. However, other modes of inheritance have also been considered.

Frequency: Not so very low; since the first description well over 100 'complete' (and probably a corresponding number of 'incomplete') cases have been described.

Course, prognosis: Apparently, the more unfavorable, the earlier the onset. Sudden deterioration and (heart or brain stem) death is possible even with the best possible cardiac care.

Comment: The group of mitochondrial encephalomyopathies is not small and includes, among others, Menkes syndrome, mitochondrial myopathy, and Zellweger syndrome.

Treatment: Symptomatic. Careful cardiac follow-up with early, possibly preventative implantation of a pacemaker. Surgical treatment of severe ptosis may be indicated. Hearing assessments. Physiotherapy and orthopedic measures. Hormone replacement if indicated. Coenzyme Q_{10} replacement appears to improve eye mobility, ptosis and, to some extent, ataxia and ECG changes. Genetic counseling.

Illustrations:

1 and 2 A 15¾-year-old girl, the fourth child of healthy parents after three healthy siblings. Primary delay of motor development; bilateral ptosis at 4 years (multiple operations). Total ophthalmoplegia, retinitis pigmentosa, hypoacusis, dysphagia, complete left bundle branch block (preventative implantation of a pacemaker), myopathy especially of the proximal limb musculature, ataxia, short stature under the third percentile, poor intellectual development, muscle wasting.

H.-R.W.

References:

Kearns, T.R. and Sayre, G.P. Retinitis pigmentosa, external ophthalmoplegia and complete heart block. *Arch. Ophthalmol.*, 60, 280 (1958).

Egger, J. and Wilson, J. Mitochondrial inheritance in a mitochondrially mediated disease. *N. Eng. J. Med.*, 309, 142–146 (1983).

Machraoui, A., Breviere, G.M. et al. Syndrome de Kearns familial. *Ann. Pédiatr.*, 32, 701–711 (1985).

Siemes, H. Mitochondriale Myopathien und Encephalomyopathien… *Monatschr. Kinderheilkd.*, 133, 798–805 (1985).

Ogasahara, S., Nishikawa, Y. et al. Treatment of Kearns–Sayre syndrome with coenzyme Q_{10}. *Neurology*, 36, 45–53 (1986).

Kleber, F.X., Park, J.-W. et al. Congestive heart failure… in Kearns–Sayre syndrome. *Klin. Wochenschr.*, 65, 480–486 (1987).

Rowland, L.P., Hausmanowa-Petrusewicz, I. et al. Kearns–Sayre syndrome in twins: lethal dominant mutation or acquired disease? *Neurology*, 38, 1399–1402 (1988).

Zeviani, M., Moraes, C.T. et al. Deletions of mitochondrial DNA in Kearns–Sayre syndrome. *Neurology*, 38, 1339–1346 (1988).

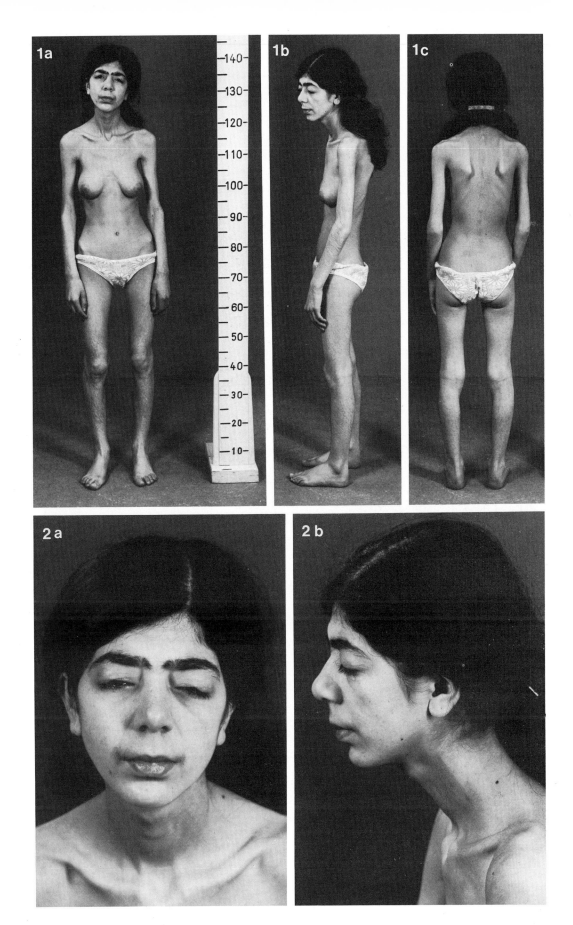

250. Myasthenia Gravis

Myasthenia is characterized by signs of abnormal muscular fatigability after physical exercise with recovery taking several minutes to hours.

Main signs:
1. Neonatal transitory form (10% of cases seen in childhood forms) in 15% of newborns of myasthenic mothers between the first and third days of life: generalized muscular hypotonia, decreased movements, weak sucking, difficulties swallowing, ptosis.
2. Neonatal persisting form (20% of childhood cases), the same signs as above, but persisting.
3. Juvenile myasthenia, the most frequent form in childhood, usually occurs after the tenth year of life. Girls:boys = 6:1. First signs usually postinfectious with uni- or bilateral ptosis. Occasionally also generalized with ophthalmoplegia and weakness of facial and limb musculature. Persistence of features until the fourth to sixth decade of life.

Supplementary findings: Myasthenic crises can be life-threatening with infections, stress, or surgery.

Manifestation:
1. The first form, at birth.
2. The second form, before the second year of life.
3. The third form, after age 10 years.

Etiology: The result of autoimmune reactions against muscle acetylcholine receptors. Other immunological disorders may also be present. Hyperplasia of the thymus, thymomas, lupus erythematosus. The demonstration of an association between HLAB8 and myasthenia gravis indicates genetic factors. In familial cases, siblings frequently affected. The rare infantile familial forms show severe respiratory distress and recurrent apneic episodes, and are probably transmitted by autosomal dominant inheritance.

Frequency: 1:15,000–1:200,000, worldwide. Familial cases rare; usually sporadic occurrence.

Course, prognosis: The neonatal transitory form (in children of myasthenic mothers) may lead to death within hours or days *post partum* if untreated. The persisting myasthenia of newborns (with healthy mothers) has a good prognosis for life once diagnosed. With the juvenile form, intervening crises must be anticipated.

Differential diagnosis: Myasthenic syndrome with disorders of thyroid function and lupus erythematosus.

Treatment:
1. Thymectomy in patients who do not respond well to cholinesterase inhibitors.
2. Cholinesterase inhibitor pyridostigmine bromide (Mestinon).
3. Immunosuppressive therapy with prednisone.
(Avoid: tranquilizers, barbiturates, narcotics, local anesthetics, antiarrhythmic agents, and certain antibiotics, including tetracycline, neomycin, colistin, lincomycin.)

Illustrations:
1a and 2a A 9½-year-old patient with recent onset of ocular myasthenia (ptosis of the upper lids, double vision).
1b and 2b The same girl immediately after intravenous administration of 10 mg edrophonium chloride (Tensilon).

J.K.

References:
Gordon, N. Congenital myasthenia. *Develop. Med. Child Neurol.*, 28, 803–813 (1986).
Haas, J. Myasthenia gravis. Aktuelle Therapie unter pathophysiologischen Aspekten. *Dtsch. Ärztebl.*, 85, C-114–C-118 (1988).
Otherwise, any pediatric or internal medicine textbook.

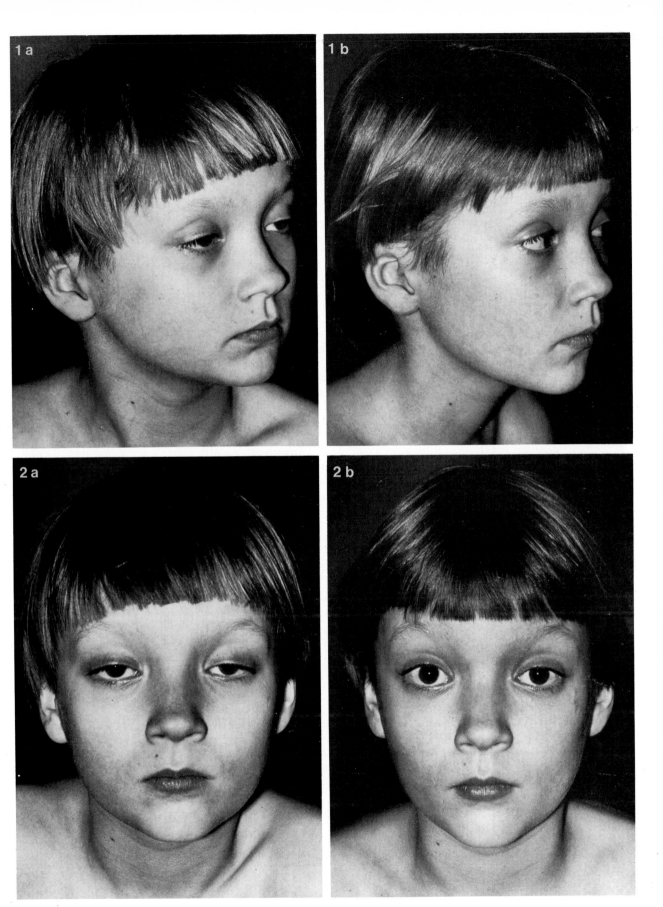

503

251. Myotonic Dystrophy Curschmann–Steinert

An autosomal dominant disorder with severe myotonic signs in newborns, transmitted by mildly affected mothers.

Main signs:
1. Neonatal form: Severe generalized muscular hypotonia with symmetric weakness of the limb muscles, triangular open ('tent-shaped') mouth and ptosis (facial diplegia). Initially, good deep-tendon reflexes. Frequently disorders of sucking, swallowing, and respiration, often life-threatening, during the first days to weeks. Global development delay common.
2. Adult form: myotonic facies, localized muscle atrophy, cataract, frontal baldness. Characteristic inability to 'bury the eyelashes' by tightly closing the lids.

Supplementary findings:
1. Neonatal form: mother with myotonic dystrophy (usually only mild signs). Frequent pes equinovarus; high palate and other minor signs. Possible edema, tendency to bleed into the skin, liver, brain. Enlarged cerebral ventricles.
2. Adult form: hollow temples, myotonic reaction on thenar percussion, rapid fatigability with repeated clenching of the fist (recuperation pauses when typewriting). Endocrinopathies. In 65% of patients, cardiac involvement. Decreased fertility in both males and females (small testes with progressive involution of the seminiferous tubules; menstrual disorders). High-risk patients for anesthesia.

Manifestation: At birth for the neonatal form—frequently after weak fetal movements during pregnancy and often with hydramnios.

Etiology: Autosomal dominant disorder. Mildly affected mothers have to expect a high risk with their children; 12% stillbirths or neonatal deaths, 9% severely affected (survival), 29% affected later. Affected fathers rarely have children with the severe neonatal form. Intrafamilial variability. New mutations very rare. Always search for affected parents (mothers), especially with severely affected newborns. Gene localized to chromosome 19.

Frequency: Differs with geographic location. Estimated 1:20,000–40,000. In Switzerland, 50 affected per 1 million general population. Estimated mutation rate 1.3×10^{-5}.

Course, prognosis: Up to 50% neonatal mortality from severe respiratory insufficiency. Subsequently muscle weakness in early childhood is barely or not progressive and myotonia scarcely or not noticeable. Motor development delayed, but the patients usually learn to walk. In later years, increasing muscle weakness and atrophy, especially in the face (flaccid, expressionless myotonic facies with open mouth), the neck (sternocleidomastoids), the distal extremities (e.g., extensors of the hands and fingers, levators of the feet), and other areas. Usually impaired articulation. Deep reflexes often reduced, moderate myotonic signs present. The endocrine features and cataracts of the adult form are not present in the first decade of life. Poor long-term prognosis: little hope of an independent existence (mental retardation, increasing muscular atrophy). In adulthood, progressive cataracts; early death from pulmonary infections or cardiac arrhythmia.

Diagnosis: In the neonate, only a clinical diagnosis possible. Close examination of the parents—inability to 'bury' the eyelashes, as mentioned above, is an unfailing sign even in those (at least 15%) not previously recognized as affected. Slit-lamp examination of the lenses (cataract) and muscle biopsy frequently confirm the diagnosis in adults. Frequent myopathic EMG. Creatine kinase often normal (with slight elevation, especially critical evaluation).

Differential diagnosis: In the newborn period, the various causes of 'floppy infants': cerebral anoxia, trauma, medication, neonatal myasthenia, Prader–Willi syndrome. Werdnig–Hoffmann, and many more.

Treatment: Difficult ethical problem in severely ill neonates with respiratory insufficiency. Genetic counseling. Molecular genetic diagnosis and prenatal diagnosis possible in informative families.

Illustrations:
1–3 Female first-born with the congenital form; in 1, as a neonate; in 2 and 3, at 4 weeks. The mother, her brother and father: myotonic dystrophy.
4 A woman, previously not known to be affected, and her typically affected newborn; the mother was unable, on request, to 'bury' her eyelashes.
5 Father and son; neither able to close his eyes tightly.

J.K./H.-R.W.

References:
Glanz, A. and Fraser, F.C. Risk ... myotonic dystrophy. *J. Med. Genet.*, 21, 186 (1984).
Rutherford, M.A. et al. Congenital myotonic dystrophy. *Arch. Dis. Child.*, 64, 191 (1989).

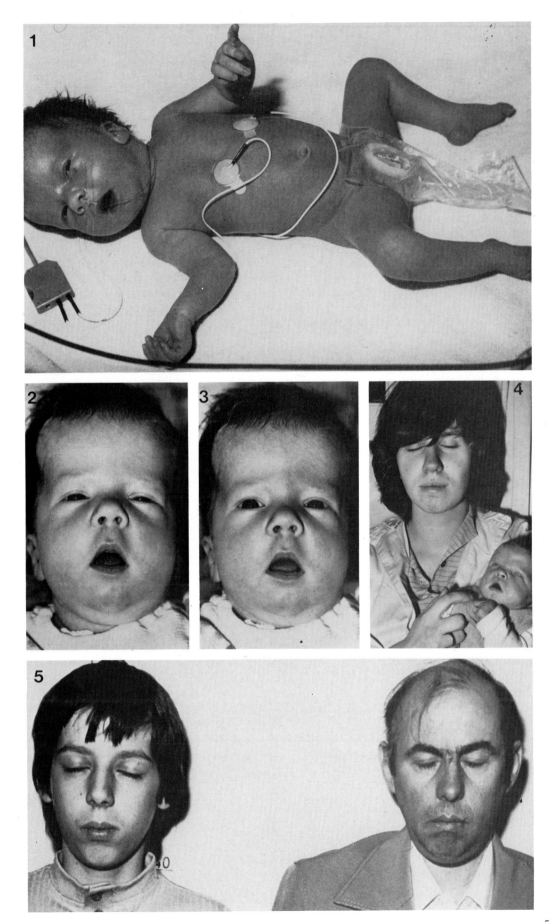

505

252. Myotonia Congenita, Becker Type

An autosomal recessive myotonia causing increasing clinical handicap and associated with distinct muscular hypertrophy.

Main signs:
1. A strong or sudden stimuli elicit a state of tonic contraction of the innervated striated muscles (especially in the extremities, but also the external eye muscles, etc.), the rigidity resolving only after a few seconds, becoming less, and finally no longer occurring when the movement is carried out repeatedly. Onset of symptoms in the legs, then the hands and arms, later the throat and masticatory muscles, etc., becoming generalized by adulthood.
2. Distinct hypertrophy of the musculature (1–3) without increase in general strength.
3. Limited dorsiflexion of the hands and feet.

Supplementary findings: Reflexes and sensation normal. Diagnostically, the patient cannot open his fist immediately after (on request) clenching it suddenly and forcefully, tapping the thenar eminence, tongue, or biceps briefly with a reflex hammer elicits a persisting contraction depression as a myotonic reaction; characteristic myotonic pattern on EMG.

Manifestation: Usually between the fourth and twelfth years of life; in males, possibly later.

Etiology: Autosomal recessive disorder.

Frequency: About 1:50,000.

Course, prognosis: A generalized progressive disorder leading to increasing weakness and atrophy of the musculature.

Differential diagnosis: In autosomal dominant myotonia congenita Thomsen type, pronounced muscle hypertrophy is an exception; the disorder runs a milder course and usually does not cause the individual to seek medical help.

Treatment: Protection from cold; avoidance of a high-calcium diet. In cases with particular complaints due to the myotonic reaction, treatment may be initiated with quinidine sulfate or procainamide, among other possibilities. Genetic counseling.

Illustrations:
1–3 A 12½-year-old boy, mentally normal, from a healthy family. Myotonia, manifest since age 8 years, was initially limited to his lower extremities (at first, disturbance of gait; difficulties with starts in sports), and is now generalized, including involvement of m. levator palpebrae and m. orbicularis oculi. Pronounced muscle hypertrophy and slightly reduced general strength. A myotonic reaction can be elicited mechanically on the tongue and thenar eminences; characteristic EMG findings.

H.-R.W.

References:
Any comprehensive pediatric, internal medicine, or neurology textbook.
Zellweger, H., Pavone, L., Biondi, A. et al. Autosomal recessive generalized myotonia. *Muscle Nerve*, 3, 176 (1980).
Sun, S.F. and Streib, E.W. Autosomal recessive generalized myotonia. *Muscle Nerve*, 6, 143–148 (1983).
Editorial: Treatment of myotonia. *Lancet*, I, 1242–1244 (1987).

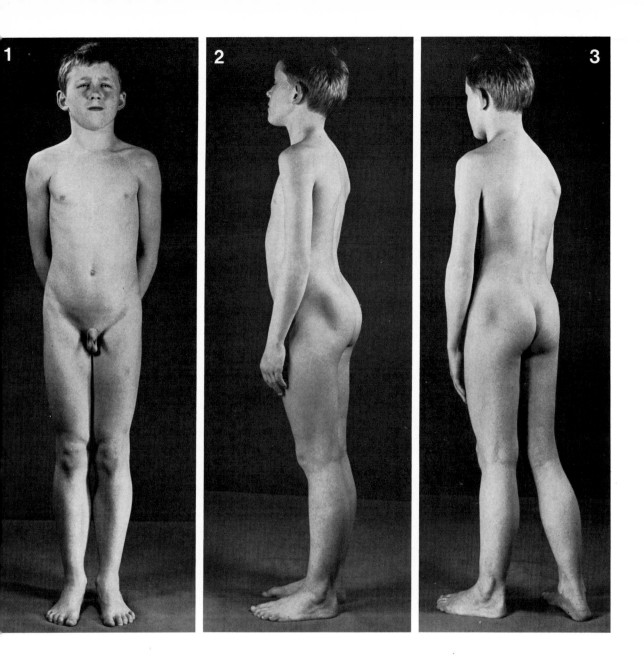

253. Catel–Schwartz–Jampel Syndrome

(Chondrodystrophic Myotonia)

A characteristic hereditary disorder with postnatal development of myotonic signs, typical facies, growth retardation, and osteoarticular changes.

Main signs:
1. Flat, full-cheeked face, which appears small in relation to the normal-sized cranium, small-appearing mouth, small chin, and fixed expression. Eyes appear deep set; narrow palpebral fissures (possibly with slight antimongoloid slant) as a result of blepharospasm of variable severity. Tightly closed, puckered mouth which is difficult to open. The facial expression may be described as 'a frozen smile', but also 'sad' or 'as when crying' and rarely relaxes.
2. Increasing growth retardation of intrauterine onset; linear growth often below the third percentile. 'Truncal dwarfism', i.e., a short trunk with relatively overlong extremities (3, 4).
3. Poor motor function, rapid fatigability due to 'stiffness' of the palpably firm, sometimes hypertrophic musculature of the trunk and extremities. (Myotonic reaction usually readily elicited on the thenar eminences.) Early flexion contractures of most large joints; corresponding gait and posture. Hyporeflexia.
4. Early onset of pain, especially in the legs. On X-ray, dysplasia especially of the femoral head (6); all in all a picture of moderately severe spondyloepimetaphyseal dysplasia. Osteoporosis.

Supplementary findings: Horizontal wrinkling of the brow and raised eyebrows due to the contracted facial musculature. Large, low-set ears (2). Possible distichiasis; ptosis in some cases; frequent, possibly severe myopia. Alae nasi sometimes hypoplastic; high palate; possible dimpled chin. High nasal voice (occasionally stridor).

Short neck; elevated shoulders (3); pectus carinatum; increased dorsal kyphosis and lumbar lordosis; scoliosis also. Possibly retarded bone age.

Myotonia on EMG. No biochemical abnormalities. Mental development normal in 80% of cases.

Manifestation: Slowing of growth and motor development, facial changes and motor impairment usually become distinct in the second year of life or later; onset of pain and rapid fatigability at about the same time. Manifestation at birth (to date, 8 observations) or in infancy is unusual.

Etiology: Autosomal recessive disorder with very variable expression. Basic defect unknown.

Frequency: Low; about 60 cases described up to 1987.

Course, prognosis: Life expectancy apparently not affected. The myotonic manifestations may remain stationary soon after appearing in early childhood; motor function may improve. However, further slow progression over years is also possible.

Diagnosis, differential diagnosis: Growth retardation and conspicuous osteoarticular signs with 'peculiar facies' may so dominate the clinical picture that the myotonia and, thus, the diagnosis are overlooked. Myotonia must be confirmed electromyographically.

The Freeman–Sheldon syndrome (p.46) shows considerable overlap with this syndrome. However, the former, present at birth, does not show multiple bony dysplasias or a myotonic EMG, and as a rule is transmitted by autosomal dominant inheritance.

Easily delineated from myotonia congenita (p.506), paramyotonia, and myotonic dystrophy (p.504).

Treatment: Antimyotonic agents are apparently ineffective. Remedial orthopedic measures; ophthalmological attention; psychological care. Increased risk with anesthesia. Genetic counseling. Prenatal diagnosis.

Illustrations:
1–5 A boy as a toddler, before the characteristic facies were distinctly manifest (1), and at 6½ years, with the full clinical picture (2–5; on his back, a pigmented nevus).
6 Typical hip findings in this boy. The first child of healthy parents. Disorder manifest at age 2 years (eyes closed slowly). Smooth, shiny facial skin with taut musculature. Blepharophimosis right > left; marked difficulty in opening his contracted, snout-like mouth. High narrow palate. Stiffness, impaired mobility, and contractures; leg pain. Typical EMG findings. Small stature. Normal intellect. Some improvement of function later.

H.-R.W.

References:
Rütt, A. Ein Beitrag zum Krankheitsbild der Chondrodystrophia tarda. Z. Orthop., 83, 609 (1953).
Seay, A.R. et al. Malignant hyperpyrexia in ... Schwartz–Jampel syndrome. J. Pediatr., 93, 83 (1983).
Farrell, S.A. et al. Neonatal Schwartz–Jampel syndrome. Am. J. Med. Genet., 27, 799–805 (1987).
Hunziker, U.A. et al. Prenatal diagnosis ... Prenat. Diag., 9, 127 (1989).

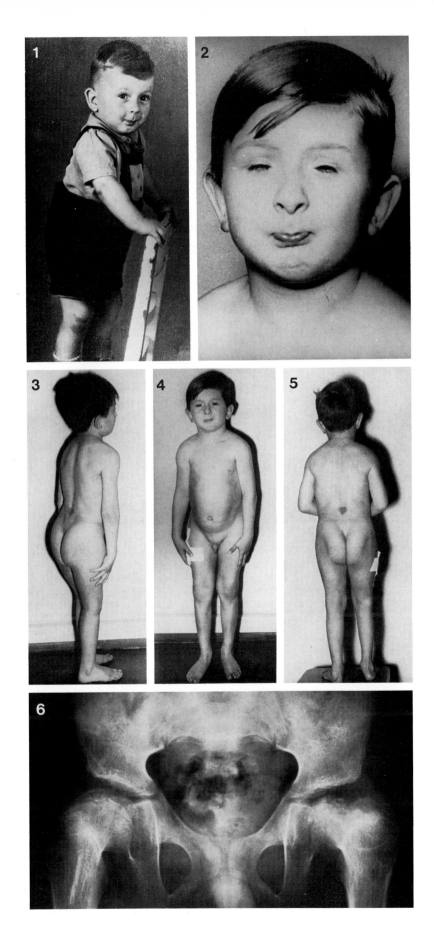

254. Syndrome of Blepharophimosis, Pterygium Colli, Flexion Contractures of the Fingers and Toes, and Osteodysplasia

A syndrome of unusual facies, short neck with mild pterygium, development of flexion contractures of fingers and toes, and of spondyloepiphyseal dysplasia.

Main signs:
1. Facies: round with blepharophimosis, broad nasal root, epicanthus and small mouth with very narrow prolabium (1). 'A congenital strabismus syndrome of microstrabismus convergens with bilateral dissociated vertical squint and rotary nystagmus'. Left-sided amblyopia.
2. Short neck; nuchal hairline somewhat low; slight pterygium colli (1, 2).
3. Flexion contractures of the—very long—second to fifth fingers bilaterally, especially of the proximal interphalangeal joints, and of all toes (3, 4) with subluxation of the distal joints of the second to fifth bilaterally.
4. Somewhat small stature (around the tenth percentile) with the extremities being relatively too long. Dysgenesis of vertebral bodies and epiphyses (5), see below.

Supplementary findings: Freely mobile large joints. Winging of the scapulae. Mild pectus carinatum; S-form scoliosis. Genu valgum. Flat feet.

On X-ray, slight flattening of the vertebral bodies dorsally, causing slightly ovoid configuration. Flattening of both femoral heads with both irregularly honeycombed and markedly sclerotic changes, left > right (5), both resembling the changes seen in Perthes disease. Coxa vara. Slight flattening of the epiphyses of the knee joints; somewhat plaque-like structure of the patellae. Varus deformity of the toes bilaterally (6).

Normal intellectual development. No evidence of a neurological or muscular disorder. Normal biochemical findings. Normal female karyotype.

Manifestation: Partly at birth (facies); partly later in infancy and early childhood (flexion contractures of fingers and toes; osteodysplasia).

Etiology: Not clear. Genetic basis assumed. (The unusual appearance with narrow palpebral fissures and narrow lips is also present in the child's mother and maternal grandfather; on the other hand the deceased paternal grandmother and her mother are said to have suffered from severely twisted toes. The child's father is quite unremarkable.)

Comment: The clinical picture presented here shows certain similarities to disorders as diverse as arthro-ophthalmopathy (Stickler syndrome, p.532), chondrodystrophic myotonia (Schwartz–Jampel syndrome, p.508), and Ullrich–Turner syndrome (p.192), none of which is present here.

Illustrations:
1–6 The proband at 9 years. The second child of young, healthy, nonconsanguineous parents; older brother unremarkable. Birth and early development unremarkable. Later in early childhood, manifestation of finger and toe contractures, which have not progressed since then and do not handicap the patient. At about the same time, clinical manifestation of hips dysplasia—especially on the left—with pain in the left leg, which tired easily and which she favored. Subsequent surgery of the hip joint by bilateral intertrochanteric osteotomy with realignment. Patient now free of pain.

H.-R.W.

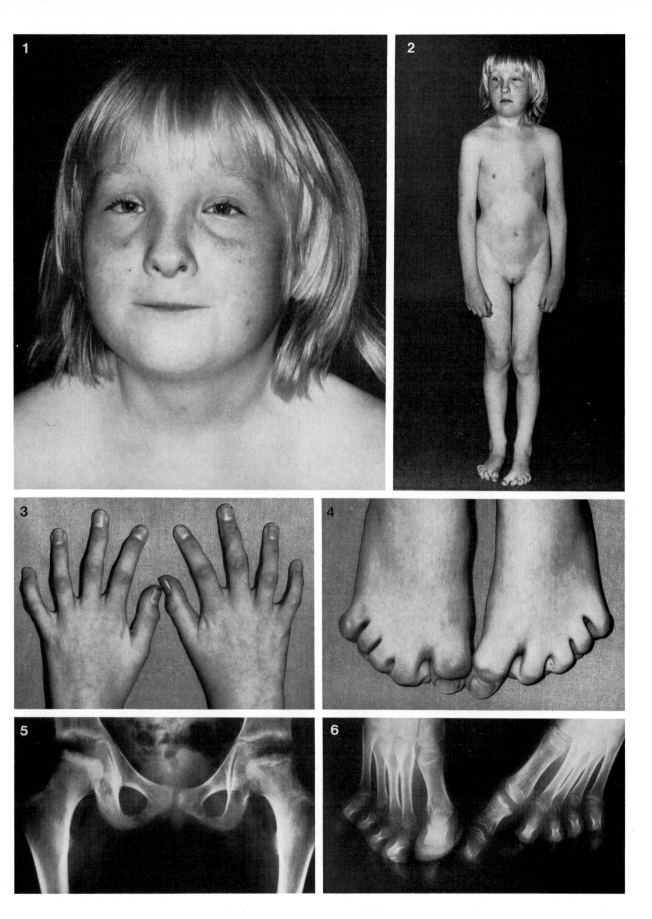

255. Lowe Syndrome

(Oculo-Cerebro-Renal Syndrome)

An X-linked recessive syndrome with congenital cataract, muscular hypotonia, areflexia, severe psychomotor retardation, tubular proteinuria, and aminoaciduria.

Main signs:
1. Male patients. Bilateral central cataracts, occasionally with glaucoma, buphthalmos, corneal clouding, enophthalmos.
2. Severe progressive psychomotor retardation; disturbance of growth; high shrill cry.
3. Muscular hypotonia, areflexia; myopathic electromyogram.
4. Tubular proteinuria, aminoaciduria.

Supplementary findings: Prominent forehead, thin hair, pale skin. Adiposity in the first year of life, later wasting. Cryptorchidism. Hyperphosphaturia with hypophosphatemic rickets; metabolic acidosis, intermittent glycosuria. Often constant low-grade fever. Elevated creatine kinase values.

Manifestation: Eye signs and muscular hypotonia at birth. Later, distinct motor and intellectual deterioration.

Etiology: X-linked recessive disorder. Female carriers may show cataracts or corneal clouding on slit-lamp examination.

Frequency: More than 100 cases have been described.

Course, prognosis: Most patients die in childhood, in the first decade. Few, severely handicapped, attain adulthood.

Treatment: Correction of eye anomalies, of acidosis, of hypophosphatemia, and of rickets.

Differential diagnosis: Zellweger cerebro-hepatorenal syndrome.

Illustrations:
1 A 6-year-old boy; enophthalmos on the left, corneal clouding on the right.
2 A 17-year-old; bilateral corneal clouding.

J.K.

References:

Abassi, V., Lowe, C.U., Calcagno, P.L. Oculo-cerebro-renal syndrome. A review. *Am. J. Dis. Child.*, 115, 145 (1968).
Pallisgaard, G. and Goldschmidt, E. The oculo-cerebro-renal syndrome of Lowe in four generations of one family. *Acta Pediatr. Scand.*, 60, 146–148 (1971).
Gardner, R.J.M. and Brown, N. Lowe's syndrome: identification of carriers by lens examination. *J. Med. Genet.*, 13, 449–454 (1976).
Hanefeld, F., Stephani, U., Lennert, T. et al. Congenitale Myopathie bei Kindern mit Lowe-Syndrom. In: *Fortschritte der Myologie*, vol. VI, 63–66 (1981). 'Deutsche Gesellschaft für Bekampfung der Muskelkrankheiten e.V.', Freiburg.
Tripathi, R.C., Cibis, G.W., Harris, D.J. et al. Lowe's syndrome. *Birth Defects*, 18, no. 6, 629–644 (1982).
Kownatzki, R. Das okulo-zerebro-renale Syndrom (Lowe-Syndrom). *Pädiatr. Prax.*, 32, 511–519 (1985/86).
Hodgson, S.V., Heckmatt, J.Z., Hughes, E. et al. A balanced de novo X/autosome translocation in a girl with manifestations of Lowe syndrome. *Am. J. Med. Genet.*, 23, 837–847 (1986).

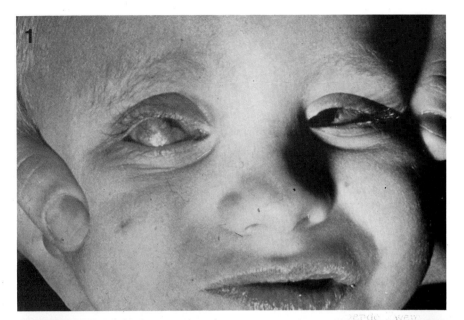

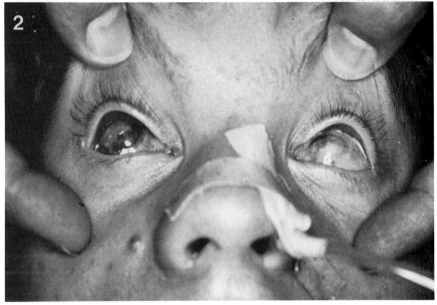

256. Zellweger Syndrome

(Cerebro-Hepato-Renal Syndrome)

An autosomal recessive, metabolic dysplasia syndrome with characteristic facies, extreme muscular hypotonia, hepatomegaly, practically absent psychomotor development, and usually early death.

Main signs:
1. Characteristic facies with high forehead, increased interocular distance, flat nasal root, possible slight mongoloid slant of the palpebral fissures and epicanthi, anteverted nares, dysplastic helices, 'full' cheeks, and micrognathia. Wide-open fontanelles and cranial sutures, persisting frontal suture; high palate (**1, 3**).
2. Extreme muscular hypotonia (**4**) with absence of deep-tendon reflexes and weak sucking and swallowing reflexes. Cerebral seizures.
3. Extremely little psychomotor development. Deafness.
4. Hepatomegaly (fibrosis, cirrhosis), occasionally also splenomegaly, liver function disorders, gastrointestinal bleeding.
5. Retarded growth.

Supplementary findings: Corneal clouding, glaucoma, cataract, nystagmus, pallor of the optic discs, retinal changes.

Cubitus valgus, contractures of the finger joints, simian crease; club feet, clitoral hypertrophy or cryptorchidism, hypospadias.

Renal cortical cysts, albuminuria, aminoaciduria. Cardiovascular anomalies.

Speckled calcifications of the skeleton (**2**), similar to those in chondrodysplasia punctata (p.220).

Anomalies of the central nervous system.

Frequently, elevated serum iron and copper levels, siderosis of the reticuloendothelial system. Elevated serum levels of long-chain fatty acids and of pipecolic and other acids, and further abnormal biochemical characteristics.

Manifestation: At birth (hepatomegaly usually later).

Etiology: Autosomal recessive disorder; peroxisomal enzyme defect ('peroxisomopathy').

Frequency: Not so very low: over 130 cases since the first case was described in 1964. Estimated: 1:50,000 newborns.

Course, prognosis: Death usually within the first half-year of life. (Apparently, elevated serum iron levels and siderosis of the reticuloendothelial system are more likely to be demonstrated in the younger patients, while fibrosis and cirrhosis of the liver are found primarily in the somewhat older patients.) Occurrence also of a milder variant.

Treatment: Treatment by diet still in the experimental stage. Genetic counseling; prenatal diagnosis possible.

Illustrations:
1–4 A female patient, death at age 6 months. Serum iron levels markedly elevated on several occasions in the first months of life; on follow-up at age 6 months, normal. The initially, markedly elevated transaminases also showed a tendency to decrease with increasing age. Hypoprothrombinemia, no icterus. Cerebral seizures. No psychomotor development. At autopsy: arhinencephalia, moderate hydrocephaly; liver fibrosis; renal cortical cysts.

H.-R.W./J.K.

References:

Danks, D.M., Tipett, P., Adams, C. et al. Cerebro-hepato-renal syndrome of Zellweger; a report of 8 cases with comments upon the incidence, the liver lesions and a fault in pipecolic acid metabolism. *J. Pediatr.*, 86, 382 (1975).

Gilchrist, K.W., Gilbert, E.F., Goldfarb, S. et al. Studies of malformation syndromes of man XI B: the cerebro-hepato-renal syndrome of Zellweger: comparative pathology. *Z. Kinderheilkd.*, 121, 99 (1976).

Hittner, H.M. and Kretzer, F.L. Zellweger syndrome. Lenticular opacities indicating carrier status... *Arch. Ophthalmol.*, 99, 1977 (1981).

Schutgens, R.B.H., Heymans, H.S.A. et al. Prenatal detection of Zellweger syndrome. *Lancet*, II, 1339–1340 (1984).

Koch, M. and Wolf, H. Zellweger syndrome... Klinik, Morphologie und biochemische Diagnostik. *Klin. Pädiatr.*, 197, 492–497 (1985).

Bleeker-Wagemaker, E.M., Oorthuys, J.W.E. et al. Long-term survival of a patient with the cerebro-hepato-renal... syndrome. *Clin. Genet.*, 29, 160–164 (1986).

Wilson, G.N., Holmes, R.G. et al. Zellweger syndrome: diagnostic assays, syndrome delineation, and potential therapy. *Am. J. Med. Genet.*, 24, 69–82 (1986).

Zellweger, H. The cerebro-hepato-renal syndrome... *Develop. Med. Child Neurol.*, 29, 821–829 (1987).

Stephenson, J.B.P. Inherited peroxisomal disorders involving the nervous system. *Arch. Dis. Child.*, 63, 767–770 (1988).

Wilson, G.N., Holmes, R.D. et al. Peroxisomal disorders... *Am. J. Med. Genet.*, 30, 771–792 (1988).

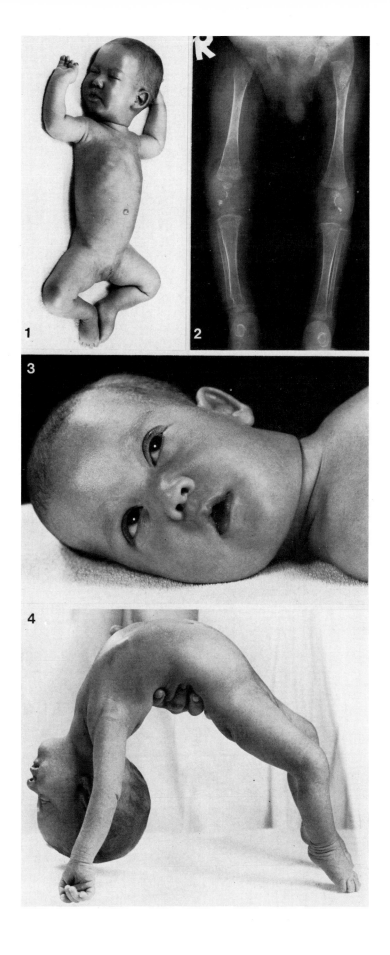

257. Werdnig–Hoffmann Spinal Muscular Atrophy

(Acute to Subacute Infantile Type of Progressive Spinal Muscular Atrophy)

A characteristic picture with onset of progressive muscular hypotonia and atrophy in infancy; loss of tendon reflexes; and appearance of further signs of denervation; with intelligence, sensorium, sensation, and sphincter function remaining unaffected.

Main signs:
1. Symmetrical hypotonia, weakness, and decreased movements, at first of the pelvic and leg muscles, then of all other major muscle regions. Lower extremities externally rotated, flaccid; upper extremities abducted, flaccid, 'handle' appearance. Almost exclusively diaphragmatic breathing; long narrow bell-shaped thorax. Little facial expression (1–3).
2. Disappearance of tendon reflexes. Sensorium intact; absence of pain. Sensation, sphincter function, and intelligence unaffected.
3. Muscle fasciculation (most readily recognized in the tongue; 5).

Supplementary findings: Abundant fatty infiltrations.
Development of contractures of the large joints, kyphoscoliosis, deformity of the thorax (4).
Neurogenic atrophy pattern on EMG.

Manifestation: During infancy. In some cases, the mother may note weak or gradual decrease of fetal movements, and the diagnosis can be established immediately after birth.

Etiology: Autosomal recessive disorder.

Frequency: Not particularly low.

Course, prognosis: Unfavorable. Death not infrequently in infancy, otherwise usually within the first years of life, often after the onset of signs of bulbar paralysis, leading to hypostatic or aspiration pneumonia. Occasional patients survive longer, eventually becoming completely paralyzed (4).

Differential diagnosis: Congenital, early form of myotonic dystrophy (p.504), Prader–Willi syndrome (p.286), Zellweger syndrome (p.514).

Treatment: Symptomatic: care by a physiotherapist; prevention of contractures. High-protein diet; prevention of obesity. Protection against infections. Intellectual stimulation. Psychological guidance. Genetic counseling.

Illustrations:
1–3 Patient 1, almost 4 months old: at 4 weeks, rapidly progressive muscle weakness and paralysis noted. Exclusively diaphragmatic respiration; thorax deformity. Contractures of the knee and hip joints. Generalized areflexia. Complete degeneration reaction. Little facial expression. Mental development normal. Soon thereafter, death from respiratory paralysis. Diagnosis confirmed histopathologically. A similarly affected sibling died at age 2 months.
4 and 5 Patient 2 at 8 and almost 11 years. Diagnosed clinically and by muscle biopsy in infancy. With optimal care, survival of multiple episodes of pneumonia. Extreme muscle atrophy, pectus excavatum, kyphoscoliosis, joint contractures; absolutely no head control; little facial expression; intellectual responses normal for age. Signs of denervation. Puffy deformity of the tongue with marked fasciculations.

H.-R.W.

References:
Any pediatric book.

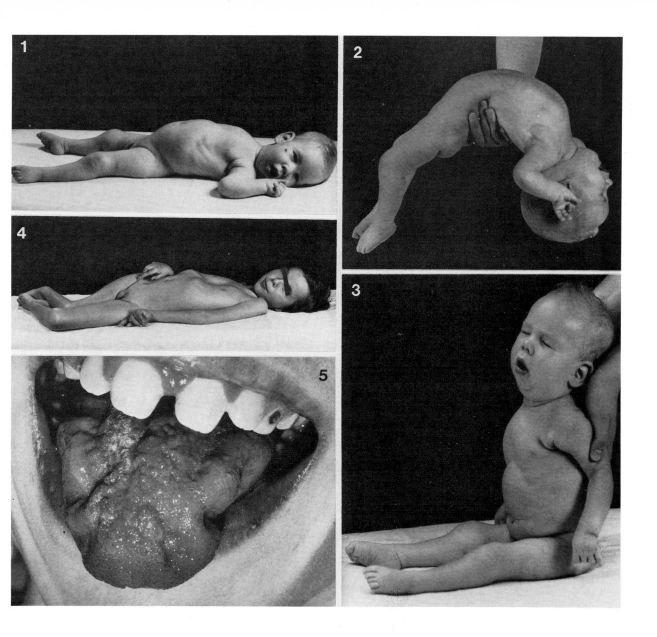

258. Duchenne Muscular Dystrophy

(Infantile Progressive Muscular Dystrophy of the Duchenne Pseudohypertrophic Type)

A characteristic hereditary syndrome in males, with onset in childhood of 'ascending' muscle atrophy beginning in the pelvis and thigh regions, at first obscured by fatty infiltration, and associated with a corresponding progressive decrease in performance (with simultaneous slowing of mental development in about one-third of cases).

Main signs:
1. After learning to walk, often poorly and with delay (with frequent falling), development of a rocking, weaving, or waddling gait; difficulty getting up from the floor, eventually 'climbing up himself' (Gower's sign; **1**).
2. Hyperlordosis with protruding abdomen (**1c, 3**). Broad-based stance (**1–3**). Prominent, 'loose' shoulders (**2, 3a**).
3. Pseudohypertrophy (fatty infiltration) especially of the calves, also of the thigh and buttock musculature (**1–3**), less frequently of other muscle regions.
4. Ascending degeneration of the musculature starting at the pelvic girdle and thighs, clinically involving the rest of the trunk, then the shoulder girdle, upper arm, and other regions. Tendency for contractures to develop, especially in the legs: relatively early tendency to develop talipes equinus and toe-walking.
5. Mental retardation in about 30% of the children.

Supplementary findings: Absence of unusual pain, disordered sensation, or denervation phenomena. Gradual weakening and eventual loss of tendon reflexes. Myocardial involvement frequently demonstrable on ECG.

Small stature. Frequent development of scoliosis; coxa valga. Secondary obesity not unusual.

Markedly increased serum creatine phosphokinase (also of some other enzyme activities to a lesser degree), especially in the initial stages of the process.

Manifestation: The first few years of life.

Etiology: X-linked recessive disorder; thus, almost exclusively boys affected. About one-third represent new mutations. Genetic defect in the short arm of the X chromosome (X p21).

Frequency: Not so very low (at least 1 in 4,000 male newborns).

Course, prognosis: Relentless progression. Invalidism (wheelchair) usually about the end of the first decade of life, and death in the course of the second.

Differential diagnosis: Other conditions in the large group of muscular dystrophies and other types of diseases ('pseudomyopathic') are usually not difficult to exclude by careful observation of onset, clinical picture, and course; in cases of doubt, EMG, enzyme, and possibly muscle biopsy findings should make differentiation possible.

Treatment: Improvement and conservation of physical mobility to the limits of possibility. Physiotherapy, swimming, prevention of contractures, avoidance of any unnecessary bed confinement or inactivity. Promotion of intellect and social contacts. Psychological guidance. Identification of female carriers possible by enzyme determination and other clinical methods; more recently by direct or indirect demonstration of the deletion. Prenatal diagnosis for such a 'carrier' during pregnancy.

Illustrations:

1–3 Three typically affected patients, aged 6, 7½, and 8 years, showing pseudohypertrophy, Gower's sign (**1**), hyperlordosis, winging of the scapulae, waddling gait, inability to climb stairs. Mental retardation in two of the boys.

H.-R.W.

References:

Stern, L.M., Caudrey, D.J. et al. Carrier detection in Duchenne muscular dystrophy using computed tomography. *Clin. Genet.*, 27, 392–397 (1985).

Hejtmancik, J.F., Harris, S.G. et al. Carrier diagnosis of Duchenne muscular dystrophy using restriction fragment length polymorphisms. *Neurology*, 36, 1553–1562 (1986).

Rabbi-Bortolini, E. and Zatz, M. Investigation on genetic heterogeneity in Duchenne muscular dystrophy. *Am. J. Med. Genet.*, 24, 111–117 (1986).

Darras, B.T., Harper, J.F. et al. Prenatal diagnosis and detection of carriers with DNA probes in Duchenne's muscular dystrophy. *N. Engl. J. Med.*, 316, 985–992 (1987).

Hyser, C.L., Doherty, R.A. et al. Carrier assessment for mothers and sisters of isolated Duchenne dystrophy cases: the importance of serum enzyme determinations. *Neurology*, 37, 1476–1480 (1987).

Sibert, J.R., Williams, V. et al. Swivel walkers in Duchenne muscular dystrophy. *Arch. Dis. Child.*, 62, 741–742 (1987).

Goodship, J., Malcolm, S. et al. Service . . . DNA analysis for genetic prediction in Duchenne muscular dystrophy. *J. Med. Genet.*, 25, 14–19 (1988).

Lindlöf, M., Kääriäinen, H. et al. Microdeletions in patients with X-linked muscular dystrophy . . . *Clin. Genet.*, 33, 131–139 (1988).

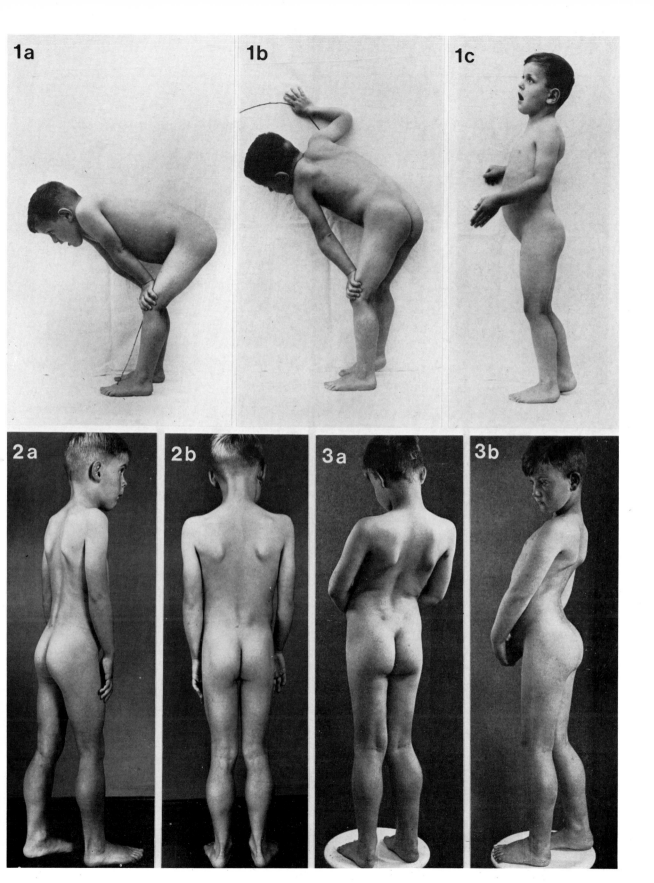

259. Progressive Diaphyseal Dysplasia

(Camurati–Engelmann Syndrome)

Hereditary systemic hyperostosis and sclerosis of the diaphyses of the long tubular bones and of the cranium associated with myopathy of the skeletal musculature.

Main signs:
1. Waddling or dragging gait and rapid fatigability, especially of the lower extremities; also complaints of limb pain after exertion.
2. Unusual proportions with relatively short trunk and overlong, very slender extremities (thin muscles, little subcutaneous fat) (1).
3. Radiologically, widening and thickening of the diaphyses of the long bones (4–8) due to endosteal and periosteal proliferation; also sclerosis of the skull (2, 3), base > calotte.

Supplementary findings: Neurologically unremarkable as a rule.

Slight—usually transitory—short stature in childhood; occipital and frontal bossing (1); and mild exophthalmos possible.

Delayed sexual maturity not unusual.

Manifestation: Very often in early childhood, but variable. Not infrequently, delay in learning to walk without support; then abnormal gait (see above) and general failure to thrive. Later, variable decrease in general vitality, with possible spontaneous remission in this respect during or after adolescence. Mild cases of this syndrome may be recognized only from an incidental finding on X-ray.

Etiology: Autosomal dominant disorder; often distinct intrafamilial differences in expression.

Frequency: Low; at least 140 cases described in the literature.

Prognosis: Life expectancy not affected. Late complications due to cranial nerve compression (impaired sight or hearing, facial paralysis) relatively infrequent.

Treatment: Definite improvement with long-term, low-dose corticosteroid treatment has been repeatedly observed. Genetic counseling.

Illustrations:
1 An 11-year-old boy.
2 and 4–7 His X-rays.
3 Skull X-ray of the same patient at age 32 years; later optic nerve damage in the optic canal.
8 and 9 Progression of the changes at 15 and 21 years.

H.-R.W.

References:
Wiedemann, H.-R. Systematisierte sklerotische Hyperostose des Kindesalters mit Myopathie. *Z. Kinderheilkd.*, 65, 346 (1948).
Hansen, H.G. Progressive diaphysäre Dysplasie. *Handbuch der Kinderheilkunde*, vol. 6. Springer, Heidelberg, 1967, (p.356ff.).
Spranger, J.W., Langer, L.O., Jr., Wiedemann, H.-R. *Bone Dysplasias. An Atlas of Consitutional Disorders of Skeletal Development.* G. Fischer and W.B. Saunders, Stuttgart and Philadelphia, 1974.
Kuhlencordt, F., Kruse, H.-P., Hellner, K.-A. et al. Diaphysäre Dysplasie (Camurati–Engelmann-Syndrom) mit fortschreitendem Visusverlust. *Dtsch. Med. Wochenschr.*, 106, 617 (1981).
Sheldon, J., Reeve, J., Clayton, B. Engelmann's disease (progressive diaphyseal dysplasia). A review and presentation of two cases with abnormal phosphate retention. *Metab. Bone Dis. Rel. Res.*, 2, 307 (1981).
Naveh, Y., Kaftori, J.K. et al. Progressive diaphyseal dysplasia . . . *Pediatrics*, 74, 399–405 (1984).
Naveh, Y., Alon, U. et al. Progressive diaphyseal dysplasia: evaluation of corticosteroid therapy. *Pediatrics*, 75, 321–323 (1985).
Naveh, Y., Ludatscher et al. Muscle involvement in progressive diaphyseal dysplasia. *Pediatrics*, 76, 944–949 (1985).
Ghosal, S.P., Mukherjee, A.K. et al. Diaphyseal dysplasia associated with anemia. *J. Pediatr.*, 113, 49–57 (1988).

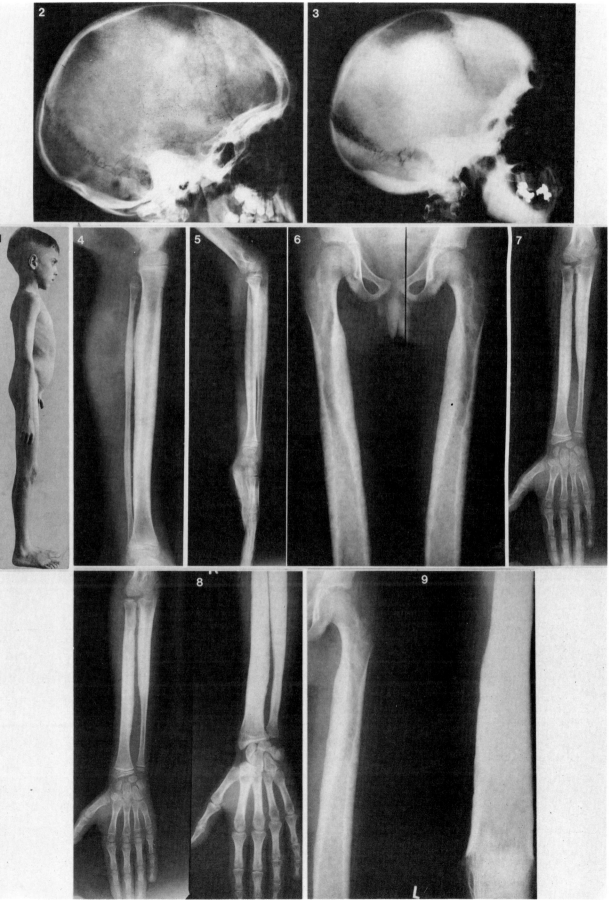

260. Lesch–Nyhan Syndrome

An X-linked recessive syndrome in males who show a cerebral disorder with dystonia, choreoathetosis, mental retardation, and a marked tendency to self mutilation, associated with hyperuricemia (and its typical sequelae).

Main signs:
1. Cerebral disorder manifest as spastic paralysis, choreoarthetoid hyperkinesia with severe dysarthria (if not anarthria), and severe mental defect (1).
2. Pathognomonic bizarre, aggressive behavior with frenzied biting and scratching especially in the form of self mutilation [biting through or picking apart the lips (2, 3), fingers, and toes, scratching the eyelids, etc., until severely damaged].
3. Development of signs of gout (with hyperuricemia, hematuria, crystalluria, urolithiasis, progressive nephropathy, and—usually not until much later—tophi and recurrent attacks of acute arthritis).

Supplementary findings: Short stature.
  Macrocytic anemia, usually of moderate severity, is a common finding.

Manifestation: First year of life and after. (Initial generalized hypotonia developing into generalized spasticity. Mental retardation. Failure to thrive. Choreoathetosis from the second year of life; and from about the third year, aggressive tendencies with frenzied biting, scratching, and self mutilation.)

Etiology: X-linked recessive disorder with variable expression. Thus, exclusively males affected, with absence of the enzyme hypoxanthine-guanine phosphoribosyltransferase (HGPRT), with corresponding effect on purine synthesis and purine base catabolism. Gene localized to the long arm of the X chromosome (X q26).

Frequency: Low.

Course, prognosis: Patients at risk of renal involvement and nutritional problems as a result of choreoathetoid dysphagia and frequent vomiting. Before the introduction of allopurinol therapy, patients rarely survived beyond the fifth year of life.

Diagnosis: In rare, exceptional cases, mental deficiency and aggressive tendencies may be absent.

Treatment: Allopurinol on a long-term basis is very effective in the treatment of hyperuricemia and all of its direct (gouty) consequences. However, it can neither prevent not mitigate the cerebral disorder. Protection from automutilation as far as possible. Genetic counseling. Identification of heterozygotes possible. Prenatal diagnosis.

Illustrations:
1–3 A 2¼-year-old boy, his parents' first child, with the typical clinical picture. Diagnosis—and heterozygosity in his mother—confirmed by determination of the rate of ^{14}C-hypoxanthine incorporation. In the second pregnancy, prenatal recognition of a male fetus as affected; confirmation of the diagnosis after interruption of the pregnancy. The third pregnancy, again with a male fetus, resulted in the birth of a healthy child after prenatal exclusion of the disorder.

H.-R.W.

References:
Leiber, B. and Olbrich, G. Lesch–Nyhan-Syndrom. *Monatschr. Kinderheilkd.*, 121, 42 (1973).
Letts, R.M. and Hobson, D.A. Special devices as aids in the management of child selfmutilation in the Lesch–Nyhan syndrome. *Pediatrics*, 55, 852 (1975).
Francke, U., Felsenstein, J., Gartler, S.M. et al. The occurrence of new mutants in the . . . Lesch–Nyhan disease. *Am. J. Hum. Genet.*, 28, 123 (1976).
Schneider, W., Morgenstern, E., Schindera, I. Lesch–Nyhan-Syndrom ohne Selbstverstümmelungstendenz. *Dtsch. Med. Wochenschr.*, 101, 167 (1976).
Manzke, H. Variable Expressivität der Genwirkung beim Lesch–Nyhan-Syndrom. *Dtsch. Med. Wochenschr.*, 101, 428 (1976).
Christie, R., Bay, C., Kaufman, I.A. et al. Lesch–Nyhan disease: clinical experience with nineteen patients. *Develop. Med. Child. Neurol.*, 24, 293 (1982).
Dempsey, J.L., Morley, A.A. et al. Detection of the carrier state for . . . the Lesch–Nyhan syndrome . . . *Hum. Genet.*, 64, 288–290 (1983).
Wilson, J.M., Young, A.B. et al. Hypoxanthine-guanine phosphoribosyltransferase deficiency. *N. Engl. J. Med.*, 309, 900–910 (1983).
Gibbs, D.A., Crawford, M. et al. First trimester diagnosis of Lesch–Nyhan syndrome. *Lancet*, II, 1180–1184 (1984).
Goldstein, M., Anderson, L.T. et al. Self-mutilation in Lesch–Nyhan disease is caused by dopaminergic denervation. *Lancet*, I, 338–339 (1985).
Mizuno, T. Long-term follow-up of ten patients with Lesch–Nyhan syndrome. *Neuropediatrics*, 17, 158–161 (1986).

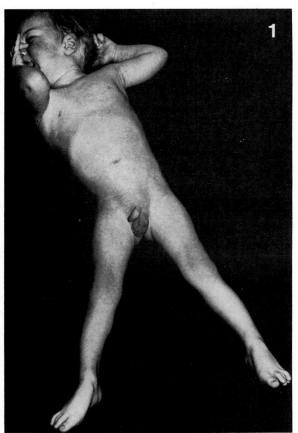

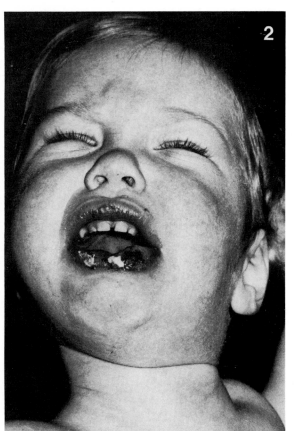

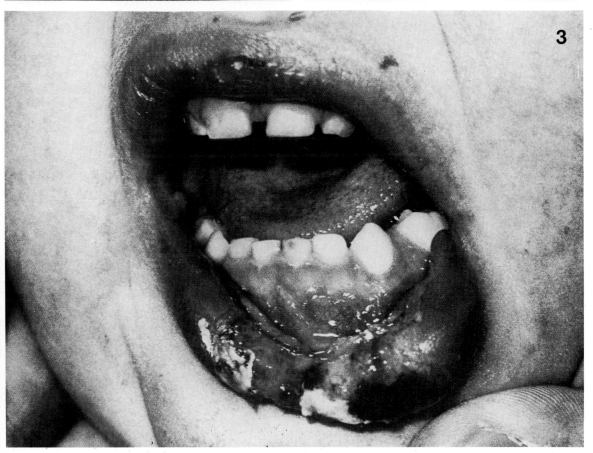

261. Ataxia Telangiectasia

(Louis–Bar Syndrome, Progressive Cerebellar Ataxia with Telangiectasia)

A characteristic hereditary syndrome with neurological, cutaneous, and immunopathological signs.

Main signs:

1. Progressive cerebellar *ataxia*, both at rest and with movement (beginning in early childhood) (1). Subsequent choreoathetosis; later, dyssynergia and intention tremor. Deterioration of speech, disturbance of eye movements; flaccid, apathetic to masklike facial expression (2) with slow development of a smile. Drooling. Stooped posture. Occasionally myoclonus. Mental involvement beginning about the end of the first decade in a proportion of cases, gradually increasing with age.

2. *Telangiectasia* (from the second half of early childhood), at first mainly in the areas of the bulbar conjunctiva exposed to light (3), later possibly on the lids, in a butterfly distribution on and alongside the nose, on the ears (4, 5), palate, back of the neck, chest, elbows, knees, and backs of the hands and feet. The vessels, which are initially delicate and attenuated, giving the impression in the eyes of mere conjunctival hyperemia, become increasingly dilated and tortuous. Preferred areas are those most exposed to sunlight. Gradually, the ears become inelastic, the facial skin stretched and taut with loss of adipose tissue. Affected skin areas develop pigmentation disorders (areas of hyper- and depigmentation side by side) and become atrophic; patients show signs of seborrheic dermatitis. Also frequently café au lait spots.

3. *Immune deficiency* (dysplasia of the thymolymphatic system), causing frequent or 'constant' signs of respiratory-tract infections (sinobronchitis, frequently progressive bronchiectasis, pneumonias).

Supplementary findings: Short stature regularly present (usually first noted in the pre-school child).

Wasting. Later, disorders of sexual maturation and other endocrinological anomalies.

Possible lymphocytopenia. Serologically, deficiency of mainly IgA and IgE, also particularly of IgG2 and IgG4. Increased levels of alphafetoprotein.

Chromosome analysis shows an increased tendency to chromosome breakage; structural aberration of the long arm of chromosome 14 in 3–5% of cells.

Patients definitely have an increased risk of developing lymphoreticular malignancies.

Manifestation: Onset of ataxia from the beginning of the second year of life or later, appearance of telangiectases usually between about age 3 and 5 years; mental impairment, when present, often first apparent at an advanced stage of the disease.

Etiology: Autosomal recessive disorder; heterogeneity. The pathogenetic relationships between the neurological disorder (primary cerebellar degeneration), the skin and mucous membrane changes, and the immunological defect are still largely unexplained.

Frequency: Relatively low (by 1983 over 300 cases were reported in the literature).

Course, prognosis: Progressive. Patients often confined to a wheelchair by the middle of the second decade of life and usually succumb to the sequelae of chronic pulmonary infections or of the neurological disorder itself or to a malignancy before the end of the third decade.

Diagnosis: Unmistakable when telangiectases are present.

Treatment: Symptomatic. Particular benefit from conservative physiotherapy; timely antibiotic therapy for acute bacterial infections. Genetic counseling. Possibility of prenatal diagnosis. Microsigns in heterozygotes? Tendency to leukosis?

Illustrations:

1–5 A 10-year-old girl, no longer able to stand alone. Completely unremarkable development until age 18 months; then, onset of progressive ataxia. Telangiectases of the conjunctiva, lids, ears, and upper arms. Mask-like fixed facial expression; frequent episodes of extrapyramidal dyskinesia, usually with torsion of the head to the right. Small stature, wasting, lymphocytopenia.

H.-R.W.

References:

Bridges, B.A. and Harnden, D.G. *Ataxia-Telangiectasia . . .* John Wiley, Chichester, 1982, 422 pp.
Jaspers, N.G.J. and Bootsma, D. Genetic heterogeneity in ataxia-telangiectasia . . . *Proc. Natl. Acad. Sci.*, 79, 2641–2644 (1982).
Oxelius, V.-A., Berkel, A.I., Hanson, L.A. IgG2 deficiency in ataxia telangiectasia. *N. Engl. J. Med.*, 306, 515 (1982).
Shaham, M., Voss, R., Becker, Y. et al. Prenatal diagnosis of ataxia telangiectasia. *J. Pediatr.*, 100, 135 (1982).
Gatti, R.A. and Swift, M. *Ataxia-Telangiectasia . . .* Alan Liss, New York, 1986.
Rosin, M.P. and Ochs, H.D. In vivo chromosomal instability in ataxia-telangiectasia homozygotes and heterozygotes. *Hum. Genet.*, 74, 335–340 (1986).
Shiloh, Y., Parshad, R. et al. Carrier detection in ataxia-telangiectasia. *Lancet*, I, 689 (1986).
Boder, E. Ataxia-telangiectasia. In: *Neurocutaneous Diseases.* Butterworths, Boston, 1987 (pp. 95–117).

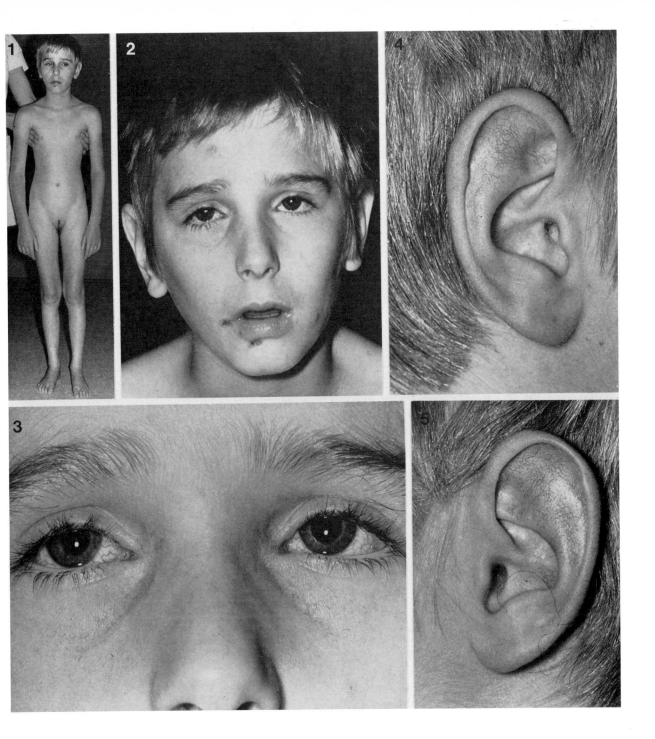

262. Marinesco–Sjögren Syndrome

(Cerebellolenticular Dystrophy with Mental Retardation)

A syndrome of early manifest cataracts, mental retardation, ataxia, myopathy, and small stature.

Main signs:
1. Cerebellar ataxia with a variable degree of motor impairment such as severe delay in and difficulty with walking.
2. Primary mental retardation of variable grades of severity.
3. 'Congenital' cataract.
4. Myopathy (with elevated serum creatine kinase), muscular hypotonia.
5. Moderate growth deficiency.

Supplementary findings: Dysarthria, strabismus, nystagmus.
Hypergonadotrophic hypogonadism.
Possible development of scoliosis, pectus carinatum, pes planovalgus.

Manifestation: The first year of life.

Etiology: Autosomal recessive disorder. Lysosomal storage disease?

Frequency: Low; about 80 cases described up to 1985.

Course, prognosis: Very dependent on the degree and progression of ataxia and on the severity of mental impairment.

Differential diagnosis: Other ataxia syndromes should be easy to differentiate, especially in view of the cataracts.

Treatment: Symptomatic. The ophthalmological care is especially important. Genetic counseling.

Illustrations:
1–3 A 15-year-old girl, the second child of healthy parents with no known consanguinity. Cataract surgery in the first year of life. Primary mental retardation. Early manifest ataxia. Height 1.56 m. Strabismus, little change of facial expression. Micrognathia; genu valgus.
4–6 The 21-year-old sister of the proband, 1.60 m tall; quite similar development, but not yet needing crutches. Both girls tend to be whiny.

H.-R.W.

References:

Anderson, B. Marinesco–Sjögren syndrome: spinocerebellar ataxia, congenital cataract, somatic and mental retardation. *Devel. Med. Child. Neurol.*, 7, 249 (1965).
Alter, M. and Kennedy, W. The Marinesco–Sjögren syndrome. *Minn. Med.*, 51, 901 (1968).
Superneau, D., Wertelecki, W. et al. The Marinesco–Sjögren syndrome described a quarter of a century before Marinesco. *Am. J. Med. Genet.*, 22, 647–648 (1985).
Walker, P.D., Blitzer, M.G. et al. Marinesco–Sjögren syndrome: evidence for a lysosomal storage disorder. *Neurology*, 35, 415–419 (1985).

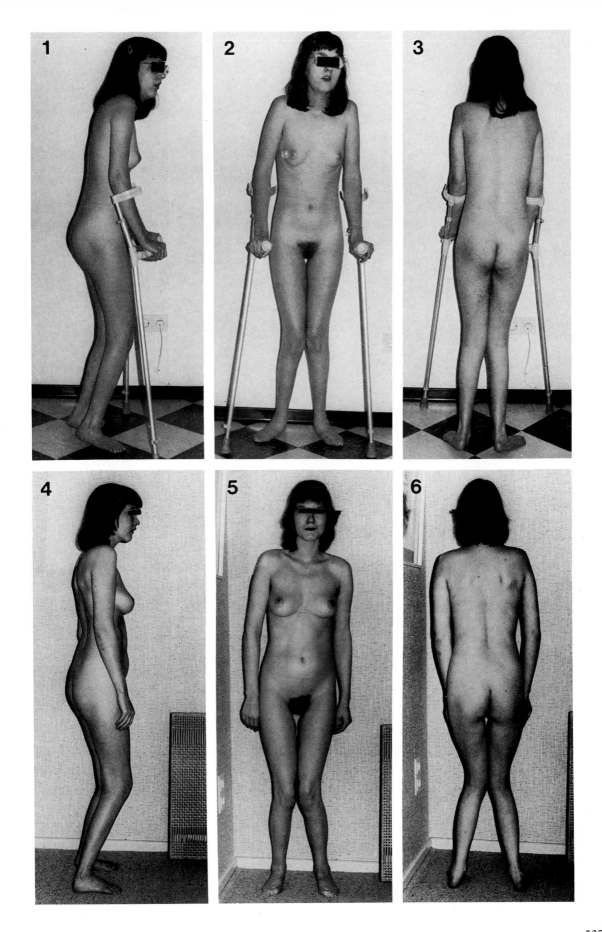

263. Rubella Embryofetopathy

(Extended Gregg Syndrome)

A characteristic picture varying in extent, of embryonal and/or fetal damage due to the rubella virus.

Main signs:

I. Syndrome of defects in older children (previously called Gregg syndrome) (1–3, 5–7, 9): Cataract, uni- or bilateral, frequently with microphthalmos (and retinitis pigmentosa). Sensorineural hearing defect or deafness, uni- or bilateral, frequently with signs of defective vestibular function. Small size, microcephaly (usually mild) in relation to linear growth, and psychomotor retardation (mild to severe, with or without neurological signs). Cardiovascular anomalies: most frequently patent ductus arteriosus (PDA) or pulmonary stenosis.

II. Spectrum of disease and damage in newborns and infants (4, 8): Usually, small size at birth, failure to thrive and problems with rearing. Cataract at birth or possibly manifest in the first weeks of life. Secondary glaucoma with corneal clouding may be present at birth or develop in the following weeks. Additional possible signs noted in 8: thrombocytopenic purpura, hepatosplenomegaly, hepatitis, myocarditis, meningoencephaloretinitis, etc.

Supplementary findings: Possible hypoplastic anemia. X-ray evidence of metaphyseal lesions of the long bones during the first months of life.

Demonstration of rubella-specific IgM in the child's serum.

It is possible to demonstrate rubella virus in tissues, body fluid (CSF), and excretions of the child for months after birth.

Manifestation: At birth and early infancy.

Etiology: Infection of the embryo and/or fetus with rubella virus.

Frequency: Variable—depending on the virulence of the organism or on the extent to which young women have been immunized. In Germany, 1 case in 2,000 births is still a possibility. Maternal rubella in the first trimester, results in defects in all children (principally of the heart and auditory organ); maternal rubella in the following period until the 16th week of pregnancy, leads to defects in up to at least one-third of children (primarily hearing impairments).

Course, prognosis: Dependent on the type and extent of damage as well as on the intensity and quality of rehabilitation. Fatal outcome in the first months not rare.

Differential diagnosis: Microphthalmos, microcephaly, central nervous signs, and deafness may also occur with embryofetal cytomegalic virus infection or fetal toxoplasmosis; and generally the signs of fetal rubella may resemble those of congenital infection from other, diverse pathogens. A hereditary syndrome of congenital cataract and cardiomyopathy should also be considered.

Treatment: Urgent treatment of glaucoma. Removal of cataracts generally after the sixth month of life. Operative correction of a cardiac defect as appropriate. Early application of hearing aids if hearing impairment present. Other appropriate handicap aids. Prednisone recommended for thrombocytopenic purpura and hypoplastic anemia. Prophylaxis: immunization against rubella of girls at age 14 years.

Illustrations:

1, 7, 9 A 4-year-old patient; maternal rubella in first and second months of pregnancy. Low birth weight, rearing problems; congenital cataracts and microphthalmos bilaterally; deafness; slight microcephaly, mental retardation, amblyopic motoricity and athetosis; small stature.

2 A 9-year-old patient; cataract, microphthalmos, mental retardation, PDA, club foot, dysodontiasis.

3 and 6 A 4-year-old patient; microphthalmos and cataract on the right, retinopathy on the left; sensorineural hearing defect; mild microcephaly, mental retardation, PDA.

4 A 6-week-old patient; cataract, microphthalmos and corneal clouding bilaterally; PDA and atrial septal defect (ASD); hepatosplenomegaly, icterus, anemia, thrombocytopenia; muscular hypotonia; prenatal dystrophy, maternal rubella in third to fourth months of pregnancy.

5 A 9-month-old patient; microcephaly, cataract, microphthalmos, amblyopia, cardiac defect, small stature.

H.-R.W.

References:

Miller, E., Craddock-Watson, J.E. et al. Consequences of confirmed maternal rubella at successive stages of pregnancy. *Lancet*, II, 781–784 (1982).

Behbehani, A.W., Westmeier, M. et al. Rötelnembryopathie mit Meningoencephalitis… *Monatschr. Kinderheilkd.*, 132, 55–57. (1984).

Daffos, F., Forester, F. et al. Prenatal diagnosis of congenital rubella. *Lancet*, II, 1–3 (1984).

Craddock-Watson, J.E., Anderson, M.J. et al. Rubella reinfection and the fetus. *Lancet*, I, 1039 (1985).

Cruysberg, J.R.M. Presumed congenital rubella syndrome: virus embryopathy or hereditary disease? *Lancet*, I, 529 (1988).

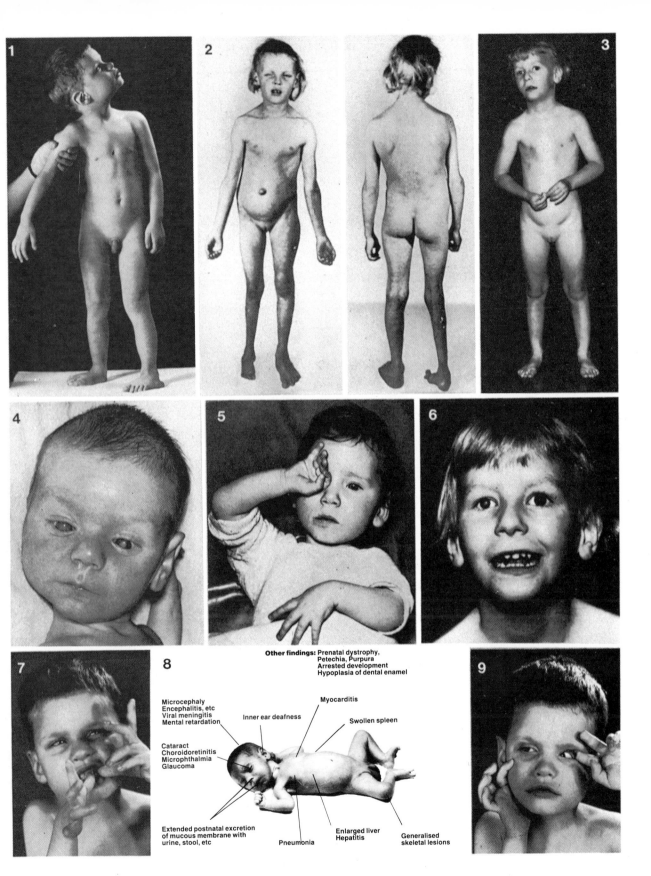

Other findings: Prenatal dystrophy,
Petechia, Purpura
Arrested development
Hypoplasia of dental enamel

Microcephaly
Encephalitis, etc
Viral meningitis
Mental retardation

Inner ear deafness

Myocarditis

Swollen spleen

Cataract
Choroidoretinitis
Microphthalmia
Glaucoma

Extended postnatal excretion
of mucous membrane with
urine, stool, etc

Pneumonia

Enlarged liver
Hepatitis

Generalised
skeletal lesions

529

264. Hallermann–Streiff–François Syndrome

(François' Dyscephalic Syndrome; Oculo-Mandibulo-Dyscrania with Hypotrichosis)

A highly characteristic syndrome of dyscrania with hypotrichosis, anomalies of the face and especially of the eyes, and short stature.

Main signs:
1. Abnormalities of the skull (frontal and/or occipito-parietal bossing, delayed closure of fontanelles and sutures; relatively small face with flat orbits, hypoplasia of the jaw and micrognathia) (1–7).
2. Microphthalmos; cataracts (congenital, or manifest in the early postnatal period).
3. Small, narrow nose, becoming increasingly 'beaklike' (3–5, 7).
4. Congenital teeth and other dental anomalies; high narrow palate.
5. Atrophy of the skin, especially over the nose and cranial sutures; hypotrichosis, especially of the scalp, brows, lashes (3–5, 7).
6. Proportionate short stature.

Supplementary findings: Mental development is normal as a rule, but exceptions are not uncommon. Frequent amblyopic nystagmus, strabismus. Blue sclerae may occur. On X-ray, hypoplasia of the ascending ramus of the mandible and anterior displacement of the temporomandibular joint. Occurrence of pectus excavatum, winged scapulae, and other skeletal anomalies. Also, right heart anomalies and hypogenitalism.

Manifestation: At birth.

Etiology: Genetic basis certain, but the causes remain unknown. Almost always sporadic occurrence (perhaps as new mutations of an autosomal dominant gene; however, evidence also of possible autosomal recessive transmission. Heterogeneity?).

Frequency: Low; over 150 cases described in the literature up to 1982.

Course, prognosis: In early infancy, glossoptosis or related anomalies may cause feeding and respiratory problems. Later, eye defects present the greatest problem (however, spontaneous resorption of the cataracts has been reported); vision often markedly decreased. Adult height in females usually greater than 150 cm and in males over 155 cm.

Differential diagnosis: Progeria and progeroid syndromes are not difficult to rule out; mandibulofacial dysostosis, cleidocranial dysostosis, and pyknodysostosis are even less difficult.

Treatment: Ophthalmological and dental care are very important. There may be indications for growth hormone. Genetic counseling.

Illustrations:
1–5 An 18-month-old boy with the complete picture of the syndrome. Congenital cataracts, congenital teeth. Mental development normal for age. Height below the third percentile. Cataract operation at age 5 months; vision well corrected with contact lenses. **6 and 7** The same patient at 10½ years. Height and weight below the third percentile. Bone-age retarded by about 3 years. Distinct partial HGH deficiency; growth hormone treatment was instituted. Mental development normal. He has one healthy sister, three years younger.

H.-R.W.

References:
Steele, R.W. and Bass, J.W. Hallermann–Streiff syndrome. *Am. J. Dis. Child.*, 20, 462 (1970).
Suzuki, Y., Fujii, T., Fukuyama, Y. Hallermann–Streiff syndrome. *Develop. Med. Child. Neurol.*, 12, 496 (1970).
Dinwiddie, R., Gewitz, M., Taylor, J.F.N. Cardiac defects in the Hallermann–Streiff syndrome. *J. Pediatr.*, 92, 77 (1978).
Ronen, S., Rozenmann, Y., Isaacson, M. et al. The early management of a baby with Hallermann–Streiff–François syndrome. *J. Pediatr. Ophthalmol. Strab.*, 16/2, 119 (1979).
François, J. François' dyscephalic syndrome. *Birth Defects*, 16, 6: 595–619 (1982).
Huber, J. Dento-alveolar abnormalities in oculomandibulodyscephaly (Hallermann–Streiff syndrome). *J. Oral Pathol.*, 13, 147–154 (1984).

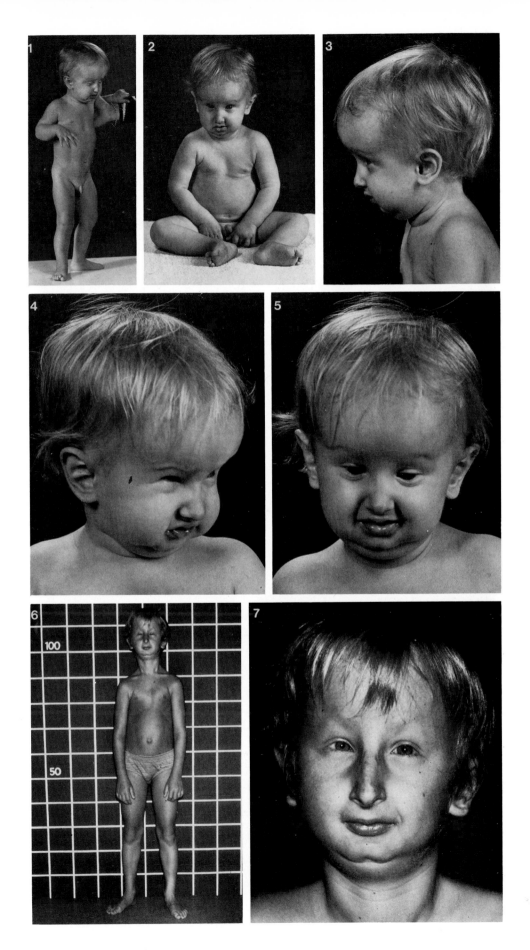

265. Arthro-Ophthalmopathy

(Stickler Syndrome)

A relatively frequent and important autosomal dominant disorder of orofacial signs with abnormalities of the eyes, skeleton, and joints.

Main signs:
1. Flat, often asymmetrical face with variably depressed nasal root and nose (**1, 4**); epicanthic folds; midface (**1, 4**) or mandibular (**3**) hypoplasia; cleft palate (hard and/or soft palate, sometimes with bifid uvula); frequently with fully expressed Robin triad (p.68).
2. Early myopia of marked to extreme severity with changes of the fundi, possible glaucoma, cataract, retinal detachment and retinoschisis leading to blindness.
3. Not infrequently, marfanoid habitus (**1, 2, 4**). Moderately developed, hypotonic musculature and hyperextensibility of large (and possibly also of small) joints; in some cases mild, rheumatoid arthropathies, even in childhood, severe arthropathies also seen occasionally. Hip and knee joints most severely affected. The arthropathies are not constant and the least important sign.

Supplementary findings: Hearing impairment not so infrequent (conductive or sensorineural defect). Dental anomalies. Possible development of kyphosis or scoliosis; thoracic deformities; genu valgus (**1**), etc.
   Prolapse of the mitral valve frequent.
   Radiologically, the picture of a mild spondyloepiphyseal dysplasia with flattening of the vertebral bodies reminiscent of the picture in Scheuermann disease, narrow diaphyses and broad metaphyses of the long bones and changes of the knee and other joints (e.g., subluxation of the hip joints).

Manifestation: At birth (orofacial signs and possible conspicuous, bony prominence of the large joints, especially of the ankle, knee and wrist joints) and later. Myopia usually manifest during early childhood; retinal detachment usually not until the second decade or later.

Etiology: Autosomal dominant disorder (generalized stromal dysplasia) with very varied expression of individual signs, even intrafamilialy, and with incomplete penetrance. Polyallelism possible.

Frequency: Not low (about 1:20,000). Stickler syndrome should be considered in every case of isolated cleft palate, Robin anomaly, or dominantly occurring myopia, and myopia should be ruled out in the former two conditions.

Course, prognosis: Usually normal life expectancy, intellectual development, and height. Handicap due to visual or joint disorders may occur, usually starting in the second decade (or even earlier).

Differential diagnosis: Marfan syndrome and homocystinuria (pp. 142, 146), spondyloepiphyseal dysplasias (e.g., p.246), osteodysplasia type Kniest (p.250), and possibly the Ehlers–Danlos syndrome (p.364) are usually easy to distinguish. A few Stickler syndrome-like combinations of signs go by other names (Marshall syndrome, Weissenbacher–Zweymüller syndrome); their classification as separate entities does not yet seem to be unequivocally settled.

Treatment: Pediatric care of a Robin anomaly. From infancy, regular check-ups by a qualified ophthalmologist; glaucoma therapy may be indicated, operation for cataracts or specific treatment for retinal detachment. Closure of cleft palate and speech therapy as required. Audiometric assessment. Avoidance of physical strain. Cardiac assessment and treatment as needed. Genetic counseling.

Illustrations:
1–4 A child and adolescents from a large sibship with Stickler syndrome.
1 and 4 Midface hypoplasia.
3 Micrognathia.

H.-R.W.

References:

Herrmann, J., France, T.D., Spranger, J.W. et al. The Stickler syndrome (hereditary arthroophthalmopathy). *Birth Defects*, XI/2, 76 (1975).
Hanson, J.W., Graham, C.B., Smith, D.W. Early diagnosis of the Stickler syndrome presenting as Robin anomalad. *Birth Defects*, 13/3, 235 (1977).
Blair, N.P., Albert, D.M., Liberfarb, R.M. et al. Hereditary progressive arthroophthalmopathy of Stickler. *Am. J. Ophthalmol.*, 88, 876 (1979).
Liberfarb, R.M., Hirose, T., Holmes, L.B. The Wagner–Stickler syndrome . . . 22 families. *J. Pediatr.*, 99, 394 (1981).
Meinecke, P. Das Stickler-Syndrom. *Pädiatr. Prax.*, 24, 705 (1980/81).
Weingeist, T.A., Hermsen, V. et al. Ocular and systemic manifestations of Stickler's syndrome. *Birth Defects*, 18/6, 539–560 (1982).
Aymé, S. and Preus, M. The Marshall and Stickler syndromes: objective rejection of lumping. *J. Med. Genet.*, 21, 34–38 (1984).
Liberfarb, R.M. Prevalence of mitral-valve prolapse in the Stickler syndrome. *Am. J. Med. Genet.*, 24, 387–392 (1986).

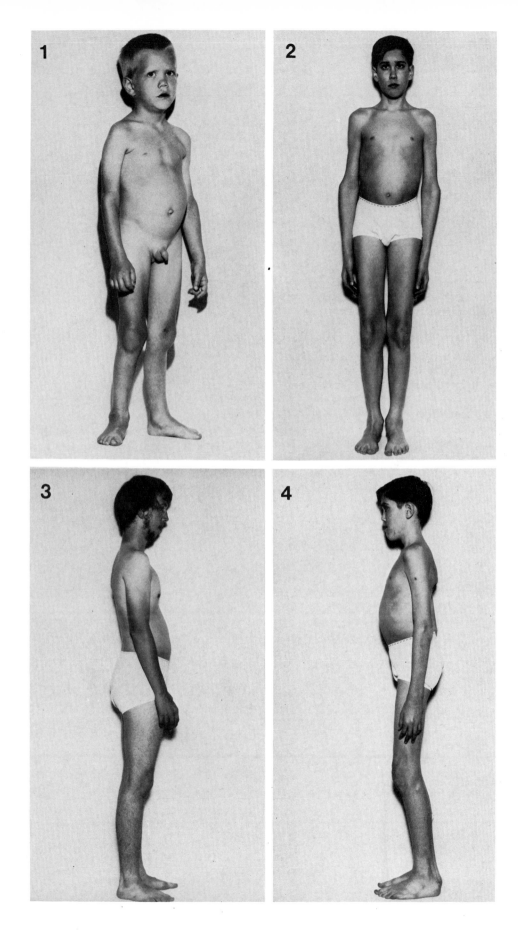

266. Unknown Malformation–Retardation Syndrome with Hemorrhagic Diathesis

A syndrome of eye and skeletal anomalies, hemorrhagic diathesis, and mental retardation.

Main signs:
1. Ptosis, more severe on the right than the left (1) with deep-set eyes and myopia on the right. Loss of roundness of the iris on the right, typical coloboma of the iris on the left. Large coloboma of the choroid below the optic disc bilaterally. Large ears of simple configuration (1, 2).
2. Scoliosis, lumbar hyperlordosis (2); clinodactyly of the little and index fingers bilaterally (3); bilateral pes cavus.
3. Hemorrhagic diathesis beginning at 6 years of age, with palm-size hematomas.
4. Psychomotor retardation (IQ 66 at 11 years)—uncertain whether primary, or as a result of unilateral akinetic cerebral focal seizures that occurred from early infancy until about 4–5 years of age.

Supplementary findings: On X-ray, somewhat coarse, poorly modeled first rays of the hands and feet (4, 5). Very coarse epiphyses of the terminal phalanges of the big toes and malformations of the ungual processes; atypical middle and terminal phalanges of the other toes (5). Mild clinodactyly of the fifth fingers, quite pronounced pseudoepiphyses of the second metacarpals (4).

Hematologically: occasionally borderline platelet counts; prolonged periods of leukopenia; normo-erythremia. Somewhat cell-poor bone marrow, picture, without definite pathological findings. Good global thrombocyte function. No evidence of defective clotting factors. (Hemoglobin analysis negative. No erythrocyte enzyme defects demonstrable.)

Manifestation: Birth and later.

Etiology: Unknown.

Course, prognosis: Apart from the mental deficiency, apparently favorable. At 14½ years, no further bleeding, platelet count normal; still slight 'constitutional' leukopenia.

Comment: The patient has no cardiac defect (see Ho), no basis for Fanconi anemia syndrome (p.440), nor for cat-eye syndrome (p.66), etc.

Treatment: Symptomatic.

Illustrations:
1–5 The same boy, at 7 years (4), and at 9 years (1–3, 5), the third child of healthy, young, nonconsanguineous parents after two healthy brothers. Pregnancy and delivery normal (3600 g; 51 cm). No hyperpigmentation. Normal linear growth (at 14½ years, 11 cm above average height). Normal head circumference. Normal genitalia and normal sexual maturation for age. Heart normal; renal pyelogram normal. Normal male karyotype and no increased chromosome breakage.

H.-R.W.

Reference:
Ho, C.K., Kaufman, R.L., Podos, S.M. Ocular colobomata, cardiac defect, and other anomalies. A study of seven cases including two sibs. *J. Med. Genet.*, 12, 289 (1975).

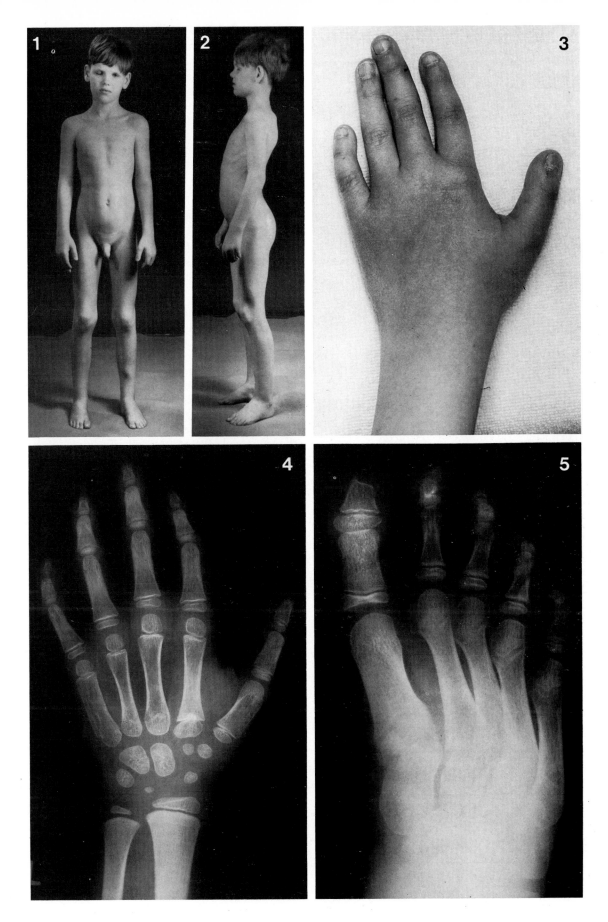

535

267. Adrenogenital Syndrome, Salt-Losing Type

A disorder of adrenal steroid biosynthesis (21-hydroxylase defect) with increased production of adrenal androgens causing virilization (or intersex in females), salt loss, and hyperkalemia.

Main signs:
1. Intersex of XX individuals: female pseudohermaphroditism with clitoral hypertrophy to complete masculinization (Prader stages I–V). Patients with stages I and II still have separate urethral and vaginal openings; with stages III–V, only one urogenital opening, which, however, may separate distally into urethra and vagina. XY patients show precocious pseudopuberty with enlargement of the penis and pigmented scrotum.
2. Failure to thrive from the second week of life, with marked vomiting, fever, weight loss. Renal cortical hyperplasia. Without treatment, death in the first weeks of life.

Supplementary findings: Increase of 17-ketosteroids and pregnanetriol in the urine, and demonstration of pregnanetriolone, which is not normally present.

Manifestation: In females, at birth; in males (in the absence of salt-losing syndrome), diagnosis in later years. At least 40% of children with precocious puberty appear to be heterozygotes for the defective 21-hydroxylase gene.

Etiology: Autosomal recessive 21-hydroxylase defect of adrenal steroid biosynthesis in the zona fasciculata and glomerulosa. The defective gene is linked with the HLA locus on chromosome 6.

Frequency: Most frequent congenital disorder of steroid biosynthesis (about 90% of all cases). Worldwide regional differences, e.g., 1:500 in the Eskimos of south-western Alaska, 1:5,000 in Switzerland, and 1:67,000 in the USA. Corresponding heterozygote frequencies between 1:11, 1:35, and 1:128.

Course, prognosis: Rapid growth, accelerated skeletal maturity, appearance of pubic hair at age 2–3 years, and pronounced muscle contours. In girls, increased clitoral hypertrophy; in boys, signs of puberty with small testicles (androgen production in the adrenals, no increase of gonadotropins). With continued absence of therapy, premature closure of the epiphyses (eighth year of life). Adult height about 145 cm. Men with AGS on appropriate therapy have no fertility problems. Complications with febrile illnesses, surgical procedures, and trauma due to increased demand for (unavailable) cortisol, producing: hypoglycemia, tachycardia, respiratory difficulties, seizures, somnolence, profuse sweating.

Prenatal diagnosis: This is important, since prenatal therapy appears possible. *Either*: diagnosis by determining 17-OH progesterone levels in amniotic fluid in the 16th week of pregnancy (beware the mother who is homozygous for the 21-hydroxylase defect); *or* HLA typing after a first child with AGS (HLABw47).

Treatment: With the onset of acute vomiting, electrolyte replacement, aldosterone, and prednisone parenterally. Long-term replacement therapy with hydrocortisone during childhood. After cessation of growth, prednisone. Fludrocortisone as mineralocorticoid. Individual adjustment of dosage. With treatment, normal adult heights are attained. Operative correction of XX individuals and rearing as females (Prader types I–IV). Management of type V needs to be thoroughly discussed with all concerned. Prenatal treatment with dexamethasone to prevent virilization appears possible.

Illustrations:
1a–1d The 3-year-old sister of a boy who also has AGS.
1b The penis-like clitoris.
1c Fusion of the labia majora, urogenital sinus, and clitoral hypertrophy.
1d Appearance at age 4½ years.
2 The 18-month-old sister of a boy with AGS; clitoral hypertrophy.
2b Scrotum-like hyperpigmented labia, urogenital sinus, clitoral hypertrophy.
3 A 4½-year-old with thoroughly boyish appearance. Salt-losing AGS; female pseudohermaphroditism (46 XX) with maximal virilization (Prader type V). Gonadectomy, hysterectomy, and implantation of prosthetic testes performed when the patient was 12 years old.

J.K.

References:

David, M. and Forest, M.G. Prenatal treatment of congenital adrenal hyperplasia resulting from 21-hydroxylase deficiency. *J. Pediatr.*, 105, 799–803 (1984).
Knorr, D. Das congenitale adrenogenitale Syndrom. *Monatschr. Kinderheilkd.*, 133, 327–335 (1985).
Miller, W.L. and Levine, L.S. Molecular and clinical advances in congenital adrenal hyperplasia. *J. Pediatr.*, 111, 1–17 (1987).
Schwab, K.O., Kruse, K. et al. Effekt einer mütterlichen Dexamethasonbehandlung … bei AGS … *Monatschr. Kinderheilkd.*, 137, 293–296 (1989).

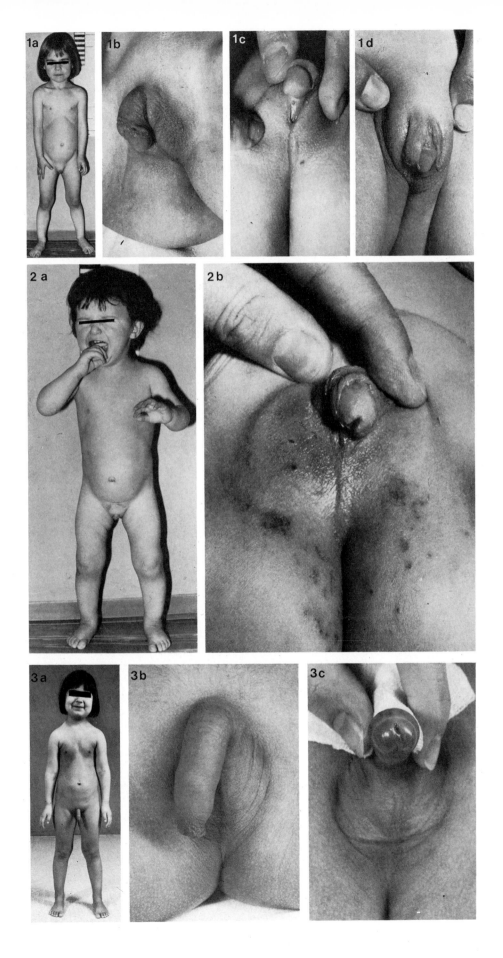

268. Incomplete Testicular Feminization Syndrome

An X-linked pseudohermaphroditism syndrome with bilateral testes; ambiguous genitalia; short, blind-ending vagina; absent uterus; and XY constitution.

Main signs:
1. Inguinal or intra-abdominal testes, short blind-ending vagina, absence of uterus and tubes, clitoral hypertrophy. Only partially differentiated wolffian ducts; müllerian derivatives absent.
2. Chromosomal status: 46 XY.

Supplementary findings: At puberty, various degrees of masculinization and breast development. Phenotypic variability within a female. Sterility.

Manifestation: Intersex at birth.

Etiology: X-linked recessive inheritance. Gene defect with variable expression. Unremarkable carrier mothers. Incomplete resistance to androgen: defect of the cytosol androgen receptors, which normally transport testosterone and other androgens from the cell membrane to the nucleus.

Frequency: All forms of male pseudohermaphroditism together, about 1:10,000. The ITF syndrome is correspondingly less frequent.

Course, prognosis: Various degrees of masculinization and breast development during puberty. The risk of testicular neoplasm in the first two decades of life is low.

Differential diagnosis: Easily differentiated from complete testicular feminization (normal female external genitalia, inguinal hernias containing testes, primary amenorrhea, absence of secondary sexual hairgrowth). Milder forms of androgen resistance: Lubs syndrome (female phenotype, partial labioscrotal fusion, pseudovagina), Gilbert–Dreyfus syndrome (male phenotype, small phallus, pubertal azoospermia, gynecomastia), Reifenstein syndrome (perineoscrotal hypospadias, bifid scrotum, gynecomastia), Rosewater syndrome (male phenotype, sterility, gynecomastia).

Treatment: Orchidectomy after puberty. Estrogen therapy. Feminizing plastic surgery of the genitalia. In individual cases, careful differential diagnosis and psychological assessment.

Illustrations:
1a and 1b A 13-month-old child. Clitoral hypertrophy, testes in the labioscrotal folds. Karyotype: XY.
1c and 1d Same child at age 5 years.
2a and 2b Sibling, 2-days old, intersex genitalia with clitoral hypertrophy; testes in the scrotum-like labia. Karyotype: 46 XY.

J.K.

References:

Any pediatric textbook.

Pinsky, L., Kaufman, M., Summitt, L. Congenital androgen insensitivity due to a qualitatively abnormal androgen receptor. *Am. J. Med. Genet.*, 10, 91–99 (1981).

Pinsky, L. et al. Human minimal androgen insensitivity with normal dihydrotestosterone-binding capacity in cultured genital skin fibroblasts: evidence for an androgen-selective qualitative abnormality of the receptor. *Am. J. Hum. Genet.*, 36, 965–978 (1984).

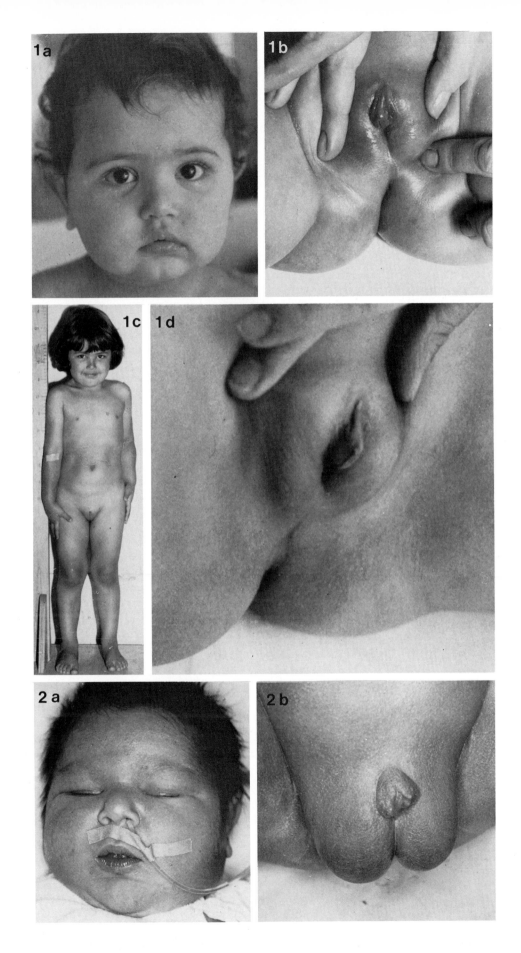

269. Complete Testicular Feminization Syndrome

(Hairless Women)

An X-linked recessive male pseudohermaphroditism with female phenotype, primary amenorrhea, decreased axillary and pubic hair, abdominal and/or inguinal testes, and a male chromosome complement.

Main signs:
1. Normal external female genitalia, no clitoral hypertrophy, labia majora and minora normal, separate urethral and vaginal openings.
2. No differentiation of the müllerian ducts: short vagina (absence of the proximal part), no cervix, no uterus, no fallopian tubes.
3. Likewise, no development of the wolffian duct: duct of epoophoron (appendix vesiculosa) and rudiments of Gartner's duct.
4. The gonads are testes. They are intra-abdominal or inguinal (hernias) or in the labia.
5. During puberty, normal mammary development, decreased pubic and axillary hair. Primary amenorrhea. Normal body proportions. Sterility.

Supplementary findings: Up to puberty, the testes are histologically normal. After puberty, absence of spermatogonia, infantile seminiferous tubules, no sperm formation. Leydig-cell hyperplasia. Unremarkable feminine psychosexuality.

Manifestation: At birth? However, may not be diagnosed until the menses fail to occur (primary amenorrhea).

Etiology: X-linked recessive inheritance. The genital tubercle and the fetal urogenital sinus cannot respond to induction by testicular androgens, and so male genital organs do not develop. Hair follicles also do not react to androgens. Carrier mothers often show a paucity of pubic and axillary hair.

Frequency: About 1:62,000 live-born male individuals.

Prognosis: In 5–20% formation of gonadal neoplasms, such as tubular adenomas and seminomas. Otherwise normal life expectancy. Normal intelligence.

Differential diagnosis: To be delineated from incomplete testicular feminization.

Treatment: Gonadal tumors do not occur before puberty. Gonadectomy after puberty is usually recommended, although some favor prepubertal removal. With prepubertal gonadectomy, an estrogen should be administered from the second decade of life; with postpubertal removal correspondingly later. Plastic surgery to construct a deeper vagina. Herniotomy with diagnostic clarification of the contents of the hernia (especially sex-chromatin diagnosis). The decision to inform the patients, who identify as females and may be married, of their male karyotype, requires very careful consideration. As a rule, patients are not told their nuclear sex.

Illustrations:
1 and 2 A 17-year-old, typically affected except for relatively little mammary development (primary amenorrhea, etc., XY constitution; androgen receptor defect demonstrated in genital skin fibroblasts).

J.K.

References:
Any gynecology or pediatric textbook.
Griffin, J.E. and Wilson, I.D. The syndromes of androgen resistance. *N. Engl. J. Med.*, 302, 198–209 (1980).

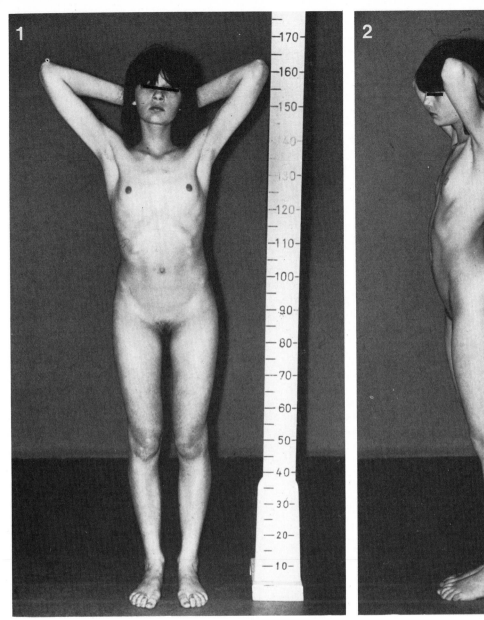
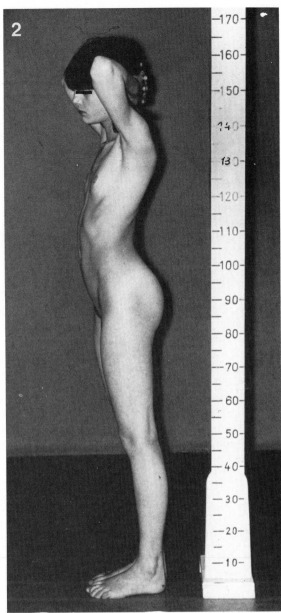

541

270. Kallmann Syndrome

Familial hypogonadotropic hypogonadism with anosmia, in both sexes.

Main signs:
1. Eunuchoid habitus with abnormally wide arm span, etc. Hypogonadotropic hypogonadism (1).
2. An- or hyposmia (seldom spontaneously reported).

Supplementary findings: Cryptorchidism and unilateral renal hypo- or agenesis (found by ultrasonography) may occur. Furthermore, color blindness, deafness. Also, cleft lip and/or palate, cardiac defect, thrombocytopathy.

Manifestation: Boys with Kallmann syndrome may come to medical attention at birth due to cryptorchidism and micropenis. Parents should be carefully examined to determine whether they are affected. Early hormonal diagnosis.

Etiology: Genetic disorder. Heterogeneity. Evidence for each of the classic modes of inheritance has been found in diverse sibships. The hormonal disorder is due to defective LHRH secretion by the hypothalamus; the disorder of smell, to absence of the anlage of the olfactory bulb and tract.

Frequency: Probably not so very low. Sporadic cases (in families with isolated cases of anosmia) and also extensive observations in sibships.

Prognosis: Hormonal replacement therapy easier in girls. Prognosis for fertility less favorable in boys than in girls.

Diagnosis, differential diagnosis: Ask specifically for a history of anosmia. Test sense of smell. Other forms of delayed puberty and hypogonadism must be ruled out.

Treatment: Adequate hormonal treatment to induce puberty and for maintenance therapy. Recently, LHRH administered in pulsatile form, has been added to the usual HCG/HMG treatment to improve fertility, at least for women who wish to have children.

Illustrations:
1 A 13¾-year-old patient; eunuchoid proportions, pubes and secondary hair, testes and penis markedly underdeveloped.
2 The same patient after 2 years of LHRH treatment in pulsatile form.

H.-R.W.

References:

Evain-Brion, D., Gendrel, D., Bozzala, M. et al. Diagnosis of Kallmann's syndrome in early infancy. *Acta Pediatr. Scand.*, 71, 937–940 (1982).
Brämswig, J.H., Schellong, G., König, A. et al. Familiarer Hypogonadismus mit Anosmie: Kallmann-Syndrom. *Monatsch. Kinderheilkd.*, 131, 232–234 (1983).
Hermanussen, M. and Sippell, W.G. Heterogeneity of Kallmann's syndrome. *Clin. Genet.*, 28, 106–111 (1985).
Partsch, C.-J., Hermanussen, M., Sippell, W.G. Differentiation of male hypogonadotropic hypogonadism and constitutional delay of puberty by pulsatile administration of gonadotropin-releasing hormone. *J. Clin. Endocrin. Metab.*, 60, 1196–1203 (1985).
Pawlowitzki, I.H., Diekstall, P., Miny, P. et al. Abnormal platelet function in Kallmann syndrome. *Lancet*, II, 166 (1986).
Schwanzel-Fukuda, M. and Pfaff, D.W. Origin of lutenizing hormone releasing hormone neurons. *Nature*, 338, 161–164 (1989).

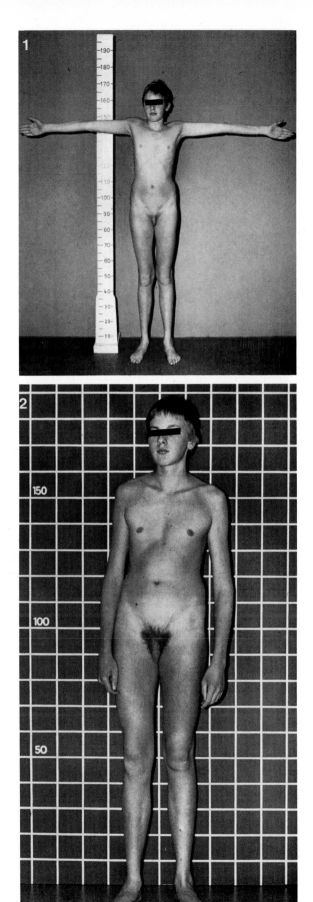

543

271. Klinefelter Syndrome

(XXY Syndrome)

A hypogonadism syndrome in males with an additional X chromosome.

Main signs:
(A) *In Childhood:*
1. Frequently tall stature with mildly eunuchoid body proportions (unusually long lower extremities).
2. Slightly below average intelligence, IQ below 80 in about 15–20% of cases, possibly with behavioral disorders. (Relatively late onset of speech. Tendency to mild intention tremor. Increased disposition to epilepsy.)
3. Possibly delayed onset of puberty, gynecomastia.
(B) *In Adolescence and Adulthood:*
1. Eunuchoid proportions with (moderate) tall stature. Variable degree of gynecomastia in about 40% of cases. Frequent development of obesity.
2. Slightly below average intelligence with infantile tendencies, possible impulsive behavior, or other psychological signs (anxiety, avoidance of social contact, difficult social adjustment).
3. Normally developed penis but small firm testes of about 2.5 ml and possible poor development of secondary sexual characteristics (female distribution of pubic hair; sparse growth of beard).

Supplementary findings: Increased disposition to varicosities of the lower legs and leg ulcers.
   (Below average libido and potency; azoospermia; infertility.)
   X-chromatin positive on screening (buccal smear); confirmation of anomalous sex-chromosome constitution by chromosomal analysis: XXY in about 80%; different types of mosaicism in about 20%.

Manifestation: Clinically by tall stature with relatively long legs (possibly combined with slightly below average intelligence) in early childhood. Most patients are diagnosed after their 14th year of life.

Etiology: The syndrome expresses a chromosomal aberration in the form of an extra X resulting from abnormal chromosome separation during oogenesis or spermatogenesis.

Frequency: About 1:500 male newborns.

Course, prognosis: Probably normal life expectancy. Poor social adjustment not infrequent. Infertility.

Differential diagnosis: Other forms of male hypogonadism.

Treatment: If endocrinological testicular insufficiency is demonstrated, androgen therapy beginning in the 15th year of life. Surgical treatment of marked gynecomastia may be indicated. Psychological guidance. Prevention of obesity.

Illustrations:
1 A proband at 8½ years: height excess, 18.5 cm; mental retardation; marked psychological signs; anomalous EEG.
4, 5, and 8 The same case at 26 years.
2, 3, 6 and 7 A 14¼-year-old: 176.5 cm (above the 97th percentile); left testis 2 ml, right 3 ml, firm; moderate mental retardation.
   Both cases confirmed by chromosomal analysis.

H.-R.W/J.K.

References:
Any comprehensive pediatric or internal medicine textbook.
Netley, C.T. Summary overview of behavioural development in individuals with neonatally identified X and Y aneuploidy. *Birth Defects*, XXII, 3, 293–306 (1986).
Editorial: Klinefelter's syndrome. *Lancet*, I, 1316–1317 (1988).

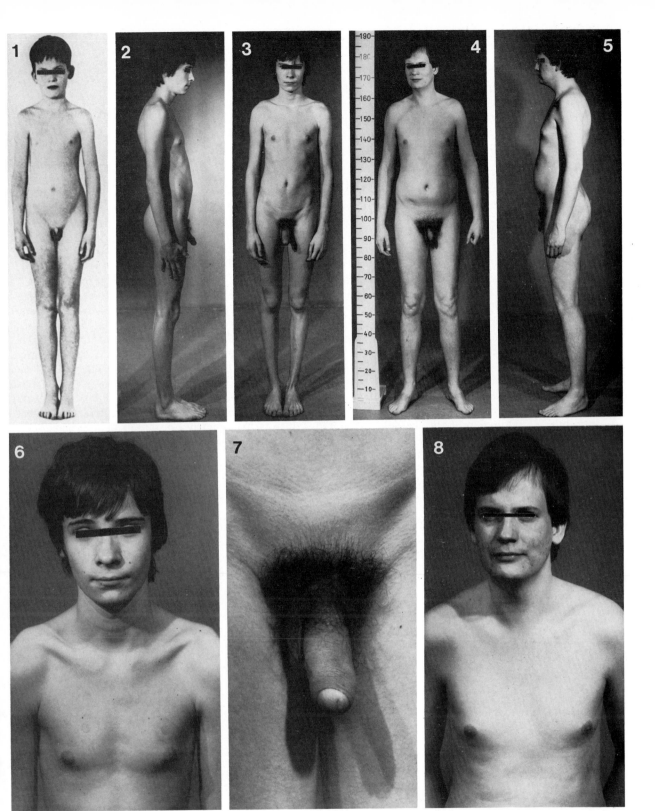

272. Idiopathic Hemihypertrophy

(Hemigigantism, Congenital Asymmetry)

Congenital hypertrophy of unknown etiology, which may be unilateral or partial and may occur together with involvement of the paired internal organs.

Main signs:
1. Hemihypertrophy of one half of the body or only a part thereof (face, upper and/or lower extremity, mandible, tongue, or other area); right more frequently involved than left.
2. Involvement of the internal paired organs (urogenital tract).
3. Mental retardation in 10–20% of patients.
4. Increased risk of Wilms' tumor (3%), adrenocortical neoplasia, and hepatoblastoma; possible contralateral occurrence of these.
5. Radiologically, possibly accelerated bony growth on the affected side.

Manifestation: At birth; sometimes first diagnosed in the early months of life.

Etiology: Unknown, probable heterogeneity. Different chromosomal changes described in isolated cases. Sporadic occurrence, only isolated familial observations. Pathogenetically, probably a disorder of early embryogenesis; histologically, increased numbers of cells without increased size of individual cells.

Frequency: 1:14,300 in a series of children up to 6 years old; according to other authors 1:100,000. Males are said to be more frequently affected; however, other reports speak of a 1:1 distribution.

Course, prognosis: The prognosis varies, depending on the extent of the hypertrophy; no compensatory growth of the unaffected side. Increased risk of tumors (corresponding diagnostic procedures when suspected).

Differential diagnosis: Hemihypertrophy as a feature of: von Recklinghausen neurofibromatosis, hemi 3M syndrome, Klippel–Trenaunay syndrome, von Hipple–Lindau angiomatosis, Silver–Russell syndrome, Proteus syndrome, Maffucci syndrome, Wiedemann–Beckwith syndrome, McCune–Albright syndrome, Langer–Giedion syndrome, F.P. Weber syndrome, Ollier enchondromatosis. Distinguish from progressive hemiatrophy. Hemihypertrophy associated with angiomatous, lipomatous, and lymphomatous malformations or tumors or with hamartomas (see also above) can be secondary.

Treatment: Dependent on the associated problems.

J.K.

References:

Ringrose, R.E., Jabbour, J.T., Keele, D.K. Hemihypertrophy. A review. *Pediatrics*, 36, 434–448 (1965).
Viljoen, D., Pearn, J., Beighton, P. Manifestations and natural history of idiopathic hemihypertrophy: a review of 11 cases. *Clin. Genet.*, 26, 81–86 (1984).

273. Currarino Triad

(Anterior Sacral Menigocele; Presacral Neurenteric Cyst; Congenital Anal Stenosis with Presacral Teratoma)

A combination of anorectal malformations, sacrococcygeal defect, and presacral tumor, with familial occurrence.

Main signs:
1. Anal atresia or anal stenosis and/or perineal anus.
2. Sacrococcygeal defect with 'Turkish saber' sacral deformity ('Scimitar' sacrum).
3. Anterior meningocele, lipoma, hamartoma, teratoma, dermoid cyst, cystic duplication of the intestines possibly with a fistula between the spinal canal and the rectum.

Supplementary findings: Chronic constipation.
Urogenital complications: urinary tract infections, vesicoureteric reflux, neurogenic bladder, gynecological and obstetric complications.
Meningitis.
Malignancy.
Malformations of the lower extremities, A-V fistula in the knee-joint region, ambiguous genitalia, tethered cord syndrome (i.e., club feet and neurological defects as with manifest myelocele, while only myelodysplasia, associated with an abnormally low level of the conus medullaris, is present).

Manifestation: At birth (anal obstruction) to adulthood (constipation).

Etiology: Mostly autosomal dominant inheritance; occasionally X-linked dominant inheritance and sporadic cases.

Frequency: Almost 100 cases known.

Prognosis: With timely diagnosis and surgical intervention, normal life expectancy. *Caveat:* malignant degeneration.

Treatment: Surgical.

J.K.

References:
Yates, V.D., Wilroy, R.S., Whitington, G.L. et al. Anterior sacral defects: an autosomal dominantly inherited condition. *J. Pediatr.*, 102, 239–242 (1983).
Welch, J.P. and Atermark, K. The syndrome of caudal dysplasia: a review, including etiologic considerations and evidence for heterogeneity. *Pediatr. Radiol.*, 2, 313–327 (1984).
Janneck, C. and Holthusen, W. Die Currarino-Trias . . . *Z. Kinderchir.*, 43, 112–116 (1988).

274. VATER Association

(Vacterl Syndrome: vertebral defects, anorectal atresia, cardiac anomalies, tracheoesophageal fistula with esophageal atresia, renal anomalies, and upper limb defects)

Main signs:
1. Renal dysplasia, agenesis, and other renal anomalies (167/220 = 73%).
2. Congenital cardiac defect (161/220 = 73%).
3. Defects of the vertebral bodies (133/220 = 60%).
4. Tracheoesophageal malformation (137/230 = 60%).
5. Anal stenosis and other anal malformations (128/229 = 56%).
6. Radial dysplasia and other malformations of the upper extremities (96/217 = 44%).

Supplementary findings: Malformations of the lower extremities (43%), genital and gonadal anomalies (43.5%), rib anomalies (40%), ear anomalies (39%), ureteral anomalies (36%), single umbilical artery (33%), scoliosis/kyphosis/lordosis (32%), inguinal hernia (23.5%), anomalies of the small intestines (22%), cleft lip and palate (13%), choanal atresia (11%).

Manifestation: At birth.

Etiology: Distinct preponderance of male patients (0.698). Birth weight on average decreased to 2250 g with a gestation of about 35.5 weeks. A history of a prolonged period of infertility, prior to becoming pregnant, is found in 10% of cases. No causative genetic factors demonstrable. Sporadic occurrence.

Frequency: 1.6 in 10,000 live births. Approximately 200 published cases.

Prognosis: Of those born alive, 50–85% die within the first year of life; 12% stillborn.

Differential diagnosis: Three or more components of the VACTERL complex occur in patients with trisomies 18 and 13 and in the cri du chat syndrome. Furthermore, consider the Meckel syndrome, Zellweger syndrome, sirenomelia, Potter sequence, amniotic bands syndrome, and the Goldenhar syndrome.

Treatment: Surgery as indicated.

J.K.

References:

Khoury, M.J., Cordero, J.F., Greenberg, F. et al. A population study of the VACTERL association: evidence for its etiologic heterogeneity. *Pediatrics*, 71, 815–820 (1983).
Czeizel, A. and Ludanyi, I. An aetiologic study of the VACTERL-association. *Eur. J. Pediatr.*, 144, 331–337 (1985).
Weaver, D.D., Mapstone, C.L., Yu, P.-L. The VATER association. *Am. J. Dis. Child.*, 140, 225–229 (1986).
Fernbach, S.K. and Glass, R.B.J. The expanded spectrum of limb anomalies in the VATER association. *Pediatr. Radiol.*, 18, 215–220 (1988).

275. SHORT Syndrome

(Short stature, hyperextensibility of joints and/or hernia, ocular depression, Rieger anomaly, delayed teething)

Main signs:
1. Short stature with intrauterine growth retardation.
2. Hyperextensibility of the joints and/or inguinal hernias.
3. Deep-set eyes.
4. Rieger anomaly (irido-dental syndrome = Axenfeld syndrome).
5. Delayed dentition.

Supplementary findings: Slow weight gain after birth, recurrent infections, triangular face, telecanthus, broad nasal root, hypoplastic alae nasi, micrognathia, deficient subcutaneous tissue (lipoatrophy), hearing impairment, delayed bone age, delayed development of speech, normal intelligence.

Manifestation: At birth and early childhood.

Etiology: Autosomal recessive inheritance. Thus, to be differentiated from the autosomal dominant syndrome of partial lipoatrophy with small stature and insulin dependent diabetes.

Frequency: To date four observations, only once in siblings.

Course, prognosis: Good prognosis, normal intelligence.

Treatment: Symptomatic.

J.K.

References:
Toriello, H.V., Wakefield, S., Komar, K. et al. Report of a case and further delineation of the SHORT syndrome. *Am. J. Med. Genet.*, 22, 311–314 (1985).

276. HARD + E Syndrome

(Warburg Syndrome; Chemke Syndrome; Pagon Syndrome; Walker–Warburg Syndrome; Cerebro-Ocular Dysplasia = COD)

A lethal familial disorder comprising *h*ydrocephalus, *a*gyria, *r*etinal *d*ysplasia, and *e*ncephalocele.

Main signs:
Hydrocephalus, usually due to aqueduct stenosis.
   Agyria.
   Retinal dysplasia.
   Encephalocele (not obligatory).

Supplementary findings: Cataracts, microphthalmos, hypoplasia of the iris, coloboma of the optic nerve. Severe developmental retardation, cerebellar dysplasia, agenesis of the corpus callosum, hypoplasia of the white matter of the brain.

Manifestation: At birth. Hydrocephalus can be demonstrated prenatally by ultrasonography.

Etiology: Autosomal recessive inheritance.

Frequency: About 35 observations; of these, one-third familial.

Course, prognosis: All patients have died within the first year of life. Severe developmental delay.

Differential diagnosis: Lissencephaly.

J.K.

References:

Ayme, S. and Mattei, J.F. HARD (plus or minus) E syndrome: report of a sixth family with support for autosomal-recessive inheritance. *Am. J. Med. Genet.*, 14, 759–766 (1983).

Whitley, C.B., Thompson, T.R., Mastri, A.R. et al. HARD syndrome: a lethal neurodysplasia with autosomal recessive inheritance. *J. Pediatr.*, 102, 547–552 (1983).

Williams, R.S., Swisher, C.N., Jennings, M. et al. Cerebro-ocular dysgenesis (Walker–Warburg) syndrome: neuropathologic and etiologic analysis. *Neurology*, 34, 1531–1541 (1984).

Crowe, C., Jassani, M., Dickerman, L. The prenatal diagnosis of Warburg syndrome (abstract). *Am. J. Hum. Genet.*, 37, A214 (1985).

Crowe, C., Jassani, M., Dickerman, L. The prenatal diagnosis of Walker–Warburg syndrome. *Prenat. Diagn.*, 6, 177–185 (1986).

Burton, B.K., Dillard, R.G., Weaver, R.G. Brief clinical report: Walker–Warburg syndrome with cleft lip and cleft palate in two sibs. *Am. J. Med. Genet.*, 27, 537–541 (1987).

Dobbyns, W.B., Pagon, R.A. et al. Diagnostic criteria for Walker–Warburg syndrome. *Am. J. Med. Genet.*, 32, 195–210 (1989).

277. CHARGE Association

(CHARGE Complex, CHARGE Syndrome: coloboma, heart disease, atresia of choanae, retarded mental development, genital hypoplasia, ear anomalies, and deafness)

Main signs:
1. Bi- or unilateral coloboma of the iris, retina, and/or the optic nerve. Less frequently, micro- or anophthalmia. Found in 80% of the patients.
2. In 32% of all patients with choanal atresia, cardiac defects are found: patent ductus arteriosus, atrial septal defect, ventricular septal defect, tetralogy of Fallot, atrioventricular canal, combined defects.
3. Up to two-thirds of all patients have bilateral choanal atresia. Look for further malformations!
4. Somatic or psychomotor retardation in 87% and 94% respectively of all patients. Probably due to hypoxic damage.
5. In 74% of patients, signs of genital hypoplasia without secondary problems. Females are fertile. Males frequently show cryptorchidism and/or hypospadias.
6. Normal or quite dysplastic helices, may be unilateral, with sensorineural and conductive hearing impairment of various grades of severity.

Supplementary findings: Orofacial clefts, high palate; esophageal atresia, tracheoesophageal fistula; renal malformations and dysplasia (agenesis, hypoplasia, heterotopia, hydronephrosis).

Facial dysmorphism: micrognathia, antimongoloid slant of the palpebral fissures, pug nose.

Manifestation: At birth.

Etiology: Usually sporadic occurrence. Occasionally, autosomal dominant mode of inheritance (then called CHARGE syndrome). Affected siblings with healthy parents have also been observed. A similar clinical picture is seen with various chromosomal abnormalities.

Disturbance of embryological differentiation between the 35th and 38th days.

Frequency: About 200 cases documented.

Course, prognosis: Choanal atresia a life-threatening complication *post partum*. Mental impairment of various grades of severity, but may have normal intelligence.

Diagnosis: According to some authors, the combination of characteristic ear malformations (increased width and decreased length of the ear, 'snipped off' helix, absent lobulus auriculae, prominent antihelix, triangular concha) with 'wedge-shaped' audiogram (loss of low frequencies of bone conduction and loss of high frequencies of air conduction) are key to the diagnosis.

Treatment: Hearing aids are essential.

J.K.

References:

Koletzko, B. and Majewski, F. Congenital anomalies in patients with choanal atresia: CHARGE association. *Eur. J. Pediatr.*, 142, 271–275 (1984).

Davenport, S.L.H., Hefner, M.A., Mitchell, J.A. The spectrum of clinical features in CHARGE syndrome. *Clin. Genet.*, 29, 298–310 (1986).

Metlay, L.A., Smythe, P.S., Miller, M.E. Familial CHARGE syndrome: clinical report with autopsy findings. *Am. J. Med. Genet.*, 26, 577–581 (1987).

Lin, A.E., Chin, A.J., Devine, W. et al. The pattern of cardiovascular malformation in the CHARGE association. *Am. J. Dis. Child.*, 141, 1010–1013 (1987).

Oley, C.A., Baraitser, M., Grant, D.B. A reappraisal of the CHARGE association. *J. Med. Genet.*, 25, 147–156 (1988).

Meinecke, P., Polke, A., Schmiegelow, P. Limb anomalies in the CHARGE association. *J. Med. Genet.*, 26, 202–203 (1989).

278. GAPO Syndrome

(Growth retardation, alopecia, pseudoanodontia, progressive optic atrophy)

Main signs:
Severe growth retardation with retarded bone age.
  Alopecia, severe hypotrichosis.
  Pseudoanodontia (failure of tooth eruption)
  Progressive optic atrophy beginning in early childhood.

Supplementary findings: Characteristic facial appearance with high prominent forehead, midface dysplasia, prominent eyes with flat orbits. Delayed closure of the wide-open anterior fontanelle. Micrognathia. Low, depressed nasal root. Umbilical hernia.

Manifestation: Usually after the first year of life.

Etiology: Autosomal recessive inheritance.

Frequency: Ten published cases.

Course, prognosis: Good. Normal mental development.

Treatment: Symptomatic.

Differential diagnosis: Progeria.

J.K.

References:

Tipton, R.E. and Gorlin, R.J. Growth retardation, alopecia, pseudoanodontia, and optic atrophy—the GAPO syndrome: report of a patient and review of the literature. *Am. J. Med. Genet.*, 19, 209–216 (1984).

Gagliardi, A.R.T., Gonzales, C.H., Pratesi, C.H. GAPO syndrome: report of three affected brothers. *Am. J. Med. Genet.*, 19, 217–223 (1984).

Manouvrer-Hanu, S., Largilliere, C., Bernalioua, M. et al. Brief clinical report: the GAPO syndrome. *Am. J. Med. Genet.*, 26, 683–688 (1987).

279. Alagille Syndrome

(Anteriohepatic Dysplasia)

A familial syndrome with characteristic facies, chronic cholestasis, posterior embryotoxon, butterfly-like anomalies of the vertebral arches, peripheral pulmonary stenosis, and cardiac defect.

Main signs:
1. Facial dysmorphism in 95%: prominent forehead; slight hypertelorism; deep-set eyes; prominent, narrow chin; saddle nose or accentuated, straight nasal bridge.
2. Chronic cholestasis in 91% of patients, beginning in the first three months of life in 50% and between the fourth month and the third year of life in the remainder. Splenomegaly in somewhat fewer than half of the patients; one-fifth develop portal hypertension. Xanthomata on the extensor sides of the finger joints, on the back of the neck, the anal folds, and the popliteal space, from the fourth year of life (progressive).
3. Posterior embryotoxon: visible by slit lamp in 89% of patients.
4. Defects of the vertebral arches; failure of the arches to fuse, leading to a butterfly-like appearance.
5. Cardiovascular disorders in 85%: frequently asymptomatic isolated, nonprogressive peripheral stenosis of one or both pulmonary arteries. One-sixth of all patients have additional cardiac defects (such as tetralogy of Fallot).

Supplementary findings: Growth retardation in 50% of the patients, increasing with age. Mesangial lipidosis in 17/23 with only mild clinical renal signs. IQ below 80 in 16/80. Occasionally, high-pitched voice.

Manifestation: From birth to the sixth month or third year of life.

Etiology: Autosomal dominant inheritance with variable penetrance. Genetic counseling is difficult due to variable clinical expression.

Frequency: Over 100 families have been reported.

Course, prognosis: Recurrent episodes of cholestasis, often associated with respiratory infections, especially in the first year of life. Malnutrition with severe cholestasis. One-fourth of all patients have died between 3 months and 23 years of age. Hepatic complications were causally involved in only 5%, severe cardiac anomalies in 7.5%. Death from respiratory infections in 30%. Delayed puberty. Retarded linear growth.

Treatment: Low-fat diet with medium-chain triglycerides. Intramuscular administration of fat-soluble vitamins. Phenobarbital to reduce pruritis. Liver transplantation should be considered.

J.K.

References:
Alagille, D., Estrada, A., Hadchouel, M. et al. Syndromic paucity of interlobular bile ducts (Alagille syndrome or arteriohepatic dysplasia): review of 80 cases. *J. Pediatr.*, 110, 195–200 (1987).

280. Hydrolethalus Syndrome

(Salonen–Herva–Norio Syndrome)

A hereditary syndrome with severe malformations of the brain, polydactyly, pulmonary hypoplasia, and facial clefts.

Main signs:
1. Hydrocephalus (93%), absence of the corpus callosum and septum pallucidum, Dandy–Walker malformation, olfactory aplasia, and many others.
2. Polydactyly (88%): always preaxial in the feet, occasionally additional postaxial hexadactyly of the toes. Polydactyly of the hands; when present, always postaxial.
3. Cleft lip and palate (56%).
4. Micrognathia (84%), tongue small or absent.
5. Malformations of the tracheobronchial tree (65%).
6. Abnormal lobation of the lungs (50%).
7. Cardiac defect (58%): VSD, atrioventricular canal.
8. Hydramnios (100%), still birth or death immediately *post partum.*

Supplementary findings: Simply modeled nose, microphthalmos, adrenal hypoplasia in children with absent hypophysis (midline defect), no intestinal rotation, cryptorchidism, double or septate uterus. Normal kidneys.

Manifestation: Pre- and postnatally.

Etiology: Autosomal recessive inheritance. The syndrome has been observed relatively frequently in Finland, but also in Arabic families and in Africans.

Frequency: About 50 cases described, usually with affected siblings.

Prognosis: Always lethal.

Differential diagnosis: Patients with Meckel–Gruber syndrome always have dysplastic cystic kidneys. The Smith–Lemli–Opitz syndrome and trisomy 13 can be clearly differentiated.

J.K.

References:

Salonen, R., Herva, R., Norio, R. The hydrolethalus syndrome: delineation of a 'new' lethal malformation syndrome based on 28 patients. *Clin. Genet.*, 19, 321–350 (1981).
Anyane-Yeboa, K., Collins, M., Kupsky, W. et al. Hydrolethalus (Salonen–Herva–Norio) syndrome: further clinicopathological delineation. *Am. J. Med. Genet.*, 26, 899–907 (1987).

281. Pena–Shokeir Phenotype

(Pena–Shokeir Syndrome I; Pseudotrisomy 18; Fetal Akinesia/Hypokinesia Sequence)

An etiologically heterogeneous clinical picture with trisomy 18-like phenotype.

Main signs:
1. Intrauterine growth retardation of length and weight.
2. Craniofacial anomalies: ocular hypertelorism, micrognathia, short neck, low-set and simply modeled ears, depressed tip of the nose.
3. Anomalies of the extremities: retardation of growth, ankylosis of the large joints, abnormally formed fingers and toes (cylindrical), slender extremities, overlapping fingers as in trisomy 18, equinovarus positioning of the feet, rocker-bottom feet, deficient calcification of the bones.
4. Pulmonary hypoplasia.
5. Short umbilical cord.
6. Hydramnios (important presenting sign).
7. Disorders of the central nervous system and peripheral nerves: thin cortex, dilated ventricles, polymicrogyria, neurogenic muscular atrophy.

Supplementary findings: Telecanthus, epicanthic folds, microstomia, high palate, cleft palate, mandibular hypoplasia, camptodactyly, nuchal hygroma.

Manifestation: At birth. Prenatal diagnosis by ultrasonography is possible with a positive history.

Etiology: Heterogeneity. Mostly autosomal recessive inheritance or sporadic cases. X-linked recessive cases also known. Even intrafamilial heterogeneity has been described. Risk of recurrence 10–15%.

Frequency: About 75 cases published. The syndrome is under-diagnosed: Shokeir estimates one case in 12,000 newborns.

Course, prognosis: 30% stillbirths; 40% die within the first 14 days; demise of almost all further patients by the 16th week of life. Occasional survival. Weak suck, failure to thrive.

Differential diagnosis: Trisomy 18 can be excluded cytogenetically. Patients with the cerebro-oculo-facio-skeletal (COFS) syndrome (previously called Pena–Shokeir syndrome II) survive birth, but then show severe, progressive psychomotor deterioration with no development of speech, and death in the third year of life. Phenotypically identical with Pena–Shokeir syndrome I, suggesting different expression.

Treatment: Symptomatic.

J.K.

References:

Shokeir, M.H.K. Multiple ankyloses, camptodactyly, facial anomalies and pulmonary hypoplasia (Pena–Shokeir I syndrome). In Vinken, P.J. and Bruyn, G.W. (eds.). Handbook of Clinical Neurology, vol. 43. *Neurogenetic directory*, part II. North-Holland Publishing, Amsterdam, 1982 (pp. 437–439).

Lindhout, D., Hageman, G., Beemer, F.A. et al. The Pena–Shokeir syndrome: report of nine Dutch cases. *Am. J. Med. Genet.*, 21, 655–688 (1985).

Hunt-MacMillan, R., Harbert, G.M., Davis, W.D. et al. Prenatal diagnosis of Pena–Shokeir syndrome type I. *Am. J. Med. Genet.*, 21, 279–284 (1985).

Hall, J.G. Invited editorial comment: analysis of Pena–Shokeir phenotype. *Am. J. Med. Genet.*, 25, 99–117 (1986).

Hageman, G., Willemse, J., van Ketel, B.A. et al. The heterogeneity of the Pena–Shokeir syndrome. *Neuropediatrics*, 18, 45–50 (1987).

Ohlsson, A., Fong, K.W., Rose, T.H. et al. Prenatal diagnosis of Pena–Shokeir syndrome type I, or fetal akinesia deformation sequence. *Am. J. Med. Genet.*, 29, 59–65 (1988).

282. Cerebro-Oculo-Facio-Skeletal (COFS) Syndrome

(Pena–Shokeir II Syndrome)

An autosomal recessive clinical picture with lethal course, severe progressive psychomotor retardation, facial dysmorphism, skeletal anomalies, and flexion contractures of the large joints.

Main signs:
1. Microcephaly, muscular hypotonia, hyperreflexia, areflexia, progressive psychomotor decline, no development of speech.
2. Microphthalmos, anophthalmia, cataract, blepharophimosis.
3. Prominent nasal root, micrognathia, large ears.
4. Camptodactyly, overlapping fingers, flexion contractures of the elbow and knee joints, kyphosis, dysplastic acetabula, coxa valga, rocker-bottom feet, osteoporosis.

Supplementary findings: Indistinct border between the grey and white matter, lissencephaly, agenesis of the corpus callosum, reduction of neurons in the cerebrum, cerebellum, spinal cord, and retina (as with neuronal destruction resulting from fetal anoxia). In older children, dilated ventricles, decrease of the white matter of the brain.

Manifestation: Birth to the sixth month of life.

Etiology: Autosomal recessive inheritance. Parental consanguinity frequently demonstrable.

Frequency: About 1 in 10,000 newborns among Caucasians, Asians, and Blacks.

Course, prognosis: No sign of prenatal growth retardation at birth. Postnatal course of severe general developmental retardation with no development of speech. Death in the third year due to respiratory infection.

Differential diagnosis: Pena–Shokeir syndrome I.

Treatment: Symptomatic.

J.K.

References:

Shokeir, M.H.K. Cerebro-oculo-facio-skeletal (COFS) syndrome (Pena–Shokeir II syndrome). In: Vinken, P.J. and Bruyn, G.W. (eds.) Handbook of Clinical Neurology, vol. 43. *Neurogenetic directory*, part II. North-Holland Publishing, Amsterdam, 1982, (pp.341–343).
Silengo, M.C., Davi, G., Bianco, R. et al. The NEU–COFS (cerebro-oculo-facio-skeletal) syndrome: report of a case. *Clin. Genet.*, 25, 201–204 (1984).

Index

Page numbers in *italics* refer to illustrations.